AMERICAN JOURNAL OF HEMATOLOGY

Volume 45, 1994

Ananda S. Prasad
Editor

605 Third Avenue
New York, NY 10158-0012

AMERICAN JOURNAL OF HEMATOLOGY

Volume 45, Number 1 **January 1994**

ORIGINAL ARTICLES

Characteristics of Zinc Binding to Human Red Blood Cell Membranes
José Brandão-Néto and William R. Bell 1

Quantitative Defect of Glycoprotein Ib in Severe Cirrhotic Patients
María J. Sánchez-Roig, José Rivera, José M. Moraleda, and Vicente Vicente García 10

Direct Evidence for Systemic Fibrinogenolysis in Patients With Acquired α_2-Plasmin Inhibitor Deficiency
Kenji Okajima, Isao Kohno, Gilbu Soe, Hiroaki Okabe, Kiyoshi Takatsuki, and Bernd R. Binder 16

Peripheral Neuropathy in IgM Monoclonal Gammopathy and Wäldenstrom's Macroglobulinemia: A Frequent Complication in Elderly Males With Low MAG-Reactive Serum Monoclonal Component
Luca Baldini, Edoardo Nobile-Orazio, Andrea Guffanti, Sergio Barbieri, Marinella Carpo, Lilla Cro, Bruno Cesana, Isabella Damilano, and Anna T. Maiolo 25

Detection of Tumor Necrosis Factor-α in Bone Marrow Plasma and Peripheral Blood Plasma From Patients With Aplastic Anemia
John C. Schultz and Nasrollah T. Shahidi 32

Splenic Lymphoma With Circulating Villous Lymphocytes: Report of Seven Cases and Review of the Literature
Tsieh Sun, Myron Susin, Judith Brody, Klaus Dittmar, Saul Teichberg, Robert Weiner, Jen H. Lin, and Norbert Felber 39

Polymorphic Pattern of the $(AT)_X(T)_Y$ Motif At −530 5′ to the β-Globin Gene in Over 40 Patients Homozygous for Various β-Thalassemia Mutations
A.J. Dimovski, A.D. Adekile, V. Divoky, E. Baysal, and T.H.J. Huisman 51

CASE REPORTS

Cytokine Profile During High-Dose rhG-CSF Therapy in Severe Congenital Neutropenia
Toshiji Shitara, Shin-ichiroh Yugami, Hiroko Ijima, Manabu Sotomatu, and Takayoshi Kuroume 58

Dyshematopoiesis in Combined Immune Deficiency With Congenital Neutropenia
Cristina Gasparetto, Clay Smith, Meri Firpo, Dieter Dennig, Trudy Small, Alfred P. Gillio, Robert Lichtenberg, Richard J. O'Reilly, and Malcolm A.S. Moore 63

CLINICAL STUDIES IN HEMOSTASIS AND THROMBOSIS AT TEMPLE UNIVERSITY SCHOOL OF MEDICINE

Factor XI Deficiency and Hemostasis
Robert W. Colman, A. Koneti Rao, and Ronald N. Rubin, Editors
Discussant: Peter N. Walsh 73

BRIEF REPORTS

Autoimmune-Thrombocytopenia and SLE in a Patient With 5q-Anomaly and Deletion of the c-fms Oncogene
Ulrich Jaeger, Simon Panzer, Claus Bartram, Oskar Haas, Beatrix Volc-Platzer, Wolfgang Graninger, Klaus Geissler, Thaddaeusz Radaszkiewicz, and Klaus Lechner 79

A Novel Mediterranean "δβ-Thalassemia" Determinant Containing the δ^+27 and $\beta^\circ39$ Point Mutations in Cis
Lina Oggiano, Luciana Guiso, Laura Frogheri, Georgios Loudianos, Paola Pistidda, Elena Rimini, Mario Pirastu, Antonio Cao, and Maurizio Longinotti 81

Laboratory Monitoring of Warfarin Therapy in Utah
Susan B. Garr and George M. Rodgers 85

Production of Parathyroid Hormone-Related Protein by Cultured Human Myeloma Cells
Akira Suzuki, Takayuki Takahashi, Yoshiaki Okuno, Reiko Tsuyuoka, Yutaka Sasaki, Manabu Fukumoto, Hideki Katakami, Kenkichi Kita, and Tsunefumi Shibuya 88

Quantities of α^Q Chain Variants in Heterozygotes With and Without a Concomitant β-Thalassemia Trait
W.-B. Qin, E. Baysal, K.F. Wong, T.P. Molchanova, D.D. Pobedimskaya, S. Sharma, J.B. Wilson, and T.H.J. Huisman 91

LETTERS AND CORRESPONDENCE

Acute Lymphoblastic Leukemia in Fanconi's Anemia
Sevgi Yetgin, Murat Tuncer, Ertuğrul Güler, Feride Duru, and Mehmet Ali Kaşifoğlu 94

Standard Ph Chromosome, t(9;22)(q34;q11) as an Additional Change in a Patient With Acute Myelomonocytic Leukemia (M4Eo) Associated With inv(16)(p13q22)
I. Miura, H. Takatsu, A. Yamaguchi, K. Hashimoto, T. Nimura, T. Nishinari, H. Niitsu, and A.B. Miura 94

Iron Deficiency Anemia in Hemoglobinopathy
Şinasi Özsoylu 96

β^S-Gene-Cluster Haplotypes in Sickle Cell Anemia Patients From Two Regions of Brazil
F.F. Costa, V.R. Arruda, M.G. Gonçalves, S.R.P. Miranda, M.H. Carvalho, M.F. Sonati, S.O.T. Saad, F. Gesteira, D. Fernandes, M.L. Nascimento, and I.L. Queiroz 96

Burkitt's Lymphoma Presenting as Ophthalmoplegia in an Elderly Male
Sheryl A. Russ and Omar H. Yumen 97

Intracranial Hemorrhage in an Adult With Factor-VII Deficiency
Barbara J. Seaborg, C. Patrick Burns, John D. Olson, Beverly J. Pennell, and Kenneth A. Follett 98

High-Dose Human Immunoglobulins in Thrombotic Thrombocytopenic Purpura
Camillo Porta and Enrico Bobbio-Pallavicini 99

HTLV-I Associated Adult T-Cell Leukaemia/Lymphoma in Hong Kong
Raymond Liang 100

INSTRUCTIONS TO AUTHORS 102

Volume 45, Number 2 **February 1994**

ORIGINAL ARTICLES

Hemophilic Pseudotumor: Multicenter Experience Over a 25-Year Period
M. Magallón, J. Monteagudo, C. Altisent, A. Ibáñez, A. Rodríguez-Pérez, J. Riba, J. Tusell, and J. Martín-Villar 103

Von Willebrand Factor Availability in Platelet Concentrates Stored for 5 Days
Jesús M. Cesar, Angel García-Avello, Juán Monteagudo, José I. Espinosa, José C. Lodos, Ricardo Castillo, and José L. Navarro 109

Changes in Longevity and Causes of Death Among Persons With Hemophilia A
Terence L. Chorba, Robert C. Holman, Tara W. Strine, Matthew J. Clarke, and Bruce L. Evatt 112

Varying Populations of CD59-Negative, Partly Positive, and Normally Positive Blood Cells in Different Cell Lineages in Peripheral Blood of Paroxysmal Nocturnal Hemoglobinuria Patients
Seitoku Fujioka and Teruo Yamada 122

Topical Thrombin and Acquired Coagulation Factor Inhibitors: Clinical Spectrum and Laboratory Diagnosis
Thomas L. Ortel, Linda A. Charles, Frank G. Keller, P. Kelly Marcom, H. Newland Oldham, Jr., William H. Kane, and B. Gail Macik 128

Transgenic Mouse Model of Pharmacologic Induction of Fetal Hemoglobin: Studies Using a New Ribonucleotide Reductase Inhibitor, Didox
B.S. Pace, H.L. Elford, and G. Stamatoyannopoulos 136

Continuous Infusion of Monoclonal Antibody-Purified Factor VIII: Rational Approach to Serious Hemorrhage in Patients With Allo-/Autoantibodies to Factor VIII
Erlinda M. Gordon, Fatma Al-Batniji, and Jonathan C. Goldsmith 142

Prevalence of Abnormal Iron Studies in Heterozygotes for Hereditary Hemochromatosis: An Analysis of 255 Heterozygotes

Paul C. Adams . . . 146

CD21 Antigen in T-Lineage Neoplastic Lymphoid Cells: Characteristic Expression at Thymic Stage
Eiji Tatsumi, Noriko Yoneda, Seiji Kawano, and Nobuo Yamaguchi . . . 150

Hypofibrinolysis: A Common, Major Cause of Osteonecrosis
Charles J. Glueck, Richard Freiberg, Helen I. Glueck, Clyde Henderson, Michael Welch, Trent Tracy, Davis Stroop, Tracey Hamer, Felix Sosa, and Mark Levy . . . 156

Skin Manifestation of Agnogenic Myeloid Metaplasia
Gabriel Loewy, Anna Mathew, and Ariel Distenfeld . . . 167

CASE REPORTS

Primary Amyloidosis Associated With a Novel Heavy-Chain Fragment (AH Amyloidosis)
Alan Solomon, Deborah T. Weiss, and Charles Murphy . . . 171

Treatment of Refractory Undifferentiated Acute Myelogenous Leukemia With All-*Trans*-Retinoic Acid
Jennifer J. Griggs, Susan E. Henley, and Jacob M. Rowe . . . 177

BRIEF REPORTS

Expression of the Thrombospondin Receptor (CD36) on the Cell Surface in Megakaryoblastic and Promegakaryocytic Leukemias: Increment of the Receptor by Megakaryocyte Differentiation In Vitro
Nobutaka Imamura, Hiromi Ota, Kazuhiro Abe,and Atsushi Kuramoto . . . 181

Molecular Abnormality of a Unique Japanese Glucose-6-Phosphate Dehydrogenase Variant (G6PD Kobe) With a Greatly Increased Affinity for Galactose-6-Phosphate
Akira Hirono, Shiro Nakayama, Hisaichi Fujii, and Shiro Miwa . . . 185

Reversible Encephalopathy After Cryopreserved Peripheral Blood Stem Cell Infusion
Madhav Dhodapkar, Stuart L. Goldberg, Ayalew Tefferi, and Morie A. Gertz . . . 187

A Possible Survival Advantage in Adults With Acute Leukemia Receiving ABO-Identical Platelet Transfusions
Joanna Mary Heal, Naomi Kenmotsu, Jacob M. Rowe, and Neil Blumberg . . . 189

LETTERS AND CORRESPONDENCE

Acquired Ichthyosis as a Manifestation of Abdominal Recurrence of Non-Hodgkin's Lymphoma
Jun'ichi Tamura, Masahiko Shinohara, Takafumi Matsushima, Morio Sawamura, Hirokazu Murakami, and Kazuo Kubota . . . 191

Cyclosporin Therapy for Pure Red Cell Aplasia in Patients With Chronic Lymphocytic Leukemia
M. Sivakumaran and M. Bhavnani . . . 192

Serum and Red Cell Ferritin: Diagnostic Tools and Pathophysiologic Clues
Gerard Vreugdenhil . . . 192

Author's Reply
Ed Balaban, Richard Sheehan, and Eugene P. Frenkel . . . 193

Antiphospholipid Antibodies in Sickle Cell Disease
Munther A. Khamashta and Graham R.V. Hughes . . . 193

Author's Reply
M.P. Westerman . . . 194

Circulating Late-Stage Erythroid Progenitors in a Patient With Agnogenic Myeloid Metaplasia
Hua-Kang Wu, Shigeru Chiba, Ken Inamori, Hiroyuki Mano, Tsuyoshi Tange, Yoshio Yazaki, Hisamaru Hirai, and Mark D. Minden . . . 194

Translocation (3;3)(q21;q26)
Vesna Najfeld . . . 195

Author's Reply
Ram S. Verma . . . 196

Factor VIIa Levels Are Decreased in Patients With Hemophilia B
Juzo Matsuda, Noriko Saitoh, Kengo Gohchi, Miyo Tsukamoto, Moritaka Gotoh, Hideji Hanabusa, and Minoru Inagaki . . . 196

Announcement . . . 199

Instructions to Authors . . . 200

Volume 45, Number 3 March 1994

ORIGINAL ARTICLES

A New Deletional α-Thalassemia Detected in Yemenites With Hemoglobin H Disease
Lea Shalmon, Chava Kirschmann, and Rina Zaizov 201

von Willebrand's Disease: Use of Collagen Binding Assay Provides Potential Improvement to Laboratory Monitoring of Desmopressin (DDAVP) Therapy
Emmanuel J. Favaloro, Mark Dean, Linda Grispo, Tom Exner, and Jerry Koutts 205

Detection of PML-Retinoic Acid Receptor-α Fusion Transcripts in Acute Promyelocytic Leukemia With Trisomy 8 But Without t(15;17)
Kazuma Ikeda, Kazunori Sasaki, Taizo Tasaka, Masami Nagai, Koichi Kawanishi, Jiro Takahara, and Shozo Irino 212

Stability of Factor VIII Concentrates After Reconstitution
Sam Schulman, Sanford Gitel, and Uri Martinowitz 217

Effects of Interleukin-2 Administration on Platelet Function in Cancer Patients
Leslie Oleksowicz, Dina Zuckerman, Zbigniew Mrowiec, Elena Puszkin, and Janice P. Dutcher 224

Elevated Plasma Tissue Factor Antigen Level in Patients With Disseminated Intravascular Coagulation
Hideo Wada, Tsutomu Nakase, Ryusuke Nakaya, Kouzou Minamikawa, Yoshihiro Wakita, Toshihiro Kaneko, Michiaki Ohiwa, Katsumi Deguchi, and Shigeru Shirakawa 232

CASE REPORTS

Erythropoietin in the Treatment of Delayed Immune Hemolysis of a Major ABO-Incompatible Bone Marrow Transplant
J. López, J.L. Steegmann, G. Pérez, M.J. Otero, M. Berberana, R. Cámara, M. Lamana, M.J. Fernández Villalta, and J.M. Fernández-Rañada 237

Spontaneous Factor VIII Inhibitor Occurring in Association With Chronic Graft-Versus Host Disease
Christopher W. Seidler, Letha E. Mills, Mary E.D. Flowers, and Keith M. Sullivan 240

Malignant Histiocytosis Associated With Autoimmune Thrombocytopenia
Tatsuharu Ohno, Tateo Sugiyama, Hiroo Furukawa, Takafumi Ishibashi, and Minoru Okuma 244

α-Interferon Treatment for Idiopathic Hypereosinophilic Syndrome
Paula L. Bockenstedt, John T. Santinga, and Steven F. Bolling 248

Pentosan Polysulfate-Induced Thrombocytopenia and Thrombosis
Brigitte Tardy-Poncet, Bernard Tardy, Françoise Grelac, Jacqueline Reynaud, Patrick Mismetti, Jean Claude Bertrand, and Denis Guyotat 252

BRIEF REPORTS

Thrombocytopenia Following Acute Acetaminophen Overdose
Michael Fischereder and Jeffrry P. Jaffe 258

Hereditary Hemochromatosis and Red Cell Aplasia
Paul C. Adams 260

IgE Plasma Cell Leukemia Successfully Treated With Combination of VAD (Vincristine, Doxorubicin, Dexamethasone) and MP (Melphalan, Prednisolone) Followed by Interferon-α
Noboru Yamagata, Chihiro Shimazaki, Hideo Goto, Toshiyuki Hirata, Eishi Ashihara, Naritoshi Oku, Tohru Inaba, Naohisa Fujita, and Masao Nakagawa 262

Mild $\beta^{+}(-87)$-Thalassemia CACCC Box Mutation Is Associated With Elevated Fetal Hemoglobin Expression in Cis
John G. Gilman, Laura Manca, Laura Frogheri, Paola Pistidda, Luciana Guiso, Maurizio Longinotti, and Bruno Masala 265

LETTERS AND CORRESPONDENCE

Lung Perfusion Scaning in Two Patients With Malignant Histiocytosis
Hideyo Natori, Ken Tanaka, Kaori Shiraishi, Seishi Osabe, Hiroto Jojima, Kotaro Oizumi, and Masatoshi Ishibashi 268

Good Response to High Dose Intravenous Immunoglobulin in Patients With Alveolar Hemorrhage Refractory to Platelet Transfusion
M.E. Purucker and M. Cottler-Fox 269

Normal Pregnancy and Delivery in Essential Thrombocythemia Even Without Interferon Therapy
Maria Luigia Randi, Ersilia Barbone, and Antonio Girolami 270

Author's Reply
José Petit 271

Common Acute Lymphoblastic Leukemia Antigen (CD10)-Positive Sézary's Syndrome
Akihiko Chubachi, Takako Ishino, Noriko Satoh, and Akira B. Miura 271

Acquired Platelet Storage Pool Deficiency Due to Severe Valvular Disease Corrected by Prosthetic Valve Replacement
Rolando E. Rumbaut, Michael H. Kroll, Ferenc Gyorkey, and Andrew I. Schafer 272

Detection of Human T Lymphotropic Virus Type I Proviral DNA in Fresh Cells From Ascitic Fluid in a Patient With Adult T-Cell Leukemia
Masahito Iwahashi, Maki Otsuka, Makoto Matsumoto, Shigemi Shimotakahara, and Nobuyuki Kobayashi . . . 273

Parvovirus B19 Infection Causing Severe Peripheral Blood Thrombocytopenia and Persistent Viremia
Eiichi Oeda, Kenji Shinohara, Hirofumi Inoue, and Jun Nomiyama 274

Leishman's Stain, A Romanowsky Stain Suboptimal for Demonstration of Auer Rods
K.F. Wong, S.K. Ma, J.K.C. Chan, and J.S.L. Chung 275

ANNOUNCEMENT 277

INSTRUCTIONS TO AUTHORS 278

Volume 45, Number 4 **April 1994**

ORIGINAL ARTICLES

Alpha Thalassemia and Stroke Risk in Sickle Cell Anemia
Robert J. Adams, Abdullah Kutlar, Virgil McKie, Elizabeth Carl, Fenwick T. Nichols, Jin Cai Liu, Kathleen McKie, and Anthony Clary 279

Autologous Peripheral Stem Cell Transplantation of the Blastic Phase of Chronic Myeloid Leukemia Following Sequential High-Dose Cytosine Arabinoside and Melphalan
Ursula A. Matulonis, James D. Griffin, and George P. Canellos 283

Serum Transferrin Receptor in Hereditary Hemochromatosis and African Siderosis
Roy D. Baynes, James D. Cook, Thomas H. Bothwell, Brian M. Friedman, and Theo E. Meyer 288

Molecular Basis and Hematological Characterization of Hb H Disease in Southeast Asia
Ta-Chih Liu, Shyh-Shin Chiou, Sheng-Fung Lin, Tyen-Po Chen, Wen-Ping Tseng, Pao-Huei Chen, and Jan-Gowth Chang 293

Intravenous Extended Infusion of Recombinant Human Soluble Thrombomodulin Prevented Tissue Factor-Induced Disseminated Intravascular Coagulation in Rats
Mitsunobu Mohri, Michiko Oka, Yoshikazu Aoki, Yasunori Gonda, Sigeto Hirata, Komakazu Gomi, Takao Kiyota, Taisuke Sugihara, Shuji Yamamoto, Torao Ishida, and Ikuro Maruyama 298

Thrombotic Microangiopathy and Retroviral Infections: A 13-Year Experience
Antonio Ucar, Hugo F. Fernandez, John J. Byrnes, Eric C-Y Lian, and William J. Harrington, Jr. 304

Lineage Determination of CD7+ CD5− CD2− and CD7+ CD5+ CD2− Lymphoblasts: Studies on Phenotype, Genotype, and Gene Expression of Myeloperoxidase, CD3ε, and CD3δ
Noriko Yoneda, Eiji Tatsumi, Keisuke Teshigawara, Shigekazu Nagata, Takahiro Nagano, Yuji Kishimoto, Takashi Kimura, Koujiro Yasunaga, and Nobuo Yamaguchi 310

Prevalence of Antithrombin Deficiency in Healthy Blood Donors: A Cross-Sectional Study
Philip S. Wells, Morris A. Blajchman, Penny Henderson, Michael J. Wells, Christine Demers, Ron Bourque, and Ann McAvoy 321

CASE REPORTS

Disseminated *Mycobacterium avium*-Intracellulare Infection in a Patient With Myelodysplastic Syndrome (Refractory Anemia)
Hiroko Tsukada, Takaaki Chou, Yasuo Ishizuka, Osamu Ogawa, Takako Saeki, Satoshi Ito, Masaya Wakabayashi, Naoki Hayashi, and Masaaki Arakawa **325**

Deep Vein Thrombosis in a 13-Year-Old Boy With Hereditary Protein S Deficiency and a Review of the Pediatric Literature
A. Blanco, M. Bonduel, L. Peñalva, M. Hepner, and M. Lazzari **330**

Myelomonocytic Crisis With t(5;17) and a p53 Mutation in a Patient With Chronic Myelogenous Leukemia
Hitoshi Nakagawa, Hiroshi Fujii, Hiroyuki Nakai, Johji Inazawa, and Shinichi Misawa **335**

REVIEW

Impact of Reinduction Regimens for Relapsed and Refractory Acute Lymphoblastic Leukemia in Adults
Jeanna L. Welborn **341**

BRIEF REPORT

Two Different Mutations in Codon 68 Are Observed in Hb G-Philadelphia Heterozygotes
T.P. Molchanova, D.D. Pobedimskaya, Z. Ye, and T.H.J. Huisman **345**

LETTERS AND CORRESPONDENCE

Rearrangement of the BCR/ABL and TCR-β Genes in Lymph Node Blast Crisis Diagnosed of Chronic Myeloid Leukemia
A. Villegas and F.A. González **347**

Gaucher's Disease and Acquired Coagulopathy
John E. Humphries and Charles E. Hess **347**

Megadose Methyprednisolone for Pure Red Cell Aplasia
Şinasi Özsoylu **348**

Essential Thrombocythemia and Pregnancy
Naomi Rahimi-Levene, Zion Hagay, Uriel Elchalal, and Alain Berrebi **348**

Hodgkin's Disease in a Patient With Neurofibromatosis
Hideyo Natori, Ken Tanaka, Kaori Shiraishi, Seishi Osabe, Hiroto Jojima, Junichi Honda, Kazuhiko Matsuo, Osamu Nakashima, and Kotaro Oizumi **349**

Splenic Infiltrates in Acute Lymphoblastic Leukemia
Ashwin P. Patel, Kirti M. Patel, Shilin N. Shukla, Bipin N. Savani, N. Gopal, Ketan N. Bavishi, P.L. Madan, Asha Anand, Bharat J. Parikh, and Pankaj M. Shah **349**

Aspergilloma Formation in a Pneumatocele in a Patient With Acute Lymphoblastic Leukemia
Ken Satoh, Akihiko Chubachi, Hidetaka Niitsu, Takashi Nimura, and Akira B. Miura **351**

Acute Monoblastic Leukemia (M5a) Presenting Numb Chin Syndrome
Tatsuharu Ohno, Yuzuru Yasuda, and Hiroo Furukawa **352**

Hirulog® Therapy for Heparin-Associated Thrombocytopenia and Deep Venous Thrombosis
Thomas Reid III and Barbara M. Alving **352**

Author's Reply
Sucha Nand **353**

Author Index to Volume 45 . . . . **355**

Subject Index to Volume 45 . . . . **359**

American Journal of Hematology 45:1–9 (1994)

Characteristics of Zinc Binding to Human Red Blood Cell Membranes

José Brandão-Néto and William R. Bell

Division of Endocrinology and Metabolism, Department of Medicine, Universidade Estadual Paulista (J.B.-N.), Botucatu, São Paulo, Brasil, and Division of Hematology, Department of Medicine, The Johns Hopkins University School of Medicine (W.R.B.), Baltimore, Maryland

The objective of the present study was to standardize the analysis of zinc binding on human red blood cell (RBC) membranes in 20 normal adults. The displacement studies revealed that at the maximal stable zinc concentration tested (600 μM), 57% (mean) of the bound ^{65}Zn was displaced and to displace half maximal ^{65}Zn, the stable zinc concentration was 300 μM. Scatchard plots revealed two classes of binding sites for zinc on RBC membranes: one with higher affinity, Kd = 1.20×10^{-5} M (site I), and the other with lower affinity, Kd = 2.77×10^{-4} M (site II). Binding sites occupancy was 97% means and 58.5% means for sites I and II, respectively. The displacement was affected by temperature, membrane protein concentration, freezing, thawing, and dialysis. Other metal cations, including Co^{++}, Fe^{++}, and Mn^{++}, had very little effect on ^{65}Zn displacement, in contrast copper displaced ^{65}Zn from its binding sites on RBC membranes. Zinc binding to RBC membranes was rapid and readily reversible in a dynamic equilibrium with its binding sites. It is anticipated that this method will be applicable to studies of a wide variety of diseases specifically related to zinc metabolism in humans as well as in animals.

Key words: erythrocyte ghost, zinc binding sites, trace elements, normal individuals

INTRODUCTION

Zinc is an essential trace element for the functional activity of over 200 metalloenzymes and is required for lipid, carbohydrate, protein, and nucleic acid metabolism [1]. It has been indicated as an important metal for the proper maintenance and stabilization of cells and biomembranes [2]. There is a small but critical concentration of zinc in biomembranes which varies according to the levels of plasma zinc. For example, the membrane is protected and stabilized by increased zinc levels and the inverse occurs when zinc levels are decreased [3]. This trace element is important for the structural and functional integrity of the membrane and these functions cannot be performed by other ions [2,3]. Thus, it is crucial to cellular physiology and, for this reason, it has been suggested that many of the pathological clinical signs of zinc deficiency can be explained by a loss of zinc from the plasma membrane [3,4]. Indeed, total zinc content in erythrocytes from zinc-deficient rats was similar to that in erythyrocytes from zinc-adequate controls but membrane zinc contents was significantly reduced in the RBC of zinc-deficient animals [5].

On the basis of these reports, which have established the structural and functional relationship between zinc and biomembranes, the present investigation was undertaken to standardize the features of ^{65}Zn binding on human RBC membranes.

MATERIALS AND METHODS

This study was conducted on 20 adult normal individuals, 14 males and 6 females, aged 21–43 years (33.9 ± 7.76) who were not taking any medications. Blood samples were collected in the morning and 10–20 ml of whole blood were collected by sterile atraumatic venepuncture from each subject and placed in vacutainer tubes containing EDTA.

Received for publication July 7, 1992; accepted May 13, 1993.

Address reprint requests to Dr. J. Brandão-Néto, Departamento de Clínica Médica, Faculdade de Medicina, Universidade Estadual Paulista, Botucatu, São Paulo 18610, Brasil.

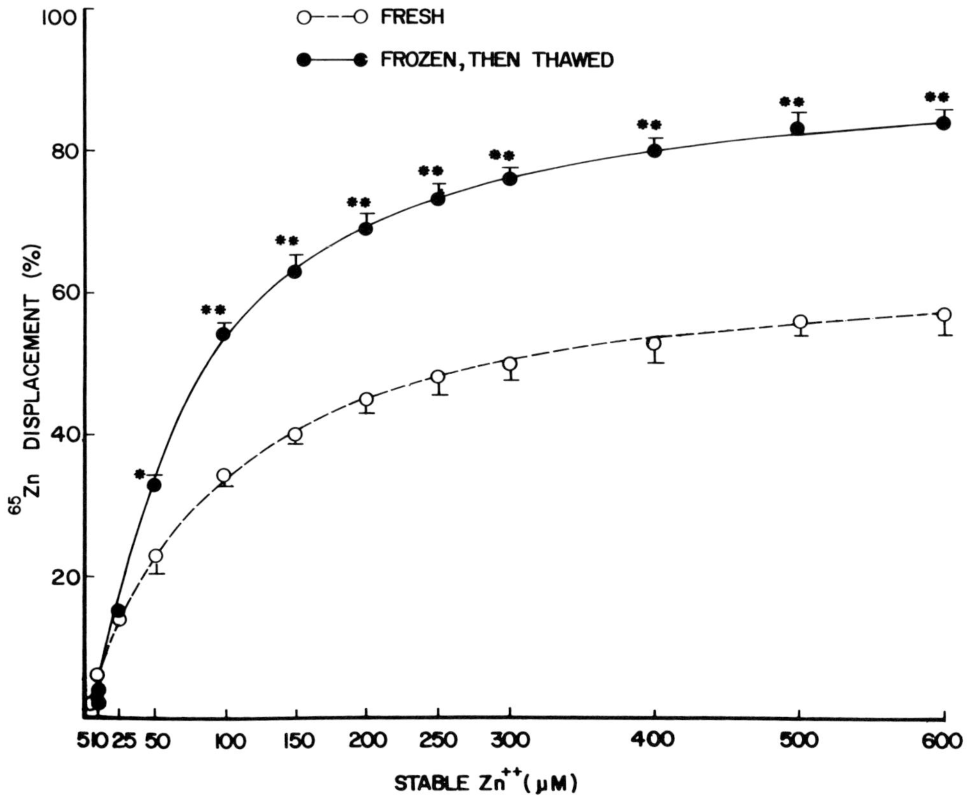

Fig. 1. Displacement of ^{65}Zn binding to RBC membranes by stable Zn^{++}. Values are mean ± SD of duplicate samples from fresh and frozen and then thawed membranes from eight experiments. Values significantly different from fresh membranes are indicated by the following superscripts: *$P < 0.001$ and **$P < 0.0001$, by Student's t test [8]. Experimental procedures are described in Materials and Methods.

Membrane Preparation

The procedure was carried out by the method of Steck and Kent [6]. Blood was centrifuged at 2,500 rpm for 10 min at 5°C. The plasma, white blood cells, and platelets were removed. One milliliter of remaining red blood cells (RBC) was transferred to a 50 mL polypropylene round bottom centrifuge tube and washed three times with 40 mL PBS-EDTA, pH 7.4 (5 mM sodium phosphate, 150 mM NaCl, and 0.1 M NaEDTA) at 2,500 rpm for 5 min at 5°C. The supernatant was discarded after each centrifugation. In the same test tube(s), the washed RBC were then lysed with lysing buffer, pH 7.4 (5 mM sodium phosphate, 0.1 M NaEDTA). Erythrocyte ghosts were centrifuged (19,000 rpm for 10 min at 5°C) in a Sorvall centrifuge with an SS-34 rotor and washed six times with the same buffer until they were white and the supernatant was clear. A very small viscous pellet was removed each time. Phenylmethylsulfonyl fluoride (35 mg in 1 mL dimethyl sulfoxide) was used immediately before cell lysing at the concentration of 40 μL/tube. To reseal membranes outside-out, the ghosts were washed twice more in TBS (pH 7.4, 10 mM Tris-HCl, 150 mM NaCl) and incubated overnight at 5°C.

Protein Determination

Soluble protein was measured by a Bio-Rad dye-binding procedure based on the method of Bradford [7], and the membranes were adjusted to 1.0 mg membrane protein/mL TBS, pH 7.4.

Protocol for ^{65}Zn Binding to RBC Membranes

^{65}Zn retention and displacement. One milligram membrane protein/mL TBS, pH 7.4, was incubated with 1 μCi $^{65}ZnCl_2$ at 37°C (reaction mixture), for 60 min, in a water bath shaker. One hundred microliters of reaction mixture was added at 30 sec intervals to 900 μL stable Zn^{++} (5 to 600 μM) in TBS, pH 7.4, in duplicate, at 37°C, for 15 min, using a water bath shaker. Incubation was stopped exactly after 15 min by the addition of ice-cold buffer (1 mL TBS pH 7.4). Ghosts were washed twice with 1 mL cold TBS, pH 7.4, and centrifuged twice at 10,000 rpm for 15 min at 5°C. The supernatants were discarded and the pellet was counted in a gamma counter Gamma 8000, Beckman Scientific Instruments, Fullerton, CA. Retention of ^{65}Zn was calculated as the amount of ^{65}Zn bound to RBC membranes after displacement with stable zinc (or other cations) and expressed as per

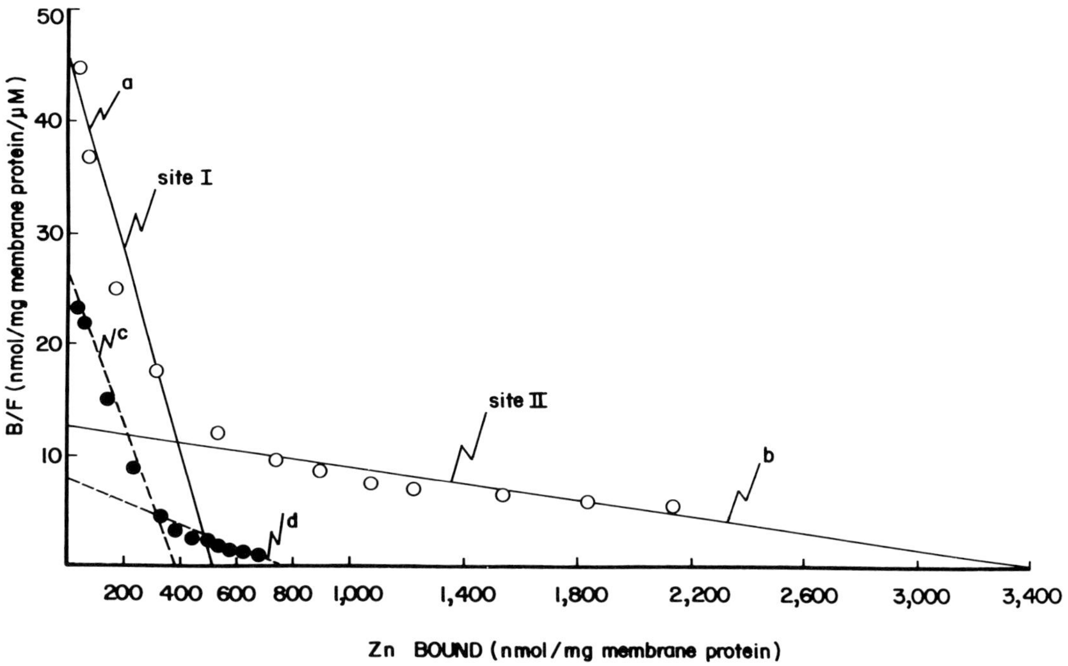

Fig. 2. Scatchard plot of ^{65}Zn binding to RBC membranes. A curvilinear Scatchard plot was generated by a mixture of binding sites in the samples: site I represents high affinity and site II represents low affinity. Lines a and b (fresh membranes) and c and d (frozen and thawed membranes) were determined by computer analysis [9,10].

cent ^{65}Zn bound to the membranes at a given concentration of added stable cation. Per cent displacement is calculated by subtracting per cent retention from 100. Maximal displacement was the value obtained after the addition of the highest concentration of stable cation. Using the above protocol we examined following a) freezing and thawing of RBC membranes, using the same amount and batch of fresh membranes, thawed 24 hr later; b) temperature dependence, altering the temperature from 37 to 4, 25 and 45°C; c) protein dependence, testing the values of 0.05 mg and 0.25 mg membrane protein/100 μL TBS, pH 7.4, against the usual protein concentration (0.1 mg/100 μL); and d) cations and histidine on zinc specificity, testing Cu^{++}, Co^{++}, Fe^{++}, Mn^{++}, and histidine on the same stable zinc molarity (5 to 600 μM).

^{65}Zn Reversibility evaluated with two different sets of conditions. 1) Three hundred micromolars of stable zinc was added 60 min after incubation of ^{65}Zn with RBC membranes, under the conditions described in the previous paragraph. The incubation times were 30 sec, and 1, 2, 4, 6, 8, 10, 20, 30, 40, 50, and 60 min, using tubes in duplicate. 2) Membranes (0.1 and 1.0 mg protein/mL) were dialyzed against 1 L TBS, pH 7.4, at room temperature, and duplicate samples were taken to measure ^{65}Zn in a gamma counter at times 1, 2, 3, 4, 5, 6, 7, 8, 12, and 24 hr. A molecular porous membrane (Spectra/Por; Spectrum Medical Industries, Inc., USA) with mw exclusion limit (6.000–8.000) was employed.

Radioactive zinc (^{65}Zn) was purchased from DuPont (USA). All reagents were of analytical grade and metal ions were obtained from Sigma Chemical Co, St. Louis, and all other chemicals from Pharmacia Fine Chemicals, Piscataway, NJ. Plastic ware was used and washed with 3 N HCl along with deionized water in all experiments.

RESULTS

^{65}Zn Retention and Displacement

Displacement was prompt at low concentrations of added zinc (5 to 150 μM) and decreased rapidly up to 600 μM concentration. This indicates that zinc binding to and displacement from RBC membranes occurred at a specific rate in relation to a specific concentration of added stable zinc (Fig. 1). A Scatchard plot of these data is shown in Figure 2, indicating that there are two binding sites for zinc on RBC membranes. Zinc bound tightly to site I and loosely to site II. When the curves for fresh membranes were compared with the curves for frozen and thawed membranes, displacement was found to be more pronounced in thawed membranes (Fig. 1). The competitive results of K_d (M), binding sites occupancy (%), and maximal zinc displacement (%) are indicated in Table I and Figure 2.

TABLE I. Zinc Binding Characteristics to Human RBC Membranes*

Membrane conditions	Fresh		Frozen and thawed	
binding sites	I	II	I	II
Correlation coefficient	−0.97 ± 0.01	−0.91 ± 0.00	−0.99 ± 0.01	−0.94 ± 0.06
Slope	−0.09 ± 0.04	−0.004 ± 0.00	−0.07 ± 0.01	−0.01 ± 0.00
Y intercept	45.87 ± 13.33	12.46 ± 1.00	26.34 ± 4.09	7.67 ± 0.94
X intercept	509.11 ± 69.02	3418.21 ± 347.61	373.88 ± 34.50	771.89 ± 131.69
K_d (M)	120×10^{-5} ± 00.43	2.77×10^{-4} ± 0.46	1.46×10^{-5} ± 0.37	1.03×10^{-4} ± 0.33
Binding sites occupancy (%)	96.97 ± 1.10	58.45 ± 4.37	97.33 ± 0.64	83.82 ± 4.46
Maximal zinc displacement (%)	57.00 ± 2.48		84.38 ± 1.80	

*Mean ± SD of duplicate samples in four experiments for each kind of membrane. See Figure 2.

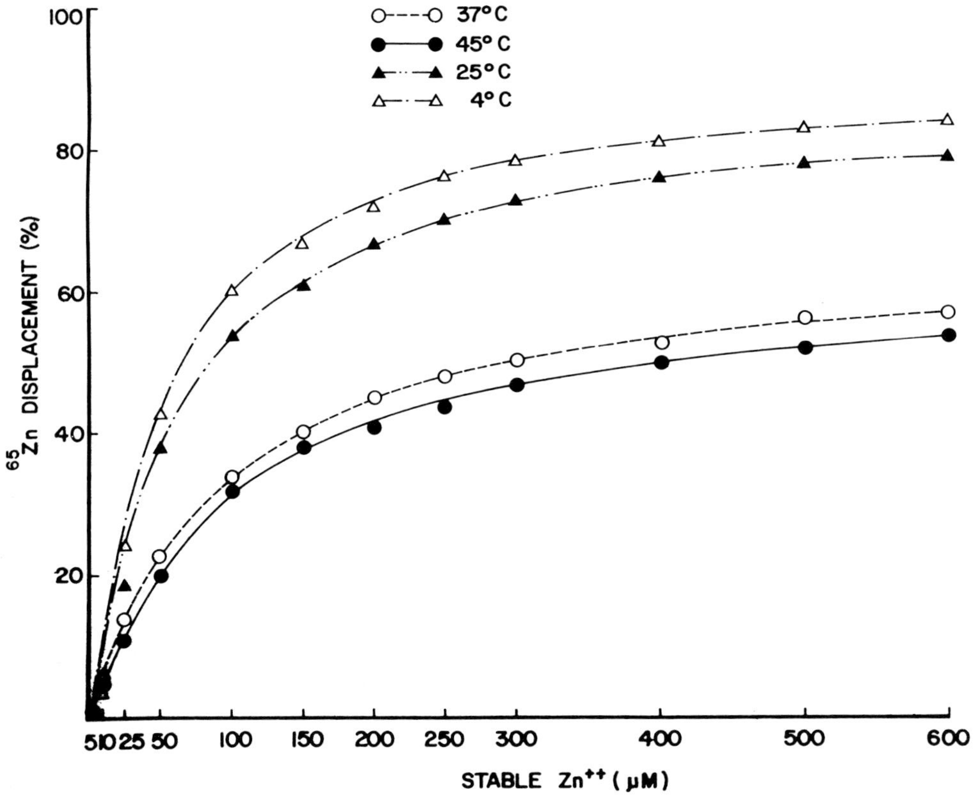

Fig. 3. Effect of temperature on ^{65}Zn displacement. Data are means of duplicate samples. The data obtained at 37°C are from four experiments and those obtained at all other temperatures are from one experiment each. See Table II and Materials and Methods for details.

Effect of the Temperature on ^{65}Zn Displacement

Figure 3 shows that ^{65}Zn displacement was practically equal at temperatures of 25 and 4°C and at 37 and 45°C, although there was a clear difference between these two temperature sets. This observation was confirmed by analysis of the results of K_d (M), binding sites occupancy (%), and maximal zinc displacement (%) in Table II. Thus, for the temperatures of 25 and 4°C, the K_d and binding sites occupancy at site I and site II, were similar, the same occurring with maximal zinc displacement. When these data are compared with those obtained at 37 and 45°C, clear differences can be observed.

Effect of Membrane Protein Concentration on ^{65}Zn Displacement

Three distinct curves were obtained for membrane protein concentrations ranging from 0.05 mg to 0.25 mg. By inspection at 150 μM on the abscissa (Fig. 4), it can be observed that the increase in displacement velocity is proportional to the fall in protein concentration. The re-

TABLE II. Effect of Temperature on Zinc Binding Characteristics of Human RBC Membranes*

Membrane condition	Fresh							
Temperatures	4°C		25°C		37°C		45°C	
binding sites	I	II	I	II	I	II	I	II
Correlation coefficient	−0.98	−0.92	−0.99	−0.90	−0.97	−0.91	−0.99	−0.91
Slope	−0.20	−0.007	−0.20	−0.006	−0.09	−0.004	−0.10	−0.004
Y intercept	53.67	6.70	62.44	7.66	45.87	12.46	55.64	15.24
X intercept	267.54	912.94	313.01	1356.96	509.11	3418.21	554.65	3695.67
K_d (M)	0.50×10^{-5}	1.36×10^{-4}	0.50×10^{-5}	1.77×10^{-4}	1.20×10^{-5}	2.77×10^{-4}	1.00×10^{-5}	2.42×10^{-4}
Binding sites occupancy (%)	99.05	79.27	99.00	73.51	96.97	58.45	97.32	59.87
Maximal zinc displacement (%)	84.00		79.00		57.00		54.00	

*Values for 37°C are the means of four experiments performed in duplicate. Values for 4°C, 25°C, and 45°C are the means of duplicate samples in one experiment. See Figure 3.

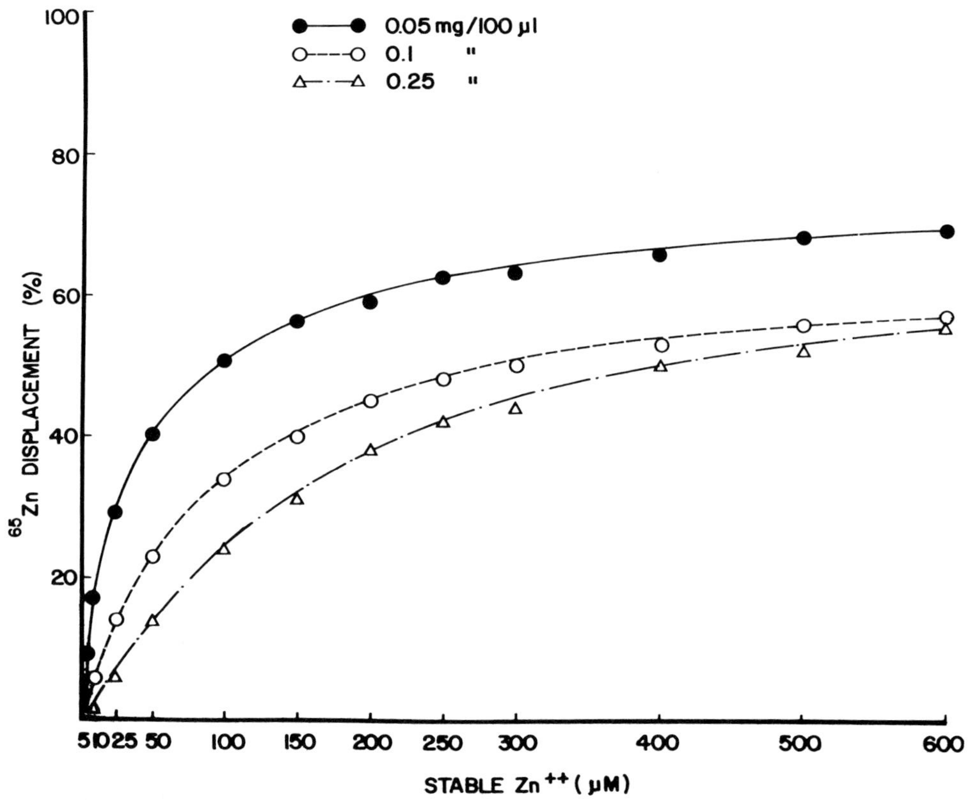

Fig. 4. Effect of membrane protein concentration on ^{65}Zn displacement. Values are means of duplicate aliquots from four experiments. See Table III and Materials and Methods for details.

sults of the ^{65}Zn binding characteristics are presented in Table III.

Effect of Cu^{++}, Co^{++}, Fe^{++}, and Mn^{++} on ^{65}Zn Displacement

The curves for the four elements were totally different from the zinc displacement curve (Fig. 5) and could be divided into two classes: one including Cu^{++} which induced marked ^{65}Zn displacement and the other including Co^{++}, Fe^{++}, and Mn^{++} which induced very little zinc displacement. On the other hand, the chelate structure of histidine also removed the ^{65}Zn from the RCB membranes.

Reversibility of ^{65}Zn Binding to RBC Membranes

To examine this reversibility, stable zinc (300 µM) was added 60 min after the incubation of ^{65}Zn with RBC membranes. ^{65}Zn displacement was rapid, 57% within 30

TABLE III. Effect of Membrane Protein Concentration on Zinc Binding Characteristics of Human RBC Membranes*

Membrane condition	Fresh					
protein concentrations	0.05 mg		0.1 mg		0.25 mg	
binding sites	I	II	I	II	I	II
Correlation coefficient	−0.96	−0.93	−0.97	−0.91	−0.99	−0.91
Slope	−0.06	−0.002	−0.09	−0.004	−0.14	−0.007
Y intercept	37.93	11.56	45.87	12.46	36.03	9.14
X intercept	665.24	4727.45	509.11	3418.21	247.36	1214.06
K_d (M)	1.75×10^{-5}	4.09×10^{-4}	1.20×10^{-5}	2.76×10^{-4}	0.69×10^{-5}	1.33×10^{-4}
Binding sites occupancy (%)	96.37	53.25	96.97	58.45	98.13	73.06
Maximal zinc displacement (%)	69.00		57.00		55.00	

*Values for 0.1 mg are the means of four experiments performed in duplicate. Value for 0.05 mg and 0.25 mg are the means of duplicate aliquots in one experiment. See Figure 4.

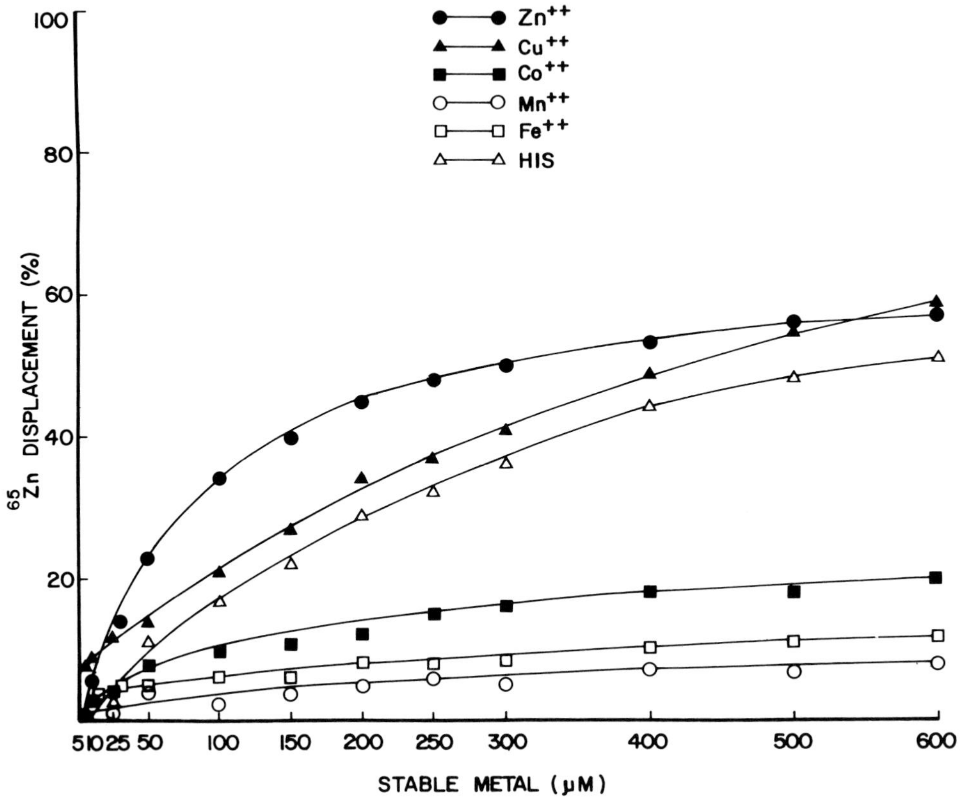

Fig. 5. Displacement of ^{65}Zn binding to RBC membranes by stable Zn^{++} and other metal cations. For Zn^{++} each point represents the mean of duplicate determinations of four experiments. For all other cations (and histidine) each point represents the mean of duplicate determinations of one experiment. Experimental procedures are described in Materials and Methods.

sec, and plateaued at this level for 8 min. After 10 min, zinc levels decreased to 75% within 60 min (Fig. 6). In another study, membranes were dialyzed against TBS, pH 7.4, after incubation with ^{65}Zn. As shown in Figure 7, about 50% of bound ^{65}Zn was dissociated from binding sites on the membranes during the first hour for 0.1 mg membrane protein/mL and within 5 hr for 1.0 mg membrane protein/mL. After 24 hr of dialysis, about 95% ^{65}Zn was displaced at both membrane protein concentrations.

DISCUSSION

The experiments performed suggest that the total amount of ^{65}Zn displaced from its binding sites depended partially on the concentrations of stable zinc used. As

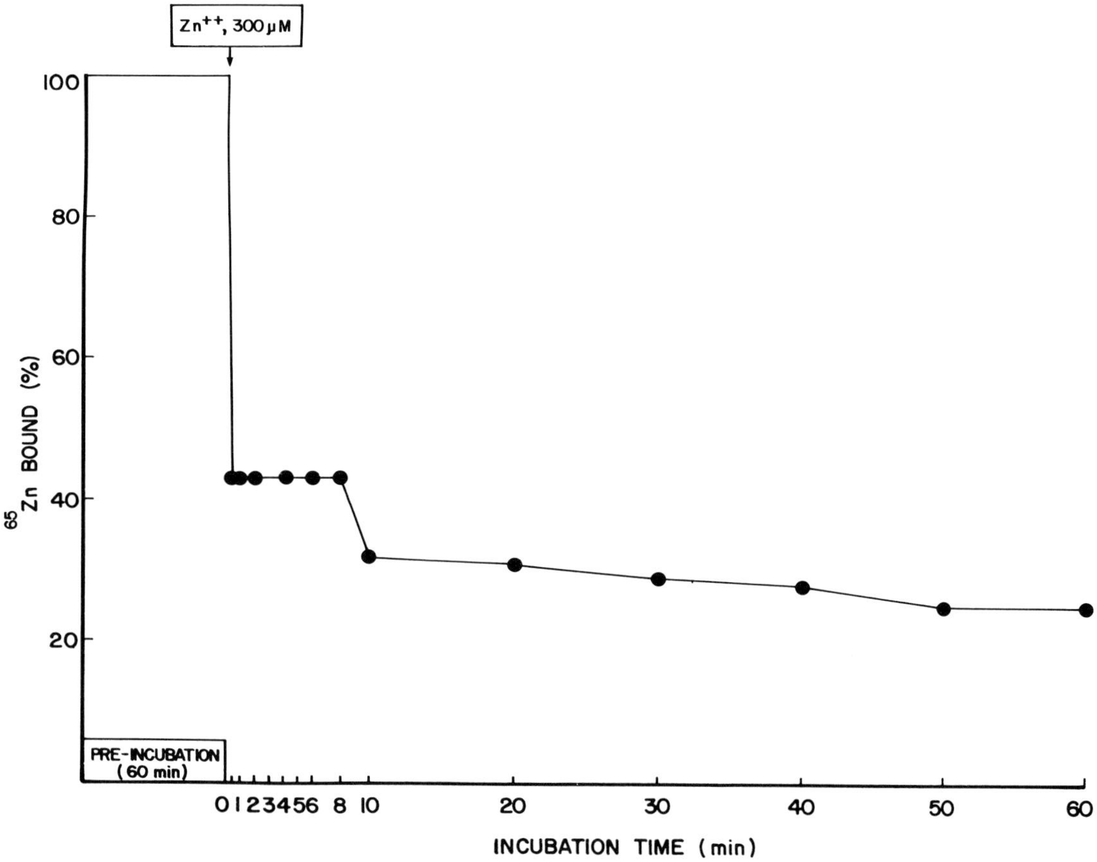

Fig. 6. Reversibility of ^{65}Zn binding to RBC membranes by 300 μM Zn^{++}. Each point represents the mean of duplicate samples from one experiment and is representative of two others under identical conditions. See Materials and Methods for details.

shown in Figure 1, ^{65}Zn displacement increased with increasing stable zinc concentration reaching a plateau at about 300 μM concentration. The maximum ^{65}Zn concentration (600 μM) displaced only 57% ^{65}Zn. This 43% retention can be undestood by observing Figure 2 and Table I. Two binding sites for zinc were detected on human RBC membranes: zinc bound more tightly to site I than to site II. The 43% retention may be explained by K_d which may reflect an equilibrium state between ^{65}Zn retention and displacement at site II.

This retention of ^{65}Zn by binding sites was also affected by other conditions. Freezing and thawing (Fig. 1 and 2; Table I) significantly affected the functional integrity of membranes and probably altered their physical state [6], demonstrating that this procedure is inappropriate for studies with erythrocyte ghost membranes. Temperature (Fig. 3; Table II), membrane protein concentration (Fig. 4; Table III), and the effect of other ions (Fig. 5) also influenced retention. The displacement curves for ^{65}Zn versus stable Cu^{++}, Co^{++}, Fe^{++}, and Mn^{++} were completely different when compared with the curve for stable Zn^{++}, except for Cu^{++} with a curve similar to that of stable Zn^{++}. A possible explanation is that the Cu^{++}-binding site is very close to the Zn^{++}-binding site but slightly different in terms of geometric configuration. Zinc is usually found in a tetrahedral configuration and Cu^{++} in square planar geometry [11]. Zinc is an integral part of the erythrocyte membrane [12], has preferential affinity for its lipoproteins and proteins [3], and the presence of cysteine and histidine residues is required for the binding of this metal [11,13]. The removal of ^{65}Zn by histidine as shown in Figure 5 illustrates this phenomenon. Finally, a rapid and ready reversibility of ^{65}Zn bound to its binding sites was clearly demonstrated when excess stable zinc (300 μM) was added 60 min after incubation of ^{65}Zn with membranes (Fig. 6) and during dialysis against TBS, pH 7.4, at room temperature (Fig. 7). All of these results demonstrate the specificity and reversibility of the zinc binding sites on RBC membranes.

Human RBC contain 150–200 μM Zn/L^{-1} cells [14], while human plasma contains about 15 μM Zn^{++} [15]. These values are within the range established for the variation of stable zinc concentrations when K_d was de-

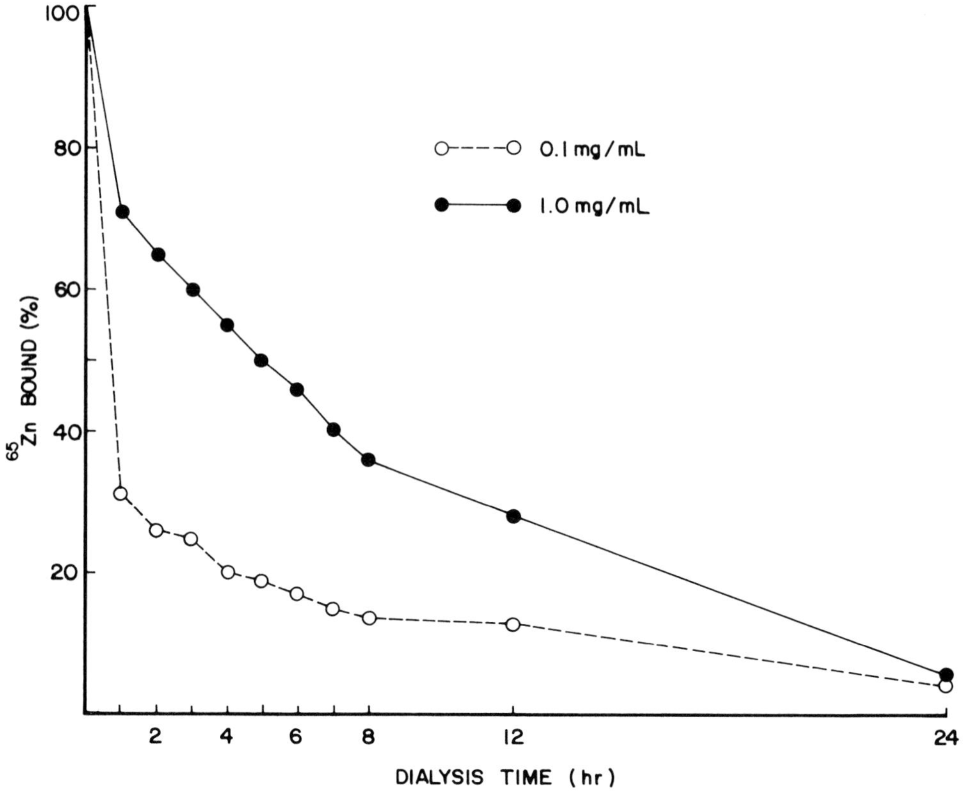

Fig. 7. Reversibility of ^{65}Zn binding to RBC membranes. Dialysis was performed using 0.1 and 1.0 mg membrane protein against 1 L of TBS, pH 7.4, at room temperature for 24 hr. Fifty percent of bound ^{65}Zn represents 30 min and 5 hr for 0.1 mg and 1.0 mg membrane protein, respectively. Values given are means of duplicate samples. See Materials and Methods for details.

termined. These data suggest that zinc may be found in a state of dynamic equilibrium with its concentration in plasma and RBC and with the K_d of the binding sites.

In summary, we believe that this method, based on the evidence that zinc has an important role in the structure and function of biomembranes [4,16], may greatly contribute to a more complete understanding of the pathophysiology of zinc deficiency.

ACKNOWLEDGMENTS

We thank CNPq (number 201412/88.8) and FUNDUNESP (number 413/91) for supporting this work and Dr. Richard A. Anderson from Beltsville Human Nutrition Research Center—USDA for his critical review of this paper, and Mario Augusto Dallaqua for help in the preparation of the manuscript. This work was supported in part by Grants HL36260, HL24898, and HL07525 from NHLBI of the NIH of the Department of Health Education and Welfare, Bethesda, Maryland 20892.

REFERENCES

1. Hambidge KM, Casey CE, Krebs NF: Zinc. In Mertz W (ed): "Trace Elements in Human and Animal Nutrition." Orlando: Academic Press, Inc., 1986, p 1.
2. Chvapil M: Effect of zinc on cells and biomembranes. Med Clin North Am 60:799, 1976.
3. Bettger WJ, O'Dell BL: A critical physiological role of zinc in the structure and function of biomembranes. Life Sci 28:1425, 1981.
4. Jay M, Stuart SM, McClain CJ, Palmieri DA, Butterfield DA: Alterations in lipid membrane fluidity and the physical state of cell-surface sialic acid in zinc-deficient rat erythrocyte ghosts. Biochim Biophys Acta 897:507, 1987.
5. Bettger WJ, Fernandez MS, O'Dell BL: Effect of zinc deficiency on the zinc content of rat red cell membranes. Fed Proc 39:896, 1980.
6. Steck TL, Kant JA: Preparation of impermeable ghosts and inside-out vesicles from human erythrocyte membranes. Methods Enzymol 31:172, 1974.
7. Bradford MM: A rapid and sensitive method for the quantification of microgram quantities of protein utilizing the principle of protein-dye binding. Anal Biochem 72:248, 1976.
8. Snedecor GW, Cochran WG: "Statistical Methods." Ames: The Iowa State University Press, 1967, p 135.
9. Scatchard G: The attractions of proteins for small molecules and ions. Ann NY Acad Sci 51:660, 1949.

10. Bolander FF: Receptors. In Bolander FF (ed.): "Molecular Endocrinology." San Diego: Academic Press, Inc., 1989, p. 61.
11. Vallee BL, Wacker WEC: Metalloproteins. In Nuerath H (ed): "The Proteins: Composition, Structure, and Function." New York: Academic Press, Inc., 1970, p 61.
12. Chvapil M, Montgomery D, Ludwig JC, Zukoski CF: Zinc in erythrocyte ghosts. Proc Soc Exp Biol Med 162:480, 1979.
13. Lee MS, Gippert GP, Soman KV, Case DA, Wright PE: Three-dimensional solution structure of a single zinc finger DNA-binding domain. Science 245:635, 1989.
14. Ohno H, Doi R, Yamamura K, Yamashita K, Iizura S, Taniguchi N: A study of zinc distribution in erythrocytes of normal humans. Blut 50:113, 1985.
15. Foote JW, Delves HT: Albumin bound and alpha-2-macroglobulin bound zinc concentration in the sera of healthy adults. J Clin Pathol 37:1050, 1984.
16. Bettger WJ, O'Dell BL: A critical physiological role of zinc in the structure and function of biomembranes. Life Sci 28:1425, 1981.

American Journal of Hematology 45:10–15 (1994)

Quantitative Defect of Glycoprotein Ib in Severe Cirrhotic Patients

María J. Sánchez-Roig, José Rivera, José M. Moraleda, and Vicente Vicente García
Division of Hematology, Hospital General Universitario, Avda Intendente Palacios, Murcia, Spain

A decrease of platelet agglutination induced by ristocetin has been described in cirrhotic patients. In order to investigate the relationship of such phenomenon with a putative defect on platelet membrane glycoprotein Ib, we have studied the quantitative and functional status of Gp Ib in eleven severe alcoholic cirrhotic patients, and the ability of their formalin-fixed platelets to agglutinate in the presence of normal plasma plus ristocetin. Interestingly, we found a significant decrease of immunoreactive GP Ib molecules (9,978 ± 1,534 vs. 17,064 ± 404 molecules per platelet) and ristocetin-dependent binding of vWF (9,113 ± 1,338 vs. 13,992 ± 1,968 molecules per platelet) ($P < 0.01$) in comparison to the levels found in a control group of healthy subjects. Immunoblotting analysis of platelet lysates confirmed the reduction of GP Ib level in cirrhotic patients, but showed no modification on the precipitation pattern of this glycoprotein. The ristocetin-induced platelet agglutination (light transmission %) was also significantly lower in patients with cirrhosis (48 ± 7.6 vs. 92 ± 3.6, $P < 0.01$), and correlated with the binding of normal vWF ($r = 0.863$, $P = 0.0013$). Patients with bleeding times longer than 7 min and/or clinical history of bleeding episodes showed the lowest values of platelet agglutination and GP Ib level. In conclusion, our present results indicate that liver cirrhosis is associated with a relevant decrease of functional GP Ib molecules on the platelet surface. This reduction might be related to the prolongation of bleeding time and to the bleeding diathesis observed in cirrhotic patients.

Key words: glycoprotein Ib, liver cirrhosis

INTRODUCTION

Bleeding is a frequent complication in patients suffering from severe liver cirrhosis. Several mechanisms have been proposed to explain the hemostatic defects in these patients, including abnormalities of the platelet function [1,2]. In fact, the attachment of platelets to the vessel wall is a critical step in the regulation of hemostasis. This step is mainly mediated by the interation of the von Willebrand factor (vWF) present at the subendothelium with the platelet glycoprotein Ib/IX (GP Ib/IX) complex, the most relevant vWF receptor [3]. The importance of this interaction is emphasized by the hemorragic complications observed in patients with Bernard-Soulier's syndrome, in which the GP Ib/IX is defective [4], or with von Willebrand's disease, in which vWF is abnormal [5].

Taking into account that the GP Ib/IX complex can be readily degradated or modulated by a number of proteases [6], it is not surprising that the platelet function becomes altered in pathological conditions where the fibrinolytic activity rises. In patients with severe liver cirrhosis an increased thrombin activation rate and fibrinolytic activity has been shown [7], which might be responsible for the proteolytic fragmentation of vWF and GP Ib/IX observed in vivo [8,9].

In order to gain further insight into the role of GP Ib/IX in the pathogenesis of the hemostatic disorders present in liver cirrhosis, we have investigated the functional status of this complex in eleven severe cirrhotic patients and correlated the data to the bleeding time (BT) and bleeding tendency of these patients.

Received for publication December 31, 1992; accepted May 13, 1993.

Address reprint requests to Prof. Dr. Vicente Vicente García, Servicio de Hematología-Centro Regional de Hemodonación, Hospital General Universitario, Avda Intendente Palacios, Murcia, Spain.

TABLE I. Clinical and Laboratory Data of Cirrhotic Patients Enrolled Into the Study

Patient	Bleeding history	Bleeding time	Platelet count (10^9/l)	Ristocetin cofactor (%)	MPV (fL)
1	Yes	17	51	558	8.9
2	No	10	195	505	8.2
3	No	4	247	137	8.8
4	No	6	201	166	8.7
5	No	6	363	549	8.5
6	Yes	9	179	455	8.6
7	No	—	51	234	9.3
8	No	—	70	412	9.4
9	Yes	7	83	739	9.4
10	No	4	262	352	8.9
11	Yes	—	51	575	10.1
Normal values	No	3–7[a]	197–329[a]	65–150[a]	8.1–10.2[a]

[a]Normal values were obtained from fifty healthy volunteers.

MATERIALS AND METHODS

Monoclonal Antibodies (MAbs), vWF, and Other Reagents

The anti GP Ib MAbs, LJ-P19 and LJ-Ib10 were generously provided by Dr. ZM Ruggeri (Research Institute of Scripps Clinics, CA). The purification and immunochemical properties of both antibodies have been extensively detailed elsewhere [3,10]. Normal vWF was purified from a pool of blood bank cryoprecipitates essentially as reported by Newman et al. [11]. The final vWF preparation had more than 100 U/mg of protein of ristocetin cofactor activity and a multimeric structure like that of plasma vWF [3]. Ristocetin was obtained from Menarini Diagnostics (Italy). All other reagents were commercially available and were of the highest purity grade.

Patients and Control Group

Eleven patients were involved in the study (eight men and three women, mean age 52 years, range 38–69 years) with biopsy-proven liver cirrhosis. In all the patients the pathogenic cause was chronic alcohol consumption. Four patients had a clinical history of bleeding complications (Table I). For comparisons, we also studied seven age and sex matched healthy individuals without a bleeding history who had been tested to have normal liver function. Patients and healthy volunteers were fully informed of the aims and procedures involved in the experimental study, which was performed according to the Declaration of Helsinki as amended in Venice in 1983.

Blood Collection, Bleeding Time, and RiCof

Blood samples of patients and normal volunteers were collected by venipuncture through a 19-gauge needle into one-sixth final volume of acid/citrate/dextrose (ACD), pH 4.5, and immediately centrifuged at 160g for 10 min to obtain platelet-rich plasma (PRP). Unless otherwise stated, platelets from PRP were washed by the albumin density-gradient technique [12], fixed with formalin as described [13], and finally resuspended in 20 mmol/L hepes buffer, pH 7.35, also containing 137 mmol/L NaCl. Platelet count and size were determined using a Coulter Counter, Model STKS (Coulter Electronics, Hialeah, FL). No agglutination of platelet suspensions occurred upon addition of ristocetin (1 mg/ml) unless normal plasma or purified vWF was added. The skin bleeding times were obtained on the volar part of the forearm using a commercial template method (Simplate II, General Diagnostics, NJ) as recommended by Mielke [14]. Results were expressed as the average bleeding time from two vertical incisions. All bleeding times were performed by a single trained nurse, unaware of the purpose of the study. Ristocetin cofactor activity assays (RiCof) were performed in formalin-fixed platelets as described [15].

Measurement of Platelet Agglutination Induced by Ristocetin

Studies of formalin-fixed platelets agglutination were performed according to the method of Sloand et al. [16], with minor modifications. Briefly, fixed-platelets (2×10^5 cells/μL) were mixed (v/v) with normal plasma (a pool of 15 normal blood donors) in a cuvette, which was placed into an aggregometer (Aggrecorder II, Menarini Diagnostics, Italy) previously set up at 37°C and continuous stirring at 1,000 rpm. After warming for 5 min,platelet agglutination was induced by the addition of ristocetin at a final concentration of 1 mg/mL and the light transmission recorded for 7 min.

TABLE II. Values of Ristocetin Agglutination and Binding of LJ-P19 and vWF for Patients and Controls

	LJ-P19		vWF		Ristocetin agglutination
	Bmax (mol/pl)	Kd (range,nM)	Bmax (mol/pl)	Kd (range,nM)	Light transmission (%)
Patients (n = 11)	9,978 ± 1534**	16.9 ± 2.2	9,113 ± 1338*	11.1 ± 2.1	48 + 7.6***
Controls (n = 7)	17,064 ± 404	12.1 ± 3.4	13,992 ± 1968	9.7 ± 0.6	92 ± 3.6

*P = 0.05 with respect to control values.
**P = 0.007 with respect to control values.
***P = 0.0004 with respect to control values.

Radioiodination of Proteins

LJ-P19 and vWF to be used in binding assays were radiolabeled with carrier-free Na-1251 (Amersham International, Oxford, England) using Iodogen (Pierce Chemical Rockford, IL), as described by Fraker and Speck [17]. Specific activities ranged between 0.2 and 0.9 mCi/mg of protein. Polyacrylamide gel electrophoresis of radiolabeled proteins showed no structural alteration as compared to the unlabeled counterparts.

Binding Studies

The methods used to measure the binding of monoclonal IgG and vWF (ristocetin-dependent binding) to platelets have been previously described [3]. Briefly, formalin-fixed platelets (1×10^8 cells/ml) were incubated with increasing concentrations of radiolabeled LJ-P19 (0–50 μg/ml) or vWF (0–40 μg/ml) plus ristocetin (1 mg/ml), for 30 min at RT. Platelet-bound and free radioactivity were separated by centrifugation and counted in a gamma-scintillation counter (LKB, Multigamma, Pharmacia, Sweden). Binding parameters, including the estimate of nonspecific binding, were derived from scatchard type analysis using the computer-assisted program LIGAND [18].

SDS-PAGE and Immunoblotting

The procedures for the obtaining of platelet lysates, SDS-PAGE, and immunoblotting analysis of GP Ib have been described in detail in a previous publication [3]. Bands containing GP Ib were identified by autoradiography (X-omat AR film, Kodak, Rochester, NY), following incubation of nitrocellulose membranes with the anti-GP Ib MAb LJ-Ib10 and with rabbit anti-mouse IgG labeled with ^{125}I.

Statistical Analysis

Results are given as mean values ± SEM. All data were subjected to a test of normal distribution. Differences in variables between the different groups of patients and the controls were evaluated by the one-way analysis of variance (ANOVA) and the Student's unpaired t test. To estimate a correlation between variables, Pearson's product moment correlation coefficients were calculated.

RESULTS

An overall picture of the BT, platelet count, plasma levels of RiCof, and MPV are given in Table I. Most cirrhotic patients showed high plasma levels of RiCof, and in four the BT was longer than 7 min. Binding studies with the anti-GP Ib MAb LJ-P19 (Table II) demonstrated a significant reduction in the level of this glycoprotein (Bmax values) in platelets of cirrhotic patients as compared to controls, whereas no differences were observed in the antigen-antibody affinity (Dissociation constant values, Kd). With respect to the functional status of the GP Ib, the ristocetin-induced binding of vWF was significantly decreased in platelets of patients with liver cirrhosis in comparison to controls, but the affinity of the vWF-GP Ib interaction was similar in both groups (Table II). In addition to these data, the ristocetin-induced agglutination of formalin-fixed platelets was also significantly reduced in cirrhotic patients (mean agglutination rate, light transmission, and %) (Table II). Interestingly, the ristocetin-induced binding of vWF and platelet agglutination had a good correlation in the group of patients with cirrhosis ($r = 0.863$, $P = 0.0013$). Therefore, the significant correlations between GPIb molecules per platelet, ristocetin agglutination, and vWF binding were found ($r = 0.845$, $P = 0.0083$ and $r = 0.807$, $P = 0.0155$, respectively).

No significant correlation could be demonstrated between platelet count vs. GPIb molecules per platelet ($r = 0.182$, $P = 0.665$), platelet count vs. ristocetin agglutination ($r = 0.518$, $P = 0.125$), bleeding time vs. GPIb molecules per platelet ($r = 0.186$, $P = 0.724$), and bleeding time vs. ristocetin agglutination ($r = 0.169$, $P = 0.639$).

TABLE III. Binding of LJ-P19 and vWF to Platelets From Control and Patients With Bleeding Time <7 and Bleeding Time >7 Min and Values of Ristocetin Agglutination

	LJ-P19		vWF		Ristocetin agglutination
	Bmax (mol/pl)	Kd (range,nM)	Bmax (mol/pl)	Kd (range,nM)	Light transmission (%)
Patients with BT <7 min (n = 4)	12,166 ± 2577	16.2 + 2.8	9,984 ± 1791	14.1 ± 2.1	63 ± 8**
Patients with BT >7 min (n = 4)	8,329 ± 1452***	12.8 ± 1.8	8,390 ± 2422*	8.8 ± 5.0	38 ± 11***
Controls (n = 7)	17,064 ± 40	12.1 ± 3.4	13,992 ± 1968	9.7 ± 0.6	92 ± 3.6

$^*P < 0.05$, $^{**}P < 0.005$, $^{***}P < 0.0005$ with respect to control values.

TABLE IV. Binding of LJ-P19 and vWF to Platelets From Patients With Bleeding History or Patients Without Bleeding History and Values of Ristocetin Agglutination for Both Groups

	LJ-P19		vWF		Ristocetin agglutination
	Bmax (mol/pl)	Kd (range,nM)	Bmax (mol/pl)	Kd (range,nM)	Light transmission (%)
Patients with bleeding history (n = 4)	9,639 ± 2252	16.3 ± 2.3	8,752 ± 2739	9.9 ± 4.7	35 ± 9
Patients without bleeding history (n = 7)	10,203 ± 2238	17.4 ± 3.5	9,319 ± 1590	11.7 ± 2.1	56 ± 10

As presented in Tables III and IV, when compared, cirrhotic patients with BT shorter and longer than 7 min and patients with or without bleeding clinical history, we found lower levels of LJ-P19/vWF binding (Bmax values) and ristocetin agglutination in those patients with longer bleeding times and in those with bleeding clinical history.

Finally, immunoblotting analysis of platelet lysates with the anti-GP Ib MAb LJ-Ib10 confirm a relevant decrease of GP Ib level in cirrhotic patients in comparison to controls, and revealed no other modification of this glycoprotein (Fig. 1).

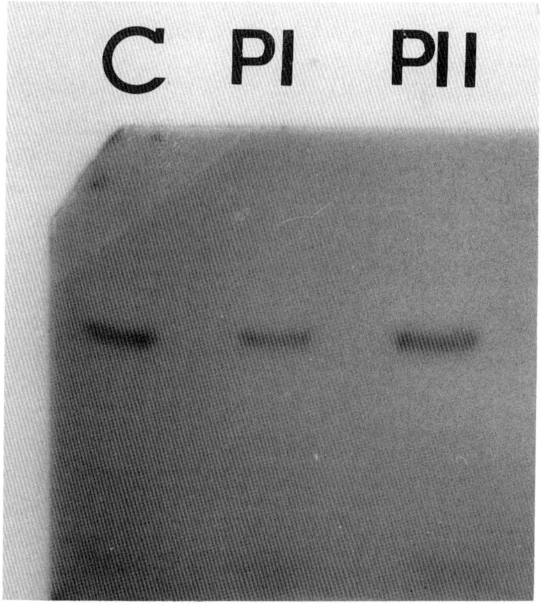

Fig. 1. Immunoblotting analysis of platelet GP Ib in control and cirrhotic patients. Lysates of ≈7 × 107 platelets of control (C) and cirrhotic patients (P) were analyzed by immunoblotting with the anti-GP Ib Mab LJ-Ib10 as described in Methods. The figure is a representative example of patients showing low level of GP Ib (PI and PII). An identical electrophoretic pattern of the GP Ib was observed in all the patients and the controls.

DISCUSSION

This paper describes new data indicating that patients affected by severe liver cirrhosis had decreased platelet agglutination induced by ristocetin in the presence of normal pooled plasma, and a reduced expression GP Ib on the platelet surface membrane. The mechanism(s) responsible for this defect of glycoprotein remains to be elucitated. Much evidence suggests that an increased proteolytic activity in the plasma of cirrhotics can induce proteolysis of circulating von Willebrand factor [8]. In addition, plasmin has been implicated in the reduction of GP Ib level in malignancies [19], uremia [16], and liver cirrhosis [9]. It has also been suggested that a loss of GP Ib in patients undergoing cardiopulmonary bypass or thrombolytic therapy might be due to the "peeling" of the platelet membrane by proteases [20]. Indeed, various proteolytic enzymes have been shown to cut the GP Ib releasing a 140 KD m.w. polypeptide from the amino terminal region, namely, glycocalicin [21]. This fragment contains functionally active binding sites for vWF and thrombin, and it is consequently involved in platelet adhesion and aggregation [10,22].

In our group of cirrhotic patients we have found a marked reduction of GP Ib levels on the platelet surface, by means of binding studies using both the specific anti-GP Ib MAb LJ-P19 and purified vWF. In addition, they have a defective platelet agglutination induced by ristocetin in the presence of normal plasma, which correlated with the vWF binding level. These findings are unlikely to be due to an internalization of GP Ib or to an abnormal GP Ib in the surface membrane, since immunoblotting analysis of platelet lysates with LJ-Ib10, which detects both membrane-bound and intracellular pools of GP Ib [23], confirms a decrease in the total platelet level of the glycoprotein and demonstrated a normal electrophoretic pattern of GP Ib in cirrhotic patients. Since the ristocetin-mediated binding of vWF to normal platelets depends on the integrity of GP Ib, it seems reasonable to speculate that the quantitative changes in GP Ib in these patients are related to a membrane glycoprotein fragmentation, as a result of an increased proteolytic activity generated under this clinical condition. The reason(s) why some cirrhotic patients have a prolonged bleeding time is unknown. Despite the fact that mild or moderately severe thrombocytopenia could be implicated in that prolongation in some of these patients, we have found evidence indicating, as previously suggested [15], that the platelet count is unrelated to bleeding time in liver cirrhosis. Furthermore, it seems rather unlikely that these patients are undergoing abnormalities at the level of the plasmatic vWF that may prolong the bleeding time, since we found high levels of RiCof, and we have previously described a normal multimeric structure of plasma vWF in liver cirrhosis [15]. Quantitative or qualitative alterations of the GP Ib/IX at the platelet membrane might be another explanation for the prolongation of the bleeding time in some cirrhotic patients because this complex plays a major role in the platelet adhesion to the vascular subendothelium. As mentioned above, in this study we found no apparent structural modification of the glycoprotein in liver cirrhosis, but significantly lower than normal level of GP Ib. Interestingly, we observed a tendency for those patients with bleeding times above 7 min, and those with history of bleeding episodes, to have decreased anti-GP Ib MAb/vWF binding and ristocetin induced agglutination. Although this decrease, in comparison to patients with shorter bleeding times and/or those without history of bleeding, failed to reach statistical significance, it also might be useful for the understanding of the hemostatic disorders in cirrhotic patients.

CONCLUSION

In patients suffering from liver cirrhosis, there is a significant reduction in the level of total and functional glycoprotein Ib in platelet that might be implicated in their hemostatic disorders.

ACKNOWLEDGMENTS

We thank Dr. Z.M. Ruggeri (Scripps Research Institute, La Jolla, CA) for providing MAbs against GP Ib/IX. This work was supported by research grants from Programa Sectorial de Promoción del Conocimiento en el área de Biomedicina y Ciencias de la Salud (PM 89-0070), Ministerio de Educación y Ciencia, and Fundación Ramón Areces. MJ Sánchez is a research fellow from MEC.

REFERENCES

1. Huber K, Kirchheimer JC, Korninger C, Binder BR: Hepatic synthesis and clearance of components of the fibrinolytic system in healthy volunteers and in patients with different stages of liver cirrhosis. Thromb Res 62:491, 1991.
2. Ingeberg S, Jacobsen P, Fischer E, Bentsen KD: Platelet aggregation and release of ATP in patients with liver cirrhosis. Scand J Gastroenterol 20:285, 1985.
3. Vicente V, Houghten RA, Ruggeri ZM: Identification of a site in the alpha-chain of platelet glycoprotein Ib that participates in von Willebrand factor binding. J Biol Chem 265:274, 1990.
4. De Marco L, Mazzucato M, Fabris F, De Roia D, Coser P, Girolami A, Vicente V, Ruggeri ZM: Variant Bernard-Soulier Syndrome type-Bolzano: A congenital bleeding disorder due to a structural and functional abnormality of the platelet glycoprotein Ib/IX complex. J Clin Invest 86:25, 1990.
5. Ruggeri ZM. Structure and function of vWF: Relationship to von Willebrand's disease. Mayo Clin Proc 66:847, 1991.
6. Cramer EM, Lu H, Caen JP, Soria C, Berndt MC, Tenza D: Differential redistribution of platelet glycoproteins Ib and IIb/IIIa after plasmin stimulation. Blood 77:694, 1991.
7. Paramo JA, Rifon J, Fernandez J, Cuesta B, Rocha E: Thrombin activation and increased fibrinolysis in patients with chronic liver disease. Blood Coag Fibrinol 2:227, 1991.
8. Lombardi R, Mannucci PM, Seghatchian MJ, Vicente V, Coppola R: Alterations of Factor VIII von Willebrand Factor in clinical conditions associated with an increase in its plasma concentration. Br J Haematol 49:61, 1981.
9. Ordinas A, Maragall S, Castillo R, Nurden AT: A glycoprotein I defect in the platelets of three patients with severe cirrhosis of the liver. Thromb Res 13:297, 1978.
10. Murata M, Ware J, Ruggeri ZM: Site-directed mutagenesis of a soluble fragment of platelet glycoprotein Ib-alpha demonstrating negatively charged residues involved in von Willebrand factor binding. J Biol Chem 266:15474, 1991.
11. Newman J, Johnson AJ, Karpatkin MH, Puszkin S: Methods for the production of clinically effective intermediate and high-purity factor-VIII concentrates. Br J Haematol 21:1, 1971.
12. Walsh PN, Mills DCB, White JG: Metabolism and function of human platelets washed by albumin density gradient separation. Br J Haematol 36:281, 1977.
13. Allain JP, Cooper HA, Wagner RH, Brinkhous KM: Platelets fixed with paraformaldehyde: A new reagent for assay of von Willebrand factor and platelet aggregating factor. J Lab Clin Med 85:318, 1975.

14. Mielke CH: Measurement of the bleeding time. Thromb Haemostas 52:210, 1984.
15. Mannucci PM, Vicente V, Vianello L, Cattaneo M, Alberca I, Coccato MP, Faioni E, Mari D: Controlled trial of desmopressin in liver cirrhosis and other conditions associated with a prolonged bleeding time. Blood 67:1148, 1986.
16. Sloand EM, Sloand JA, Prodouz K, Klein HG, Yu MW, Harvath L, Fricke W: Reduction of platelet glycoprotein Ib in uremia. Br J Haematol 77:375, 1991.
17. Fraker DJ, Speck JC: Protein and cell membrane iodinations with a sparingly-soluble-chloroamide, 1,3,4,6-tetrachloro,3a,6a-diphenylglycoluril. Biochem Biophys Res Commun 80:849, 1978.
18. Munson PJ, Rodbard D: LIGAND: A versatile computerized approach for characterization of ligand binding system. Anal Biochem 107:220, 1980.
19. Sloand EM, Kenney DM, Chao FC, Lawler J, Tullis J: Platelet antithrombin defect in malignancy: Platelet protein alterations. Blood 69:479, 1987.
20. Coller B: Platelets and thrombolytic therapy. N Engl J Med 322:33, 1990.
21. Handa M, Titani K, Holland LZ, Roberts JR, Ruggeri ZM: The Von Willebrand factor-binding domain of platelet membrane glycoprotein Ib: Characterization by monoclonal antibodies and partial amino acid sequence analysis of proteolitic fragments. J Biol Chem 261:12579, 1986.
22. De Marco JL, Mazzucato M, Masotti A, Fenton JW, Ruggeri ZM: Function of glycoprotein Ib-alplha in platelet activation induced by alpha thrombin. J Biol Chem 266:23776, 1991.
23. Michelson AD, Adelman B, Barnard M, Carrol E, Handin R: Platelet storage results in redistribution of glycoprotein Ib molecules: Evidence for a large intraplatelet pool of glycoprotein Ib. J Clin Invest 81:1734, 1988.

American Journal of Hematology 45:16–24 (1994)

Direct Evidence for Systemic Fibrinogenolysis in Patients With Acquired α_2-Plasmin Inhibitor Deficiency

Kenji Okajima, Isao Kohno, Gilbu Soe, Hiroaki Okabe, Kiyoshi Takatsuki, and Bernd R. Binder

Departments of Laboratory Medicine (K.O., H.O.) and Medicine (K.T.), Kumamoto University Medical School, Kumamoto, Japan; Research Division, Iatron Laboratories (I.K., G.S.), Tokyo, Japan; and Department of Medical Physiology (K.O., B.R.B.), University of Vienna, Vienna, Austria

To examine whether or not acquired α_2-plasmin inhibitor deficiency is associated with systemic fibrinogenolysis, we analyzed the fibrin and fibrinogen degradation products in eight patients with this condition in various disease states. The underlying disease was gastric cancer in three patients, metastatic prostatic cancer in two, acute promyelocytic leukemia in two, and abdominal aortic aneurysm in one patient. In all eight patients, the α_2-plasmin inhibitor level was reduced to less than 50% of normal, and plasmin-α_2-plasmin inhibitor complex levels were increased. Immunoblotting of serum using an anti-fibrinogen antibody detected a 250 kDa protein (corresponding to fragments X or DY) in all eight patients. Fragment Y and D monomer were detected in seven of the eight patients, indicating the occurrence of systemic fibrinogenolysis. However, they were not detected in one patient with metastatic prostatic cancer. To determine whether or not fibrinogen degradation was also occurring in the patient without fragment Y, we characterized the 250 kDa protein in all eight patients. The protein was found to be fragment X in the metastatic prostatic cancer patient without fragment Y, while it was fragment DY in the other seven patients. Thus, systemic fibrinogenolysis was present in all eight patients. In the two patients with metastatic prostatic cancer, the level of α_2-plasmin inhibitor gradually increased with the reduction of tumor size by treatment. Fragment X, fragment Y, and D monomer were not detected when the α_2-plasmin inhibitor level exceeded 60% of normal in both patients. In the other six patients fragment Y and D monomer also disappeared when the α_2-plasmin inhibitor level exceeded 60% of normal.

These findings suggest that systemic fibrinogenolysis only occurs when the plasma levels of α_2-plasmin inhibitor falls below 60% of normal due to activation of the fibrinolytic system by various pathological conditions.

Key words: α_2-plasmin inhibitor, systemic fibrinogenolysis, fibrin and fibrinogen degradation products, disseminated intravascular coagulation, bleeding tendency, antifibrinolytic therapy

INTRODUCTION

The fibrinolytic system plays an important role in controlling the dissolution of thrombus. The system consists of a plasminogen activator and plasminogen (which is converted to plasmin), and their inhibitors: plasminogen activator inhibitors and α_2-plasmin inhibitor (α_2PI). A balance between the serine proteases and the inhibitors is important in determining the function of the fibronolytic system. Pathological conditions involving the system include both hemorrhagic disorders resulting from excessive fibrinolysis and thrombosis resulting from inadequate fibrinolysis. Some useful molecular markers are available for evaluating the activity of fibrinolytic system; the plasma levels of plasmin-α_2PI complex, fibrin and fibrinogen degradation products, and cross-linked fibrin degradation products are increased as plasmin generation increases, while the levels of plasminogen and α_2PI are concomitantly decreased. Moreover, when excessive fibrinolysis occurs (i.e., fibrinogenolysis), fibrin-

Received for publication December 31, 1992; accepted May 13, 1993.

Address reprint requests to Dr. Kenji Okajima, Department of Laboratory Medicine, Kumamoto University Medical School, Honjo 1-1-1, Kumamoto 860, Japan.

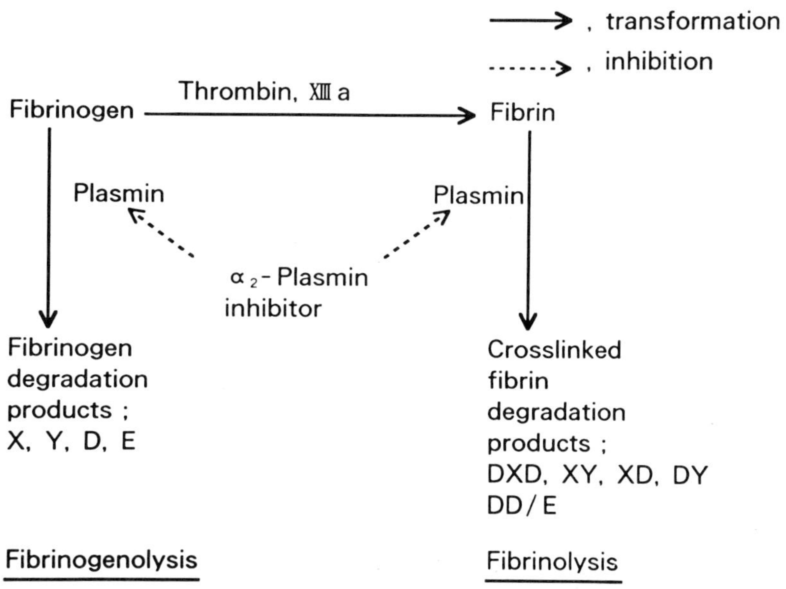

Fig. 1. Degradation of fibrinogen and fibrin by plasmin.

ogen degradation products (fragments X, Y, D, and E) can be detected in the plasma (Fig. 1).

The most important inhibitor of plasmin is α_2PI, which was isolated by Moroi and Aoki [1], and the molecular mechanisms by which α_2PI regulates fibrinolysis have also been elucidated [2,3]. Patients with congenital α_2PI deficiency develop a bleeding tendency as a result of accelerated fibrinolysis [4], suggesting that α_2PI may have an important influence on the fibrinolytic system in various disease states. However, direct evidence of accelerated fibrinolysis in patients with acquired α_2PI deficiency has been lacking.

In the present study, to investigate the role of α_2PI in various conditions which activate the fibrinolytic system, we determined whether or not systemic fibrinogenolysis was present in patients with acquired α_2PI deficiency.

MATERIALS AND METHODS

Reagents

All chemicals were purchased from commercial sources. Thrombin and urokinase were obtained from Mochida Pharmaceutical Co. (Osaka, Japan). Sodium dodecyl sulfate-polyacrylamide gel electrophoresis (SDS-PAGE) showed that the thrombin preparation contained only α-, β-, and γ-thrombin, with the major band being α-thrombin. Reptilase was purchased from Iatron Co. (Tokyo, Japan) and fibrinogen was purchased from KabiVirtum (Stockholm, Sweden). Analysis using SDS-PAGE demonstrated that the purity of the fibrinogen preparation was >95%. Although some minor bands with a higher molecular weight than that of fibrinogen were detected by SDS-PAGE, they did not react with an anti-human fibrinogen antibody upon immunoblotting. Alkaline phosphatase-conjugated goat anti-mouse immunoglobulin, alkaline phosphatase-conjugated goat anti-rabbit immunoglobulin, nitrocellulose membranes, and molecular weight standards [soybean trypsin inhibitor (21,500), carbonic anhydrase (31,000), ovalbumin (45,000), bovine seruma ablumin (66,200), phosphorylase b (92,500), β-galactosidase (116,250), and myosin (200,000)] were obtained from BioRad (Richmond, CA). In addition, 5-bromo-4-chloro-3-indolyl phosphate and nitro-blue tetrazolium were purchased from Sigma Chemical Co. (St. Louis, MO), while CNBr-activated Sepharose 4B was obtained from Pharmacia Fine Chemicals (Uppsala, Sweden). The monoclonal antibodies JIF-25 and JIF-23 were kindly supplied by Dr. Gilbu Soe (Research Division, Iatron, Inc., Chiba, Japan). Purified fragment E (E1,2) was kindly supplied by Dr. Michio Matsuda (Division of Hemostasis and Thrombosis Research, Institute of Hematology, Jichi Medical School, Tochigi, Japan). All other reagents used were of analytical grade.

Patient Profile and Definition

We studied eight patients with acquired α_2PI deficiency due to various underlying diseases (gastric cancer in three, metastatic prostatic cancer in two, acute promyelocytic leukemia in two, and abdominal aortic aneurysm in one). The results of coagulation and fibrinolysis studies in the eight subjects are shown in Table I. A diagnosis of disseminated intravascular coagulation (DIC) was made in seven patients on the basis of the following criteria: 1) the presence of an underlying disease fre-

TABLE I. Laboratory Findings of Coagulation and Fibrinolysis in Patients With Acquired α_2-Plasmin Inhibitor Deficiency

	Patients								
	Metastatic prostatic cancer		Acute promyelocytic leukemia		Gastric cancer				
Tests[a]	1	2	1	2	1	2	3	Abdominal aortic aneurysm	Normal values (mean ± S.D.)
Soluble fibrin monomer complex	−	+++	+	+	+	++	++	+	−
FDP (D) (ng/ml)	20930	86120	57370	31420	17320	28450	87520	27730	487 ± 105
Cross-linked fibrin degradation products (μg/ml)	3.3	88.1	7.7	28.9	5.3	29.2	65.4	14.1	0.18 ± 0.16
α_2-PI (% of normal)	36	39	39	46	44	49	48	42	101.0 ± 9.4
Plasmin-α_2 PI complex (μg/ml)	2.6	13.2	14.1	10.3	6.7	2.6	9.2	5.0	0.22 ± 0.1

[a] α_2 PI, α_2-plasmin inhibitor; FDP (D), fibrin and fibrinogen degradation products (D).

quently associated with DIC, 2) the presence of clinical bleeding or organ dysfunction, and 3) detection of soluble fibrin monomer complex and an increase of the fibrin and fibrinogen degradation products (E) [FDP(E)] level > 500 ng/ml. A diagnosis of acquired α_2PI deficiency was made according to the following criteria: 1) α_2PI activity decreased to less than 50% of normal, 2) increased plasma levels of FDP(E) and plasmin-α_2PI complex, and 3) absence of liver failure (no clinical and laboratory evidence for hepatic impairment. After the diagnosis of acquired α_2PI deficiency and/or DIC was made, the patients were treated as follows. One patient with gastric cancer (a 45-year-old man, patient 1) underwent gastrectomy, while the other two gastric cancer patients (a 51-year-old man, patient 2, and a 42-year-old woman, patient 3) received chemotherapy and administration of heparin (10,000 U/day). Both of the patients with metastatic prostatic cancer (a 56-year-old man, patient 1, and a 60-year-old man, patient 2) received castration and hormonal therapy. In addition, the two patients with acute promyelocytic leukemia (a 48-year-old man, patient 1, and a 39-year-old woman, patient 2) were treated with heparin (10,000 U/day) and chemotherapy, while the 72-day-old man with an abdominal aortic aneurysm underwent aneurysectomy. Gingival bleeding was observed in the patients with metastatic prostatic cancer and aortic aneurysm, while gingival bleeding and petechiae were observed in the leukemia patients. Gastrointestinal bleeding was observed in all three gastric cancer patients. Antifibrinolytic agents were not administered to any patients.

Blood Collection and Assays

Blood samples were collected with a 1/10 volume of 3.8% sodium citrate and centrifuged at 2,000g for 10 min at 4°C. The plasma thus obtained was stored at −70°C prior to laboratory analysis. To obtain serum samples, plasma was incubated for 30 min at room temperature with a 1/10 volume of saline containing 40 IU/ml of bovine thrombin, 5 mM $CaCl_2$, and 5.7 trypsin inhibitor units/ml of aprotinin for 30 min at room temperature followed by centrifugation at 15,000g for 30 min at 4°C. The resultant supernatant was used as serum. Blood samples for the determination of FDP(D) fractions were collected into evacuated SPLI-tubes (Diagnostica Stago, France), which contained reptilase, aprotinin, and $CaCl_2$. After being allowed to stand for 30 min at room temperature, the blood samples were centrifuged at 2,000g for 20 min at room temperature, and the resultant supernatant was used for the determination of FDP(D).

The FDP(D) fraction was determined by a latex agglutination method, using anti-human fibrinogen antibody-coated particles and an automatic analyzer (LA-2000; Eiken Chemical Co., Japan), as described previously [5]. Plasma levels of cross-linked fibrin degradation products were determined by a latex agglutination assay, using latex particles coated with a monoclonal antibody (JIF-23) against the plasmic fragment DD derived from human cross-linked fibrin [6]. Measurement was performed with an automatic analyzer (LPIA-100; Iatron Co., Tokyo, Japan). The level of α_2PI was determined from the residual plasmin activity after incubation of diluted plasma with excess plasmin by using a chromogenic substrate (S-2251; Kabi Diagnostica, Sweden) [7]. Plasmin-α_2PI complex levels were determined by a one-step sandwich enzyme immunoassay using polyclonal anti-plasminogen antibody-coated polystyrene balls and a peroxidase-conjugated monoclonal anti-α_2PI antibody (Teijin Co. Tokyo, Japan) [8]. Soluble fibrin monomer complex levels were determined by the fibrin monomer-coated erythrocyte agglutination method [9].

Preparation and Purification of the Plasmic Degradation Products of Fibrinogen and Cross-Linked Fibrin

For the purification of fragment D, human fibrinogen (12 mg/ml) was dissolved in 50 mM sodium phosphate buffer (pH 7.5) containing 150 mM NaCl, 5 mM $CaCl_2$, and 0.05% NaN_3, and then was incubated for 3 hr at 37°C with a mixture of 1.5 U/ml of plasminogen and 1,000

IU/ml of urokinase. After the addition of 100 trypsin inhibitor units/ml of aprotinin, plasmic digests were subjected to gel filtration on a 2.6 × 67 cm Sephacryl S300 column (Pharmacia) in a buffer containing 50 mM Tris-HCl (pH 7.4), 28 mM sodium citrate, 0.1 M NaCl, 0.02% NaN_3, and 0.028 trypsin inhibitor units/ml of aprotinin. Fractions containing fragment D were pooled and dialyzed against 10 mM Na_2HPO_4 (pH 9.1), after which they were applied onto a 2.5 × 18 cm DEAE-cellulose column (Whatman, DE-52) equilibrated with 10 mM NaH_2PO_4 (pH 9.1) followed by 320 mM KH_2PO_4 (pH 4.4). Preparation of cross-linked fibrin and its plasmic digest was performed according to the method of Olexa [10]. Human fibrinogen (grade L, KabiVirtum) was enriched with factor XIII and clotted as described by Terukina [11]. Cross-linked fibrin (1 g) was suspended in 20 ml of 0.15 M Tris-HCl (pH 7.8), containing 5 mM $CaCl_2$ and 0.02% NaN_3. Plasmin (0.53 IU/ml) was added to this solution, which was then incubated for 2 hr at 37°C. At the end of incubation, 500 μl of aprotinin (100 trypsin inhibitor units/ml) was added to terminate the reaction. Plasmic digests of cross-linked fibrin were then applied to a lysine Sepharose 4B column (Pharmacia) to remove plasmin. Plasmic digests of cross-linked fibrin were subjected to gel filtration using Sephacryl S300 (Pharmacia) to separate FDP fragments with a high molecular weight (higher than that of DY/YD or YY/DXD) from those with a low molecular weight (mainly DD/E). These high molecular weight FDP fragments [FDP(A)] and the low molecular weight FDP fragments [FDP(B)] were used as standards in the present experiments. For the purification of DD/E, FDP(B) was re-chromatographed on a Sephacryl S300 column to remove contaminating high molecular weight FDP fragments.

Plasmic Digestion of Serum Samples

Serum samples were incubated with 1,000 IU/ml of urokinase and 10 casein units/ml of plasminogen in 0.15 M NaCl for 90 min at 37°C. Aprotinin (20 trypsin inhibitor units/ml) was added to terminate the reaction. After being let stand for 30 min at room temperature, the serum samples were subjected to immunoblotting.

SDS-PAGE and Protein Extraction

SDS-PAGE with 4% and 10% gels or a 3.5–9% linear gradient gel in 0.1% SDS was performed as described previously [12]. Gels were subjected to silver-staining using a commercially available kit (Daiichi Pure Chemicals Co., Tokyo, Japan). After SDS-PAGE, each gel was cut into 5 mm strips between 2.5 cm and 7.5 cm from the upper edge. Protein was extracted by incubating each strip with a solution of 0.02 M Tris-HCl, 0.15 M NaCl, and 0.1% SDS (pH 7.6) for 72 hr at 25°C, and then the solubilized protein was precipitated with acetone. The precipitate was evaporated to dryness and dissolved in a buffer containing 0.0625 M Tris-HCl (pH 6.8), 1.8% SDS, 6.4% glycerol, and 0.005% bromophenol blue with or without 0.58 M 2-mercaptoethanol. The samples thus obtained were subjected to further SDS-PAGE as was done above and immunoblotting.

Immunoblotting

For the separation and identification of fibrin and fibrinogen degradation products, immunoblotting was performed using a rabbit anti-human fibrinogen antibody (Dako, Inc.) or a monoclonal antibody against the γ-remnant (residues 86–302) of fibrinogen (JIF-25) [11] as the primary antibody. After separation by SDS-PAGE, proteins were electrophoretically transferred from the gel onto nitrocellulose membrane (20 mA/cm^2 for 2 hours) using an electroblot apparatus (Holizeblot AE-6670, Atto Co. Tokyo) according to the method described previously [12]. The transfer buffer consisted of 0.1 M Tris-HCl (pH 8.3), 0.192 M glycine, 20% methanol, and 0.02% SDS. After transfer, the nitrocellulose membranes were soaked in 0.02 M Tris-HCl (pH 7.6) containing 0.15 M NaCl and 1% (w/v) gelatin for 1 hr at room temperature, and then incubated for 3 hr at room temperature with either 50 μg/ml rabbit anti-fibrinogen antibody or JIF-25 in the same buffer. After three washes with 0.02 M Tris-HCl (pH 7.6) containing 0.15 M NaCl and 0.1% Tween 20, the membranes were incubated for 1 hr at room temperature with alkaline phosphatase-conjugated goat anti-rabbit IgG or anti-mouse IgG (BioRad, Inc.). They were finally washed four times with the same buffer and incubated with 100 mM 5-bromo-4-chloro-3-indolyl phosphate and 100 mM nitro-blue tetrazolium in 100 mM diethanolamine and 5 mM $MgCl_2$ buffer (pH 9.5) for color development.

Adsorption of Plasma Samples by Immuno-Affinity Gel

The F(ab′)^2 fragment of the monoclonal antibody JIF-23 was coupled to CNBr-activated Sepharose 4B according to the manufacturer's instructions. Ten microliters of plasma was incubated with 200 μl of the gel suspension (50% v/v) in 0.05 M Tris-HCl (pH 8.0) with 0.15 M NaCl for 13 hr at 4°C. Then the mixture was centrifuged at 10,000g for 10 min at 20°C. The resultant precipitate was resuspended and subjected to 3 cycles of incubation in 0.02 M Tris-HCl (pH 7.6), 150 mM NaCl, and 0.05% Tween-20 for 30 min at 25°C, followed by centrifugation at 10,000g for 10 min at 20°C. The precipitate was incubated with 0.02 M Tris-HCl (pH 7.6) containing 150 mM NaCl and 2% SDS, followed by centrifugation with acetone precipitation, and was then subjected to SDS-PAGE.

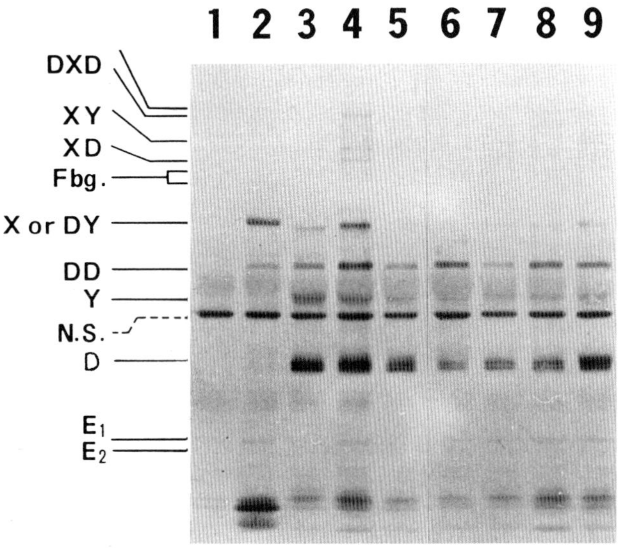

Fig. 2. Immunoblotting of FDP in patient serum using anti-human fibrinogen antibody. After being subjected to SDS-PAGE with 3.5% to 9% linear gradient gel, serum samples from normal human subjects and the patients with acquired α_2PI deficiency were analyzed by immunoblotting using a rabbit anti-human fibrinogen antibody as described in Materials and Methods. Lane 1, serum sample from normal human subjects; lanes 2–9, serum samples from the patients with acquired α_2PI deficiency. Normal human subject, lane 1; metastatic prostatic cancer, lane 2 (patient 1 without DIC) and lane 4 (patient 2 with DIC); acute promyelocytic leukemia, lane 3 (patient 1) and lane 7 (patient 2); abdominal aortic aneurysm, lane 5; gastric cancer, lane 6 (patient 1), lane 8 (patient 2), and lane 9 (patient 3). N.S., non-specific band.

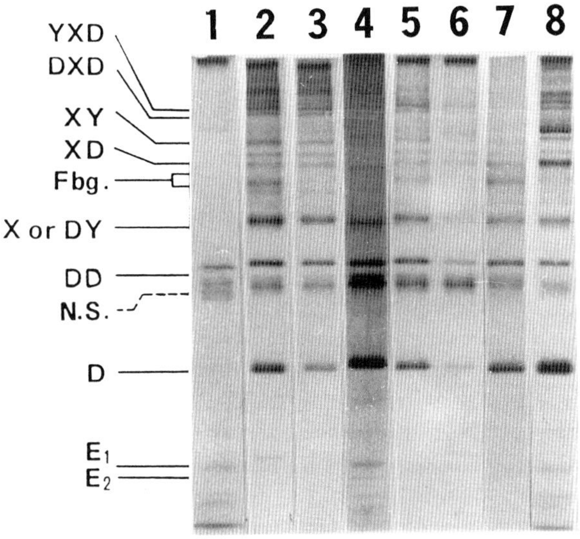

Fig. 3. SDS-PAGE of patient FDP bound to Sepharose 4B-conjugated monoclonal antibody, JIF 23. Plasma samples from the patients with acquired α_2PI deficiency were incubated with Sepharose 4B to which the monoclonal antibody JIF-23 was conjugated. The gels were then treated with 0.2% SDS to dissociate the bound proteins as described in Materials and Methods. Recovered proteins derived from the serum samples of these patients were analyzed by SDS-PAGE with 10% gel according to the method of Laemmli [12]. SDS-PAGE of the recovered proteins from patients with metastatic prostatic cancer (lane 1, patient 1 without DIC; lane 3, patient 2 with DIC), acute promyelocytic leukemia (patient 1, lane 2; patient 2, lane 6), abdominal aortic aneurysm (lane 4), and gastric cancer (patient 1, lane 5; patient 2, lane 7; patient 3, lane 8) are shown.

RESULTS

Coagulation and Fibrinolysis in Acquired α_2PI Deficiency

The eight patients in this series all had acquired α_2PI deficiency and their coagulation and fibrinolysis parameters are shown in Table I. Common characteristic findings other than a marked decrease of the α_2PI level were a significant increase of FDP(D) and plasmin-α_2PI complex levels. DIC was present in seven of the eight patients and fibrinogen levels were decreased in three patients (two with leukemia and one with gastric cancer). No clinical and laboratory evidence for hepatic impairment was observed. These findings suggested that the decrease of α_2PI levels might be due to consumption as a consequence of plasmin generation.

Analysis of FDP by Immunoblotting

Since determination of plasma immunoreactive FDP levels using anti-fibrinogen antibody does not allow a distinction between the degradation products of fibrinogen and fibrin, immunoblot analysis of FDP was performed to detect fibrinogenolysis. As shown in Figure 2, immunoblot analysis of serum samples using anti-human fibrinogen antibody revealed a 250 kDa protein (corresponding to fragments X or DY) in all the patients as well as detecting fragment Y and D monomer in the seven patients with DIC. DD fragments were also observed in all of the patients with DIC. These findings suggested that fibrinogenolysis was occurring in the DIC patients in addition to the degradation of cross-linked fibrin.

Adsorption of Plasma Samples by JIF-23-Conjugated Sepharose 4B

To determine whether or not fibrinogenolysis was also occurring in the patient without DIC (patient 1 with metastatic prostatic cancer), we investigated whether this patient's 250 kDa protein was fragment X. To distinguish fragment X from fragment DY, we examined the 250 kDa proteins detected in all eight patients using JIF 23, a monoclonal antibody that recognizes the N-terminus of fragment D [6]. After the incubation of plasma samples or various standard samples of FDP with JIF 23-conjugated Sepharose 4B, the protein was eluted with a buffer containing 2% SDS. The eluted protein was then analyzed by SDS-PAGE. As shown in Figure 3, the 250 kDa

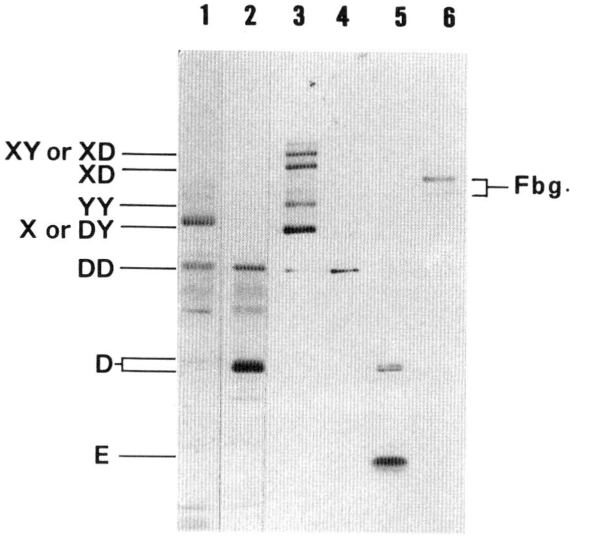

Fig. 4. Immunoblotting of serum sample from patient 1 with metastatic prostatic cancer before and after plasmin treatment. The serum sample from patient 1 with metastatic prostatic cancer was incubated with urokinase (1,000 IU/ml) and plasminogen (10 casein units/ml) as described in Materials and Methods. Serum samples thus treated were subjected to immunoblotting using anti-human fibrinogen antibody, according to the method described in Figure 2. Immunoblotting of serum samples from patient 1 with metastatic prostatic cancer before (lane 1) and after plasmin treatment (lane 2). Immunoblotting of FDP(A) (lane 3) and FDP(B) (lane 4) and fragments D, E1, and E2 (lane 5), and fibrinogen (lane 6) are also shown.

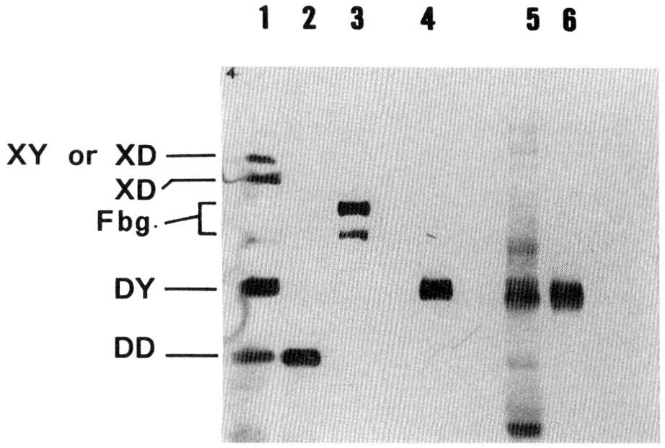

Fig. 5. Immunoblotting of the Mr 250 kDa protein detected in patient 1 with metastatic prostatic cancer and fragment DY after extraction from SDS-PAGE gel using anti-human fibrinogen antibody. After SDS-PAGE of the patient 1 serum sample and FDP(A) with 3.5–9% linear gradient gel, the Mr 250 kDa protein and DY fragment were extracted from the gel as described in Materials and Methods. Immunoblottings, using anti-human fibrinogen antibody of FDP(A) (lane 1), FDP(B) (lane 2), fibrinogen (lane 3), the extracted DY fragment (lane 4), serum sample of the patient 1 (lane 5), and the extracted Mr 250 kDa protein in the patient 1 (lane 6), are shown.

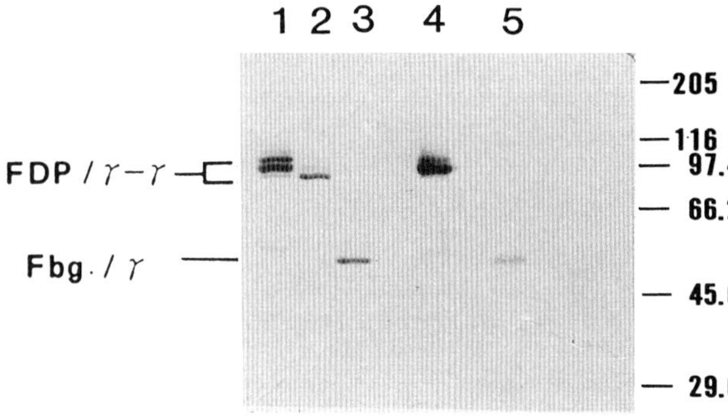

Fig. 6. Immunoblotting of the Mr 250 kDa protein and fragment DY after reduction with 2-mercaptoethanol using monoclonal antibody JIF-25. The Mr 250 kDa protein detected in patient 1 with metastatic prostatic cancer and standard DY fragment which had been extracted from SDS-PAGE gel were reduced with 2-mercaptoethanol. The resultant metabolites were analyzed by immunoblotting using the monoclonal antibody JIF-25, as described in Materials and Methods. Immunoblottings of FDP(A) (lane 1), FDP(B) (lane 2), fibrinogen (lane 3), the extracted DY fragment (lane 4), and the extracted Mr 250 kDa protein after reduction (lane 5) are shown. Molecular weight values (kDa) are shown at the right side of the figure.

proteins as well as the DD fragments and D monomer detected in the seven patients with DIC were adsorbed by JIF 23-conjugated Sepharose-4B, while the 250 kDa protein detected in the patient without DIC was not adsorbed, suggesting that it was fragment X while the proteins found in the other seven patients were fragment DY.

Plasmic Digestion and Reduction of the 250 kDa Protein

To further examine whether the 250 kDa protein detected in the patient without DIC was fragment X or DY, we performed plasmic digestion of serum and subsequent immunoblot analysis. As shown in Figure 4, the 250 kDa protein disappeared after the plasmic digestion of serum samples and D monomer was detected by immunoblotting using an anti-fibrinogen antibody. We also examined the effect of reduction of the 250 kDa protein with 2-mercaptoethanol to confirm that it was fragment X. After SDS-PAGE of serum, the 250 kDa protein was extracted from the gel with 0.1% SDS. The extracted protein revealed a single band upon immunoblotting using anti-human fibrinogen antibody (Fig. 5). The extracted protein was reduced with 2-mercaptoethanol and analyzed by immunoblotting using JIF-25, a monoclonal antibody against the γ-remnant of fibrinogen [11]. As shown in Figure 6, the γ-chain of fibrinogen (47 kDa) was demonstrated after reduction of the 250 kDa protein. In contrast, γ-γ dimer was detected after reduction of the standard DY fragment and immunoblotting using JIF-25 (Fig. 6). These findings indicated that the 250 kDa protein was not

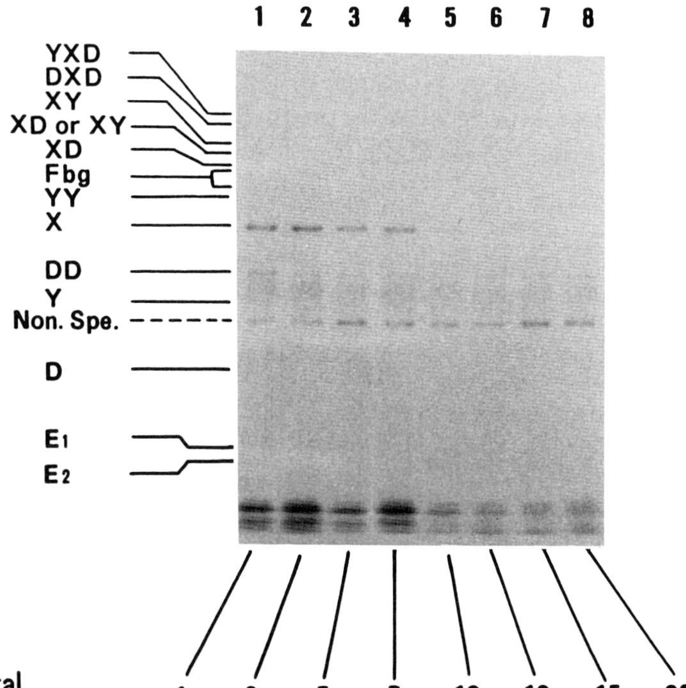

Hospital day	1	3	5	7	10	12	15	29
α_2PI (%)	36	34	37	34	45	58	64	71
Plasmin-α_2PI complex (μg/ml)	2.6	4.3	3.0	2.4	2.1	1.8	2.2	2.8
FDP (D) ($\times 10^{-3}$ ng/ml)	20.9	25.7	23.3	21.7	18.8	15.6	7.7	3.4
Cross-linked fibrin degradation products (μg/ml)	3.32	2.08	2.46	2.73	1.67	2.17	2.20	1.90

Fig. 7. Relationship between systemic fibrinogen degradation and plasma levels of α_2PI in the clinical course of patient 1 with metastatic prostatic cancer. Immunoblot analysis of FDP of patient 1 with metastatic prostatic cancer was performed using anti-human fibrinogen antibody. Immunoblotting was performed with the serum samples of day 1 (lane 1), day 3 (lane 2), day 5 (lane 3), day 7 (lane 4), day 10 (lane 5), day 12 (lane 6), day 15 (lane 7), and day 29 (lane 8). Plasma levels of plasmin-α_2PI complex, FDP(D), and cross-linked fibrin degradation products, as well as levels of α_2PI are shown on the same days of this patient's clinical course. Non. Spe., non-specific band.

fragment DY but fragment X, and further indicated that systemic fibrinogenolysis was also occurring in the patient without DIC.

Relationship Between Fibrinogen Degradation and the α_2PI Level

To investigate whether or not the plasma α_2PI level was linked to fibrinogen degradation, we examined the relationship between these two parameters in the patients during their clinical courses. Plasma levels of α_2PI and FDP in patients 1 and 2 with metastatic prostatic cancer are shown in Figures 7 and 8, respectively. In the patient 1, castration and hormonal therapy gradually decreased the size of the prostatic tumor. With the reduction of the tumor size, as assessed by a decrease of the serum acid phosphatase level, plasma α_2PI levels gradually increased. Fragment X was only detected when the plasma α_2PI level was under 50% of normal and was not detected when α_2PI level rose above 50% of normal. FDP(D) levels also decreased with the increase of α_2PI levels, while the changes in cross-linked fibrin degradation products levels were significantly smaller than those of FDP(D), suggesting that the difference between these two parameters on days 1 to 12 was mainly due to the

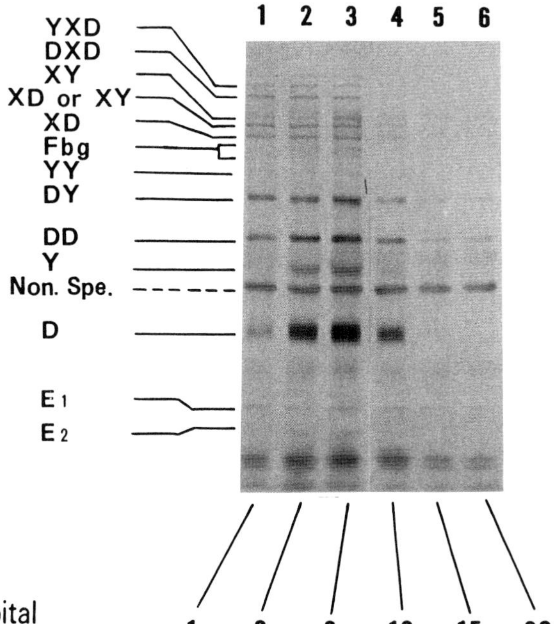

Hospital day	1	6	8	10	15	20
α_2PI (%)	72	58	39	55	68	87
Plasmin-α_2PI complex (μg/ml)	8.9	16.0	13.2	9.2	2.7	2.5
FDP (D) ($\times 10^{-3}$ ng/ml)	43.0	55.6	86.1	28.8	5.8	5.0
Cross-linked fibrin degradation products (μg/ml)	72.6	73.6	88.1	20.5	10.5	9.2

Fig. 8. Relationship between systemic fibrinogen degradation and plasma levels of α_2PI in the clinical course of patient 2 with metastatic prostatic cancer. Immunoblot analysis of FDP of patient 2 with metastatic prostatic cancer was performed using anti-human fibrinogen antibody. Immunoblotting was performed with the serum samples of day 1 (lane 1), day 6 (lane 2), day 8 (lane 3), day 10 (lane 4), day 15 (lane 5), and day 20 (lane 6). Plasma levels of α_2PI and other parameters for evaluation of the fibrinolytic state were determined in each serum sample as described in Figure 7. Non. Spe., non-specific band.

presence of fibrinogen degradation products (i.e., fragment X). In patient 2, both fragment Y and D monomer were detected from days 6 to 10, when the plasma α_2PI level was below 60% of normal. After day 10, α_2PI levels increased along with the reduction of tumor size brought about by effective hormonal therapy and fragment Y and D monomer were no longer detected when the α_2PI level rose above 60% of normal. In the other six patients, fragment Y and D monomer were also only detected when α_2PI levels were less than 60% of normal (data not shown).

These findings indicate that systemic fibrinogenolysis (enhanced fibrinolysis) only occurred when the plasma α_2PI level was under 60% of normal.

DISCUSSION

In the present study, systemic fibrinogenolysis was clearly demonstrated in patients with acquired α_2PI deficiency. This abnormal fibrinogenolysis was found to be transient, i.e., it was observed only when the plasma levels of α_2PI were reduced below 60% of normal due to consumption. Our findings indicate the potential physiological importance of α_2PI in regulating the fibrinolytic system in various disease states, as has already been suggested by the observation of a bleeding tendency due to accelerated fibrinolysis in congenital α_2PI deficiency [4]. These findings are consistent with the notion that the decrease of α_2PI levels to under 60% of normal might be a prerequisite for the occurrence of fibrinogenolysis in patients administered with thrombolytic agents, as suggested by Collen and Verstraete [14].

The α_2PI levels in our patients gradually increased after treatment of their underlying diseases, indicating that the occurrence of accelerated fibrinolysis was closely related to these disorders. The following mechanisms may have induced accelerated fibrinolysis in these patients. In acute promyelocytic leukemia, enhanced fibrinolysis and a marked decrease of α_2PI levels are frequently observed [5,15,16], and this has been suggested to be due to release of plasminogen activator from leukemic cells upon their destruction [17]. Activation of the fibrinolytic system is also frequently associated with metastatic prostatic cancer [18], probably due to the abundance of urokinase type-plasminogen activator in these tumor cells [19]. Systemic fibrinogenolysis was also demonstrated in patients with gastric cancer in the present study. Elevated levels of urokinase type-plasminogen activator have been demonstrated in human malignancies, such as colon carcinoma [20], lung cancer [21], and breast cancer [22]. Thus, urokinase type-plasminogen activator might possibly also be produced by gastric cancer cells and its release might contribute to systemic fibrinogenolysis. We also detected systemic fibrinogenolysis in one patient with abdominal aortic aneurysm, but the mechanism involved is unclear at present. Booth et al. [25] reported accelerated fibrinolysis in two patients with abdominal aortic aneurysm and speculated that plasminogen activator might have been released from the damaged aortic lining or from the endothelium of the veins occluded by a large abdominal aneurysm.

DIC was also found in seven patients in the present study. It is important to distinguish between fibrinolysis and fibrinogenolysis in patients with DIC, since antifibrinolytic therapy should only be considered when there is both a bleeding tendency and systemic fibrinogenolysis. Otherwise, the inappropriate administration of antifibrinolytic agents may exacerbate DIC by inhibiting the dissolution of microthrombi. Therefore, it is important to simultaneously determine the plasma levels of α_2PI, plasmin-α_2PI complex, cross-linked fibrin degradation products, and FDP in order to evaluate the fibrinolytic state.

D monomer was detected in seven of the eight patients with acquired α_2PI deficiency (i.e., all except patient 1 with metastatic prostatic cancer). It was not detected in patient 2 with metastatic prostatic cancer when the α_2PI level exceeded 60% of normal. Whether the D monomer detected in these patients was derived from fibrinogen or non-cross-linked fibrin is not known, but its presence in plasma implies premature clot lysis and also suggests the enhancement of fibrinolysis in the patient.

REFERENCES

1. Moroi M, Aoki N: Isolation and characterization of α_2-plasmin inhibitor form human plasma: A novel proteinase inhibitor which inhibits activator-induced clot lysis. J Biol Chem 251:5956, 1976.
2. Moroi M, Aoki N: Inhibition of plasminogen binding to fibrin by α_2-plasmin inhibitor. Thromb Res 10:581, 1977.
3. Sakata Y, Aoki N: Cross-linking of α_2-plasmin inhibitor to fibrin by fibrin-stabilizing factor. J Clin Invest 65:290, 1980.
4. Aoki N, Saito H, Kamiya T, Koie K, Sakata Y, Kobakura M: Congenital deficiency of α_2-plasmin inhibitor associated with severe hemorrhagic tendency. J Clin Invest 63:877, 1979.
5. Okajima K, Koga S, Okabe H, Inoue M, Takatsuki K: Characterization of fibrinolytic state by measuring stable cross-linked fibrin degradation products in disseminated intravascular coagulation associated with acute promyelocytic leukemia. Acta Haematol 81:15, 1989.
6. Matsuda M, Terukina S, Yamazumi K, Maekawa H, Soe G: A monoclonal antibody that recognizes the NH_2-terminal conformation of fragment D. In Matsuda M, Iwanaga S, Takada A, Henschen A (eds): "Fibrinogen 4. Current Basic and Clinical Aspects." Amsterdam: Elsevier, 1990, p 43.
7. Matsuda T, Ogawara M: Selective determination of plasmin inhibitor activity in plasma using chromogenic substrate. Thrombos Res 33:379, 1984.
8. Mimuro J, Koike Y, Sumi Y, Aoki N: Monoclonal antibodies to discrete regions in α_2-plasmin inhibitor. Blood 69:446, 1987.
9. Largo R, Heller V, Straub W: Detection of soluble intermediates of the fibrinogen-fibrin monomers. Blood 47:991–1002, 1976.
10. Olexa SE, Burdzynski AZ: Primary soluble plasmic degradation product of human cross-linked fibrin: Isolation and stoichiometry of the (DD)E complex. Biochemistry 18:991, 1979.
11. Terukina S, Matsuda M, Hirata H, Takeda Y, Miyata T, Takao T, Shimonisi Y: Substitution of Arg-275 by Cys in an abnormal fibrinogen, "Fibrinogen Osaka II." J Biol Chem 263:13579, 1988.
12. Laemmli UK: Cleavage of structural proteins during the assembly of the head of bacteriophage T4. Nature 227:680, 1970.
13. Towbin H, Staehelin T, Gordon J: Electrophoretic transfer of proteins from polyacrylamide gels to nitrocellulose sheets: procedure and some applications. Proc Natl Acad Sci USA 76:4350, 1979.
14. Collen D, Verstraete M: α_2-Antiplasmin consumption and fibrinogen breakdown during thrombolytic therapy. Thrombos Res 14:631, 1979.
15. Schwartz BS, Williams EC, Conlan MG, Mosher DF: Epsilon-aminocaproic acid in the treatment of patients with acute promyelocytic leukemia and acquired α_2-plasmin inhibitor deficiency. Ann Intern Med 61:116, 1976.
16. Avvisati G, ten Cate JW, Sturk A, Lamping R, Petti MC, Mandelli F: Acquired alpha-^{2}-antiplasmin deficiency in acute promyelocytic leukemia. Br J Haematol 70:43, 1989.
17. Wilson EL, Jacobs P, Dowdle EB: The secretion of plasminogen activators by human myeloid leukemiac cells in vitro. Blood 61:568, 1982.
18. Booth NA, Bennett B: Plasmin-α^2-antiplasmin complexes in bleeding disorders characterized by primary or secondary fibrinolysis. Br J Haematol 56:545, 1984.
19. Kirchheimer JC, Pfluger H, Ritschal P, Hienert G, Binder BR: Plasminogen activator activity in bone metastasis as compared to primary tumors. Invasion Metastasis 5:344, 1985.
20. Burtin PG, Chavanel G, Andre-Bougaran J, Gentile A: The plasmin system in human adenocarcinomas and their metastases: A comparative immunofluorescence study. Int J Cancer 39:170, 1987.
21. Markus G, Takita H, Camiolo SM, Corasanti JG, Evers JL, Hobika GH: Content and characterization of plasminogen activators in human lung tumors and normal lung tissue. Cancer Res 40:841, 1980.
22. Costantini V, Zacharski LR, Memoli VA, Kisiel W, Kudryk BK, Hunt J, Roousseau SM, Stump DC: Occurrence of component of fibrinolysis pathways in situ in neoplastic and non-neoplastic human breast tissues. Cancer Res 51:354, 1991.
23. Kwaan HC, Keer HL, Radosevich JA, Cajot J-F, Ernst R: Components of the plasminogen-plasmin system in human tumor cell lines. Semin Thromb Hemost 17:175, 1991.
24. Zacharski LR, Wojtukiewicz MZ, Costantini V, Ornstein DL, Memoli VA: Pathways of coagulation/fibrinolysis activation in malignancy. Semin Thromb Hemost 18:104, 1992.
25. Booth NA, Buckler PW, Dawson AA, AH-See AK, Bennett B: Haemorrhage associated with large abdominal aortic aneurysms. Clin Lab Haemat 6:123, 1984.

American Journal of Hematology 45:25–31 (1994)

Peripheral Neuropathy in IgM Monoclonal Gammopathy and Wäldenstrom's Macroglobulinemia: A Frequent Complication in Elderly Males With Low MAG-Reactive Serum Monoclonal Component

Luca Baldini, Edoardo Nobile-Orazio, Andrea Guffanti, Sergio Barbieri, Marinella Carpo, Lilla Cro, Bruno Cesana, Isabella Damilano, and Anna T. Maiolo

G. Marcora Centre for Blood Diseases, Hematology Service (L.B., A.G., L.C., A.T.M.), Dino Ferrari Centre for Neuromuscular Diseases, Institute of Clinical Neurology (E.N-O., S.B., M.C.), Epidemiologic Laboratory, Scientific Affairs Department (B.C., I.D.), University of Milan, Ospedale Maggiore IRCCS, Milan, Italy

Peripheral neuropathy (PN) is a frequent complication during primary macroglobulinemia (PM), whose immunological genesis has been suggested by various authors. This study involved 65 PM patients (44 men and 21 women aged 35–78), diagnostically divided into MGUS (31 cases), and indolent (IWM, 24 cases) or symptomatic (WM, 10 cases) Waldenstrom macroglobulinemia groups. All patients underwent neurological examination, including electrodiagnostic evaluation and the determination of the serum titre of antimyelin-associated glycoprotein (MAG). An evaluation was made of the prevalence of PN and its correlation with a series of hematological variables.

The prevalence of PN was 31.6%: of those with PN, 73.1% manifested both clinical and electrophysiological signs of PN, primarily of the demyelinating type. Significant correlations emerged between the presence of PN and sex (M vs. F $P = 0.0001$), advanced age ($P = 0.049$), low MC levels ($P = 0.025$), high anti-MAG titres ($P = 0.001$) and high Hb levels ($P = 0.001$). No significant correlation with the diagnostic definition of PM was found, although the majority of cases with (particularly demyelinating) PN were MGUS or IWM. At multivariate analysis, the presence of PN significantly correlated with sex ($P = 0.0001$), age ($P = 0.019$), and anti-MAG titre ($P = 0.001$).

Ten of the 26 PN cases showed no MAG reactivity. Significant correlations between PN and low serum MC levels/high MAG reactivity support the hypothesis of the antibody-mediated origin of many PN, and that the presence of PN depends on the characteristics of the proliferating pathological B clone, rather than on the tumor burden of the form of macroglobulinemia. Clinically, our data reconfirm the frequency of PN during PM and indicate simple clinicohematological variables useful for identifying patients at high neuropathic risk.

Key words: peripheral neuropathy, Wäldenstrom's macroglobulinemia, monoclonal gammopathies of undetermined significance, MAG-antibodies

INTRODUCTION

It has been noted that peripheral neuropathy (PN) is one of the most frequent complications occurring during the course of IgM monoclonal gammopathy or primary macroglobulinemia (PM) [1–3]. In most cases, this is a slowly progressive and predominantly sensory symmetric PN, which spares the cranial nerves [4–7]. In these cases, electrodiagnostic and pathological features are consistent with a demyelinating form [8–11].

Over recent years, the pathogenesis of this complication has been partially clarified: IgM deposits have been frequently found in the nervous tissue of patients [12–

Received for publication February 2, 1993; accepted May 13, 1993.

Address reprint requests to Dr. Luca Baldini, Centro "G. Marcora," Università di Milano, Ospedale Maggiore IRCCS, Via F. Sforza, 35 20122 Milano, Italy.

14]; and monoclonal component (MC) antibody reactivity with nerve structures has often been demonstrated [15,16], particularly with the carbohydrate epitope expressed by myelin-associated glycoprotein (MAG) [4,6,17–21]. There have also been less frequent findings that MC is capable of binding with nerve glycolipids [22–25] or with chondroitin sulfate C and the endoneurium, which would determine a more heterogeneous neruopathological picture [18,26]. In a varying but not negligible number of cases, no MC reactivity with nerve components has been observed [27], indicating that the neurological damage is probably not of homogeneous pathogenesis.

While the neuropathology of PN associated with PM has been widely studied, the same cannot be said for the relationships between PN and the clinicopathological aspects of the hematological disease underlying the IgM monoclonal gammopathy [16,20,21].

With the aim of bridging this gap in our knowledge, we evaluated peripheral nervous system involvement in 65 consecutive patients admitted to a single Institution with PM of various degrees of severity, diagnostically reclassified from a hematological point of view according to contemporary criteria.

Analysis of the data seems to indicate that PN is a frequent complication of PM which particularly affects male subjects over the age of 60 years with a low tumor burden, a slow evolutionary trend, and high MAG reactivity.

MATERIALS AND METHODS

Patients

The present study involved a group of 65 consecutive patients (21 women and 44 men) aged between 35 and 78 years (mean age 61.7 years), with IgM monoclonal gammopathy; in 8 of these patients, the hematological diagnosis was made after the appearance of polyneuropathic symptoms.

On the basis of hematological variables and the criteria described by Kyle and Garton [28,29] and by Bergsagel [30], as well as the criteria elaborated by reviewing our patient population, the 65 patients were divided into three pathological groups: monoclonal gammopathies of undetermined significance (MGUS), and indolent (IWM) or symptomatic (WM) Wäldenstrom's macroglobulinemia.

The MGUS group included patients with the following characteristics:

MC < 30 g/L;

Bence Jones proteinuria < 0.5 g/24 hr, as revealed by immunofixation;

Lymphocytic/lymphoplasmacytic bone marrow (BM) infiltrate $< 30\%$;

Normal or nodular bone marrow histologic pattern;

Absence of organomegaly;

Absence of anemia (Hb $\geqslant 11$ g/dl), thrombocytopenia (platelets $\geqslant 100{,}000$ per μl) and peripheral monoclonal lymphocytosis (evaluated as light chain surface immunoglobulin restriction in those patients with lymphocytosis $> 4000/\mu l$);

Absence of a significant reduction in serum IgG and IgA (IgG < 6 g/L and IgA < 0.5 g/L);

Absence of clinical and laboratory evolution for at least 2 years (the absence of MGUS-related clinical symptoms and a variation in laboratory parameters of $<25\%$).

The WM group was defined as follows:

MC often, but not necessarily, >30 g/L and anemia (Hb <11 g/dl);

AND/OR

Thrombocytopenia (platelets $<100{,}000$ per μl);

AND/OR

Peripheral monoclonal lymphocytosis (evaluated as above);

AND/OR

Symptomatic splenomegaly;

Lymphocytic/lymphoplasmacytic BM infiltrate $>30\%$;

A diffuse bone marrow histologic pattern;

Patients who fell into neither of these two groups were classified as IWM.

The characteristics of the study population are given in Table I.

Patients with macroglobulinemia secondary to chronic lymphocytic leukemia (CLL) or histologically defined non-Hodgkin's lymphoma (NHL) were excluded from the study, as were those with cryoglobulinemia.

Clinical evaluation of PN was made as previously reported [6], and its severity was graded according to the following disability scale: 0, normal; 1, symptomless clinical and/or electrophysiological signs of neuropathy (subclinical neuropathy); 2, mild motor and/or sensory symptoms with or without mild functional anomalies; 3, moderately severe motor or sensory disturbances, including ataxia; 4, patients requiring assistance in eating or dressing, or needing ambulatory support; 5, nonambulatory patients [31].

Electrodiagnostic examinations, including needle electromyogram and nerve conduction studies, were performed as previously described [6] and, in agreement with Kelly [32], the results were classified as being prevalently suggestive of demyelination or axonal degeneration, or both.

TABLE I. Characteristics of 65 Patients With Primary Macroglobulinemia*

	MGUS	IWM	WM
No. of patients	31	24	10
Sex (M/F)	21/10	14/10	9/1
Age (mean ± SD)	61.3 ± 7.9	57.5 ± 12.1	62.1 ± 8.8
Follow up in months:			
Median	76.3	80.2	62.7
Min–max	24–123	24–180	24–149
Serum MC (g/L):			
mean ± SD	13.8 ± 4.4	22.0 ± 9.3	37.7 ± 17.4
⩾3 (No. pts)	0	4	7
BJ proteinuria (no. pts)	2	7	5
Hb (g/L):			
Mean ± SD	14.1 ± 1.1	13.2 ± 1.4	9.8 ± 2.0
<11 (no. pts)	0	1	8
Platelets (per μl)			
<100,000 (No. pts)	0	0	3
Monoclonal lymphocytosis (no. pts)	0	0	3
BM infiltration			
Mean ± SD	13.8 ± 5.0	30.8 ± 12.6	56.2 ± 15.9
BM histology (no. pts)			
Normal	16	3	0
Nodular	15	10	0
Diffuse	0	11	10
Splenomegaly (no. pts)	0	3	4
Lymphadenopathy (no. pts)	0	3	3

*MGUS, monoclonal gammopathies of undetermined significance; IWM, indolent Wäldenstrom's macroglobulinemia; WM, Wäldenstrom's macroglobulinemia.

Diagnosis of PN was made on the basis of the presence of symptoms accompanied by at least two bilateral and symmetrical signs and two altered electrophysiological parameters. If no sure signs or symptoms of polyneuropathy were observed in the presence of at least two abnormal nerve conduction velocities, a diagnosis of subclinical polyneuropathy was made (grade 1 on the disability scale).

All of the patients underwent clinical and laboratory examinations in order to identify the presence of any concomitant cause of neuropathy.

Immunological Studies

The reactivity of the IgM monoclonal component with peripheral nervous system (PNS) myelin and non-myelin fractions and central nervous system myelin was evaluated by means of previously reported immunoblotting techniques [27].

The serum of each patient was immunoblotted against central nervous system myelin at an initial dilution of 1:200. The sera reacting with MAG were further tested at twofold dilutions until the results were negative.

Statistical Analysis

The baseline characteristics of the two groups (with and without PN) are reported as mean ± SD; minimum and maximum values for quantitative variables and absolute and relative frequencies for qualitative variables are also given. For proportions, 95% confidence limits were calculated.

The 8 patients in whom the hematological diagnosis was subsequent to the diagnosis of neuropathy were obviously not included in the analysis of prevalence, but they were included in the analysis of correlations with the other blood disease variables.

Univariate analysis of the prognostic relevance of baseline quantitative variables was carried out using parametric or nonparametric one-way analysis of variance (ANOVA) in order to avoid having to refer to the Gaussian law of distribution: qualitative variables were analyzed by means of the chi-square test without Yates' correction [33].

Multivariate analysis was performed using multiple logistic regression for evaluating the importance of the influence of different variables in establishing the probability of developing a neuropathy [34]. This analysis was made by dichotimising the population into age groups (⩽60/>60 years) and MC values (⩽15.0/>15.0 g/L), and taking the natural logarithm of the anti-MAG titres.

RESULTS

On the basis of the adopted diagnostic criteria, peripheral nervous system involvement was established in 26 patients (40%; 95% CL = 27–53%); 19 (73.1%; 95% CL = 54–92%) presented clinical and electrophysiological signs of PN, the remaining 7 patients (26.9%; 95% CL = 8–46%) only electrophysiological signs. In 8 patients, the clinical onset was prevalently neurological; in the other 18, PN was diagnosed after a routine neurological examination performed as part of an overall diagnostic procedure. Consequently, the prevalence of PN in this mainly hematological population was 31.6% (95% CL = 19–45%).

Grade 1, 2, and 3 neuropathies were generally silent at onset and characterised by a slowly progressive course with a symmetric distal involvement mainly affecting the lower limbs. No symptoms or signs of autonomic involvement were reported in any of the patients.

As shown in Table II, there was no significant difference in the known period of the presence of MC between the patients with or without PN, although there was a significant difference in terms of age and sex: both the mean age and the number of patients older than 60 years was higher in the group with PN ($P = 0.0491$ and 0.0191, respectively), and there was a significantly

TABLE II. Demographic Variables of Patients With and Without Neuropathy, and Neuropathy Characteristics

Variable	Neuropathic	Non-neuropathic
No. of patients	26	39
Mean age (years)	62.9*	58.1*
SD	7.9	10.6
No. aged >60 years	19**	17**
Sex (M/F)	24/1†	19/20†
Months since MC findings		
Median	66	60
Min/max	24–118	24–112
No. symptomatic pts	19	
Neuropathy severity		
Mild	10	
Moderate	13	
Severe	3	
Neuropathy type		
Axonal	4	
Demyelinating	18	
Mixed	4	

$^*P = 0.0491$; $^{**}P = 0.0191$; $^\dagger P = 0.0001$.

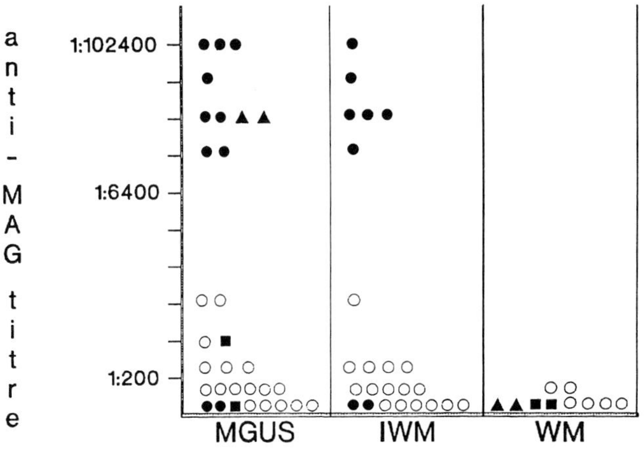

Fig. 1. Distribution and type of neuropathy (○, no PN; ●, demyelinating PN; ▲, mixed; ■, axonal) in relation to diagnostic definition (MGUS, IWM, and WM) and anti-MAG titre.

greater prevalence of men ($P = 0.0001$). In 16/26 patients (61.5%; 95% CL = 41–82%), the clinical severity of PN was medium-high and, in 19/26 patients, there was a clear prevalence of a demyelinating-type neuropathy (73.1%; 95% CL = 54–92%).

The 31 patients with MGUS included 10 with demyelinating PN, 2 with axonal PN and 2 with both (45.2%; 95% CL = 26–64%); 8/24 patients with IWM presented the demyelinating type; and there were 2 cases of the axonal and 2 cases of the mixed type among the 10 WM patients (40%; 95% CL = 5–75%) (Fig. 1).

Statistically significant differences in serum MC levels, Hb concentrations and anti-MAG titres were found between patients with and without PN. There were no

TABLE III. Hematologic Characteristics in Relation to the Presence of Peripheral Neuropathy

Variable	Neuropathic	Non-neuropathic
No. of patients	26	39
MC at diagnosis (g/L)		
Mean	15.7*	32.4*
SD	7.5	13.6
No. pts with MC <15.0	17**	11**
No. pts with MC >15.0	9**	28**
MC kappa/lambda	19/7	29/10
BJ proteinuria (No. pts)	6	8
Hb (g/dl)		
Mean	14.2†	11.8†
SD	1.3	2.0
Lymphoplasmacytic infiltration >30%	8	13
Bone marrow histology (no. pts)		
Normal	7	12
Nodular	12	13
Diffuse	7	14
Anti-MAG titre (logarithm)		
Mean	8.493‡	5.493‡
SD	2.589	0.654

$^*P = 0.00259$; $^{**}P = 0.0247$; $^\dagger P = 0.0012$; $^\ddagger P = 0.0001$.

significant differences between the two groups in terms of the diagnostic definition of PM, the presence of splenomegaly and/or lymphadenomegaly, the number of circulating lymphocytes, platelet count, the degree of bone marrow involvement, or the evolution of the hematological disease. As shown in Table III, univariate analysis revealed that mean serum MC concentrations in patients without neuropathy were significantly higher than in patients with PN ($P = 0.00259$), the majority of whom (17/26; 65.4%; 95% CL = 45–86%) presented MC <15.0 g/L ($P = 0.0247$). Mean Hb levels and mean anti-MAG titres were both higher in patients with PN ($P = 0.0012$ and $P = 0.001$, respectively).

Immunoblotting and ELISA revealed the presence of IgM anti-MAG antibodies isotypic with MC in the serum of 27 patients (41.5%; 95% CL = 29–54%): 12 with low anti-MAG titres (from 1:200 to 1:800 on immunoblotting) and 16 with high titres (>1:6,400). As shown in Table IV, all of the patients with high titres presented PN ($P = 0.0001$) which, in 14/16 cases (87.5%; 95% CL = 66–107%) was of the demyelinating type. Of the remaining cases with PN, 2 had low anti-MAG titres and 8 were anti-MAG negative; in these cases, the PN type was more heterogeneous (axonal in 4; demeylinating in 6; mixed in 2) (Fig. 1). No correlation was found between MAG titres and the severity of PN.

Analysis of the correlations between the different anti-MAG titres (negative/low or high) and the considered hematologic variables revealed a statistically significant correlation with serum MC levels. Patients with negative

TABLE IV. Relationship Between Anti-MAG Titre and the Characteristics of the Peripheral Neuropathy and Other Hematologic Variables

Variable	Negative/low (<:800)	High (>1:6400)
No. of patients	49	16
No. pts		
With neuropathy	10*	16*
Without neuropathy	39*	0*
Neuropathy type		
Axonal	4	0
Demyelinating	4	14
Mixed	2	2
MC at diagnosis (g/L)		
Mean	31.5**	13.6**
SD	12.8	5.7
No. pts with MC <15.0	16†	12†
No. pts with MC >15.0	33†	4†
Diagnostic classification[a]		
MGUS	21	10
IWM	19	6
WM	10	0

*P = 0.0001; **P = 0.00247; †P = 0.0164.
[a]MGUS, monoclonal gammopathies of undetermined significance; IWM, indolent Wäldenstrom's macroglobulinemia; WM, Wäldenstrom's macroglobulinemia.

or low anti-MAG titres had higher mean serum MC levels than patients with high anti-MAG titres (P = 0.00247); furthermore, 12/16 cases with high anti-MAG titres (75.0%; 95% CL = 47–99%), had MC levels <15.0 g/L (P = 0.0164). At multi-variate analysis, the subset of variables significantly correlating with the presence of PN included sex (P = 0.0001), age (P = 0.0190) and anti-MAG (P = 0.0001). The odds for developing neuropathy (with their 95% confidence intervals) were 29.0 (3.1–271.3) for male vs. female patients, 4.9 (1.2–19.3) for patients >60 years old vs. younger ones, and 3.2 (1.01–10.38) for each twofold dilution in MAG reactivity.

By taking into account the logistic score, it was possible to obtain the probability of developing PN for each patient (more or less than 0.50). The sensitivity of this logistic index against true status (the diagnosis of PN or not) was 0.96 (25/26 patients); its specificity was 0.82 (32/39 patients).

DISCUSSION

Over recent years, considerable progress has been made in the study of the pathogenetic mechanisms of peripheral neuropathies associated with primary macroglobulinemia [3,6,22].

However, very few in-depth epidemiological studies of PN provide an adequate statistical analysis of the weight of the hematological variables at onset [35–41]. Our analysis was restricted to a group of patients who, at bone marrow and/or spleen level, all presented the clonal expansion of an IgM-secreting B cell with immunocytomorphological characteristics of a lympholymphoplasmacytic nature. We excluded PN forms associated with cryoglobulinemia because of their probably different mechanism of neurological involvement [42]. In our population, the prevalence of PN was 31.6%, the characteristics of the neuropathies being very similar to those described by other authors [5,20].

As far as demographic variables are concerned, the prevalence of males in the group of patients with PN was confirmed even more clearly than in other studies [20], as was the greater frequency of PN in subjects over the age of 60 years (the predilection for the male sex is supported by the fact that the study population included 21 female patients). These observations are of clinical/practical importance and suggest the need for a more complete neurological evaluation in male PM patients.

Another interesting finding was the demonstration of a particular correlation between the presence of PN and some of the characteristics of serum MC concentrations and reactivity towards the myelinic components of the nerve. PN, mainly of the demyelinating type, was more frequent in patients with low serum MC levels and a high degree of MAG reactivity. These data, together with the results of immunological nerve biopsy [6,16] and a large number of immunoneurobiological studies [43–45], globally support the immuno-mediated nature of many PNs during the course of PM.

Therefore, the presence of PN seems to be conditioned not so much by high levels of serum MC, but rather by its particular antibody reactivity toward nerve structures. This, as well as the absence of any correlation between PN and the other hematologic variables used by us to define the diagnosis of PN, suggests that the presence of PN depends on the characteristics of the proliferating pathological B clone, rather than on the tumoral burden of the different forms of macroglobulinemia.

Our conclusion is in partial disagreement with that of Dellagi et al. [16] who, in a smaller population of 25 cases, were unable to demonstrate a relationship between serum MC levels (more or less than 10 q/L) and the presence of PN. On the other hand, our results agree in terms of the relationship between the high degree of reactivity of MC towards myelinic antigens and low levels of M protein and the low clinical grade of the blood disease.

It is worth noting that 8 of the 26 patients with PN (6 demyelinating, 2 mixed; 2 with grade 1, 2 with grade 2, and 4 with grade 3) were characterised by a minimum follow-up of 72 months, the absence of signs of blood disease progression, serum MC levels of <15.0 g/L and a high level of anti-MAG reactivity. This suggests the existence of a particular pathological condition whose main clinical manifestations derive from the involvement of a target apparatus (the peripheral nervous system) in an IgM immunomediated process. An analogy can be made with chronic cold agglutinin disease. In this pathology, a monoclonal IgM autoantibody produces hemolytic anemia, which is frequently the main clinical manifestation of an otherwise indolent B-cell neoplasm.

Finally, it is worth repeating that 10/26 cases of PN showed no MAG reactivity. The fact that many of them had a low MC titre and non-demyelinating PN suggests the existence of a possible antibody-mediated mechanism with different antibody reactivity. Although we found no serum reactivity against GM1 gangliosides or sulfatides (data not shown), further studies are necessary before the possibility of an antibody-mediated pathogenesis can be excluded.

In conclusion, our results identify a subset of variables (sex, age, serum MC level), and anti-MAG titre) that correlate significantly with the presence of PN, and which allow the clinician to make an early selection of those patients who should undergo in-depth neurological evaluation. An early diagnosis of PN makes it possible to intervene therapeutically, regardless of the state of the hematological disease.

ACKNOWLEDGMENTS

We would like to thank Kevin Smart (LINK srl, Milan) for his help in the preparation of the English version of this text.

REFERENCES

1. Logothetis J, Silverstein P, Coe J: Neurological aspects of Wäldenstrom's macroglobulinaemia: Report of a case. Arch Neurol 3:564–73, 1960.
2. Arfman M, Harbs H, Deicher H, et al. Polyneuropathie bei Makroglobulinamie Waldenstrom. Aktuel Neurol 11:7–12, 1984.
3. Steck AJ, Murray N, Dellagi K, Brouet JC, Seliqman M: Peripheral neuropathy associated with monoclonal IgM autoantibody. Ann Neurol 22:764–67, 1987.
4. Latov N: Immunological abnormalities associated with chronic peripheral neuropathies: Plasma cell dyscrasia and neuropathy. In Behan P, Spreafico F (eds): "Neurology." New York: Raven Press, pp 261–273, 1984.
5. Kelly JJ Jr: Peripheral neuropathies associated with monoclonal proteins: A clinical review. Muscle Nerve 8:138–150, 1985.
6. Nobile-Orazio E, Marmiroli P, Baldini L, et al: Peripheral neuropathy in macroglobulinemia: Incidence and antigen specificity of M proteins. Neurology 37:1506–1514, 1987.
7. Latov N, Hays AP, Sherman WH: Peripheral neuropathy and anti-MAG antibodies. Crit Rev Neurobiol 3:301–332, 1988.
8. Dalakas MC, Engel WK: Polyneuropathy with monoclonal gammopathy: Study of 11 patients. Ann Neurol 10:45–52, 1981.
9. Stefansson K, Marton L, Antel JP, et al: Neuropathy accompanying IgM lambda monoclonal gammopathy. Acta Neuropathol Berl 59:255–261, 1983.
10. King RH, Thomas PK: The occurrence and significance of myelin with unusually large periodicity. Acta Neuropathol Berl 63:319–329, 1984.
11. Mendell JR, Sahenk Z, Whitaker JN, et al: Polyneuropathy and IgM monoclonal gammopathy: Studies on the pathogenetic role of anti-myelin-associated glycoprotein antibody. Ann Neurol 17:243–254, 1985.
12. Julien J, Vital C, Vallat JM, Lagueny A, Deminier C, Darriet D: Polyneuropathy in Waldenstrom's macroglobulinemia. Arch Neurol 25:423–425, 1978.
13. Propp RP, Means E, Deibel R, Sherer G, Barren K: Waldenstrom's macroglobulinaemia and neuropathy. Deposition of M component on myelin sheaths. Neurology 25:980–988, 1975.
14. Takatsu M, Hays AP, Latov N, et al: Immunofluorescence study of patients with neuropathy and IgM M-proteins. Ann Neurol 18:173–181, 1985.
15. Kahn SN, Smith IS, Eames RA, Thomas PK, Lacey BW: Paraproteinemia and autoimmune peripheral neuropathy. (Letter.) N Engl J Med 304:1430, 1981.
16. Dellagi K, Duponey P, Bronet JC, et al: Waldenstrom's macroglobulinaemia and peripheral neuropathy: A clinical and immunologic study of 25 patients. Blood 62:280–285, 1983.
17. Nobile-Orazio E, Hays AP, Latov N, et al: Specificity of mouse and human monoclonal antibodies to myelin-associated glycoprotein. Neurology 34:1336–1342, 1984.
18. Freddo L, Ariga T, Saito M, et al: The neuropathy of plasma cell dyscrasia: Binding of IgM M proteins to peripheral nerve glycolipids. Neurology 35:1420–1424, 1985.
19. Ilyas AA, Quarles RH, McIntosh TD, et al: IgM in a human neuropathy related to paraproteinemia binds to a carbohydrate determinant in the myelin-associated glycoprotein and to a ganglioside. J Neuroimmunol 11:131–136, 1986.
20. Latov N: Waldenstrom's macroglobulinemia and nonmalignant IgM monoclonal gammopathies. In Kelly JJ Jr, Kyle RA, Latov N (eds): "Polyneuropathies Associated With Plasma Cell Dyscrasias." Boston: Martinus Nijhoff, pp 51–72, 1987.
21. Kelly JJ, Adelman LS, Berkman E, Bhan I: Polyneuropathies associated with IgM monoclonal gammopathies. Arch Neurol 45:1355–1359, 1988.
22. Baba H, Miyatani N, Sato S, et al: Antibody to glycolipid in a patient with IgM paraproteinemia and polyradiculoneuropathy. Acta Neurol Scand 72:218–221, 1985.
23. Ilyas AA, Quarles RH, Dalakas M, et al: Polyneuropathy with monoclonal gammopathy: Glycolipids are frequently antigens for IgM paraproteins. Proc Natl Acad Sci USA 82:6697–6700, 1985.
24. Ilyas AA, Quarles RH, Dalakas M, et al:Monoclonal IgM in a patient with paraproteinemic polyneuropathy binds to gangliosides containing disialosyl groups. Ann Neurol 18:655–659, 1985.
25. Lieberman F, Marton LS, Stefansson K: Pattern of reactivity of IgM from sera of eight patients with IgM monoclonal gammopathy and neuropathy with components of neural tissues: Evidence for interaction with more than one epitope. Acta Neuropathol Berl 68:196–200, 1985.
26. Sherman WH, Latov N, Hayes AP, et al: Monoclonal IgM k antibody precipitating with chrondroitin sulfate C from patients with axonal polyneuropathy and epiderolysis. Neurology 33:192–201, 1983.
27. Nobile-Orazio E, Francomano E, Daverio L, et al: Antimyelin associated glycoprotein IgM antibody titres in neuropathy associated with macroglobulinemia. Ann Neurol 26:543–550, 1989.
28. Kyle RA, Garton JP: The spectrum of IgM monoclonal gammopathy in 430 cases. Mayo Clin Proc 62:719–731, 1987.
29. Kyle RA, Lust JA: Monoclonal gammopathies of undetermined significance. Semin Hematol 26:176–200, 1989.
30. Bergsagel D: Macroglobulinemia. In Williams WJ, Beutler E, Erslev AJ, Lichtman MA (eds): "Hematology." New York: McGraw-Hill, 1990.
31. Prineas J. Polyneuropathies of undetermined cause. Acta Neurol Scand 46(Suppl 44):1–72, 1970.

32. Kelly JJ: Electrodiagnostic findings in peripheral neuropathy associated with monoclonal gammopathy. Muscle Nerve 6:504–509, 1983.
33. Armitage P, Berry G. "Statistical Methods in Medical Research." 2nd Ed. Oxford: Blackwell Scientific Publications, 1987.
34. Hosmer DW, Lemeshow S: "Applied logistic regression. New York: John Wiley & Sons Inc., 1989.
35. Kelly JJ Jr, Kyle RA, O'Brien PC, et al: Prevalence of monoclonal protein in peripheral neuropathy. Neurology 31:1480–1483, 1981.
36. Melmed C, Frail D, Duncan I,et al: Peripheral neuropathy with IgM kappa monoclonal immunoglobulin directed against myelin-associated glycoprotein. Neurology 33:1397–1405, 1983.
37. Meier C, Vandevelde M, Steck AJ, et al: Demyelinating polyneuropathy associated with monoclonal IgM-paraproteinaemia. J Neurol Sci 63:353–367, 1983.
38. Vital L, Deminiere C, Bourgoin B, et al: Waldenstrom's macroglobulinemia and peripheral neuropathy: Deposition of M-component and kappa light chain in the endoneurium. Neurology 35:603–606, 1985.
39. Hafler DA, Johnson D, Kelly JJ, et al: Monoclonal gammopathy and neuropathy. Myelin associated glycoprotein reactivity and clinical characteristics. Neurology 36:75–77, 1986.
40. Osby E, Noring L, Hast R, et al: Benign monoclonal gammopathy and peripheral neuropathy. Br J Haematol 51:531–539, 1982.
41. Kahan SN, Riches PG, Kohn J: Paraproteinaemia in neurological disease: Incidence, associations and classification of monoclonal immunoglobulins. J Clin Pathol 33:617–621, 1980.
42. Nemmi R, Corbo M, Fazio R, Quattrini A, Comi G, Canal N: Cryoglobulinaemic neuropathy: A clinical, morphological and immunocytochemical study of 8 cases. Brain 111:541–546, 1988.
43. Latov N, Sherman WH, Nemni R, et al: Plasma cell dyscrasia and peripheral neuropathy with a monoclonal antibody to peripheral nerve myelin. N Engl J Med 303:618–621, 1980.
44. Latov N, Braun PE, Gross RB, et al: Plasma cell dyscrasia and peripheral neuropathy: Identification of the myelin antigens that react with the human paraproteins. Proc Natl Acad Sci USA 78:7139–7142, 1981.
45. Monaco S, Bonetti B, Ferrari S, et al: Complement-mediated demyelination in patients with IgM monoclonal gammopathy and polyneuropathy. N Engl J Med 322:649–52, 1990.

American Journal of Hematology 45:32–38 (1994)

Detection of Tumor Necrosis Factor-α in Bone Marrow Plasma and Peripheral Blood Plasma From Patients With Aplastic Anemia

John C. Schultz and Nasrollah T. Shahidi

Department of Pediatrics, University of Wisconsin, Madison

Plasma levels of interferon-gamma (IFN-γ) and tumor necrosis factor-alpha (TNF-α) were determined in healthy individuals and patients with aplastic anemia (ApAn). IFN-γ was not detected in normal peripheral blood plasma (PBP) or bone marrow plasma (BMP) and was present in PBP from only 2 of 22 patients and in BMP from 1 of 14 patients and the levels were low (<1.5 U/ml). Elevated levels of TNF-α were present in BMP and PBP from patients but not in control (healthy donor) PBP and BMP. Eleven of twenty-four patients had elevated levels of TNF-α in their PBP and 6 of 13 patients had detectable levels of TNF-α in their BMP. Only one of the 14 healthy control donors had detectable TNF-α and the level was very low (7 pg/ml), while 13 of the 27 ApAn patients had detectable TNF-α (P = .009, chi-square test). Not surprisingly, the centers of the distributions of TNF-α concentrations of the controls and ApAn patients differed significantly (P < .017 for control and patient PBP and P < .056 for control and patient BMP, Wilcoxon rank-sum test). Spontaneous production of IFN-γ and TNF-α by cultured bone marrow mononuclear cells was observed in four of seven patients but not in the six healthy controls (P = 0.026). Spontaneous production of IFN-γ and TNF-α by cultured peripheral blood mononuclear cells from patients and controls was however similar. Phytohemagglutinin (PHA)-induced production of IFN-γ and TNF-α by cultured mononuclear cells did not differ significantly between ApAn patients and normal controls. The significance of overproduction of TNF-α in the pathophysiology of ApAn is discussed.

Key words: TNF-α, interferon-γ, hematopoietic suppression

INTRODUCTION

Several lines of clinical and laboratory data have indicated that immune-mediated inhibition of hematopoiesis may be the most common mechanism leading to bone marrow failure in patients with aplastic anemia (ApAn). Each of the immune competent cells, as well as some of their soluble products, have been incriminated [for review see Ref. 1]. Growth medium conditioned by peripheral blood mononuclear cells [2] and T-cell lines [3] from patients with ApAn inhibited the growth of normal allogeneic bone marrow. Interferon-gamma (IFN-γ) produced by activated suppressor T-cells was identified as the mediator of hematopoietic suppression in the conditioned medium. Zoumbos et al. [4] have reported that the hematopoietic suppressor activity in medium conditioned by PHA-stimulated T-cells from normal peripheral blood is IFN-γ. Elevated levels of IFN-γ have been detected in the bone marrow serum and peripheral blood serum of ApAn patients [2]. The higher levels of interferon in the bone marrow serum compared to the peripheral blood serum in ApAn patients suggest that marrow is the origin of interferon. It has been shown that natural and recombinant IFN-γ inhibits proliferation of hematopoietic cells in vitro [5] and that T-cells and monocytes/macrophages may play an important part in the mediation of this effect. It is well known that the administration of interferons to humans results in transient bone marrow suppression and the development of red cell aplasia, which is responsive to immunotherapy [6–8].

The concept that IFN-γ is the mediator of hematopoietic suppression in ApAn was questioned by Torok-Storb et al. [9], who found IFN-γ above the detection limit in

Received for publication January 15, 1993; accepted June 30, 1993.

Address reprint requests to Dr. John C. Schultz, Division of Pediatric Hematology/Oncology, University of Wisconsin, 600 Highland Avenue, CSC H4/475, Madison, WI 53792-4108.

only 5 of 50 patient peripheral blood serum samples and failed to show any inhibitory effect of T-cell conditioned medium on hematopoietic progenitor cell growth despite high IFN-γ levels. Peripheral blood sera from these patients had no inhibitory effect on normal erythroid burst-forming unit (BFU-E). Torok-Storb et al. [10] reported that the inhibition of erythroid progenitor growth is mediated by cytotoxic lymphocytes and not by natural killer cells or IFN-γ. These observations are in agreement with those obtained by Nathan et al. [11] who studied a series of 15 patients and failed to demonstrate any inhibitory activity in patient peripheral blood sera. Raefsky et al. [12] reported that colony growth could be inhibited with a homogenous preparation of recombinant IFN-γ; the extent of inhibition was however influenced by culture conditions such that maximum inhibition required suboptimal concentrations of fetal bovine serum. Trinchieri and Perussia [13] have reported that even high doses of recombinant IFN-γ did not significantly inhibit colony function. Hanada et al. [14] also denied the role of IFN-γ in cases in which IFN-γ production by T-cells was within the normal range when inhibitory activity by T-cells was evident. Hinterberger et al. [15], using both the standard viral inhibition bioassay which is equally sensitive for human IFN-α, IFN-β, and IFN-γ, and the IFN-γ radioimmunoassay (Centocor), reported that IFNs and IFN-γ were not detected in the peripheral blood serum and bone marrow serum of patients with ApAn and normal controls. Spontaneous and phytohemagglutinin (PHA)-induced production of these lymphokines by peripheral blood mononuclear cells, however, was highly increased in both untreated and treated severe ApAn anemia patients. The same investigators were unable to confirm previous reports in severe ApAn on improvement of stem cell growth upon neutralization of endogenous IFN-γ, absolutely increased numbers of circulating activated T-cells, and normalization of these abnormalities subsequent to successful immunosuppression. Their data clearly supported previous reports on abnormal lymphokine production in severe ApAn, but failure to relate this phenomenon to the severity of disease states raised doubts on the pathogenetic significance of lymphokine overproduction in severe ApAn.

The involvement of another lymphokine, tumor necrosis factor-α (TNF-α), in aplastic anemia was also investigated by Hinterberger et al. [15]. TNF-α was previously shown to be a potent inhibitor of colony growth in vitro of normal human bone marrow hematopoietic progenitor cells from normal donors and patients with leukemia [16–19]. Chronic exposure to TNF in vivo preferentially inhibits erythropoiesis in nude mice [20]. Administration of TNF to cancer patients resulted in a decrease in hemoglobin levels following a month of recombinant TNF treatment [21]. A single intravenous injection of TNF into healthy humans induced a marked change in the peripheral blood counts and functional properties of leukocytes [22]. Hinterberger et al. [15], using a bioassay sensitive to both TNF-α and TNF-β, found that TNF was detectable neither in peripheral blood serum nor in bone marrow serum of treated and untreated ApAn patients and control individuals. Spontaneous and PHA-induced production of TNF, however, were highly increased in both untreated and treated severe ApAn patients. Overproduction of IFNs, IFN-γ, TNFs, and TNF-α was not related to blood transfusions. Newly diagnosed and untransfused severe aplastic anemia patients carry the abnormality. Second, cytokine overproduction was demonstrated before and after blood transfusions in the same aplastic anemia patients [23]. In a recent report, Shinohara et al. [24] described spontaneous and PHA-induced TNF-α production in the supernatants of cultured peripheral blood mononuclear cells from patients with ApAn compared to normal controls and ApAn patients who had received an allogeneic bone marrow transplant. PHA-induced TNF-α production was approximately five times higher in patients than with normal control cells. Results from ApAn patients were also significantly higher than ApAn patients receiving a bone marrow transplant. Patients with high levels of TNF-α production in vitro tend to have lower hemoglobin, platelet, and leukocyte values although this was not significant statistically. Viale et al. [25] have recently shown that T-cell clones from severe ApAn patients exhibit predominantly a $CD8^+$ phenotype, a greater cytotoxic activity, and a greater production of suppressor lymphokines (TNF-α and IFN-γ) when compared with healthy controls.

The purpose of this study was to measure IFN-γ and TNF-α production in vivo by patients with ApAn using highly sensitive, commercially available immunoradiometric assays specific for immunologically recognizable IFN-γ and TNF-α in order to establish whether or not lymphokine overproduction occurs in vivo as well as in vitro. The results are discussed in terms of the significance of these lymphokines in the pathophysiology of ApAn.

MATERIALS AND METHODS

Patients

The diagnosis of ApAn was based on morphologic examination of a bone core biopsy and blood and bone marrow smears from all 27 patients (14 females and 13 males) included in this study. The patients' ages at their first visit in the study ranged from 1 to 75 years (mean ± SD of 16.2 ± 16.5 and median of 11.5 years old). All patients were seen at least once; one was seen three times, four were seen four times, and two patients were seen two times. Those with serial measurements had at least 2 months between each blood and marrow sample. Eleven patients were tested at least once prior to treatment. Sixteen patients had already been treated by the administration of anabolic steroids, corticosteroids, ATG, or cyclosporin A, or combinations of these agents. Two patients received irradiated packed red blood cells and platelets prior to study. The length of time between the last transfusion and lymphokine measurement was 6 months for one patient and 1 year for the second patient. All of the other ApAn patients were transfusion-free at the time of study.

Fourteen normal, apparently healthy, adult volunteers (laboratory personnel and blood and/or marrow donors) served as controls, while a maximum of six were sampled for any one lymphokine measurement. In addition, six pediatric patients with anemia due to other hematologic disorders, including chronic renal disease, iron deficiency anemia, refractory megaloblastic anemia, hereditary spherocytosis, and pure red cell aplasia were also studied. None of the patients and controls were infected or ill in other ways.

Peripheral Blood and Bone Marrow

Bone marrow and peripheral blood were obtained from healthy adult volunteers after informed consent according to the guidelines of the University of Wisconsin Committee on the Use of Human Subjects in Research. Patient peripheral blood and bone marrow were obtained at the time when venipuncture and bone marrow aspiration were performed for diagnostic or prognostic purpose. Bone marrow was aspirated within minutes from the time the peripheral blood was obtained.

Peripheral blood was drawn into syringes containing preservative-free heparin (20 units per ml blood, final concentration) and centrifuged (600g) for 20 min to isolate the plasma (PBP). Bone marrow aspirate (3–5 ml) from the posterior iliac crest was collected in a 20 ml syringe containing 60 units of preservative-free heparin. The aspirate was centrifuged (600g) for 20 min to isolate the bone marrow plasma (BMP).

Following removal of the PBP and BMP, the peripheral blood mononuclear cells (PBMC) and bone marrow mononuclear cells (BMMC) were obtained by Ficoll-Hypaque density-gradient centrifugation, washed, and resuspended in RPMI-1640 medium.

Preparation and Harvest of Peripheral Blood and Bone Marrow Mononuclear Cell-Conditioned Medium

Mononuclear cells were incubated at a concentration of 0.5×10^6/ml RPMI-1640 containing 10% fetal calf serum, in the absence and presence of 2 μg/ml PHA, in a humidified atmosphere of 5% CO_2/air for 3 days at 37°C. Supernatants (conditioned media) were harvested by centrifugation (600g) for 10 min, passed through sterile 0.45 μm filters, and stored at −20°C.

Determination of IFN-γ and TNF-α

Immunologically recognizable IFN-γ and TNF-α concentrations in BMP, PBP, and mononuclear cell-conditioned medium were determined by immunoradiometry (Centocor, Malvern, PA). The sensitivity of the IFN-γ assay is 0.25 U/ml. The TNF-α assay detects levels down to 6 pg/ml and has no detectable cross-reactivity with lymphotoxin (TNF-β). TNF-α stabilizing factor, provided by Centocor, was added to blood and marrow aspirates immediately upon collection.

Statistical Analysis

Association between detection of lymphokine (TNF-α or IFN-γ) in patients vs. healthy controls was assessed using chi-square tests. Subjects having serial samples were considered positive for detection of lymphokine, if at least one of the samples had a detectable level of the lymphokine.

Actual TNF-α and IFN-γ production levels were compared between the patient and control groups using Wilcoxon rank-sum tests. For these tests, subjects having multiple samples were represented by the median value of their observations. Differences between in vitro spontaneous and PHA-induced production of TNF-α and IFN-γ were tested using paired t tests of the differences for subjects having both spontaneous and PHA-induced lymphokine production measured.

Unpaired t tests were used to compare the difference in lymphokine levels between unstimulated (minus PHA) and PHA-stimulated lymphokine production between the patient and control groups.

Correlation between TNF-α level and age of patient was determined from simple linear regression of TNF-α on age.

RESULTS

IFN-γ in Plasma

Levels of IFN-γ were measured in 37 PBP samples from 22 patients and in 21 BMP samples from 14 of the patients. Serial plasma samples were obtained from 6 of the 27 patients studied. Only 1 of 21 BMP (4.8%) and 3 of 37 PBP (8.1%) tested had detectable amounts of IFN-γ (0.25 to 1.5 U/ml) (Fig. 1). The remaining samples had either no detectable amounts of IFN-γ or less than 0.25 U/ml. Nineteen control plasma samples (nine PBP from seven donors and ten BMP from six donors; one donor was tested five times) were examined and found to contain negligible amounts of IFN-γ (Fig. 1). In summary, only one of ten healthy subjects had detectable IFN-γ and only 4 of 27 ApAn patients had detectable levels of IFN-γ ($P = 0.73$, chi-square test).

TNF-α in Plasma

Levels of TNF-α were measured in 40 PBP samples from 24 patients and 21 BMP samples from 13 patients.

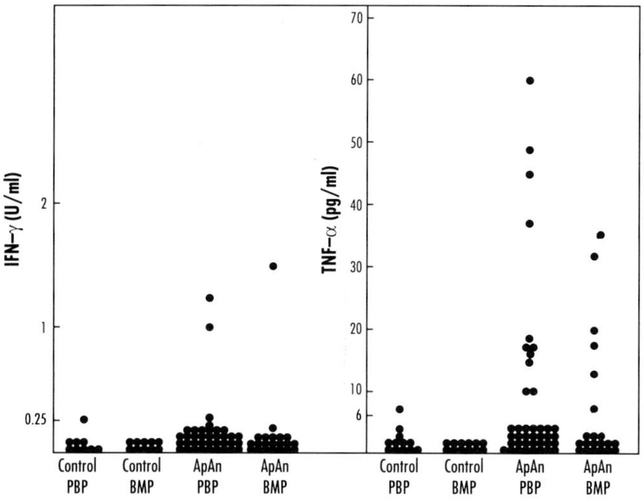

Fig. 1. Levels of IFN-γ and TNF-α in peripheral blood plasma (PBP) and bone marrow plasma (BMP) from healthy controls and patients with ApAn.

Serial plasma samples were obtained from 7 of 27 ApAn patients and 2 of 14 healthy controls. TNF-α values for all samples from the ApAn patients and healthy controls are shown in Figure 1. Eleven of twenty-four patients had elevated levels of TNF-α in the PBP and 6 of 13 patients had elevated levels in the BMP. TNF-α concentrations detected in ApAn PBP had the following characteristics (pg/ml): mean = 27.1, standard deviation = 17.2, minimum = 10, median = 18, and maximum = 59. TNF-α concentrations detected in ApAn BMP had the following characteristics (pg/ml): mean = 21.0, standard deviation = 10.8, minimum = 7, median = 19.5, and maximum = 35. The TNF-α concentration detected in the control PBP was 7 pg/ml. Not surprisingly, the centers of the distributions of TNF-α concentrations of the controls and ApAn patients differed significantly ($P < .017$ for control and patient PBP and $p < .056$ for control and patient BMP, Wilcoxon rank-sum test, where detected levels were used if there were serial samples). There was no correlation between TNF-α level and age of patient ($r = 0.003$, $P = 0.988$). Five of the thirteen ApAn patients with elevated TNF-α in the PBP and/or BMP were newly diagnosed and untreated; six were treated and two were off therapy and in remission. There was no correlation between the duration of the disease and TNF-α level ($r = 0.202$, $P = 0.509$). As mentioned above, serial plasma samples were obtained from seven ApAn patients. Three of the seven patients had no detectable TNF-α; two patients had elevated levels only once; and two patients had elevated levels on two ocassions. Four of four patients started off with undetectable levels of TNF-α at the time of diagnosis but developed elevated levels later in their course; the elevated levels did not persist in all patients. Two patients were in remission (off therapy), one patient was in remission (on therapy), and one patient was in relapse (on therapy) when TNF-α was elevated.

TNF-α and IFN-γ Levels in Patient Control Group

IFN-γ and TNF-α levels in plasma from the six anemic patients with other hematological disorders were below the sensitivity of measurement (not shown).

In Vitro Spontaneous TNF-α and IFN-γ Production

Spontaneous production of TNF-α and IFN-γ by unfractionated peripheral blood mononuclear cells (PBMC) and bone marrow mononuclear cells (BMMC) from healthy individuals and ApAn patients was examined (Table I). The association between detection of TNF-α in patients' versus healthy controls' peripheral blood mononuclear cell-conditioned medium (PBCM) did not differ significantly ($P = 0.194$, chi-square test). The centers of distributions of TNF-α levels for the two groups did not differ significantly ($P = 0.4608$, Wilcoxon rank-sum test). Patient bone marrow mononuclear cell-conditioned medium (BMCM) contained detectable TNF-α but was not detectable in normal BMCM ($P = 0.026$, chi-square test). The amounts of TNF-α detected in the patient BMCM were not significantly different from that present in medium conditioned by their PBMC ($P = 0.1005$, Wilcoxon rank-sum test). The association between detection of IFN-γ in patients' versus healthy controls' PBCM did not differ significantly ($P = 0.763$, chi-square test). The centers of distributions of the IFN-γ levels did not differ significantly ($P = 0.763$, Wilcoxon rank-sum test). Patients BMCM contained detectable IFN-γ but was not detectable in normal BMCM ($P = 0.026$, chi-square test). The centers of distribution of the IFN-γ levels did not differ significantly ($P = 0.4628$, Wilcoxon rank-sum test).

PHA-Stimulated Production of TNF-α and IFN-γ

As seen in Table II, levels of detectable IFN-γ and TNF-α in PBCM varied greatly for both groups, but there was no significant difference observed between the centers of distribution of the two groups for TNF-α ($P = 0.9778$, Wilcoxon rank-sum test) and IFN-γ ($P = 0.4855$, Wilcoxon rank-sum test).

Comparison of In Vitro Spontaneous and Lectin-Induced Production of IFN-γ and TNF-α by PBMC and BMMC

Data for both spontaneous and PHA-induced production of TNF-α and IFN-γ were available for 7 ApAn patients and 18 healthy controls. Difference in production of the lymphokine was analyzed using the paired differences of PHA-stimulated production minus spontaneous production for these 25 subjects. No significant differences were observed in TNF-α or IFN-γ production

TABLE I. Summary Statistics for Spontaneous Production of IFN-γ and TNF-α In Vitro

	Number of subjects producing lymphokine	Mean ± SD[a]	Minimum	Median	Maximum
TNF-α (pg/ml)					
Normal controls					
PBCM	6 of 19 (31%)	227 ± 220	15	185.5	534
BMCM	0 of 6 (0%)	—	—	—	—
ApAn patients					
PBCM	9 of 17 (53%)	59 ± 59	10	33.5	198
BMCM	4 of 7 (57%)	178 ± 141	18	179	334
IFN-γ (U/ml)					
Normal controls					
PBCM	5 of 20 (25%)	5.6 ± 6.0	1	3	15
BMCM	0 of 6 (0%)	—	—	—	—
ApAn patients					
PBCM	5 of 17 (29%)	2.6 ± 4.1	0.3	1	10
BMCM	4 of 7 (57%)	3.9 ± 4.4	0.6	2.5	10

[a]Only conditioned medium containing detectable levels of TNF-α and IFN-γ are included in the statistical analyses shown above.

TABLE II. Summary Statistics for PHA-Stimulated Production of IFN-γ and TNF-α In Vitro

	Number of subjects responding to PHA[a]	Mean ± SD	Minimum	Median	Maximum
TNF-α (pg/ml)					
Normal controls					
PBCM	18/18	1,160 ± 971	56	888	2,597
ApAn patients					
PBCM	8/8	1,660 ± 1,576	36	1,737	4,100
BMCM	2/2	788 ± 1,044	49	788	1,526
IFN-γ (U/ml)					
Normal controls					
PBCM	18/18	39.4 ± 32.1	1	29	100
ApAn patients					
PBCM	6/8	24.1 ± 22.5	15	32.5	50
BMCM	2/2	18.7 ± 25.9	0.4	18.7	37

[a]Number of patients (or controls) showing increased production of TNF-α or IFN-γ in the presence of PHA compared to levels produced spontaneously per total number of patients (or controls) studied.

($P = 0.2506$, TNF-α; $P = 0.3309$, IFN-γ). Since no significant difference were observed between the control and patient groups, both groups were combined to test for the overall difference between PHA-stimulated and spontaneous lymphokine production. PHA-stimulated production was significantly higher than spontaneous production in these 25 subjects ($P = 0.0001$ TNF-α production, $P < 0.0001$ IFN-γ production; paired t-tests).

DISCUSSION

The results of the present study show that elevated levels of TNF-α are present in PBP and BMP from patients with ApAn. The significance of this finding is emphasized by the consistently undetectable values obtained in normal control PBP and BMP. This is the first report of detectable levels of TNF-α in the circulation and bone marrow of patients with ApAn. The inability of Hinterberger et al. [15] to detect TNF-α in untreated severe ApAn patients may be due to the sensitivity of the assay. The Hinterberger group used a bioassay which is sensitive to 88 pg/ml of TNF (TNF-α or TNF-β) [26]. The highest concentration of TNF-α found in plasma in our studies was 69 pg/ml. The Centocor radioimmunoassay used in our studies detects TNF-α at levels down to 6 pg/ml. A lack of correlation between results obtained with bioassays and immunologically based assays of TNF-α have been described by other workers as well [27].

Our inability to detect IFN-γ in BMP and PBP from patients with ApAn and healthy controls is, however, consistent with the results of Hinterberger et al. [15] who failed to detect interferon activity in the serum of normal individuals and both treated and untreated severe ApAn patients using both a biologic assay sensitive to all types of human IFN (α, β, and γ) and the Centocor radioimmunoassay utilized in our studies which is specific for IFN-γ. The radioimmunoassay is 10–100 times more sensitive than the biological microcytopathic assays used to measure human IFN-γ. In our studies, elevated IFN-γ was present in only 3 of 58 plasma samples and the levels were low (<2 U/ml).

We did, however, observe spontaneous production of TNF-α and IFN-γ in vitro by PBMC from patients and normal controls; the difference in level of production between the patient and control group was not significant. Very interestingly, spontaneous production of IFN-γ and TNF-α was obtained with BMMC from ApAn patients but not with normal BMMC. PHA-induced production of IFN-γ and TNF-α by ApAn patient and control mononuclear cells in vitro did not differ significantly.

In the course of our investigation of lymphokine overproduction in acquired ApAn and its possible association with suppressed hematopoiesis, we had the opportunity to extend our studies to include patients with Fanconi's anemia (FA). Elevated levels of TNF-α are present in BMP and PBP from patients with FA; IFN-γ levels are negligible [28]. The abnormality of TNF-α overproduction is thus exhibited in both congenital (Fanconi's anemia) and acquired ApAn. Various in vitro and clinical observations suggest that FA patients are unable to adequately detoxify superoxide anions (O_2^-) [29]. Recent studies have shown that certain lymphokines such as TNF-α, which is secreted by activated macrophages/monocytes and lymphocytes, can enhance the respiratory burst and secretion of reactive oxygen intermediates including O_2^- by phagocytes [30] in addition to inhibiting hematopoietic progenitor cell growth in vitro. It is tempting to speculate that the overproduction of TNF-α in vivo in FA and ApAn arises via a cyclic mechanism as follows. Free radical production including O_2^- may provide a positive signal for release of TNF-α by the monocytes and/or lymphocytes. There is circumstantial evidence that generation of free radicals is closely connected with the generation of TNF-α [31]. The TNF-α, in turn, further enhances free radical production by the activated phagocytes, and TNF-α induces production of O_2^- by nonphagocytic cells as well [32]. In other words, there is an amplification of generation of both toxic oxygen products and TNF-α. Incubation of neutrophils with TNF-α is known to enhance release of O_2^- [33,34]. Reduction in the ability to detoxify the DNA damaging oxygen reduction products in patients with congenital and acquired ApAn may explain the elevated levels of circulating TNF-α in these patients in the absence of any overt infection or inflammation. The elevated level of TNF-α may contribute to the pathogenesis of the progressive hematopoietic suppression in bone marrow failure in FA and ApAn by its enhancing effect on production of reactive oxygen intermediates.

In a recent review article, Nissan [1] indicated that it is unlikely that one cell type or one lymphokine causes aplastic anemia. IFN-γ and TNF-α overproduction occurs with any viral infection. In the vast majority, these patients do not develop aplasia; therefore an abnormal sensitivity of ApAn precursor cells to these lymphokines would have to be assumed. TNF-α overproduction has also been described in patients with a wide variety of non-viral diseases and inflammatory conditions [35], indicating that lymphokine production is not unique to aplasia related diseases. TNF-α overproduction in patients with ApAn and FA may arise as a product of the patient's immune system attempting to destroy the abnormal tissue. Elevated TNF-α levels enhance free radical production which in turn causes further elevation of TNF-α. This cyclic process thus results in a sustained generation of factors detrimental to progenitor and mature cells. Consequently, endogenous lymphokine overproduction or the administration of IFN-γ and/or TNF-α to FA patients, and possibly to ApAn patients for therapeutic purposes may result in excessive O_2^- production leading to cellular damage.

In summary, the elevated level of TNF-α may contribute either directly or indirectly to the pathogenesis of the progressive hematopoietic suppression in bone marrow failure in aplastic anemia.

ACKNOWLEDGMENTS

This work was financially supported by the Aplastic Anemia Research Fund. We thank Centocor, Inc. for generously providing the IFN-γ and TNF-α RIA test kits. We would also like to thank Rebecca Langhough-Koscik and Gary Lensmeyer for their assistance with the statistical analysis of our data.

REFERENCES

1. Nissen C: The pathophysiology of aplastic anemia. Semin Hematol 28:313–318, 1991.
2. Zoumbos NC, Gascon P, Djeu JY, Young NS: Interferon is a mediator of hematopoietic suppression in aplastic anemia in vitro and possibly in vivo. Proc Natl Acad Sci USA 82:188–192, 1985.
3. Herrmann F, Griffin JD, Meuer SC, Meyer zum Büschenfelde K-H: Establishment of an interleukin 2-dependent T cell line derived from a patient with severe aplastic anemia, which inhibits in vitro hematopoiesis. J Immunol 136:1629–1634, 1986.
4. Zoumbos NC, Djeu JY, Young NS: Interferon is the suppressor of hematopoiesis generated by stimulated lymphocytes in vitro. J Immunol 133: 769–774, 1984.

5. Mamus SW, Beck-Schroeder S, Zanjani ED: Suppression of normal human erythropoiesis by gamma interferon in vitro. Role of monocytes and T lymphocytes. J Clin Invest 75:1496–1503, 1985.
6. Quesada JR, Talpaz M, Rios A, Kurzrock R, Gutterman JU: Clinical toxicity of interferons in cancer patients: A review. J Clin Oncol 4:234–243, 1986.
7. Mangan KF, Zidar B, Shadduck RK, Zeigler Z, Winkelstein A: Interferon-induced aplasia: Evidence for T-cell-mediated suppression of hematopoiesis and recovery after treatment with horse antihuman thymocyte globulin. Am J Hematol 19:401–413, 1985.
8. Gutterman JU, Blumenschein GR, Alexanian R, Yap H-Y, Buzdar AU, Cabanillas F, Hortobagyi GN, Hersh EM, Rasmussen SL, Harmon M, Kramer M, Pestka S: Leukocyte interferon-induced tumor regression in human metastatic breast cancer, multiple myeloma, and malignant lymphoma. Ann Intern Med 93:399–406, 1980.
9. Torok-Storb B, Johnson GG, Bowden R, Storb R: Gamma-interferon in aplastic anemia: Inability to detect significant levels in sera or demonstrate hematopoietic suppressing activity. Blood 69:629–633, 1987.
10. Torok-Storb B, Graf L, Shankar P: Inhibition of erythroid progenitor growth is mediated by cytotoxic lymphocytes and not by natural killer cells or IFN-γ. J Immunol 143:1837–1842, 1989.
11. Nathan C, personal communication cited in reference 15.
12. Raefsky EL, Platanias LC, Zoumbos NC, Young NS: Studies of interferon as a regulator of hematopoietic cell proliferation. J Immunol 135:2507–2512, 1985.
13. Trinchieri G, Perussia B: Immune interferon: A pleiotropic lymphokine with multiple effects. Immunol Today 6:131–136, 1985.
14. Hanada T, Yamamura H, Ehara T, Iwasaki N, Shin R, Nakahara S, Takita H: No evidence for gamma-interferon mediated haematopoietic inhibition by T cells in aplastic anemia: An observation in the course of immunosuppressive therapy. Br J Haematol 67:123–127, 1987.
15. Hinterberger W, Adolf G, Aichinger G, Dudczak R, Geissler K, Höcker P, Huber C, Kalhs P, Knapp W, Köller U, Lechner K, Volc-Platzer B: Further evidence for lymphokine overproduction in severe aplasic anemia. Blood 72:266–272, 1988.
16. Degliantoni G, Murphy M, Kobayashi M, Francis MK, Perussia B, Trinchieri G: Natural killer (NK) cell-derived hematopoietic colony-inhibiting activity and NK cytotoxic factor: Relationship with tumor necrosis factor and synergism with immune interferon. J Exp Med 162:1512–1530, 1985.
17. Broxmeyer HE, Williams DE, Lu L, Cooper S, Anderson SL, Beyer GS, Hoffman R, Rubin BY: The suppressive influences of human tumor necrosis factors on bone marrow hematopoietic progenitor cells from normal donors and patients with leukemia: Synergism of tumor necrosis factor and interferon-γ. J Immunol 136:4487–4495, 1986.
18. Murase T, Hotta T, Saito H, Ohno R: Effect of recombinant human tumor necrosis factor on the colony growth of human leukemia progenitor cells and normal hematopoietic progenitor cells. Blood 69:467–472, 1987.
19. Beran M, McCredie KB, Keating MJ, Gutterman JU: Antileukemic effect of recombinant tumor necrosis factor α in vitro and its modulation by α and γ interferons. Blood 72:728–738, 1988.
20. Johnson RA, Waddelow TA, Caro J, Oliff A, Roodman GD: Chronic exposure to tumor necrosis factor in vivo preferentially inhibits erythropoiesis in nude mice. Blood 74:130–138, 1989.
21. Blick M, Sherwin SA, Rosenblum M, Gutterman J: Phase 1 study of recombinant tumor necrosis factor in cancer patients. Cancer Res 47:2986–2989, 1987.
22. van der Poll T, van Deventer SJH, Hack CE, Wolbink GJ, Aarden LA, Büller HR, ten Cate JW: Effects on leukocytes after injection of tumor necrosis factor into healthy humans. Blood 79:693–698, 1992.
23. Hinterberger W, Adolf G, Bettelheim P, Geissler K, Huber C, Irschick E, Kalhs P, Köller U, Lechner K, Meister B, Woloszczuk W: Lymphokine overproduction in severe aplastic anemia is not related to blood transfusions. Blood 74:2713–2717, 1989.
24. Shinohara K, Ayame H, Tanaka M, Matsuda M, Ando S, Tajiri M: Increased production of tumor necrosis factor-α by peripheral blood mononuclear cells in the patients with aplastic anemia. Am J Hematol 37:75–79, 1991.
25. Viale M, Merli A, Bacigalupo A: Analysis at the clonal level of T-cell phenotype and functions in severe aplastic anemia patients. Blood 78:1268–1274, 1991.
26. Kramer SM, Carver ME: Serum-free in vitro bioassay for the detection of tumor necrosis factor. J Immunol Methods 93:201–206, 1986.
27. Cavallo MG, Pozzilli P, Bird C, Wadhwa M, Meager A, Visalli N, Gearing A JH, Andreani D, Thorpe R: Cytokines in sera from insulin-dependent diabetic patients at diagnosis. Clin Exp Immunol 86:256–259, 1991.
28. Schultz JC, Shahidi NT: Tumor necrosis factor-α overproduction in Fanconi's anemia. Am J Hematol 42:196–201, 1993.
29. Porfirio B, Dallapiccola B, Mokini V, Alimena G, Isacchi G, Mandelli F, Gandini E: Effects of oxidants and autoxidants on chromosome breaks in Fanconi's anemia. Pathologica 75 (Suppl): 296–300, 1983.
30. Nathan C, Sanchez E: Tumor necrosis factor and CD11/CD18 (β2) integrins act synergistically to lower cAMP in human neutrophils. J Cell Biol 111:2171–2181, 1990.
31. Clark IA, Thumwood CM, Chaudhri G, Cowden WB, Hunt NH: Tumor necrosis factor and reactive oxygen species: Implications for free radical induced tissue injury. In Halliwell B (ed.): "Oxygen Radicals and Tissue Injury Symposium." Bethesda, MD: Federation of American Societies for Experimental Biology, 1988.
32. Radeke HH, Meier B, Topley N, Flöge J, Habermehl GG, Resch K: Interleukin 1-α and tumor necrosis factor-α induce oxygen radical production in mesangial cells. Kidney Int 37:767–775, 1990.
33. Tanaka H, Ogura H, Yokota J, Sugimoto H, Yoshioka T, Sugimoto T: Acceleration of superoxide production from leukocytes in trauma patients. Ann Surg 214:187–192, 1991.
34. Berkow RL, Wang D, Larrick JW, Dodson RW, Howard TH: Enhancement of neutrophil superoxide production by preincubation with recombinant human tumor necrosis factor. J Immunol 139:3783–3791, 1987.
35. Remick DG: Significance of in vivo detection of tumor necrosis factor (editorial). Lab Invest 65:259–261, 1991.

American Journal of Hematology 45:39–50 (1994)

Splenic Lymphoma With Circulating Villous Lymphocytes: Report of Seven Cases and Review of the Literature

Tsieh Sun, Myron Susin, Judith Brody, Klaus Dittmar, Saul Teichberg, Robert Weiner, Jen H. Lin, and Norbert Felber

Departments of Laboratories (T.S., M.S., J.B., S.T.) Medicine (K.D., R.W.), and Pediatrics (S.T.), North Shore University Hospital-Cornell University Medical College, Manhasset, New York; Department of Pathology, Nassau County Medical Center, East Meadow, New York (J.H.L.); and Department of Medicine, Winthrop University Hospital, Mineola, New York (N.F.)

Splenic lymphoma with villous lymphocytes (SLVL) is a relatively new entity with only a few reports published. We report seven cases of SLVL with detailed clinicopathologic and comprehensive immunophenotypic studies to further characterize this lymphoma, which is frequently confused with hairy cell leukemia and other low-grade B-cell lymphoid neoplasms. The diagnostic criteria we used include 1) prominent splenomegaly, 2) insignificant or no lymphadenopathy, 3) lymphocytosis without leukopenia, 4) presence of circulating villous lymphocytes, 5) characteristic cytologic and histologic features, and 6) specific phenotypic and cytochemical findings. Our studies show that SLVL does not represent a pure entity but rather a morphologically heterogeneous group of low-grade lymphomas with various cytologic and histologic features. Although immunophenotyping is helpful in differential diagnosis, multiparameter studies are necessary to confirm the diagnosis. In our series, only two patients died of SLVL, who probably developed transformation to a higher-grade lymphoma.

Key words: splenic lymphoma, villous lymphocytes, low-grade B-cell lymphoma, hairy cell leukemia

INTRODUCTION

Splenic lymphoma is usually divided into primary and secondary types. Primary splenic lymphoma is defined as a lymphoma confined to the spleen, while secondary splenic lymphoma includes those originating from lymph nodes with splenic involvement [1]. In secondary splenic lymphoma, peripheral blood and bone marrow are also frequently involved. Currently, Melo et al. coined the term "splenic lymphoma with villous lymphocytes (SLVL)" for a clinicopathologic entity in which the spleen is primarily involved but the neoplasm also spreads to the peripheral blood and bone marrow without significant lymphadenopathy [2,3]. SLVL fits neither the strict definition of primary splenic lymphoma because blood and bone marrow are involved, nor that of secondary splenic lymphoma as lymph nodes are not involved initially. The importance of identifying this entity is due to its resemblance to hairy cell leukemia (HCL), but their treatment is different.

Although several series of SLVL were published under different names other than SLVL [4–8] before the reports of Melo et al., only a few cases were published recently [9–15]. We report seven cases of SLVL diagnosed in the past 4 years on the basis of 1) prominent splenomegaly, 2) insignificant or no lymphadenopathy, 3) lymphocytosis without leukopenia, 4) presence of circulating villous lymphocytes, 5) characteristic cytologic and histologic features, and 6) specific phenotypic and cytochemical findings.

MATERIALS AND METHODS

Light Microscopy

Seven peripheral blood specimens, five bone marrow aspirates, six bone marrow biopsies, five splenectomy specimens, three lymph nodes, and two liver (specimens) were examined by light microscopy. All tissue sections

Received for publication January 22, 1993; accepted June 30, 1993.

Address reprint requests to Dr. Tsieh Sun, Department of Laboratories, North Shore University Hospital-Cornell University Medical College, Manhasset, NY 11030.

TABLE I. Monoclonal Antibodies Used in Immunohistochemical Studies

Cluster designation	Monoclonal antibodies	Cell identified
CD 2	Leu 4 (BD)[a]	Pan T-cell
CD 3	Leu 5 (BD)	Pan T-cell
CD 20	Leu 16 (BD)	Pan B-cell
CD 45RO	UCHL-1 (Dako)	T-cell
CD 74	LN-2 (ICN)	B-cell, monocyte
CDw 75	LN-1 (ICN)	B-cell

[a]Manufacturers are in parentheses.

TABLE II. Monoclonal Antibodies Used for Flow Cytometric Studies

Cluster designation	Monoclonal antibodies[a]	Cell identified
CD 3	Leu 4	Pan T-cell
CD 4	Leu 3	T-helper/inducer
CD 5	Leu 1	Pan T-cell, B-CLL
CD 7	Leu 9	Pan T-cell, NK cell
CD 8	Leu 2	T-cytotoxic/suppressor
CD 11c	Leu M5	Monocyte
CD 13	Leu M7	Myelomonocytic cell
CD 14	Leu M3, My4	Monocyte
CD 19	Leu 12	Pan B-cell
CD 20	Leu 16	Pan B-cell
CD 22	Leu 14	B-cell (hairy cell)
CD 25	IL-2R	Tac positive cell
CD 33	Leu M9	Myelomonocytic cell
—	HLA-DR	B-cell, activated T-cell, myelomonocyte
—	Surface immunoglobulins[b]	B-cell

[a]My4 was from Coulter Immunology, other products were from Becton Dickinson.
[b]Surface immunoglobulin antibodies were polyclonal.
CLL, chronic lymphocytic leukemia.

were stained with hematoxylin and eosin, the bone marrow biopsies were also stained for reticulin.

Electron Microscopy

Tissues from two splenectomy specimens and two peripheral blood samples were fixed in 2.5% 0.1 M cacodylate buffered (pH 7.3) gluteraldehyde and submitted for electron microscopic studies. The cell diameter and number of cytoplasmic projections per cell profile were measured in tumor cells with a complete nucleus and a relatively symmetrical configuration. Cells from a typical case of hairy cell leukemia were also measured for comparison. A minimum of 20–25 cells/case were examined.

Immunohistochemistry

Immunohistochemical studies of paraffin and frozen sections from four splenectomy specimens were performed with the three-step avidin-biotin-peroxidase technique [16]. A panel of monoclonal antibodies were used to characterize the tumor cells (Table I).

Flow Cytometry

Immunophenotyping was performed on 14 specimens (seven peripheral blood, four spleen, and three bone marrow specimens) from seven patients with the FACScan flow cytometer (Becton Dickinson, Mountain View, CA), using a panel of monoclonal antibodies as listed in Table II. Mononuclear cells were isolated by the standard Ficoll-Hypaque technique [17]. An isotypic control (mouse immunoglobulin IgG or IgM) was used to subtract the background staining from positive results.

Cytochemistry

Acid phosphatase and tartrate-resistant acid phosphatase were performed on all specimens described under flow cytometry using standard methodology [17].

RESULTS

Clinical Findings

The clinical findings are summarized in Table III. The initial presentation was usually abdominal discomfort caused by splenomegaly and/or the discovery of lymphocytosis in the peripheral blood. Splenomegaly was prominent in all cases. Hepatomegaly was found in only one case. Lymphadenopathy was absent or palpable in five cases, but significant lymphadenopathy was present in two cases (cases 2 and 3) with lymphomatous disseminatin. Both cases showed evidence of high-grade lymphoma transformation and died. Besides these two cases, only case 4 showed a progressive clinical course; other cases were characterized by an indolent clinical course. In four cases, patients became asymptomatic or ambulatory. One case showed marked hematologic improvement (leukocyte count and spleen size returned to normal) but died of a myocardial infarct.

Laboratory Findings

The laboratory findings are summarized in Table IV. The leukocyte counts varied from 5.8–58 × 10^9/l (mean 25.6) with a percentage of lymphocytes between 44–86 (mean 64.9). Thrombocytopenia was present in five cases and varying degrees of anemia in five cases. Monoclonal IgM-kappa gammopathy was demonstrated in one case and IgM was elevated in two cases. The lactate dehydrogenase level was increased in four cases and abnormal karyotypes were found in two cases.

Three cases had hemolysis as evidenced by a positive direct Coomb's test or high reticulocyte count. The two fatal cases (cases 2 and 3) showed highest leukocyte counts, % lymphocytes, and lactate dehydrogenase levels, lowest platelet counts, and abnormal karyotypes. The two clinically mild cases (cases 5 and 6) revealed only

TABLE III. Clinical Findings

Case number	1	2	3	4	5	6	7
Age (years)	57	56	71	55	65	78	46
Race	White	Black	White	White	White	White	White
Sex	Female	Female	Male	Female	Female	Male	Female
Presentation	Splenomegaly, fatigue	Splenomegaly, lymphocytosis	Left flank pain	Fever, abdominal fullness	Abdominal pain, fever	Lymphocytosis	Weakness, left flank pain
Splenomegaly (LCM) (cm)	22	12	9	6	7	6	10
Hepatomegaly (RCM)	Palpable	6 cm	No	No	No	No	No
Lymphadenopathy (LN)	No	Cervical, axillary	Axillary	No	No	No	Axillary, inguinal
Computed tomography	Splenomegaly	N/D	Abdominal lymph adenopathy	N/D	N/D	N/D	N/D
Splenectomy	Yes	Yes	Yes	Yes	No	No	Yes
Chemotherapy[a]	No	No	Yes	Yes	No	Leukeran	Prednisone
Clinical course	Indolent	Progressive	Progressive	Progressive	Indolent	Indolent	Indolent
Observation period	3 years	6 months	3 years	6 years	1½ years	1 year	2 years
Outcome	Asymptomatic	Death	Death	Ambulatory	Ambulatory	Hematologic improvement	Asymptomatic
Cause of death	N/A	Lymphomatous dissemination	Lymphomatous dissemination	N/A	N/A	Died of MI	N/A

[a]Chemotherapy: case 3, adriamycin, vincristine, prednisone, bleomycin; case 4, cytoxin, vincristine, prednisone. LCM, left costal margin; RCM, right costal margin; LN, lymph node; MI, myocardial infarct; N/D, not done; N/A, not applicable.

TABLE IV. Laboratory Findings*

Case number	1	2	3	4	5	6	7
Leukocyte count (10^9/l)	22.3	48	58	7.8	14	23	5.8
% lymphocyte	80	62	86	52	60	70	44
Platelet count (10^9/l)	129	109	78	138	156	135	200
Hemoglobin (g/dl)	9.2	8.9	14.9	10.7	13	13.8	7.1
Hematocrit (%)	30	27	44.5	32.8	38.5	39.3	21.1
Serum IgG (mg/dl) (normal 540–1480)	1070	N/D	823	750	770[a]	950[a]	N/D
Serum IgA (mg/dl) (normal 65–180)	126	N/D	176	52	330[a]	326[a]	N/D
Serum IgM (mg/dl) (normal 45–200)	691	N/D	143	150	860[a]	400[a]	N/D
Electrophoresis	Monoclonal IgM-kappa	Normal	Normal	Normal	Normal	Normal	Normal
LD (U/l) (normal 60–200)	807	2838	1360	384	201	176	427
Cytogenetics	Normal	1p−, 14q+	Abnormal[b]	N/D	N/D	N/D	N/D
Other finding	No	AP 564 U/l	Retic count 7.5%	Direct Coombs+	No	No	Direct Coombs+

*AP, alkaline phosphatase (normal 30–115 U/l); LD, lactate dehydrogenase; N/D, not done.
[a]The immunoglobulin quantitation in cases 5 and 6 was performed in another laboratory where the normal range for IgG was 600–1700 mg/dl, IgA 70–450 mg/dl, and IgM 56–550 mg/dl.
[b]Abnormal karyotype in case 3: 45–46,X,−Y,del(1p),t(1q;12q),del(2p),+random marker, +random loss.

lymphocytosis, but other laboratory tests were all within normal limits.

Pathologic Findings

Grossly, all spleens examined were markedly enlarged weighing 780, 2,232, 2,340, 2,974, and 3,970 g, respectively. The cut surfaces of the spleens were congested and studded with grayish-white nodules suggestive of lymphomatous infiltration except for one case which showed only accentuation of the Malpighian corpuscles.

Microscopic examination of the splenectomy specimens showed mainly white pulp involvement by small lymphocytes in three cases (cases 1, 4, and 7) (Fig. 1). The white pulp was moderately expanded and formed confluent nodules in some areas. In these three cases, the red pulp was also infiltrated to a lesser degree. In the

TABLE V. Results of Monoclonal Antibody (in %) and Acid Phosphatase Reactions*

Case number	1	2	3	3	3	4	4	5	6	7	7	7
Specimen source	PB	PB	PB	PB	BM	PB	Spleen	PB	PB	BM	PB	Spleen
Date performed	1/88	8/88	1/89	5/90	5/90	7/89	12/89	3/90	7/90	9/90	10/90	3/91
CD 3	15	10	6	12	13	56	44	6	27	32	28	36
CD 4	/	/	/	7	5	/	/	/	/	18	/	/
CD 5	9	8	6	10	10	55	42	6	90	28	29	34
CD 7	9	9	7	9	12	55	40	6	24	30	28	36
CD 8	/	/	/	8	7	/	/	/	/	13	/	/
CD 11c	70	92	92	81	83	0	/	94	58	25	32	20
CD 13	/	85	/	/	/	/	/	/	/	/	/	/
CD 14	/	86	16	9	7	/	9	2	12	/	17	/
CD 19	88	96	95	93	91	41	49	89	67	67	65	51
CD 20	91	94	93	94	92	41	45	92	65	63	70	53
CD 22	83	91	88	87	90	0	/	87	63	60	65	64
CD 25	/	/	1	2	5	0	/	2	/	0	/	2
CD 33	/	87	/	/	/	/	/	/	/	/	/	/
HLA-DR	78	86	95	97	97	40	79	91	82	64	64	55
PV Ig	88	82	95	88	73	45	54	91	67	/	/	50
IgG	16	20	1	6	0	4	3	2	8	/	/	4
IgA	11	12	2	2	0	2	0	1	4	/	/	2
IgM	85	63	90	86	76	44	51	90	40	/	/	52
Kappa	86	73	89	81	65	43	50	7	40	2	3	9
Lambda	14	16	0	3	6	4	1	84	4	58	66	45
ACP	+	+	+	+	+	+	+	+	+	+	+	+
TRAP	+	+	+	+	+	−	−	+	−	−	−	−

*PB, peripheral blood; BM, Bone marrow; PV Ig, polyvalent immunoglobulin; ACP, acid phosphatase; TRAP, tartrate-resistant acid phosphatase; /, not done.

TABLE VI. Comparison of Markers for Four Related Low-Grade B-Cell Neoplasms

	CD5	CD11c	CD19	CD20	CD22	CD25	TRAP
Splenic lymphoma with villous lymphocytes	−	±	+	+	+	−	±
Hairy cell leukemia	−	+	+	+	+	+	+
Chronic lymphocytic leukemia	+	−	+	+	±	−	−
Prolymphocytic leukemia	±	−	+	+	±	−	−

other two cases (cases 2 and 3), red pulp infiltration was more prominent than that of the white pulp (Fig. 2). The infiltrate involved both the red pulp cords and sinuses and no pseudosinus pattern was demonstrated.

The tumor cells in the three cases which showed predominant white pulp infiltration were well-differentiated small lymphocytes with round nuclei, clumped chromatin, scanty cytoplasm, and low mitotic rate. In the two cases with predominant red pulp infiltration, the tumor cells were of intermediate size, with oval or indented nuclei, clumped to reticular chromatin, small nucleoli, and moderate amount of cytoplasm. The mitotic rate was higher in these two cases than in the other three. Various numbers of prolymphocytes were consistently present and intermingled with the tumor cells in all cases, while small numbers of plasma cells were seen only in two cases (cases 4 and 7).

Lymph node involvement was seen in three cases (cases 1, 2, and 4); all showed diffuse effacement of the normal architecture by the tumor cells. Liver sections were available from cases 1 and 2, in which the portal areas were mainly involved, while mild sinusoidal infiltration was also present.

Hematologic Examination

The circulating lymphocytes in cases 4, 5, 6, and 7 were the size of large lymphocytes with round to ovoid eccentric nuclei, clumped and smudged chromatin and moderate amount of variably basophilic cytoplasm (Fig. 3). Case 1 showed single distinct nucleoli, eccentric nuclei, occasional nuclear convolutions, and a lower nucleocytoplasmic ratio, mimicking prolymphocytes. In cases 2 and 3, the cells were slightly larger than in other cases with central nuclei and cytoplasmic vacuoles (Fig. 4). Case 3 also showed nuclear convolutions. In general, the nucleocytoplasmic ratio in these cases except case 1 was consistently higher than that seen in hairy cells. In all

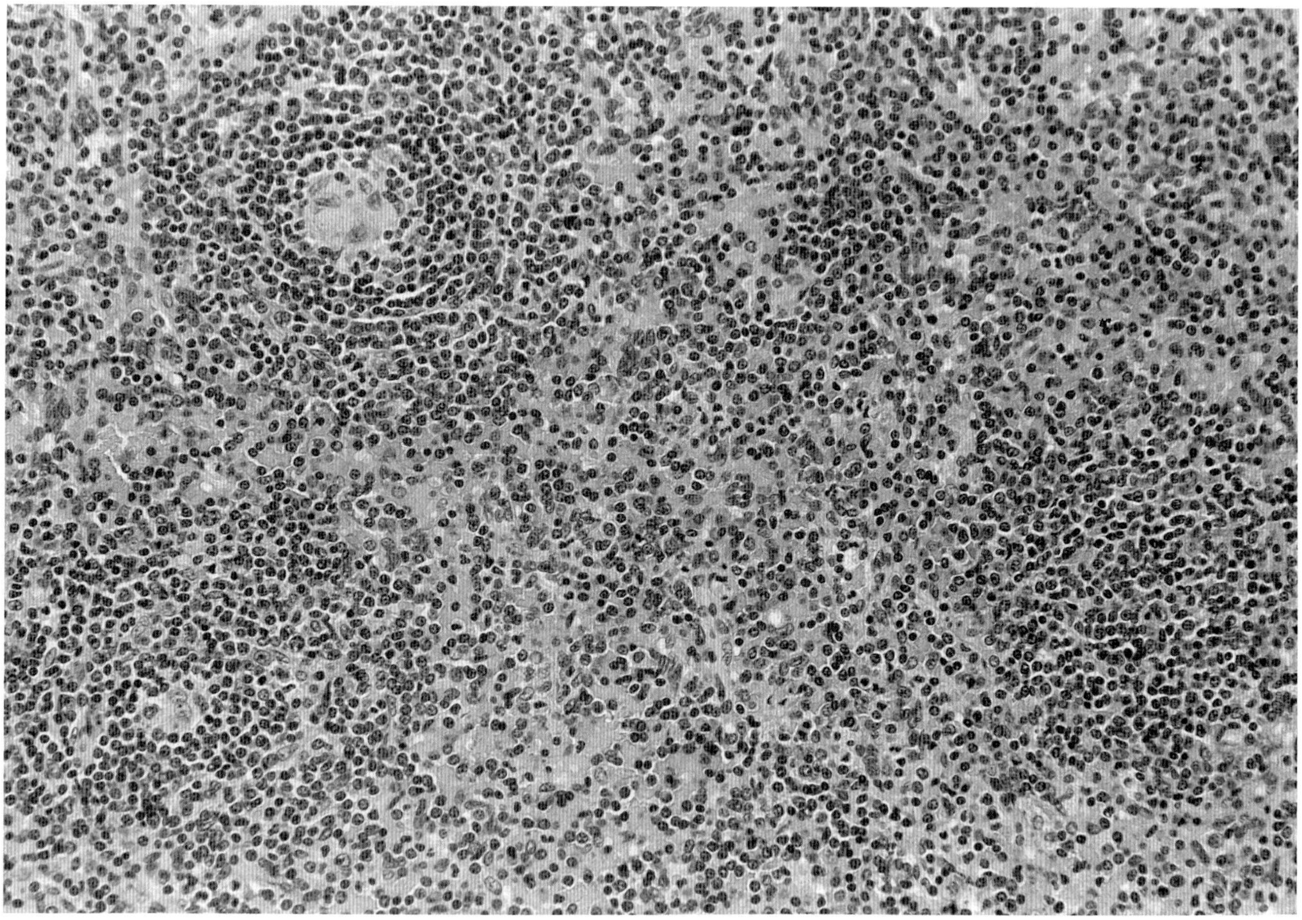

Fig. 1. Spleen from case 7 showing expansion of white pulp and infiltration of red pulp by small well-differentiated lymphoid cells (H&E, ×250).

cases, peripheral fine to coarse cytoplasmic projections, less prominent than those seen in hairy cells, were demonstrated in some but not all cells. The projections or villi were unevenly distributed; polar distribution was seen in cases 2, 4, 6, and 7.

The bone marrow aspirates in cases 3, 4, 5, 6, and 7 showed an interstitial lymphocytosis of cells cytologically similar to those seen in the peripheral blood (Fig. 3). The bone marrow biopsies in cases 4, 5, and 7 were cellular to hypercellular and showed multiple non-paratrabecular lymphoid nodules composed of loosely packed small lymphoid cells (plasma cells were also noted in case 4). In case 1, there was a diffuse and nodular small lymphocytic infiltrate. In cases 2 and 3, non-paratrabecular nodules composed of larger lymphoid cells admixed with smaller cells and histiocytes (in case 2) were present (Fig. 5). The pattern in all cases was clearly not that of hairy cell leukemia; rather it was similar to the infiltrate of chronic lymphocytic leukemia or well-differentiated lymphocytic lymphoma with slightly wider spacing of the lymphoid cells within the nodules. Reticulin stain showed a slight increase in reticulin fibers in four of five cases examined, similar to the background of reticulin usually seen in a lymphoid aggregate.

Electron Microscopy

Electron microscopic examination of two cases (cases 3 and 4) showed higher nucleocytoplasmic ratio, and shorter and fewer surface cytoplasmic projections (villi), as compared to the control case of hairy cell leukemia (Fig. 6). The distribution of the villi was uneven, but a polar distribution pattern was not a consistent finding in our two cases. The average number of villi per cell in case 3 was 7.4 ± 2.3 (mean $\pm$ SEM, $n = 29$), case 4 was 9.4 ± 4.3 ($n = 19$), and the hairy cell control was 29 ± 3.0 ($n = 22$). The cell diameter measured from the same number of cells from cases 3 and 4 was 9.2 ± 0.2 μm and 7.2 ± 0.2 μm, respectively, while that of hairy cells was 9.3 ± 0.2 μm.

Immunohistochemistry

Kappa and lambda light chain stain for frozen sections of spleen was done on only case 7, which showed a monoclonal lambda pattern. Light chain staining of par-

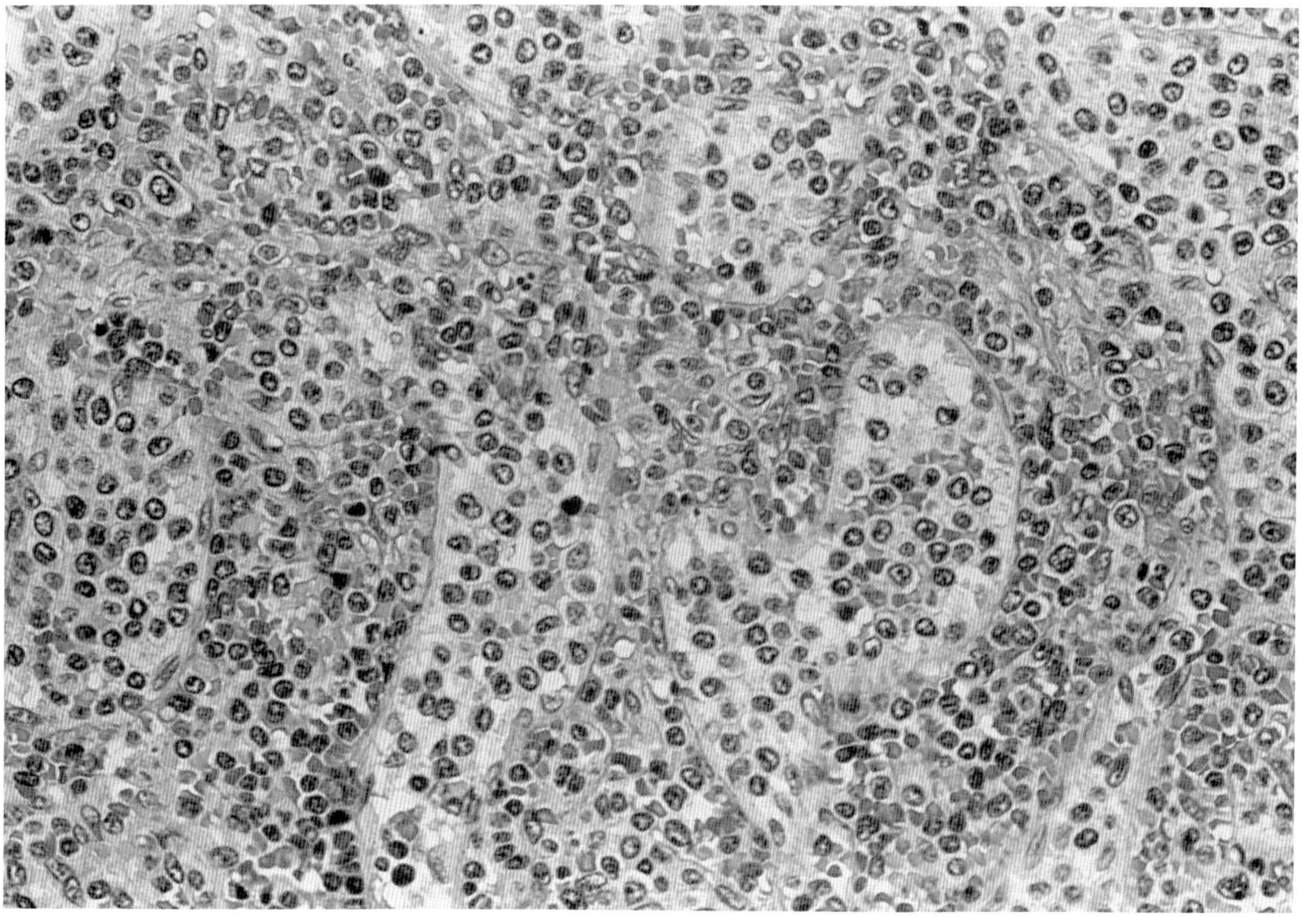

Fig. 2. Spleen from case 3 showing infiltration of red pulp cords and sinuses by small well-differentiated lymphoid cells intermingled with some intermediate-sized transformed lymphoid cells (H&E, ×400).

affin section in all five cases demonstrated only plasma cells which were polyclonal. However, most tumor cells were stained for B-cell antigens (CD 20, CD74, and CDw 75) in all five splenectomy specimens (Fig. 7). A minority of lymphocytes, which were intermingled with the tumor cells, were stained for T-cell antigens (CD 2/CD 3 and CD 45 RO).

Flow Cytometry

Of the 14 specimens studied, two splenectomy specimens (cases 2 and 3) were discarded because of low cell viability. The results of flow cytometric studies were consistent regardless of the source of specimens and the time intervals between specimen testing, as demonstrated in cases 3, 4, and 7, in which multiple specimens were collected (Table V). Essentially, all cases showed a monoclonal surface immunoglobulin pattern; five were IgM-kappa and two were IgM-lambda (cases 5 and 7). The percentage of polyvalent immunoglobulin positive cells was very close to that of B-cell antigen (CD 19, CD 20) positive and HLA-DR positive cells. The specific monoclonal antibody pair, CD 22 and CD 11c, was positive in all cases except for case 4, in which no lymphocytes from the peripheral blood and bone marrow reacted to either antigen. CD 25 was negative in all four cases examined. T-cell antigens (CD 3, CD 5, and CD 7) were positive in 6 to 56% of lymphoid cells. The number of helper and suppressor T-cells were approximately equal in the two cases tested.

Case 2 was biphenotypic showing, in addition to what has been described, high percentage (85–87%) of myelomonocytic antigen (CD 13, CD 14, and CD 33) positive cells. Case 6 was biclonal showing a population of IgG-lambda, CD 5 positive cells (consistent with chronic lymphocytic leukemia), in addition to the IgM-kappa, CD 11c positive cell population (SLVL cells).

Cytochemistry

All seven cases were positive for acid phosphatase (Table V). Four cases showed weak positivity for tartrate

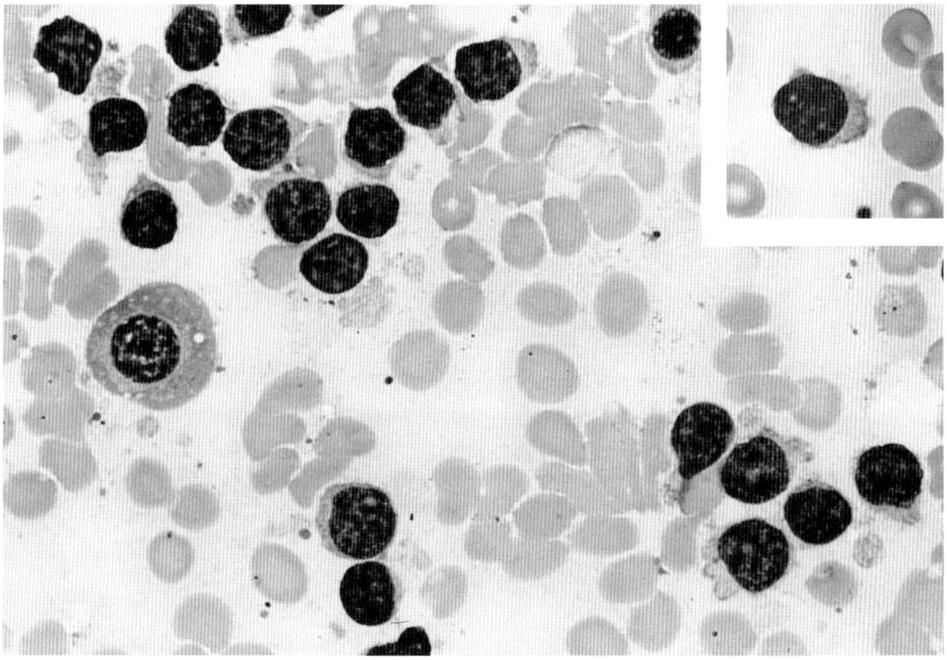

Fig. 3. Bone marrow aspirate from case 4 showing clusters of small lymphocytes and a plasma cell. The characteristic features of villous lymphocyte are usually not obvious in bone marrow smear. Inset: A villous lymphocyte from the peripheral blood of case 4 showing eccentric nuclei, homogeneous smudged chromatin, and moderate amount of cytoplasm with peripheral cytoplasmic projections (Wright-Giemsa, ×1,000).

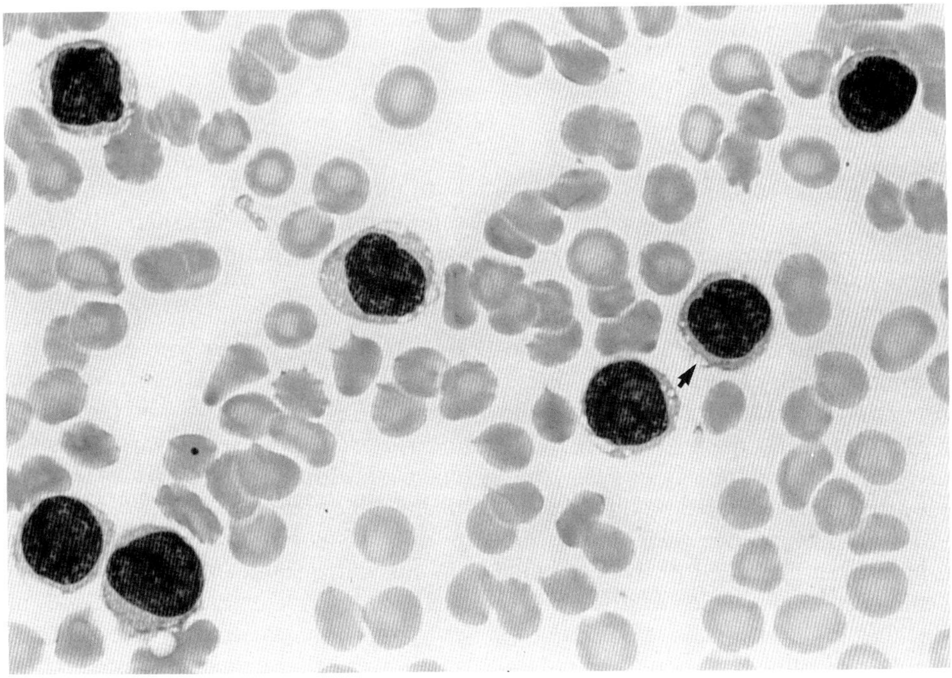

Fig. 4. Circulating villous lymphocytes from case 3 showing large size, occasional nuclear convolutions, central nuclei, and cytoplasmic vacuoles. Short villous projections (arrow) are seen on some cells (Wright-Giemsa, ×1,000).

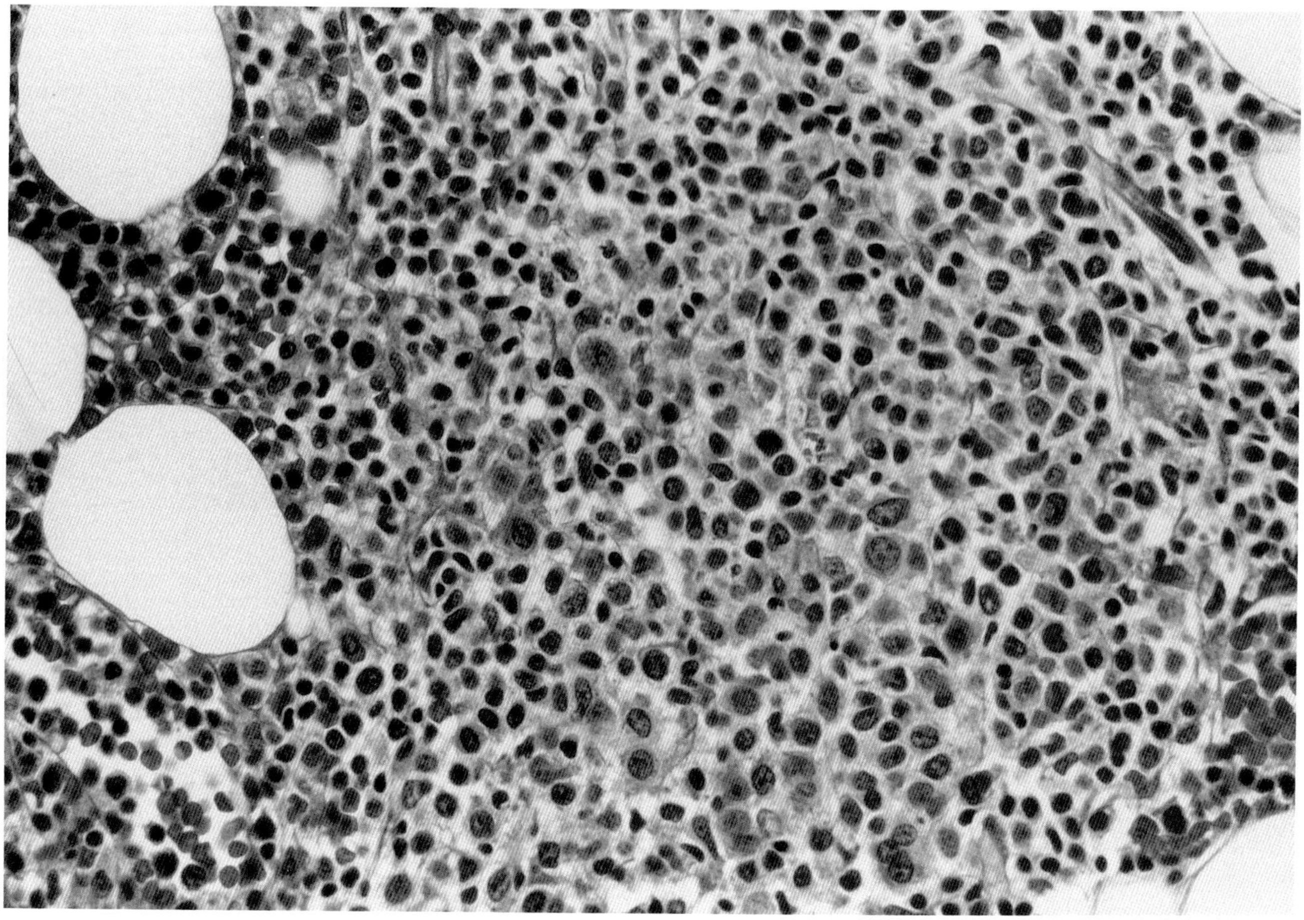

Fig. 5. Bone marrow biopsy from case 3 showing non-paratrabecular lymphoid aggregate with heterogeneous mixture of large and small lymphoid cells (H&E, ×400).

resistant acid phosphatase (TRAP). In the other three cases, the TRAP result was negative.

DISCUSSION

SLVL is not an entirely new entity, since similar cases have been reported under various names, such as splenomegalic immunocytoma [4,8], malignant lymphoma simulating leukemic reticuloendotheliosis [5], lymphocytic lymphoma simulating hairy cell leukemia [7], and chronic lymphoproliferative disorder resembling hairy cell leukemia [6]. Melo et al. first applied the term SLVL to define this entity in a more precise way in 1987 [2,3]. This terminology was promptly adopted by the FAB cooperative group in 1989 [18]. Since then only a few reports on SLVL have been published [9–14]. Detailed clinicopathologic and phenotypic studies were lacking in most reports. Its incidence was estimated to be similar to that of hairy cell leukemia, more common than prolymphocytic leukemia and hairy cell leukemia variants, but 10-fold less common than chronic lymphocytic leukemia of B-cell origin [12]. However, the incidence of SLVL in tropical West Africa seems to be higher than that in the Western world and it may be associated with or misclassified as hyper-reactive malarial splenomegaly [15].

In those 22 patients reported by Melo et al., the presenting symptoms were usually limited to mild weakness, fatigue, and abdominal discomfort caused by the enlarged spleen [2]. These were also the presenting symptoms seen in our patients except for case 2, who was at the terminal stage when medical consultation was sought. The sex ratio in four series showed male preponderance while two other series showed female predominance. The mean age in these series varied from 54 to 72 years at diagnosis. In our series, five of seven patients were female with a mean age of 62 years.

SLVL is considered a low-grade non-Hodgkin's lymphoma with a stable or slowly progressive clinical course [12]. Melo et al. stated that some patients with SLVL did not require any treatment for long periods [2]. However, in a series of 50 patients reported by Mulligan et al., 12 (24%) expired 1 month to 8 years from time of diagnosis and one third of the deaths were directly related to the progression of SLVL [12]. In our series, three patients

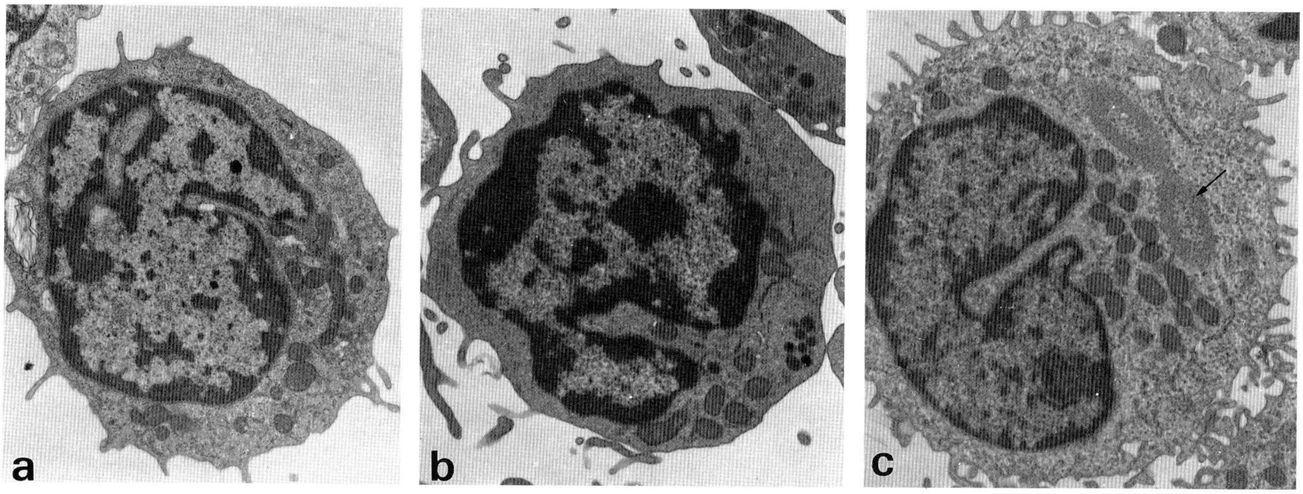

Fig. 6. Electron micrographs of typical peripheral blood lymphoid cells from case 3 (a) and case 4 (b). In (c), a cell from a patient with hairy cell leukemia is shown for comparison. In (a) and (b), the cells have small numbers of surface projections, alternating with smooth cell surface areas. In (c), the cell surface is covered with large numbers of projections and a ribosome-lamellar complex (arrow) is also seen in the cytoplasm. (a) ×6,900; (b) and (c) ×8,000.

(cases 2, 3, and 6) expired and case 6 died of an acute myocardial infarct despite the fact that his lymphoma was under control. Cases 2 and 3 showed evidence suggestive of transformation to a higher-grade lymphoma as evidenced by prominent abdominal lymphadenopathy and marked lymphocytosis. Case 2, in addition, had biphenotypic lymphoma expressing myelogenous antigens which usually carry a poor prognosis [19]. However, when a low-grade component (chronic lymphocytic leukemia) was coexistent with SLVL (case 6), it did not seem to affect the patient's prognosis.

Splenectomy was considered the treatment of choice in several reports [8,12]. In our series, case 2 died soon after splenectomy, case 3 died 1 year after splenectomy, but three other patients (cases 1, 4, and 7) did well 1 to 3 years after surgery. Chemotherapy had no effect on cases 3 and 4, but leukeran caused hematologic improvement (leukocyte count and spleen size returned to normal) in case 6. Steroid therapy helped to control hemolysis in cases 4 and 7.

As previously mentioned, it is important, although sometimes difficult, to distinguish between SLVL and hairy cell leukemia and its variants because of the differences in therapy. However, many cases of SLVL were also misdiagnosed as chronic lymphocytic leukemia (CLL) and prolymphocytic leukemia (PLL). Although lymphoma of intermediate differention (IDL) is frequently found in the spleen [20], its rarity of peripheral blood involvement makes it less likely to be confused with SLVL.

The differential diagnosis of SLVL from other B-cell lymphomas/leukemias should be made initially on the basis of the peripheral blood morphology [2]. SLVL usually shows mild peripheral lymphocytosis, with a leukocyte count between 3 and 38 $\times$ 10^9/l. HCL is characterized by pancytopenia, although leukocytosis can be seen in its variants [21]. PLL, on the other hand, is typical for its extremely high leukocyte count (more than 100 $\times$ 10^9/l) (2). The leukocyte count in CLL usually ranges between 10 and 150 $\times$ 10^9/l.

In SLVL, villous lymphocytes constitute 38–99% of all lymphocytes present in the peripheral blood [21]. A typical villous lymphocyte is larger than the small lymphocytes found in CLL and close to the size of a prolymphocyte [2,3,21]. It has a round or ovoid nucleus with clumped chromatin and, in half the cases, has a small but distinct nucleolus. The cytoplasm is usually moderate in amount and basophilic, but it may be scanty in a minority of cases. However, the striking feature of this cells is the presence of thin and short cytoplasmic villi with uneven distribution. In addition, a few long and thin cytoplasmic projections also may be observed. In contrast, hairy cells usually have numerous slender cytoplasmic villi (hairy projections) and uniformly dispersed chromatin pattern. The larger size and lower nucleocytoplasmic ratio of hairy cells also help to distinguish HCL from the villous lymphocytes of SLVL. The cells in PLL may mimic those of SLVL, but the absence or presence of cytoplasmic villi and basophilia may help to distinguish these two conditions [2]. In addition, the nucleoli in PLL cells are

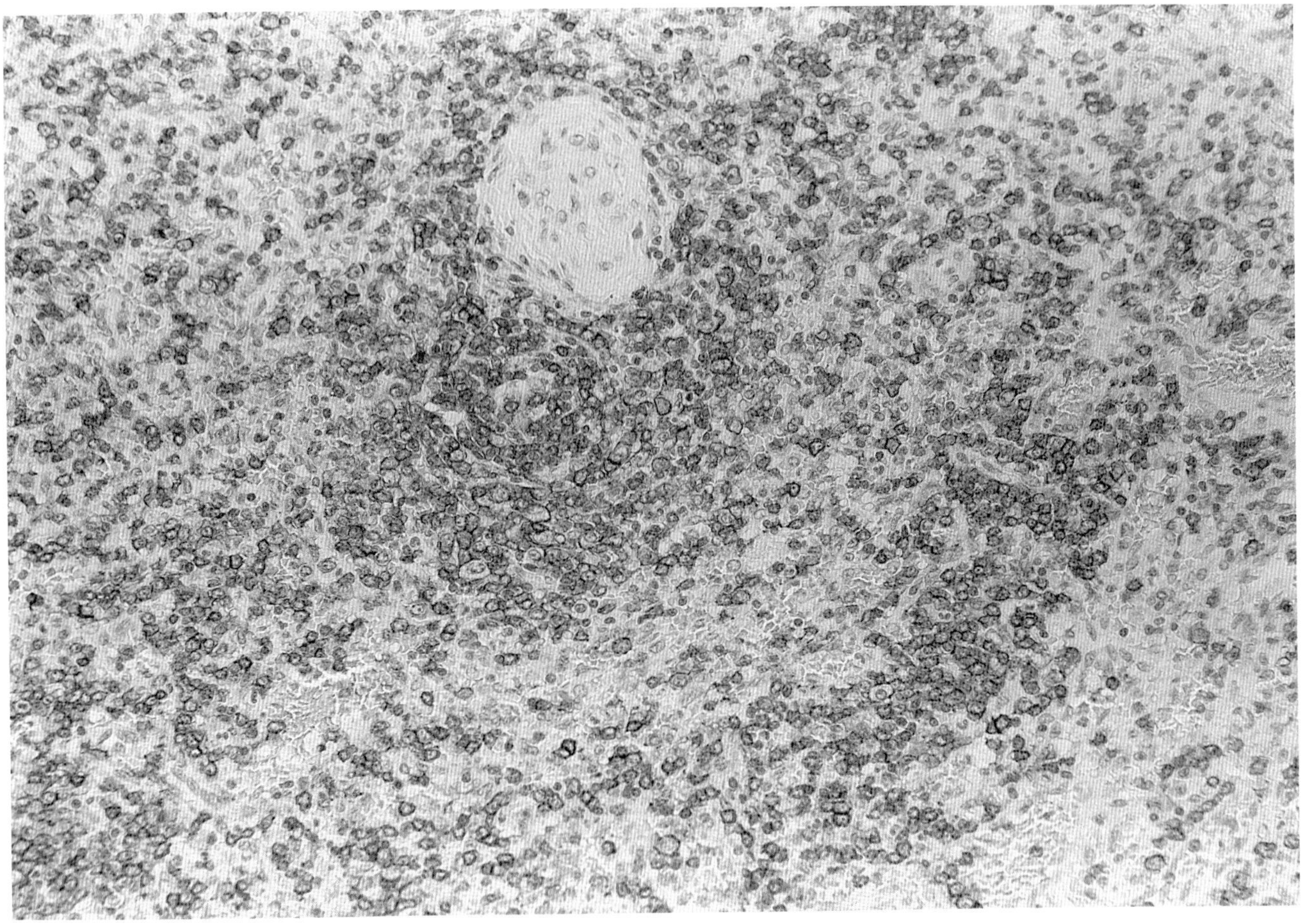

Fig. 7. Spleen from case 7. Tumor cells show strong staining for L-26 (CD20), a B-cell marker (immunoperoxidase, ×250).

more prominent than those in SLVL cells. The small cell variety of SLVL may show scanty cytoplasm and no nucleoli [21], and in those cases, CLL should be excluded by marker studies.

In addition, 3–12% of plasma cells or plasmacytoid cells may be present in the peripheral blood in SLVL [21]. Monoclonal gammopathy is also frequently demonstrated in SLVL; 60% cases were positive in one series [2]. These features, if present, are useful but not specific for differential diagnosis. However, in our series only one case showed small numbers of plasma cells in the marrow, two cases in the spleen, and only one of seven cases tested with serum electrophoresis revealed monoclonal gammopathy.

Electron microscopic examination is sometimes helpful in the differential diagnosis in equivocal cases. The demonstration of the ribosome-lamellar complex, the evenly distributed long and slender cytoplasmic projections, and large cell size may help to confirm the diagnosis of HCL [21]. However, our data suggest that the cell size in HCL and SLVL may overlap.

The examination of the spleen is instrumental for a definitive diagnosis. The spleen is usually markedly enlarged, weighing between 1,000 and 4,000 g. The cut surfaces often show grayish white nodules, a helpful clue to exclude the diagnosis of leukemia. Histologically, cells from HCL are confined to the red pulp, forming pseudosinuses [22, 23]. In SLVL, the white pulp of the spleen is usually involved with or without red pulp infiltration. Occasionally, red pulp infiltration may become predominant as seen in our series as well as others [2]. Unlike hairy cells, the tumor cells of SLVL in the red pulp are not arranged in pseudosinuses. Plasma cell infiltration is frequently seen in SLVL. In PLL, both white and red pulp are involved, as in CLL. Characteristically, the large and pale-staining PLL cells surround the white pulp, forming a "margination" or bizonal pattern.

Bone marrow aspiration is usually not as helpful as other preparations because the morphology of villous lymphocytes or hairy cells are not easily recognized in marrow smears. Bone marrow biopsy, on the other hand, is extremely useful in demonstrating the pathognomonic feature of HCL, which shows a "fried egg" pattern as tumor cells are separated from each other by a clear space because of poor staining of their abundant cytoplasm

[24]. In SLVL, the bone marrow may or may not be infiltrated and the infiltration pattern may be diffuse or nodular (3), as seen in CLL. The bone marrow infiltration by PLL cells is usually diffuse. Reticulin fibrosis is frequently seen in the bone marrow in cases of HCL, resulting in dry taps, a fact that helps to distinguish HCL from other low-grade lymphoproliferative disorders.

If morphologic features are not distinctive, marker studies can be helpful (Table VI) [25]. HCL is characterized by positive reactions to CD 22, CD 11c, CD 25, and TRAP staining, while CLL is distinctively positive for CD 5. PLL is negative in all these markers except for CD 22 and CD 5 (1/3 of cases) [21]. The distinction between HCL and SLVL is sometimes difficult because SLVL may show positivity for all HCL markers except for CD 25, as exemplified in our series, while CD 25 can also be negative in HCL cases. The high positive rate of TRAP in our series is in marked contrast to the series of Milo et al. [2,3] but is similar to that encountered in the series of Nieman et al. [5]. This discrepancy may be related to criteria of interpretation or to sensitivity of techniques [24]. However, in SLVL, the intensity of TRAP staining is usually less strong than that seen in HCL and the percentage of TRAP positive cells are usually lower.

In summary, SLVL appears to be a morphologically heterogeneous group of low-grade B-cell lymphomas, characterized by massive splenomegaly and the presence of circulating villous lymphocytes. Lymphadenopathy is either absent or insignificant unless transformation to high-grade lymphoma occurs. Bone marrow may show nodular or diffuse infiltration. Although leukopenia may occur in SLVL, most cases show mild lymphocytosis without leukopenia, a feature that helps to distinguish it from HCL. As a heterogeneous group, the SLVL cells may vary from small to medium in size, containing scanty to moderate amounts of cytoplasm with characteristic basophilia. The nuclei usually show clumped chromatin, but not as dense as those seen in CLL cells, and small nucleoli are present in one half of the cases as reported in the literature. The cytoplasmic villi are usually thin and short with uneven distribution on the cell surface which is easier to appreciate under electron microscopy. Marker studies are helpful in distinguishing SLVL from PLL and CLL but are less useful in distinguishing SLVL from HCL. However, CD 25 is consistently absent in SLVL, and CD 11c and TRAP are not as frequently demonstrated in SLVL as in HCL. The infiltration pattern in the spleen is also helpful in distinguishing SLVL, HCL, PLL, and CLL. The absence of a characteristic fried-egg pattern and reticulin fibrosis in bone marrow is useful in excluding the diagnosis of HCL. It appears that a definitive diagnosis of SLVL requires a multiparameter approach and more studies are necessary to further subclassify this heterogeneous group into better defined entities.

ACKNOWLEDGMENTS

The authors thank Joan Henshall, Joanne Cuomo, Kathy Maher, Debbie Rapp, Eleanore Boss, and Lisa Moskowitz for technical assistance and Lynn Bartholomew for secretarial help.

REFERENCES

1. Falk S, Stutte HJ: Primary malignant lymphomas of the spleen: A morphologic and immunohitochemical analysis of 17 cases. Cancer 66:2612–2619, 1990.
2. Melo JV, Hegde V, Parreira A, Thompson I, Lampert IA, Catovsky D: Splenic B-cell lymphoma with circulating villous lymphocytes: Differential diagnosis of B-cell leukemia with large spleens. J Clin Pathol 40:642–651, 1987.
3. Melo JV, Robinson DSF, Gregory C, Catovsky D: Splenic B-cell lymphoma with villous lymphocytes in the peripheral blood: A disorder distinct from hairy cell leukemia. Leukemia 1:294–299, 1987.
4. Theml H, Burger A, Keiditsch E, et al: Klinische Beobachtungen zur Charakterisierung des splenomegalen Immunozytoms. Med Klin 72:1019–1032, 1977.
5. Neiman RS, Sullivan AL, Jaffe R: Malignant lymphoma simulating leukemia reticuloendotheliosis: A clinicopathologic study of ten cases. Cancer 43:329–342, 1979.
6. Fohlmeister I, Schaefer HE, Modder B, Hellriegel KP, Fischer R: Chronische lymphoproliferative Erkrankung unter dem Bild einer Haarzell-Leukemie. Blut 42:367–377, 1981.
7. Palutke M, Tabaczka P, Mirchandani I, Goldfard S: Lymphocytic lymphoma simulating hairy cell leukemia: A consideration of reliable and unreliable diagnostic features. Cancer 48:2047–2055, 1981.
8. Spriano P, Barosi G, Invernizzi R, et al.: Splenomegalic immunocytoma with circulating hairy cells: Report of eight cases and revision of the literature. Haematologica 71:25–33, 1986.
9. Vardiman JW, Gilewski TA, Ratain MJ, Bitter MA, Bradlow BA, Golomb HM: Evaluation of Leu M5 (CD 11c) in hairy cell leukemia by the alkaline phosphatase anti-alkaline phosphatase technique. Am J Clin Pathol 90:250–256, 1988.
10. Valensi F, Durand V, Bastenaire B, Flandin G: Splenic B-cell lymphoma with villous lymphocytes (SLVL): A lymphocytic lymphoma simulating hairy cell leukemia. Nouv Rev Fr Hematol 32:409–414, 1990.
11. Kettle P, Morris TCM, Markey GM, et al.: Tartrate resistant acid phosphatase positive splenic lymphoma: A relatively benign condition occurring in a time-space cluster? J Clin Pathol 43:714–718, 1990.
12. Mulligan SP, Matutes E, Dearden C, Catovsky D: Splenic lymphoma with villous lymphocytes: Natural history and response to therapy in 50 cases. Br J Haematol 78:206–209, 1991.
13. Rousselet MC, Gardembas-Pain M, Renier G, Chevailler A, Ifrah N: Splenic lymphoma with circulating villous lymphocytes: Report of a case with immunologic and ultrastructural studies. Am J Clin Pathol 97:147–152, 1992.
14. Ribeiro I, Costa MM, Fernandes BA, et al.: Splenic lymphoma with villous lymphocytes in two sisters. J Clin Pathol 45:1111–1113, 1992.
15. Bates I, Bedu-Ado G, Rutherford T, Bevan DH: Splenic lymphoma with villous lymphocytes in tropical West Africa. Lancet 340:575–577, 1992.
16. Hsu SM, Raien L, Fanger H: Use of avidin-biotin peroxidase complex (ABC) in immunoperoxidase techniques: A comparison between ABC and PAP procedures. J Histochem Cytochem 29:577–580, 1981.
17. Sun T, Li CY, Yam LT: "Atlas of Cytochemistry and Immunochemistry of Hematologic Neoplasms." Chicago: American Society of Clinical Pathlogists Press, 1985, pp 123 and 101.
18. Bennett JM, Catovsky D, Daniel MT, et al.: Proposals for the classifi-

cation of chronic (mature) B and T lymphoid leukemias. J Clin Pathol 42:567–584, 1989.
19. Sobol RE, Mick R, Royston I, et al.: Clinical importance of myeloid antigen expression in adult acute lymphoblastic leukemia. N Engl J Med 316:1111–1117, 1987.
20. Narang S, Wolf BC, Neiman RS: Malignant lymphoma presenting with prominent splenomegaly: A clinicopathologic study with special reference to intermediate cell lymphoma. Cancer 55:1948–1957, 1985.
21. Melo JV, Robinson DSF, Catovsky D: The differential diagnosis between chronic lymphocytic leukemia and other B-cell lymphoproliferative disorders: Morphological and immunological studies. In Polliack A, Catovsky D (ed): "Chronic Lymphocytic Leukemia." Chur, Switzerland; Harwood Academic Publishers, 1988, pp 85–103.
22. Lampert IA, Thompson I: The spleen in chronic lymphocytic leukemia and related disorders. In Polliack A, Catovsky D (ed): "Chronic Lymphocytic Leukemia." Chur, Switzerland; Horwood Academic Press, 1988, pp 193–208.
23. von Krieken JHJM, Feller AC, te Velde J: The distribution of non-Hodgkin's lymphoma in the lymphoid compartments of the human spleen. Am J Surg Pathol 13:757–765, 1989.
24. Yam LT, Phyliky RL, Li CY: Benign and neoplastic disorders simulating hairy cell leukemia. Semin Oncol 11:353–361, 1984.
25. Sun T, Susin M, Shevde N, Teichberg S: Hybrid form of hairy cell leukemia and chronic lymphocytic leukemia. Hematol Oncol 8:283–294, 1990.

American Journal of Hematology 45:51–57 (1994)

Polymorphic Pattern of the $(AT)_X(T)_Y$ Motif at −530 5′ to the β-Globin Gene in Over 40 Patients Homozygous for Various β-Thalassemia Mutations

A.J. Dimovski, A.D. Adekile, V. Divoky, E. Baysal, and T.H.J. Huisman

Department of Biochemistry and Molecular Biology, Medical College of Georgia, Augusta

Nucleotide sequence analysis of the 5′ β-globin gene flanking region has been carried out for numerous homozygous β-thalassemia patients with different mutations and of various ethnic backgrounds. Four different rearrangements were found associated with numerous β-thalassemia mutations. The $(AT)_X(T)_Y$ repeat motif at −530 showed polymorphic patterns among these patients as follows: All ten IVS-II-1 (G→A) chromosomes and the two with the −87 (C→G) mutation are associated with the $(AT)_9(T)_5$ rearrangement, while the 30 IVS-I-6 (T→C), the 16 codon 39 (C→T), the six codon 8 (-AA) chromosomes, and 12 chromosomes with different promoter mutations had the $(AT)_7(T)_7$ motif. Six chromosomes with the promoter mutation at position −29 (A→G) had the $(AT)_8(T)_6$ motif, while an $(AT)_8(T)_4$ motif appears characteristic for two IVS-I-5 (G→A and G→T). No direct association between any of the $(AT)_X(T)_Y$ arrangements and an increased γ gene expression [$^G\gamma$ and fetal hemoglobin (Hb F)] levels could be demonstrated, suggesting that variations in the $(AT)_X(T)_Y$ motif are common polymorphisms.

Key words: polymorphic pattern, $(AT)_X(T)_Y$ motif, β-globin gene, β-thal mutations, fetal hemoglobin

INTRODUCTION

There have been several suggestions that the negative regulatory sequences, especially those between nucleotides (nts) −610 and −490 in the 5′ β-globin gene flanking region modulate Hb F expression and clinical severity among β-thalassemia (β-thal) and sickle cell anemia (SS) patients [1–4]. This region spans the binding site for the BP1 nuclear protein which is believed to be a negative regulatory trans-acting factor [5,6].

Of particular interest is the tandem repeat motif, $(AT)_X(T)_Y$, which has a definite haplotype-linked polymorphic pattern among β^S chromosomes [3]. It has been postulated that the $(AT)_9(T)_5$ motif is associated with a stronger binding of the BP1 protein than is seen with the more common $(AT)_7(T)_7$ motif. The former is found in the β^S Indian haplotype [3] and has also been described in several individuals with "silent β-thal" [1,2]. Ragusa et al. [4] have suggested that in patients with β°-thal this motif interacts with the C→T mutation at −158 $^G\gamma$ to generate high levels of Hb F. On the other hand, Wong et al. [7] and more recently Galanello et al. [8], proposed that the $(AT)_9(T)_5$ motif is a common polymorphism found even in normal individuals and is not necessarily associated with silent β-thal.

We have sequenced the β-globin gene 5′ flanking region in several patients with different β-thal mutations and of different ethnic backgrounds. Several aspects of the hematology and DNA sequence variations in many of these patients have been previously reported from our laboratory [9–12]. In the present study an attempt was made to correlate γ gene expression ($^G\gamma$ and Hb F levels) with the $(AT)_X(T)_Y$ motif.

MATERIALS AND METHODS

β-Thal Homozygotes

Fifteen β^+ IVS-I-6 (T→C), one β^+ IVS-I-6 compound heterozygote for the G→T and G→A substitu-

Received for publication January 22, 1993; accepted June 30, 1993.

Address reprint requests to Dr. Titus H.J. Huisman, Department of Biochemistry and Molecular Biology, Medical College of Georgia, Augusta, GA 30912–2100.

TABLE I. Summary of Hematological and Genetic Data for β-Thal Homozygotes

Mutation (Haplotype)[a]	Patient (country)[b]	Sex-age	Hb g/dl	Hb F %	Hb F g/dl	Hb A_2 %	$^G\gamma$ %	$^A\gamma^T$ %	Xmn I $-158^G\gamma$	Number of α genes	$(AT)_X(T)_Y$ X/Y	X/Y
IVS-I-6 (VI/VI)	MS (P)	F-23	7.7	23.2	1.8	4.2	60.1	39.9	−/−	4	7/7	7/7
	MH (P)	F-31	8.5	3.0	0.3	7.3	55.1	44.9	−/−	n.d.	7/7	7/7
	R-94 (M)	F-32	11.3	6.3	0.7	5.4	47.4	52.6	−/−	4	7/7	7/7
	R-95 (M)	M-30	10.9	8.4	0.9	6.6	61.0	39.0	−/−	4	7/7	7/7
	P-5 (M)	M-28	10.2	8.5	0.9	3.0	52.0	48.0	−/−	4	7/7	7/7
	4013 (T)	M-13	6.8	8.0	0.5	5.2	56.9	43.1	−/−	4	7/7	7/7
	4019 (T)	M-10	5.4	7.0	0.4	6.8	54.8	45.2	−/−	4	7/7	7/7
	4025 (T)	M-16	6.2	7.0	0.4	6.0	54.8	45.2	−/−	4	7/7	7/7
	4026 (T)	F-10	7.0	10.4	0.7	4.0	56.6	43.4	−/−	4	7/7	7/7
IVS-I-6 (VII/VII)	P-01 (M)	F-38	9.1	15.0	1.4	6.6	45.0	0	−/−	4	7/7	7/7
	P-01B (M)		9.6	35.0	3.4	4.7	52.0	0	−/−	4	7/7	7/7
	O.F. (T)	M-10	—	7.9	—	5.0	51.6	0	−/−	4	7/7	7/7
IVS-I-6 (n.d.)	P.S. (P)	F-37	8.4	23.1	1.9	4.6	74.5	0	+/+	4	7/7	7/7
IVS-I-6 (n.d.)	5412 (H)	-16	6.9	28.4	1.9	4.7	n.d.	n.d.	−/−	4	7/7	7/7
	5413 (H)	-15	9.2	17.9	1.6	5.4	n.d.	n.d.	−/−	4	7/7	7/7
IVS-I-5 (n.d.)	C.M. (T)	M-17	4.7	98.7	4.6	1.3	72.1	0	+/+	4	8/4	8/4
IVS-II-1 (III/III)	A.E. (T)	Adult	12.2	97.7	11.9	2.3	74.3	0	+/+	3	9/5	9/5
	E.O. (T)	Adult	6.2	98.6	6.1	2.3	72.2	0	+/+	4	9/5	9/5
	K. (T)	Adult	8.3	98.9	8.2	1.1	67.2	0	+/+	4	9/5	9/5
	M.K. (T)	Adult	4.3	97.4	4.2	2.6	70.0	0	+/+	4	9/5	9/5
	B.D. (T)	Adult	8.7	98.6	8.6	1.4	71.2	0	+/+	4	9/5	9/5
CD 39 (n.d.)	551 (S)	Adult	7.4		Transfused		61.6	38.4	n.d.	n.d.	7/7	7/7
	552 (S)	Adult	9.1		Transfused		58.2	18.2	n.d.	n.d.	7/7	7/7
	573 (S)	Adult	8.3		Transfused		49.8	15.8	n.d.	n.d.	7/7	7/7
	583 (S)	Adult	7.3		Transfused		n.d.	n.d.	n.d.	n.d.	7/7	7/7
	586 (S)	Adult	9.8		Transfused		66.1	0	n.d.	n.d.	7/7	7/7
	624 (S)	Adult	9.0		Transfused		n.d.	n.d.	n.d.	n.d.	7/7	7/7
	631 (S)	Adult	9.6		Transfused		70.4	26.8	n.d.	n.d.	7/7	7/7
	II-2 (S)	Adult	10.5	97.9	10.3	2.9	71.2	0	+/−	n.d.	7/7	7/7
CD 8 (IV/IV)	D.C. (T)	F-7	8.0	98.6	7.9	1.4	72.4	0	+/+	4	7/7	7/7
	K.D. (T)	F-16	10.2	98.4	10.0	1.6	73.6	0	+/+	4	7/7	7/7
	E.G. (T)[c]	F-7	11.6	36.1	4.2	1.8	72.5	0	+/+	4	7/7	7/7
-28 (n.d.)	H.B. (T)	Adult	6.3	37.4	2.4	7.2	23.8	0	−/−	4	7/7	7/7
-29 (A/A)	J.M. (A)	F-44	10.6	68.0	7.2	3.6	70.0	0	+/+	3	8/6	8/6
(A/B)	J.S. (A)	M-23	9.1	40.0	3.6	9.9	60.3	0	+/−	4	8/6	8/6
(A/B)	Jo.S. (A)	F-27	11.4	67.1	7.6	4.1	73.5	0	+/−	3	7/7	7/7
(A/$^A\gamma^T$)	L.G. (A)	F-26	9.1	43.8	4.0	8.6	66.9	0	+/−	4	8/6	8/6
-30 (n.d.)	S.S. (T)	Adult	7.0	68.0	4.8	3.2	44.8	0	−/−	4	7/7	7/7
-87 (VIII/VIII)	A.3 (T)	F-52	9.9	31.2	3.1	7.7	77.3	0	+/+	4	9/5	9/5
-88 (A1/A1)	H.G. (A)	M-80	9.4	65.2	6.1	7.1	69.3	0	+/+	4	7/7	7/7
(A1/A1)	C.W. (A)	F-24	10.7	71.7	7.7	5.9	72.0	0	+/+	4	7/7	7/7
(Y/Y)	T.M.F. (A)	M-23	11.0	56.6	6.2	5.9	34.2	0	−/−	4	7/7	7/7

[a]Haplotypes III, IV, VI, VII, and VIII according to Orkin et al. [21]; haplotypes A, A1, B, $^A\gamma^T$, and Y according to Gonzalez-Redondo et al. [9].
[b]P, Portugal; M, (Republic of) Macedonia; T, Turkey; H, Hungary; A, America; S, Sicily; n.d., not determined.
[c]Patient E.G. was transfused shortly before blood collection.

tions, five β° IVS-II-1 (G→A), eight β° codon (CD) 39 (C→T), and three β° CD 8 (-AA) patients were studied. All patients had a mild phenotype, except seven of the eight CD 39 patients who were transfusion dependent. Their countries of origin were Turkey, Macedonia, Italy, Hungary, and Portugal (Table I). Also included were three Turkish patients with a homozygosity for promoter mutations characteristic of the Mediterranean region [one each of −28 (A→C), −30 (T→A), and −87 (C→G)], and seven American Black patients with promoter mutations [four −29 (A→G) and three −88 (C→T)]. None of these ten patients was transfusion dependent.

Family Studies

Data on two illustrative families with members having a homozygosity or heterozygosity for the −88 (C→T) mutation, but with different $(AT)_X(T)_Y$ motifs and varying levels of $^G\gamma$ and Hb F, are included.

Normal Individuals

Data on the $(AT)_X(T)_Y$ motif in some Czechoslovakian individuals with normal hematology and no clinical problems are presented. Complete sequencing of the β-globin gene and gene mapping of the whole β cluster was carried

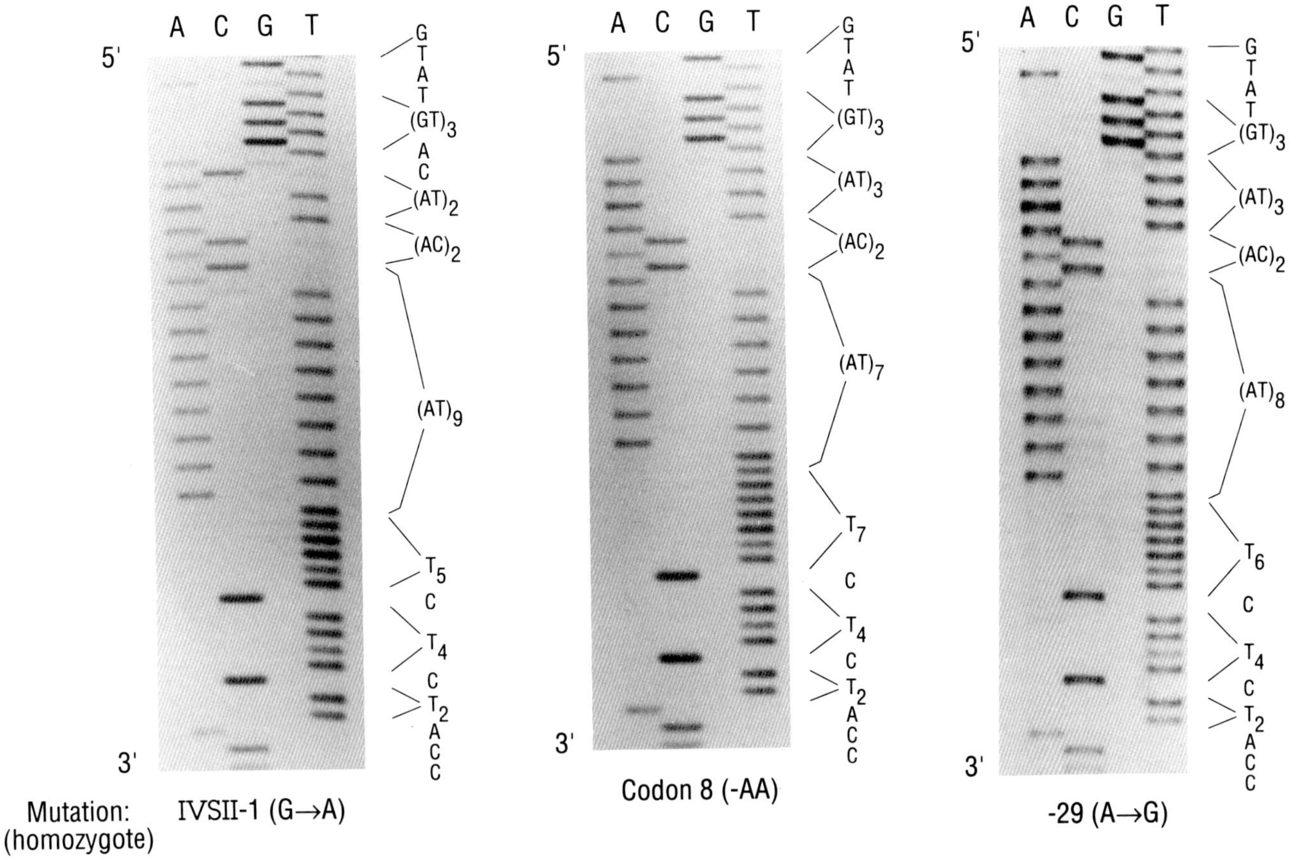

Fig. 1. Parts of sequencing gels showing the $(AT)_X(T)_Y$ motifs in three homozygous β-thal patients.

out in all these individuals and there were no detectable variations.

Blood samples were collected in vacutainers with EDTA as anticoagulant in the various centers and shipped to Augusta, GA. In some cases, DNA was isolated in the local centers before shipping. Transportation was by fast overnight air mail or by courier service.

Hematological data were obtained with automated cell counters. The Hb F and Hb A were quantified by cation exchange high-preformance liquid chromatography (HPLC) [13,14]. The relative quantities of the $^G\gamma$ and $^A\gamma$ chains were determined by reversed phase HPLC [15,16]; when necessary, Hb F was isolated from the blood samples by DEAE-cellulose chromatography [17] prior to the reversed phase HPLC analysis.

DNA was isolated by the method of Poncz et al. [18]. Sequencing analysis of PCR-amplified DNA was with the dideoxy method of Sanger et al. [19]. The amplification and sequencing primers used for the 5′ flanking region of the β-globin gene are as shown below:

Amplification primers:
5′-TCCCCAGTTAACCTCCTATT-3′
(forward), positions −823 to −804;
5′-TCTCCTTAAACCTGTCTTG-3′
(reverse), positions +178 to +159.
Sequencing primers:
5′-TAAGAGGTCTCTAGTTTTTTATCTC-3′,
positions −724 to −700;
5′-AGAATGGATGAAAACTCTACCTC-3′,
positions −446 to −468;
5′-AGAGATCCATCTACATATCC-3′,
positions −418 to −400.

Figure 1 presents the motifs obtained from three sequence analyses.

All patients were screened for the most common α-thal-2 determinants (the −3.7 kb and −4.2 kb deletions) with a PCR-based methodology, using specific oligonucleotides adjacent to the 5′ and 3′ breakpoints of each deletion. Details of this procedures are being reported separately [20].

RESULTS

Homozygous β-Thal Patients

$^G\gamma$ and Hb F levels. Among the IVS-I-6 (T→C) patients, nine were homozygous for haplotype VI and were

TABLE II. DNA Sequences From -555 to -517 of the β-Globin Gene Promoter Among β-Thal Homozygotes

Mutation Reference	Haplotype	Number of chromosomes	-551 ↓ -543 ↓ -530 ↓ -525 ↓ -521 ↓ TGTA T ATATACA C ATATATATATATAT----TTTTTTT C TTTT	$(AT)_X(T)_Y$ 7/7
IVS-I-6	VI	18	TGTA T ATATACA C ATATATATATATAT----TTTTTTT C TTTT	7/7
IVS-I-6	VII	6	TGTA T ATATACA C ATATATATATATAT----TTTTTTT C TTTT	7/7
IVS-I-6	n.d.	6	TGTA T ATATACA C ATATATATATATAT----TTTTTTT C TTTT	7/7
CD 39	n.d.	16	TGTA T ATATACA C ATATATATATATAT----TTTTTTT C TTTT	7/7
CD 8	IV	6	TGTA T ATATACA C ATATATATATATAT----TTTTTTT C TTTT	7/7
-28	n.d.	2	TGTA T ATATACA C ATATATATATATAT----TTTTTTT C TTTT	7/7
-29	B	2	TGTA T ATATACA C ATATATATATATAT----TTTTTTT C TTTT	7/7
-30	n.d.	2	TGTA T ATATACA C ATATATATATATAT----TTTTTTT C TTTT	7/7
-88	A1	4	TGTA T ATATACA T ATATATATATATAT----TTTTTTT C TTTT	7/7
-88	Y	2	TGTA T ATATACA T ATATATATATATAT----TTTTTTT C TTTT	7/7
IVS-I-5	n.d.	2	TGTA T ATATACA T ATATATATATATATAT-----TTTT T TTTT	8/4
-29	A	5	TGTA T ATATACA C ATATATATATATATAT---TTTTTT C TTTT	8/6
-29	$^{A}\gamma^{T}$	1	TGTA T ATATACA C ATATATATATATATAT---TTTTTT C TTTT	8/6
IVS-II-1	III	10	TGTA C ATATACA C ATATATATATATATATAT--TTTTT C TTTT	9/5
-87	VIII	2	TGTA C ATATACA C ATATATATATATATATAT--TTTTT C TTTT	9/5

$^{A}\gamma^{T}$ positive, three were homozygous for haplotype VII, while the haplotype was not determined in the two Hungarian and one Portuguese patients. The restriction sites used are listed in Refs. 9 and 21. The Hb F levels in these 15 patients were between 3 and 35%, and the $^{G}\gamma$ values between 45 and 74.5%. All but one were negative for the Xmn I site. The IVS-I-5 (G→T; G→A) patient had a Hb F level of 98.7% and $^{G}\gamma$ of 72.1%, and was Xmn I positive (+/+). The five IVS-II-1 (G→A) patients also had high Hb F and $^{G}\gamma$ levels and all were Xmn I positive (+/+). Hb F levels were not obtained for the seven transfusion-dependent CD 39 patients, while the one subject with a milder clinical course had high Hb F and $^{G}\gamma$ values and was an Xmn I heterozygote. Two of the three CD 8 (−AA) patients had Hb F levels of 98.6 and 98.4%, respectively, while the third had been recently transfused because of an on-going bacterial infection. The $^{G}\gamma$ values in these three patients ranged from 72.4 to 73.6%, and all were Xmn I homozygotes. The nine patients with a homozygous β°-thal and a Hb F level in excess of 97% had total Hb F values varying between 4.2 and 11.9 g/dl (average 8.0 g/dl; individual values are listed in Table I). This greatly increased synthesis of Hb F was sufficient to make these patients transfusion independent.

One of the four patients with the −29 (A→G) promoter mutation was homozygous for haplotype A (Xmn I; +/+), while the other three were heterozygotes (one with A/$^{A}\gamma^{T}$ and two with A/B). The Xmn I homozygote had a $^{G}\gamma$ level of 70% and Hb F of 68%; these values varied in the heterozygotes from 58.4 to 66.9% ($^{G}\gamma$) and from 40 to 49% (Hb F). Two of the three −88 (C→T) patients were homozygous for haplotype A_1 (Xmn I positive) and their $^{G}\gamma$ values were 69.3 and 72%, while the Hb F levels were 65.2 and 71.7%, respectively. The third patient was homozygous for haplotype Y (Xmn I negative) and had a $^{G}\gamma$ of 34.2% and Hb F of 56.6%. The haplotypes were not determined in the two patients with either the −28 (A→C) or the −30 (T→A) promoter mutations. Both were Xmn I −/− and had low $^{G}\gamma$ values. The patient with the −87 (C→G) promoter mutation was homozygous for haplotype VIII and was Xmn I +/+ with a $^{G}\gamma$ level of 77.3% but with a Hb F level of only 31.2%.

The $(AT)_X(T)_Y$ Motifs 5′ β-Globin Gene (−542 to −522). The $(AT)_7(T)_7$ arrangement was found for the following chromosomes carrying different mutations as indicated: 30 with IVS-I-6 (T→C), irrespective of their haplotypes; 16 with CD 39 (C→T); six with CD 8 (−AA); two with −28 (A→C); two with −29 (A→G); two with −30 (T→A), and six with −88 (C→T) (Table II). The chromosome with the −88 (C→T) mutation also had a C→T substitution at position −543 as described for the β^S haplotype #19 [3]. The two chromosomes carrying the IVS-I-5 mutation (either G→T or G→A) had the $(AT)_8(T)_4$ rearrangement with a C→T substitution at position −543. The six chromosomes carrying the −29 (A→G) mutation had the rare $(AT)_8$ $(T)_6$ arrangement. The $(AT)_9(T)_5$ motif was found only for the ten chromosomes with the IVS-II-1 (G→A) and for the two with the −87 (C→G) mutations. In all chromosomes studied only those with the $(AT)_9(T)_5$ motif showed the T→C mutation at position −551.

Sequences Between −302 to −294 and −275 to −263 5′ β-Globin Gene. The other potential BP1 binding site between −302 and −294 and the BP2 binding site between −275 to −263 did not reveal any differences from the reference sequence in all the patients studied (data not shown).

α-Globin Gene Status. Only three individuals were found to have an α-thal-2 trait (−3.7 kb) and the −4.2 kb deletion was absent.

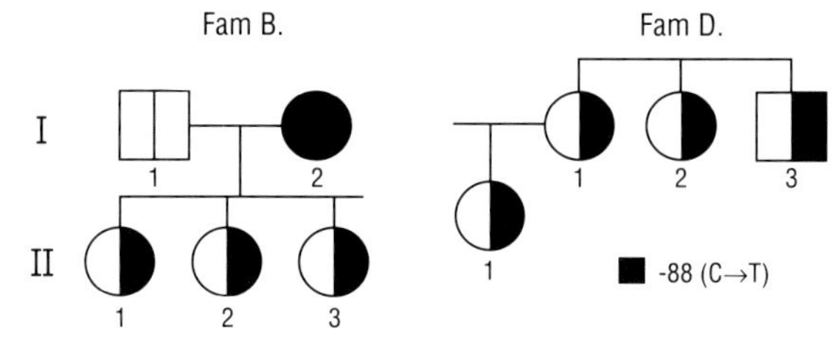

	Subject	Sex/Age	Hb (g/dl)	Hb F (%)	$^G\gamma$ (%)	Xmn I site	$(AT)_X(T)_Y$	Rsa I site
Fam B	I-1	M-48	–	–	–	+/-	9.5/7.7	+/-
	I-2	F-40	15.0	79.0	58.2	-/-	8.4/8.4	-/-
	II-1	F-20	12.7	3.0	24.9	-/-	8.4/9.5	-/-
	II-2	F-18	12.6	12.5	44.0	+/-	8.4/7.7	+/-
	II-3	F-15	13.7	12.9	39.8	+/-	8.4/7.7	+/-
Fam D	I-1	F-37	10.9	10.7	45.1	+/-	8.4/9.5	+/-
	I-2	F-25	10.2	5.2	27.7	-/-	8.4/7.7	-/-
	I-3	M-33	14.0	2.6	22.7	-/-	8.4/7.7	-/-
	II-1	F-11	10.7	9.4	39.1	-/-	8.4/7.7	+/-

Fig. 2. Pedigrees, hematology, and sequence variations for two families with the −88 (C→T) β-thal mutation.

Family Studies (Fig. 2)

Details of the hematology and sequence variations in the $^G\gamma$ and $^A\gamma$ promoters and in the locus control region (LCR) 5′ hypersensitive site-2 (HS-2) sequence of Family B have been previously reported [22]. The proband (I-2), a 40-year-old woman from Cote d'Ivoire, is homozygous for the β^+ −88 (C→T) mutation. She has had a mild clinical course, moderate microcytosis, and hypochromia, and has maintained a Hb level of 12–15 g/dl. Her Hb F level has been about 80% with a $^G\gamma$ to $^A\gamma$ ratio of 58:42. Her husband is a hematologically normal Swiss citizen. Their daughters inherited the β-thal trait with mild microcytosis, hypochromia, and elevated Hb F levels; the oldest child (II-1) had 3% Hb F with a low $^G\gamma$ value of 24.9%, and the other two children had 12.5 and 12.9% Hb F, with significantly higher $^G\gamma$ values of 44 and 39.8%, respectively. The β-globin promoter sequence analysis showed that I-2 is homozygous for the $(AT)_8(T)_4$ arrangement with a C→T mutation at −543; she is also Xmn I negative (−/−). The husband is heterozygous for the $(AT)_7(T)_7$ and the $(AT)_9(T)_5$ patterns and is heterozygous for the Xmn I site (+/−). Two children (II-2 and II-3) with the higher Hb F levels (12–13%) are heterozygous for $(AT)_8(T)_4$ and $(AT)_7(T)_7$ and are Xmn I +/−, while the other daughter (II-1) is heterozygous for $(AT)_8(T)_4$ and $(AT)_9(T)_5$, is negative for the Xmn I site, and has the lowest Hb F (3%) and $^G\gamma$ (24.5%) values among the three children.

The proband (I-1) of the second family (Family D) is a 37-year-old American Black woman being investigated because of an elevated Hb F level of 10–11%. DNA sequence studies showed that she has the −88 (C→T) mutation. Her two siblings and her daughter also inherited this β-thal trait, while her husband was not available for study. The total Hb level among these individuals ranged from 10.2 to 14 g/dl, that of Hb F from 2.6 to 10.7%, and that of $^G\gamma$ from 22.7 to 45.1%. All members of the family were Xmn I −/−, except I-1 who is +/−. All but I-1 had the $(AT)_8(T)_4/(AT)_7(T)_7$ motifs; I-1 had the $(AT)_8(T)_4/(AT)_9(T)_5$), and she had the highest $^G\gamma$ and Hb F levels.

Normal Individuals

The −530 $(AT)_X(T)_Y$ motif analysis showed that one individual was a homozygote for $(AT)_9(T)_5$ and had a C at −551; three were heterozygous for $(AT)_9(T)_5$ and $(AT)_7(T)_7$, while the remaining two were homozygous for $(AT)_7(T)_7$. One chromosome with $(AT)_7(T)_7$ had a C at −551 (Rsa I positive).

DISCUSSION

Considerable effort has been made to identify the genetic determinants of γ chain expression among patients with SS and β-thal because higher levels of Hb F ameliorate the clinical course of these diseases. The putative *cis*-acting determinants include the −158 (C→T) mutation in the $^G\gamma$ promoter [23–25], the LCR 5′HS-2 [22,26], and the negative regulatory elements in the β-globin gene promoter which suppress β chain synthesis [3–6]. While an X-linked factor has been identified [27,28], and it is also recognized that the co-existence of α-thal is associated with decreased Hb F levels [29], it is generally agreed that there are other, as yet, unidentified trans-acting factors. Of all these determinants, the −158 (C→T) mutation ($^G\gamma$), which creates a restriction site for Xmn I, appears to be the most consistently associated with increased γ gene expression (especially $^G\gamma$) in normal, SS, and β-thal individuals, and other states of erythropoietic stress.

Negative regulatory elements in the β-globin gene promoter that bind the BP1 protein have attracted considerable attention. The $(AT)_9(T)_5$ motif, in particular, has been studied with varying implications. While it has been associated with silent β-thal, and with mild phenotype and higher levels of Hb F in some homozygous β-thal patients [1–4], others have not found this association [8,29,30]. It is interesting to note that a definite haplotype-linked polymorphism of this motif exists among SS patients [3]. Only the Indian haplotype is associated with the $(AT)_9(T)_5$ rearrangement, while the Senegal haplotype, which like the Indian haplotype is Xmn I positive, has the $(AT)_8(T)_4$ motif. The Benin haplotype, which is Xmn I negative, also has the $(AT)_8(T)_4$ arrangement.

The present study of homozygous β-thal patients with mutations in the intron and coding regions shows that the $(AT)_X(T)_Y$ motif appears to have a specific polymorphic pattern. Thus, chromosomes with the IVS-I-6 (T→C), CD 39 (C→T), and CD 8 (−AA) mutations are associated with the $(AT)_7(T)_7$ motif, the IVS-I-5 (G→T and G→A) mutations with the $(AT)_8(T)_4$ pattern, while the IVS-II-1 (G→A) mutation is on a chromosome with the $(AT)_9(T)_5$ arrangement. A search of the literature [2,4] shows that at least five other IVS-II-1 chromosomes (haplotype III) have been previously studied and all had the $(AT)_9(T)_5$ motif. Promoter mutations, on the other hand, appear to be associated with various patterns. Of the eight −29 (A→G) chromosomes analyzed in this study, two with haplotype B had the $(AT)_7(T)_7$ motif, while the remaining six (haplotypes A and $^A\gamma^T$) had the $(AT)_8(T)_6$ arrangement. The −30 (T→A), −28 (A→C), and −88 (C→T) chromosomes all had $(AT)_7(T)_7$, while the −87 (C→G) mutation was associated with $(AT)_9(T)_5$. Of all these promoter mutations, only the −88 (C→T) chromosomes were associated with a C→T substitution at position −543 (Table II).

Our data also demonstrate a strong linkage between the $(AT)_X(T)_Y$ motif and the C→T mutation at −158 $^G\gamma$ (Xmn I site). All the $(AT)_9(T)_5$ chromosomes among the homozygous β-thal patients studied were Xmn I positive, while all $(AT)_7(T)_7$ chromosomes were negative except for one Portuguese IVS-I-6 patient (P.S.), the three CD 8 (−AA) patients, and several chromosomes among the Black patients with the −88 (C→T) or the −29 (A→G) mutation.

Similarly, the −551 (T→C) substitution in the β promoter exhibited a strong linkage with the $(AT)_X(T)_Y$ motif; a T at −551 was present in all chromosomes that had the $(AT)_7(T)_7$ rearrangement, while a C was found at that position in the chromosomes with the $(AT)_9(T)_5$ motif. However, in Family D, patient I-1 had one chromosome with the $(AT)_7(T)_7$ arrangement with a C at −551. The same was observed in one chromosome from a hematologically normal Czechoslovakian.

The fact that all homozygous β-thal patients with the $(AT)_9(T)_5$ motif were also Xmn I positive makes it difficult to assess the relative contributions of these two variations to any elevated γ chain expression that was observed. However, the IVS-II-1 and the CD 8 patients offer a unique opportunity for comparison. Both groups are Xmn I positive (+/+) but the former have the $(AT)_9(T)_5$ motif, while the latter is associated with the $(AT)_7(T)_7$ arrangement. The $^G\gamma$ levels in both groups are similar with an average of 71 and 72.8%, respectively. The same is true for the Hb F values, excluding the transfused CD 8 patient. Moreover, the three patients with other mutations who were homozygous for the $(AT)_7(T)_7$ motif and for the Xmn I site (P.S. with IVS-I-6, H.G. and C.W., both with the −88 promoter mutation) had high $^G\gamma$ and Hb F levels (Table I). These comparisons indeed suggest that the Xmn I site is the more important contributory factor.

The two families presented in Figure 2 also illustrate the relative contributions of the $(AT)_X(T)_Y$ motif and the Xmn I site to an enhanced γ gene expression. In Family B, for instance, subject II-1 is Xmn I negative and has the lowest values of Hb F and $^G\gamma$ among the three children (Hb F 3%; $^G\gamma$ 24.9%) but is heterozygous for the $(AT)_9(T)_5$ motif. Furthermore, subject I-1 of Family D, whose chromosomes had similar $(AT)_X(T)_Y$ motifs as seen in II-1 of Family B, but is an Xmn I heterozygote (+/−), has a considerably higher γ gene expression (Hb F 10.7%; $^G\gamma$ 45.1%). These data would indicate that the $(AT)_9(T)_5$ motif by itself probably has no influence on γ gene expression. Our finding of the $(AT)_9(T)_5$ motif in normal individuals from Czechoslovakia, without an elevation in Hb F synthesis, also supports the view that it is not a rare polymorphism.

In conclusion, therefore, while the $(AT)_X(T)_Y$ motif might indeed have a negative regulatory role on β-globin gene expression, as shown by in vitro binding studies [6], we have found no evidence that it plays an important regulatory role in γ gene expression among the β-thal patients in this study. The Xmn I site at −158 5′ to the β-globin gene shows a more positive association with γ gene expression, but its presence does not account for all the variations in $^G\gamma$ and Hb F levels observed.

ACKNOWLEDGMENTS

The authors are indebted to Dr. Ç. Altay and Dr. A. Gürgey (Turkey), Dr. G.D. Efremov (Republic of Macedonia), Dr. G.P. Tamagnini and Dr. M.L.S. Ribeiro (Portugal), Dr. G. Schiliro and Dr. B. Masala (Italy), and Dr. Ph. Beris (Switzerland) for allowing us to study their patients. Mr. E.L.D. Walker, III assisted in the collection of blood samples from several patients. This study was supported by the United States Public Health Service research grant HLB-41544.

REFERENCES

1. Semenza GL, Delgrosso K, Poncz M, Malladi P, Schwartz E, Surrey S: The silent carrier allele: β Thalassemia without a mutation in the β-globin gene or its immediate flanking region. Cell 39:123, 1984.
2. Murru S, Loudianos G, Cao A, Vaccargiu S, Pirastu M, Sciarratta GV, Agosti S, Parodi MI: A β-thalassemia carrier with normal sequence within the β globin gene. Blood 76:2164, 1990.
3. Elion J, Berg P, Lapoumeroulie C, Trabuchet G, Mittelman K, Krishnamoorthy R, Schechter AN, Labie D: DNA sequence variation in a negative control region 5′ to the β-globin gene correlates with the phenotypic expression of the β^S mutation. Blood 79:787, 1992.
4. Ragusa A, Lombardo M, Beldjord C, Ruberto C, Lombardo T, Elion J, Nagel RL, Krishnamoorthy R: Genetic epidemiology of β-thalassemia in Sicily: Do sequences 5′ to the $^G\gamma$ gene and 5′ to the β gene interact to enhance Hb F expression in β-thalassemia? Am J Hematol 40:199, 1992.

5. Berg PE, Mittleman M, Elion J, Labie D, Schechter AN: Increased protein binding to a −530 mutation in the human β globin gene associated with decreased β-globin synthesis. Am J Hematol 36:42, 1991.
6. Berg PE, William DM, Qian R-L, Cohen RB, Cao S-X, Mittelman M, Schechter AN: A common protein binds to two silencers 5′ to the human β gene. Nucleic Acids Res 17:8833, 1989.
7. Wong SC, Stoming TA, Efremov GD, Huisman THJ: High frequencies of a rearrangement (+ATA; −T) at −530 to the β-globin gene in different populations indicate the absence of a correlation with a silent β-thalassemia determinant. Hemoglobin 13:1, 1989.
8. Galanello R, Meloni A, Gasperini D, Saba L, Cao A, Rosatelli MC, Perseu L: The repeated sequence $(AT)_X(T)_Y$ upstream to the β-globin gene is a simple polymorphism. Blood 81:1974, 1993.
9. Gonzalez-Redondo JM, Stoming TA, Lanclos KD, Gu Y-C, Kutlar A, Kutlar F, Nakatsuji T, Deng B, Han IS, McKie VC, Huisman THJ: Clinical and genetic heterogeneity in Black patients with homozygous β-thalassemia from the Southeastern United States. Blood 72:1007, 1988.
10. Diaz-Chico JC, Yang KG, Stoming TA, Efremov DG, Kutlar A, Kutlar F, Aksoy M, Altay C, Gürgey A, Kilinc Y, Huisman THJ: Mild and severe β-thalassemia among homozygotes from Turkey: Identification of the types by hybridization of amplified DNA with synthetic probes. Blood 71:248, 1988.
11. Dimovski AJ, Efremov DG, Jankovic L, Juricic D, Zisovski N, Stojanovski N, Nikolov N, Petkov GT, Reese AL, Stoming TA, Efremov GD, Huisman THJ: β-Thalassemia in Yugoslavia. Hemoglobin 14:15, 1990.
12. Tamagnini GP, Goncalves P, Ribeiro MLS, Kaeda J, Kutlar F, Baysal E, Huisman THJ: β-Thalassemia mutations in the Portuguese; high frequencies of two alleles in restricted populations. Hemoglobin 17:31, 1993.
13. Bissé E, Wieland H: High-performance liquid chromatographic separation of human haemoglobins: Simultaneous quantitation of foetal and glycated haemoglobins. J Chromatogr 434:95, 1988.
14. Kutlar A, Kutlar F, Gu L-G, Mayson SM, Huisman THJ: Fetal hemoglobin in normal adults and β-thalassemia heterozygotes. Hum Genet 85:106, 1990.
15. Shelton JB, Shelton JR, Schroeder WA: High performance liquid chromatographic separation of globin chains on a large-pore C_4 column. J Liq Chromatogr 7:1969, 1984.
16. Kutlar F, Kutlar A, Huisman THJ: Separation of normal and abnormal hemoglobin chains by reversed-phase high-performance liquid chromatography. J Chromatogr 357:147, 1986.
17. Schroeder WA, Huisman THJ: "The Chromatography of Hemoglobin." Clinical and Biochemical Analysis, Vol. 9. New York: Marcel Dekker, Inc., 1980.
18. Poncz M, Solowiejczyk D, Harpel B, Mory Y, Schwartz E, Surrey S: Construction of human gene libraries from small amounts of peripheral blood: Analysis of β-like globin genes. Hemoglobin 6:27, 1982.
19. Sanger F, Nicklen S, Coulson AR: DNA sequencing with chain terminating inhibitors. Proc Natl Acad Sci USA 74:5463, 1977.
20. Baysal E, Huisman THJ: PCR-Based methodology for the detection of common α-thal-2 determinants. Abstract, 5th International Conference on Thalassaemias and the Haemoglobinopathies, Cyprus, April, 1993.
21. Orkin SH, Kazazian HH Jr, Antonarakis SE, Goff SC, Boehm CD, Sexton JP, Waber PG, Giardina PJV: Linkage of β-thalassaemia mutations and β-globin gene polymorphisms with DNA polymorphisms in human β-globin gene cluster. Nature 296:627, 1982.
22. Beris Ph, Kitundu MN, Baysal E, Öner C, Lanclos KD, Dimovski AJ, Kutlar F, Huisman THJ: Black β-thalassemia homozygotes with specific sequence variations in the 5′ hypersensitive site 2 of the locus control region have high levels of fetal hemoglobin. Am J Hematol 41:97, 1992.
23. Adekile AD, Huisman THJ: Hb F in sickle cell anemia. Experientia 49:16, 1993.
24. Gilman JG, Huisman THJ: Two independent genetic factors in the β-globin gene cluster are associated with high $^G\gamma$ levels in the Hb F of β-thalassemia patients. Blood 64:452, 1984.
25. Labie D, Dunda-Belkhodja O, Rouabhi F, Pagnier J, Ragusa A, Nagel RL: The −158 site 5′ to the $^G\gamma$ gene and $^G\gamma$ expression. Blood 66: 1463, 1985.
26. Öner C, Dimovski AJ, Altay C, Gürgey A, Gu Y-C, Huisman THJ, Lanclos KD: Sequence variations in the 5′ hypersensitive site-2 of the locus control region of the β^S chromosomes are associated with different levels of fetal hemoglobin in Hemoglobin S homozygotes. Blood 79:813, 1992.
27. Miyoshi K, Kaneto Y, Kawai H, Ohchi H, Niki S, Hasegawa K, Shirakami A, Yamo T: X-linked dominant control of F-cells in normal adult life: Characterization of the Swiss type of hereditary persistence of fetal hemoglobin regulated dominantly by gene(s) on the X chromosome. Blood 72:1854, 1988.
28. Dover GJ, Smith KD, Chang YC, Purvis S, Mays A, Meyers DA, Sheils C, Serjeant GR: Fetal hemoglobin levels in sickle cell disease and normal individuals are partially controlled by an X-linked gene located at Xp22.2. Blood 80:816, 1992.
29. Galanello R, Gasperini D, Perseu L, Melis MA, Maccioni L: Heterozygous β-thalassemia with thalassemia intermedia phenotype. Abstract, 8th Conference on Hemoglobin Switching, 1992.
30. Dover GJ, Chang UT, Boyer SH, Serjeant GR, Antonarakis S, Higgs DR: The cellular basis for fetal hemoglobin levels among sickle cell individuals with two, three and four α-globin genes. Blood 69:341, 1987.

American Journal of Hematology 45:58–62 (1994)

Cytokine Profile During High-Dose rhG-CSF Therapy in Severe Congenital Neutropenia

Toshiji Shitara, Shin-ichiroh Yugami, Hiroko Ijima, Manabu Sotomatu, and Takayoshi Kuroume

Department of Pediatrics, Gunma University School of Medicine 3-39-15, Showa-machi, Maebashi City, Gunma, Japan

The effect of recombinant human granulocyte colony-stimulating factor (rhG-CSF) on cytokine profile was evaluated in a case of severe congenital neutropenia. The plasma levels of cytokines were measured before and during rhG-CSF therapy. These included G-CSF, granulocyte-macrophage colony-stimulating factor (GM-CSF), interleukin-1α, interleukin-1 β, interleukin-2 (IL-2), interleukin-3 (IL-3), interleukin-4, interleukin-6 (IL-6), and tumor necrosis factor-α. Soluble interleukin-2 receptor (sIL-2R) was measured serially during rhG-CSF therapy. Lymphocyte subpopulations including CD2, CD3, CD4, CD8, CD19, CD20, and CD25 were also measured, rhG-CSF was administered once daily as a 30-min infusion. The patient was treated with increasing dose levels of 100, 200, 400, 800, and 1,600 $\mu g/m^2$/day. The level of endogenous G-CSF was elevated to 334 pg/ml before treatment and GM-CSF, IL-2, IL-3, and IL-6 were slightly elevated. Clinically, he showed a moderate response to a high dose of rhG-CSF (1,600 $\mu g/m^2$/day). Plasma levels of G-CSF markedly increased during therapy but plasma levels of other cytokines did not show significant changes during therapy and lymphocyte subpopulations did not significantly change. A drastic increase in sIL-2R expression was observed after rhG-CSF infusion and an increase in sIL-2R expression occurred even before a major increase in granulocyte counts. These results showed that a high dose rhG-CSF therapy may influence the cytokine network as judged by the increased sIL-2R expression.

Key words: severe congenital neutropenia, cytokines, recombinant human granulocyte colony-stimulating factor, soluble interleukin-2 receptor

INTRODUCTION

Severe congenital neutropenia (SCN), is a very rare form of neutropenia in childhood and is characterized by early onset in infancy with profound neutropenia causing severe and recurrent infection [1,2]. It has been reported that patients with SCN have no defects in granulocyte colony-stimulating factor (G-CSF) production either in vitro [3] or in vivo [4] and a defective response of neutrophil precursors to endogenous G-CSF has been suspected [4]. Kyas et al. [5] showed that SCN patients are not defective in G-CSF receptor expression according to the number of G-CSF binding sites and binding affinity. Recently, we found that stem cell factor (SCF), a *c-kit* ligand, may be involved in the pathogenesis of SCN [6].

Although there are some papers about measurements of G-CSF levels in SCN patients [4], there are no papers about cytokine profile during recombinant human G-CSF (rhG-CSF) treatment in SCN patients. In this paper we studied the effect of rhG-CSF on granulopoiesis and the cytokine levels during rhG-CSF treatment in a patient with SCN.

MATERIALS AND METHODS

Patient

The patient was a 5-year-old boy with SCN. At day 15, he was seen by a physician because of otitis media. The blood count at that time showed an absence of granulocytes and SCN was suspected. The infant was transferred to Gunma University Hospital at the age of 5 months.

The peripheral blood picture was compatible with absolute neutropenia. Bone marrow aspiration showed

Received for publication September 18, 1992; accepted April 8, 1993.

Address reprint requests to Dr. Toshiji Shitara, Department of Pediatrics, Gunma University School of Medicine, 3-39-15, Showa-machi, Maebashi City, Gunma 371, Japan.

38.2% erythroid cells, 17.7% myeloid cells, 13.7% monocytoid cells, and 30.4% lymphoid cells. However, no polymorphonuclear neutrophils were noted beyond the promyelocytic stage. Antineutrophil antibody was negative. He was consequently diagnosed as having SCN. The effect of SCF on the in vitro induction of granulopoiesis in this patient has previously been reported [6].

Administration of rhG-CSF

rhG-CSF therapy was started at the age of 5 years. rhG-CSF produced using *Escherichia coli* and recombinant DNA techniques (Kirin Co. Ltd, Tokyo, Japan) was used. rhG-CSF was administered intravenously dissolved in 5% glucose over a 30-min period every day. The initial dose was 100 μg/m²/day (75 μg/day) and this dose was gradually increased over 2–3 weeks to 1,600 μg/m²/day (1,200 μg/day).

Measurement of Cytokines

The plasma levels of cytokines were measured before and during rhG-CSF therapy. These included G-CSF, granulocyte-macrophage colony-stimulating factor (GM-CSF), interleukin-1α (IL-1 α), interleukin-1β (IL-1 β), interleukin-2 (IL-2), interleukin-3 (IL-3), interleukin-4 (IL-4), interleukin-6 (IL-6), and tumor necrosis factor-α (TNF-α).

G-CSF was measured by Bio TRAK human G-CSF (Amersham International plc, Amersham, UK), and GM-CSF was measured by a human GM-CSF ELISA kit (Genzyme Corporation, Boston, MA). IL-1 α was measured by a human IL-1 α assay kit (Otsuka, Tokyo, Japan). IL-1 β was measured by human IL-1 β assay kit (Otsuka, Tokyo, Japan). IL-2 was measured by an Interleukin-2 ELISA kit (DuPont, Boston, MA). IL-3 was measured by Bio TRAK human IL-3 (Amersham International). IL-4 was measured by Bio TRAK human IL-4 (Amersham International). IL-6 was measured by a human IL-6 ELISA kit (Toray-Fuji Bionics, Inc, Tokyo, Japan). TNF-α was measured by a human TNF-α assay kit (Otsuka, Tokyo, Japan). The sensitivities of these assays were 39.1 pg/ml for G-CSF, 2.0 pg/ml for GM-CSF, 3.9 pg/ml for IL-1 α, 7.8 pg/ml for IL-1 β, 0.5 IU/ml for IL-2, 15.6 pg/ml for IL-3, 15.6 pg/ml for IL-4, 10.0 pg/ml for IL-6, and 3.9 pg/ml for TNF-α, respectively.

Assay for Soluble Interleukin-2 Receptor (sIL-2R)

sIL-2R was measured serially by enzyme immunoassay (EIA) before and during rhG-CSF therapy and was measured by an Interleukin-2 Receptor Test kit (T Cell Sciences, Cambridge, MA). The sensitivity of this assay was 50 U/ml and the normal ranges were 220–920 U/ml.

TABLE I. Cytokine Levels Before and During rhG-CSF Therapy*

Cytokines		Before rhG-CSF	During rhG-CSF[a]
G-CSF (pg/ml)	(<39.1)	334	75,000[b]
GM-CSF (pg/ml)	(<5.00)	6.25	8.85
IL-1α (pg/ml)	(<7.80)	7.80	<7.80
IL-1β (pg/ml)	(<15.6)	15.6	<15.6
IL-2 (IU/ml)	(<1.00)	2.30	1.00
IL-3 (pg/ml)	(<31.3)	40	<31.3
IL-4 (pg/ml)	(<31.3)	31.3	<31.3
IL-6 (pg/ml)	(<40.6)	80.7	51.5
TNF-α (pg/ml)	(<7.00)	7.0	<7.0

*Values in parentheses are levels in healthy volunteers. G-CSF = Granulocyte colony-stimulating factor; GM-CSF = Granulocyte-macrophage colony-stimulating factor; Il-1α = Interleukin-1α; Il-1β = Interleukin-1β; Il-2 = Interleukin-2; Il-3 = Interleukin-3; Il-4 = Interleukin-4; Il-6 = Interleukin-6; TNF-α = Tumor necrosis factor-α.
[a]Measured at 17 weeks after treatment.
[b]Measured at 24 hr after infusion.

Lymphocyte Subpopulations

Lymphocyte subpopulations were measured by flow cytometry using monoclonal antibodies including CD2, CD3, CD4, CD8, CD19, CD20, and CD25.

All diagnostic and therapeutic procedures in this study were performed after informed consent was obtained from the parents of the child.

RESULTS

Cytokine Levels Before and During rhG-CSF Treatment (Table I)

The level of endogenous plasma G-CSF was elevated to 334 pg/ml before treatment, showing that in vivo G-CSF production was not impaired. The levels of GM-CSF, IL-2, IL-3, and IL-6 were slightly elevated before treatment. During rhG-CSF therapy, increased plasma levels of rhG-CSF were observed as high as 75,000 pg/ml measured at 24 hr after infusion. Other cytokines did not show significant changes during rhG-CSF therapy although plasma levels of IL-2 slightly decreased from 2.30 pg/ml to 1.0 pg/ml.

Effects of rhG-CSF (Fig. 1)

The peripheral blood picture did not show an increase in neutrophils at a dose of 100 μg/m²/day. This dose of rhG-CSF was gradually increased and at a dose of 1,600 μg/m²/day (= 1,200 μg/day) an increase in neutrophils was obtained. The response of this patient is comparable with the least response of the SCN patients reported by Bonilla et al. [7], indicating relative refractoriness of the patient compared with other SCN patients.

sIL-2R Expression (Fig. 2)

Before rhG-CSF treatment, sIL-2R level was 485 U/ml, which was within normal range, sIL-2R expression

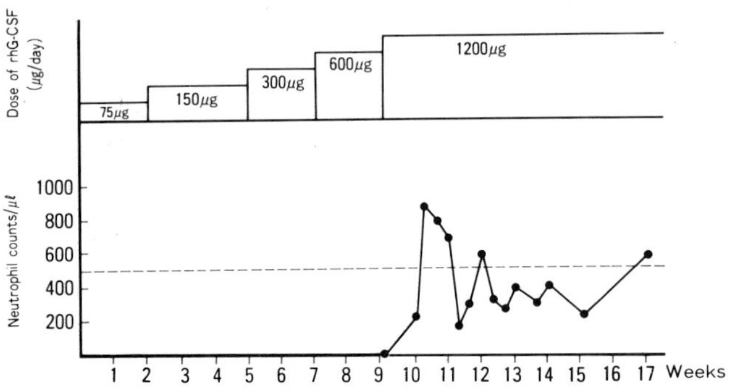

Fig. 1. Effects of recombinant human granulocyte colony-stimulating factor (rhG-CSF) on granulopoiesis. The number of neutrophils increased after dose escalation of rhG-CSF to 1,600 μg/m²/day (1,200 μg/day), indicating relative refractoriness of the patient to rhG-CSF.

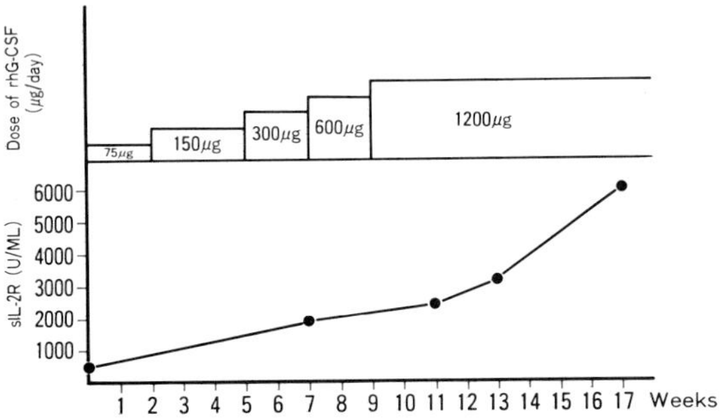

Fig. 2. Soluble interleukin-2 receptor (sIL-2R) expression during high dose rhG-CSF therapy. Before rhG-CSF treatment, sIL-2R level was 485 U/ml, which was within normal range (220–920 U/ml). sIL-2R expression increased with escalation of dose of rhG-CSF.

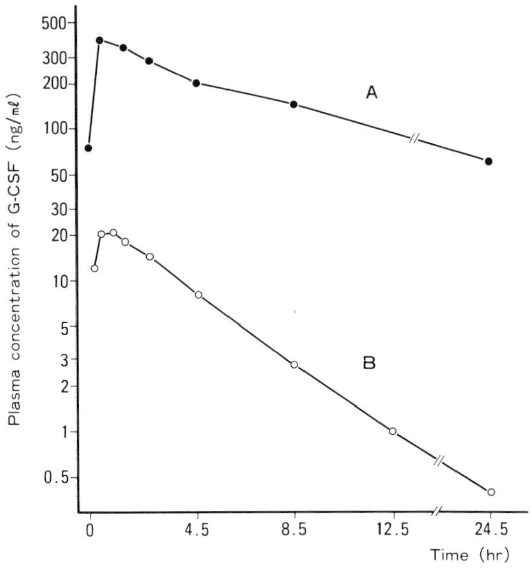

Fig. 3. Pharmacokinetic levels of recombinant human granulocyte colony-stimulating factor (rhG-CSF). A: ● = Plasma level of the rhG-CSF after intravenous infusion of 1,600 μg/m² over 30 min in a 5-year-old patient, with severe congenital neutropenia. B: ○ = Mean plasma concentration of the rhG-CSF after intravenous infusion of 3.0 μg/kg over 30 min in normal healthy volunteers (N = 5). (Cited from Azuma et al. [16] with the permission of the publisher.)

showed a drastic increase after the initiation of rhG-CSF therapy and rose as high as 6,000 U/ml at 17 weeks of treatment.

G-CSF Levels During rhG-CSF Therapy (Fig. 3)

Measurement of plasma G-CSF levels revealed an extremely high level after intravenous infusion. A high level of G-CSF was observed even 24 hr after infusion.

Lymphocyte Subpopulations

The absolute numbers of CD2, CD3, CD4, CD8, CD19, and CD20 before rhG-CSF treatment were within the normal limits and showed a slight but not significant increase after rhG-CSF treatment. The absolute numbers of CD25 showed no significant changes and the CD4/CD8 ratio did not change (data not shown).

DISCUSSION

SCN is a very rare form of neutropenia in childhood and is characterized by a maturational arrest in the bone marrow usually at the promyelocyte/myelocyte stage [1,2]. As it was reported that patients with SCN show no defects in G-CSF production either in vitro [3] or in vivo [4], a defective response of neutrophil precursors to endogenous G-CSF has been suspected [4]. However, Kyas et al. [5] recently showed that SCN patients are not defective in G-CSF receptor expression. This finding, as well as the presence of a high G-CSF concentration in vivo [4], indicates that growth factors other than G-CSF may be involved in the pathogenesis of SCN as long as defects in G-CSF receptor expression are absent [5]. We have found that SCF, a *c-kit* ligand, may be involved in the pathogenesis of SCN. As previously reported [6], SCF in combination with G-CSF significantly augmented the proliferation of granulocyte-macrophage colony-forming cells (GM-CFC), although GM-CFC was markedly depressed in the presence of G-CSF alone. This suggests that a defect at a more immature cellular level than the G-CSF level might be involved. When we examined colony-stimulating activity (CSA) in this patient using normal bone marrow cells as the target, they formed colonies and clusters, showing that peripheral blood mononuclear cells in this patient are capable of synthesizing and secreting biologically active CSA in vitro (unpublished data). A survey of literature, however, revealed no reports about cytokine profiles in SCN patients.

In spite of increased serum levels of G-CSF, administration of rhG-CSF has clinical effects in most patients with SCN. In 1989, Bonilla et al. [7] first reported the effects of rhG-CSF on neutropenia in patients with SCN. In 1990, Welte et al. [8] reported the differential effects of GM-CSF and G-CSF on SCN patients. Our patient showed a moderate response to high dose rhG-CSF with an increase in neutrophils resulting in relief of infection although endogenous G-CSF was elevated to 334 pg/ml before treatment.

The most drastic change in this study was a rise in sIL-2R. Our patient demonstrated more than a tenfold increase in sIL-2R expression compared to the pretreatment level. Although increased sIL-2R expression during therapy with rhG-CSF [9] and rhGM-CSF [10] has been reported, a survey of literature revealed no reports on the effects of rhG-CSF on an increase in sIL-2R expression in SCN patients. sIL-2R is believed to be the truncated form of the membrane-bound 55 kd chain of IL-2R and is cleaved from cells expressing IL-2R on their surface membranes [11]. Elevated sIL-2R expression is detected under several conditions including AIDS, sarcoidosis, and malignant diseases. In MDS or cancer patients, a significant correlation between sIL-2R expression and survival has been reported [12,13]. Lindemann et al. [9] reported that sIL-2R levels correlated to total WBC counts in patients receiving G-CSF and that granulocyte lineage cells might be a source of sIL-2R. However, in our patient, sIL-2R showed increase before major increase in granulocyte counts, suggesting that G-CSF could cause an increase in sIL-2R expression even in the absence of increase in granulocytes and that the source of sIL-2R might not necessarily be granulocytes in this patient with SCN. However, the possibility cannot be excluded that enhanced intramedullary myelopoiesis without releasing neutrophils into peripheral circulation is responsible for sIL-2R elevation. Although there are no significant changes in CD25+ cells, the possibility cannot be excluded either that the increased sIL-2R in our patient is released by the lymphocytes and/or monocytes/macrophages activated directly or indirectly by rhG-CSF.

Although there are many reports about the in vivo effects of rhG-CSF [7,8], there are no reports about the adverse effects of high levels of rhG-CSF in vivo. In the kinetic evaluation of plasma rhG-CSF in this patient, extremely high levels of rhG-CSF were obtained after intravenous infusion with the maximum level reaching more than 300 ng/ml. The biological effects of high and continuous serum levels of cytokines has been studied in transgenic animals and animals engrafted with retrovirus-derived expression vectors [14,15]. In both types of animals it is possible to achieve a sustained increase in growth factor levels in the serum typically 100–1,000-fold above those normally present, and as high as that were achieved in our patient. As far as possible clinical adverse effects are concerned, G-CSF might have been less likely than GM-CSF to produce adverse effects when used at high dose. The life span of animals is unchanged in the presence of elevated levels of G-CSF although the presence of grossly elevated levels of some cytokines leads to decreased animal life span [14,15]. Although there were no obvious adverse effects in our patient, further in vitro and in vivo analyses might be necessary.

As G-CSF induces sIL-2R expression as shown above, down regulation of the immune response caused by neutralization of free IL-2 cannot be excluded. Although increased sIL-2R expression results from secondary alteration of the cytokine network during high-dose rhG-CSF treatment, it remains unclear to what extent sIL-2R restricts immune responses by binding free IL-2. Even so, administration of recombinant IL-2 may be of value to compensate this down regulation. Further in vitro and in vivo studies will clarify the pathophysiology of G-CSF induced increase of sIL-2R expression.

ACKNOWLEDGMENT

We thank Mr. Fumihiko Kurimoto, Mitsubishi-Yuka Bioclinical Laboratories, for technical assistance.

REFERENCES

1. Kostmann R: Infantile genetic agranulocytosis (agranulocytosis infantalis hereditaria): A new recessive lethal disease in man. Acta Pediatr Scand 45:1, 1956 (Suppl 105).
2. Kostmann R: Infantile genetic agranulocytosis: A review with presentation of ten new cases. Acta Pediatr Scand 64:362, 1975.
3. Pietsch T, Buhrer C, Mempel K, Menzel T, Steffens U, Schrader C, Santos F, Zeidler C, Welte K: Blood mononuclear cells from patients with severe congenital neutropenia are capable of producing granulocyte colony-stimulating factor. Blood 77:1234, 1991.
4. Mempel K, Pietsch T, Menzel T, Zeidler C, Welte K: Increased serum level of granulocyte colony-stimulating factor in patients with severe congenital neutropenia. Blood 77:1919, 1991.
5. Kyas U, Pietsch T, Welte K: Expression of receptors for granulocyte colony-stimulating factor on neutrophils from patients with severe congenital neutropenia and cyclic neutropenia. Blood 79:1144, 1992.
6. Ijima H, Shitara T, Yugami S, Sotomatu M, Kuroume T: Recombinant human stem cell factor, a *c-kit* ligand, stimulates granulopoiesis in severe congenital neutropenia. Am J Hematol 42:407, 1993.
7. Bonilla MA, Gillio AP, Ruggeiro M, Kernan NA, Brochstein JA, Abboud MA, Fumagalli L, Vincent M, Welte K, Souza LM, O'Reilly RJ: Effects of recombinant human granulocyte colony-stimulating factor on neutropenia in patients with congenital agranulocytosis. N Engl J Med 320:1574, 1989.
8. Welte K, Zeidler C, Reiter A, Muller W, Odenwald E, Souza L, Riehm H: Differential effects of granulocyte-macrophage colony-stimulating factor and granulocyte colony-stimulating factor in children with severe congenital neutropenia. Blood 75:1056, 1990.
9. Lindemann A, Herrmann F, Oster W, Haffner G, Meyenburg W, Souza LM, Mertelmann R: Hematologic effects of recombinant human granulocyte colony-stimulating factor in patients with malignancy. Blood 74:2644, 1989.
10. Ho AD, Haas R, Wulf G, Knauf W, Ehrhardt R, Heilig B, Körbling M, Schulz G, Hunstein W: Activation of lymphocytes induced by recombinant human granulocyte-macrophage colony stimulating factor in patients with malignant lymphoma. Blood 75:203, 1990.

11. Rubin L, Kurman C, Fritz M, Biddison W, Boutin B, Yarchoan R, Nelson D: Soluble interleukin 2 receptors are released from activated human lymphoid cells in vitro. J Immunol 135:3172, 1985.
12. Zwierzina H, Herold M, Schöllenberger S, Geissler D, Schmalzl F: Detection of soluble IL-2 receptor in the serum of patients with myelodysplastic syndromes: Induction under therapy with GM-CSF. Br J Hematol 79:438, 1991.
13. Lai KN, Ho S, Leung JCK, Tsao SY: Soluble interleukin-2 receptors in patients with nasopharyngeal carcinoma. Cancer 67:2180, 1991.
14. Lübbert M, Jonas D, Herrmann F: Animal models for the biological effects of continuous high cytokine levels. Blut 61:253, 1990.
15. Metcalf D: The consequences of excess levels of hematopoietic growth factors. Br J Haematol 75:1, 1990.
16. Azuma J, Hamaguchi T, Seung-Eun P, Kurimoto T, Yoshida H, Seto Y, Mochizuki N, Kaneko T, Shimosaka A, Itoh H, Akahori H, Takaku F: Phase I study of KRN 8601 (rhG-CSF) in normal healthy volunteers: Safety and pharmacokinetics in single intravenous infusion. Rinsho Iyaku 5:1579, 1989.

American Journal of Hematology 45:63–72 (1994)

Dyshematopoiesis in Combined Immune Deficiency With Congenital Neutropenia

Cristina Gasparetto, Clay Smith, Meri Firpo, Dieter Dennig, Trudy Small, Alfred P. Gillio, Robert Lichtenberg, Richard J. O'Reilly, and Malcolm A.S. Moore

Bone Marrow Transplant Service (C.G., D.D., T.S., A.P.G., R.J.O.), Division of Hematologic Oncology (C.S.), James Ewing Laboratory of Developmental Hematopoiesis (M.F., M.A.S.M.), Memorial Sloan Kettering Cancer Center, New York, New York; Department of Medicine and Pediatrics, Loyola University Stritch School of Medicine, Maywood, Illinois (R.L.)

This report describes a patient with combined immune deficiency associated with congenital neutropenia (CID/CN) and reports a partial characterization of his hematopoietic abnormalities. The CID/CN syndrome described is characterized by neutropenia and by deficiencies in B-lymphoid and T-lymphoid cell number and function. Red cell and platelet counts were normal. In vitro assays indicate that the myeloid lineage was developmentally arrested at the level of the committed monocyte/granulocyte progenitor (CFU-GM), while precursors to the CFU-GM progenitor were normal. In vitro studies showed that the defect in myeloid development was not corrected with G-CSF or GM-CSF. However, combinations of cytokines present in conditioned media from the T-cell lines MO or C5MJ, or defined multiple cytokine combinations containing IL-1, IL-3, GM-CSF, kit ligand, IL-6, and IL-9, restored myelopoiesis in-vitro. In contrast, C5MJ-conditioned media did not correct deficiencies in immune function in the patient's lymphocytes and accessory cells. No abnormalities in the production of G-CSF, GM-CSF, M-CSF, or IL-1 from the patient could be identified to account for the defects in myelopoiesis orimmune function.

Key words: combined immune deficiency, congenital neutropenia, cytokine combinations

INTRODUCTION

Combined immune deficiency syndromes (CIDs) are a heterogeneous group of congenital disorders characterized by defective cellular and humoral immune function [1–3]. CID syndromes secondary to deficiencies of interleukin-1 (IL-1), IL-2, IL-1 receptors, and HLA class II determinants have been identified; however, the etiology of the immunodeficiency in the majority of CID patients remains unknown. Isolated congenital neutropenias (CNs), such as Kostmann syndrome, are a heterogeneous group of disorders characterized by variable degrees of neutropenia with normal cellular and humoral immune function [4–7]. Arrest of myeloid differentiation is observed in the bone marrow of the majority of CN patients. In most of these patients, apparently normal myelopoiesis can be restored in colony assays when bone marrow cells are incubated with granulocyte colony-stimulating factor (G-CSF) [8,9]. Correction of neutropenia in vivo in patients with CN has been demonstrated following the administration of G-CSF [8]. The underlying molecular defects in the CN disorders currently remain unknown.

Several descriptions of patients who have both combined immune deficiency and congenital neutropenia (CID/CN) have been reported [10–17]. Currently, little is known about the cellular and molecular bases of the defects in hematopoiesis or immune function occurring in CID/CN. In this report, we describe a case of CID/CN and a partial characterization of the defects in hematopoiesis and immune function in this patient.

CASE REPORT

The patient was a 3,400-g male delivered by cesarean section, following a full-term normal pregnancy. At birth, the patient was noted to have hypotonia, microcephaly, and neutropenia. A bone marrow aspiration per-

Received for publication November 9, 1992; accepted May 13, 1993.

Address reprint requests to Dr. Clay Smith, Department of Hematologic Oncology, Memorial Sloan Kettering Cancer Center, 1275 York Avenue, NY, NY, 10021.

formed at 5 days of age revealed hypercellular bone marrow with granulocytic maturational arrest. During the first 3 months of life, he experienced repeated episodes of fever and respiratory distress that responded to broad-spectrum antibiotics. At 4 months of age he developed pneumonia due to *Pneumocystis carinii* (PCP), which resolved following therapy with trimethoprim-sulfamethoxazol. At this time, he was found to have markedly decreased T-cell numbers and T-cell mitogen responses, normal natural killer (NK) cell numbers, and function, and hypogammaglobulinemia (IgG, 10 mg/dl; IgA, 7 mg/dl; IgM, 78 mg/dl). STORCH titers were negative and human immune deficiency virus (HIV) testing of the patient and his family was negative. A bone marrow aspiration and biopsy at 5 months of age revealed mild erythroid hyperplasia, eosinophilia, myeloid arrest at the promyelocyte stage, and the presence of $CD10^+$ lymphoblasts comprising 14% of the nucleated marrow elements. Cytogenetic analysis was normal, and adenosine deaminase and nucleoside phorphorylase levels were normal in parental red blood cells. At 6 months of age, direct and indirect immunofluorescence performed on the patient's serum and neutrophils at six months of age were negative for anti-IgG and IgM anti-neutrophil antibodies, and his serum did not agglutinate white cells from pooled normal donors. The patient's peripheral white blood cell (WBC) dount at this time was 1.2×10^9 cells/L with a differential of 25% polymorphonuclear cells (an absolute neutrophil count (ANC) of 0.4×10^9neutrophils/L), 10% monocytes, and 65% lymphocytes. The phenotype of his peripheral blood lymphocytes (PBL) included 21% $CD3^+$ cells, 75% $CD20^+$ cells, and 5% $CD56^+$ cells. His CD4/CD8 ratio was 9. The $CD20^+$ cells were positive for HLA-DR, CD19, CD21, CD5, and CD23 and negative for CD10. The PBL proliferative response to phytohemagglutanin (PHA) was 10–20% of normal and the PBL proliferative responses to allogeneic cells and OKT3 stimulation were both severely decreased. There was no improvement in proliferative response to PHA or OKT3 with the addition of recombinant human IL-2.

As the patient did not have an HLA-identical bone marrow donor, he was treated initially with high dose intravenous gammaglobulin; however, no increase in his neutrophil count occurred. He was subsequently maintained on monthly intravenous infusions of gammaglobulin, oral PCP prophylaxis, and intermittent parenteral hyperalimentation to supplement gastrostomy feedings. In his second year of life, his only infections were one episode of otitis media, and occasional upper respiratory tract infections, however he displayed persistent and profound failure to thrive and developmental delay. At 17 months of age, the patient was treated with GM-CSF (Schering-Plough) with escalating doses beginning at 1.5 μg/kg administered subcutaneously and advancing by 0.5 μg/kg increments every 2 days to a final dose of 4 μg/kg. No improvement in white blood cell count, absolute neutrophil count, hemoglobin concentration, or platelet count was observed, and treatment was terminated at the request of the patient's parents after 14 days. The patient expired at home at 18 months of age. No autopsy was performed.

MATERIALS AND METHODS

Bone Marrow Cells

Following informed parental consent and using ketamine anesthesia, bone marrow cells were collected into heparinized saline (1 ml heparin per 5 ml of bone marrow) from the posterior iliac crest.

Assay of Granulocyte/Macrophage Progenitors (CFU-GM Assays)

CFU-GM assays were performed as previously described [18]. Cytokines used in the colony assays included MO-conditioned media (MO-CM) (D. Golde, UCLA) [19]; C5MJ condition media (C5MJ-CM) (Genetics Institute (GI) [20], Cambridge, MA); recombinant human-Interleukin 1-β(rh-IL-1β) (Immunex, Seattle, WA); rh-Interleukin 3 (Immunex); (GI), rh-Interleukin 6 (rh-IL-6) (GI); rh-Interleukin 9 (rh-IL-9) (GI); recombinant mouse-mast cell growth factor (rm-MGF, kit-ligand) (Immunex); rh-GM-CSF (Immunex); rh-G-CSF (Amgen, Thousand Oaks, CA); and rh-M-CSF (Chiron, Emeryville, CA) at the doses indicated in the legend for Figure 1 (see also Fig. 4).

Assay for Myeloid Precursors to CFU-GM Progenitors (Pre-CFU Assay)

Assessments of precursors to CFU-GM (Pre-CFU) were performed using the Pre-CFU assay (also termed secondary CFU assay, or delta assay) exactly as previously described [18]. Briefly, the Pre-CFU assay involves two phases. First, a CFU-GM assay (primary CFU-GM assay) is performed using GM-CSF as the growth factor. Simultaneously, aliquots of marrow are placed in suspension cultures containing a variety of growth factors; then, after 7 days, cells are removed and plated in CFU-GM assays using GM-CSF as the growth factor (secondary CFU-GM assays). If no colonies are observed inthe primary CFU-GM assays, colonies arising in the secondary CFU-GM assays are presumed to derive from precursors to CFU-GM that have proliferated and differentiated under the influence of the suspension-phase cytokines. All primary CFU-GM values are colony number per 1×10^5 cells plated. Secondary CFU-GM values are the total CFU-GM colony number enumerated per 1×10^5 cells inoculated into the suspension cultures. CFU-GM assays contained 1,000 U/ml GM-CSF. Cytokine concentrations used in the suspension culture phase

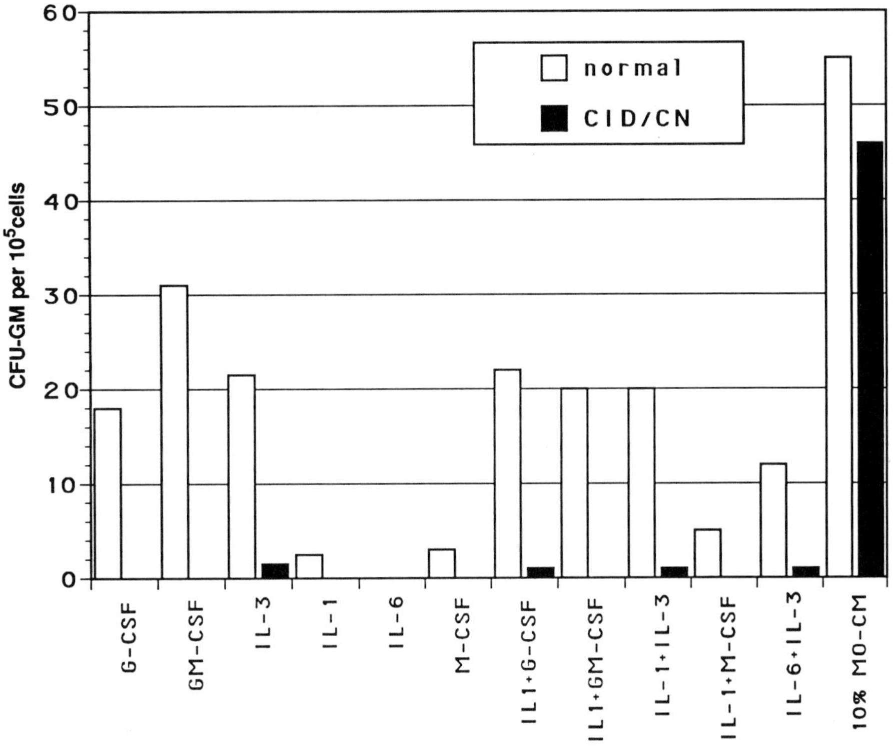

Fig. 1. CFU-GM assays of marrow obtained from the CID/CN patient at six months of age (prior to treatment with GM-CSF). CFU-GM number is per 10^5 cells plated. Cytokine concentrations included G-CSF, 1,000 U/ml; GM-CSF, 1,000 U/ml; IL-3, 50 ng/ml; IL-1, 100 U/ml; IL-6, 10U/ml; M-CSF, 1,000 U/ml. All CFU-GM values in all figures are the means of triplicate cultures.

of the Pre-CFU assay are described in the legend to Figure 2.

Antibody Inhibition Assays

Antibody inhibition assays were performed to determine the contribution of individual cytokines in supporting the growth of precursors to CFU-GM by MO-CM. Antibodies at previously determined saturating concentrations were added to the suspension phase of the secondary CFU assays with MO-CM as the suspension phase cytokine source. Antibodies to GM-CSF, G-CSF, and M-CSF were obtained as ascites from mouse recipients immunized with the appropriate purified human cytokine (David Warren, Memorial Sloan Kettering Cancer Center, NY, NY). Other antibodies were obtained from Genzyme (Boston, MA). Antibody concentrations in the suspension cultures included anti-TNF-a at 10,000 U/ml, anti-IL-1-alpha at 100 U/ml, anti-anti-IL-1-beta at 100 U/ml, anti-IL-3 at 200 U/ml, anti-IL-6 at 100 U/ml, anti-M-CSF at 100 U/ml, anti-GM-CSF at 4 μg/ml, and anti-G-CSF at 10 μg/ml. Following 7 days of suspension culture including antibodies, secondary CFU-GM were plated as described above.

Assay of Erythroid Progenitors (BFU-E Assays)

BFU-E assays utilizing erythropoietin (2 U/ml (Amgen) and rh-Interleukin 3 (50 ng/ml) were performed as previously described [21].

Assays for Cytokine Production by Bone Marrow Fibroblasts

Fibroblast cultures. One ml of unseparated bone marrow was diluted to 10 ml in minimal essential medium (MEM-alpha) (Gibco, Gaithersburg, Md) supplemented with 10% fetal bovine serum (FBS) (Hazelton) and gentamycin (50 mg/ml) (Gibco). After 5–6 passages in culture, fibroblasts were stimulated to produce colony-stimulating factors with 20 ml of medium alone or 20 ml of medium supplemented with rh-IL-1-β (50 U/ml) or rh-TNF-a (50 ng/ml, Genentech, San Francisco, CA). Fibroblast culture-conditioned media was collected after 24 hr and frozen at −70°C until assayed.

Enzyme-linked immunosorbent assay for G-CSF. Frozen serum and plasma samples from the CID/CN patient and normal donors, as well as fibroblast-conditioned media, were assayed in a h-G-CSF quantitative enzyme-

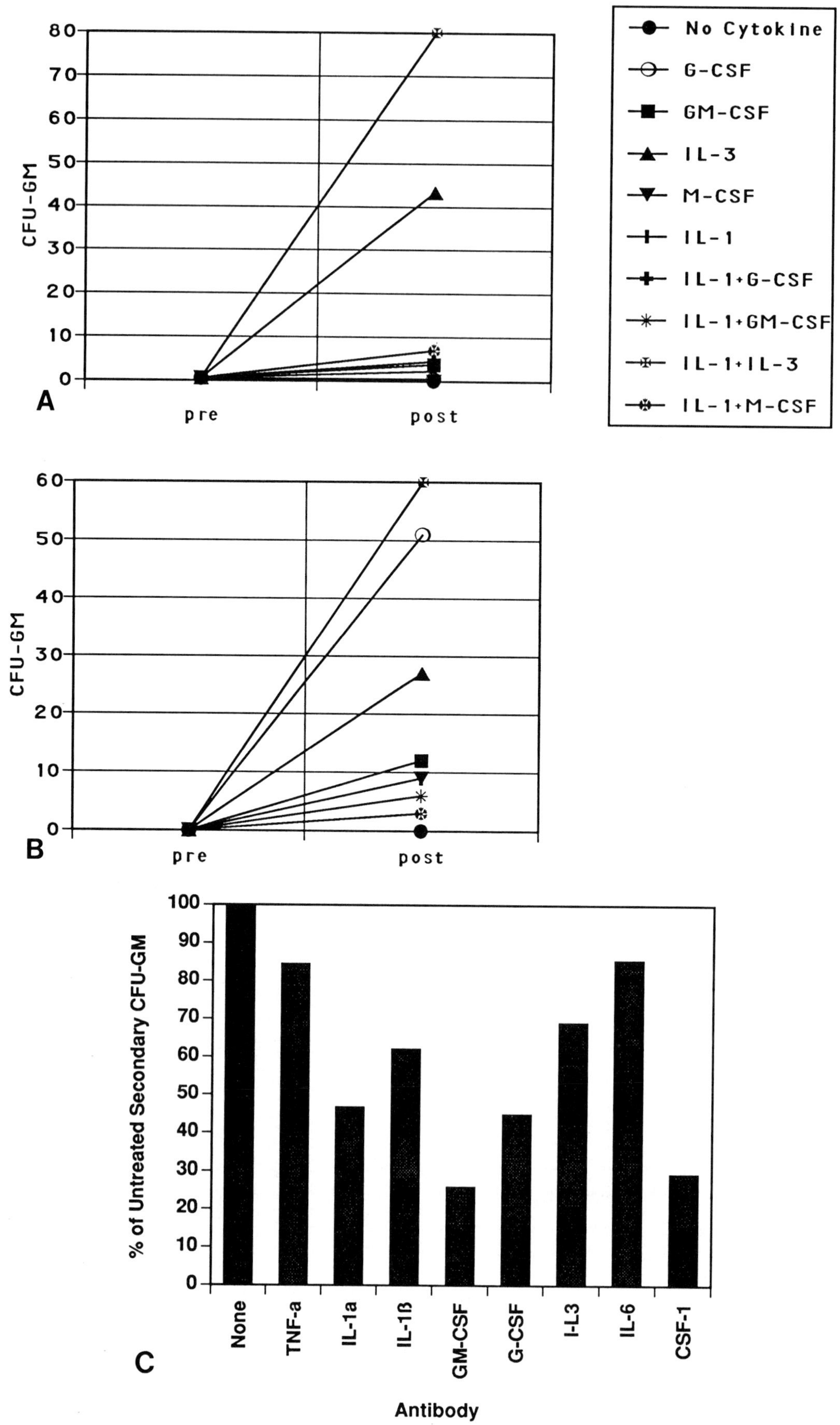

80
70
60
50
40
30
20
10
0
CFU-GM
A
pre
post
No Cytokine
G-CSF
GM-CSF
IL-3
M-CSF
IL-1
IL-1+G-CSF
IL-1+GM-CSF
IL-1+IL-3
IL-1+M-CSF
60
50
40
30
20
10
0
CFU-GM
B
pre
post
100
90
80
70
60
50
40
30
20
10
0
% of Untreated Secondary CFU-GM
None
TNF-a
IL-1a
IL-1ß
GM-CSF
G-CSF
I-L3
IL-6
CSF-1
C
Antibody

Figure 2.

linked immunosorbent assay (ELISA) kit (Oncogene Science, Uniondale, NY), according to kit instructions. ELISA plate optical densities were read on an ELISA plate reader (EIA Reader) (BioTek Instruments) at a wavelength of 405 nM.

G-CSF bioassay. NFS-60 cells maintained in IMDM supplemented with 10% FBS and 100 U/ml rhG-CSF were washed twice, then incubated for 1 hr at room temperature in RPMI-1640 with 2% FBS; 5×10^3 NFS-60 cells were then added to wells of a 96-well plate, serial dilutions of serum or fibroblast culture supernatant samples were added, and plates were incubated at 37°C for 24 hr. After pulsing for 4 hr with 0.5 mCi/well ^{3}H-TdR (NEN, Boston, MA), plates were harvested using a cell harvester, equilibrated in scintillation fluid, and counted in a β-counter for 1minper sample. Biological activity was determined by comparing results to test samples containing dilutions of standard concentrations of rhG-CSF. Assay medium was used as a negative control, and all measurements were performed in triplicate. To establish that measured activities were not due to other growth factors, assays were repeated following pre-incubation for 1 hr at 37°C with an inhibiting monoclonal antibody to human G-CSF.

RNA blot analysis. Whole-cell RNA was prepared by the method of Chomczynski and Sacchi [22] and mRNA was isolated using a Fast Track kit (Invitrogen, San Diego, CA), according to kit instructions. Twenty mg of whole cell RNA was heated to 60°C for 5 min and electrophoresed on a1% agarose/6% formaldehyde gel, then transferred to a nylon membrane and hybridized with a ^{32}P-labeled cDNA probe for 18 hr at 65°C. Blots were washed and exposed to X-ray film for autoradiography. Blots were stripped and rehybridized several times with cDNA probes to G-CSF, M-CSF, IL-1, and β-actin.

Immune Function Assays

Preparation of mononuclear cell subpopulations. Peripheral blood mononuclear cells (PBMNCs) were obtained via Ficoll-Hypaque (density 1.077 g/ml) centrifugation of 1:2 diluted heparinized, freshly drawn venous blood. PBMNCs were fractionated by adherence to plastic tissue culture dishes for 1 hr at 37°C. After collecting the supernatant that contains the nonadherent cells (peripheral blood lymphocytes, PBL), adherent cells were removed by scraping, and irradiated (3,000 cGy) prior to examination of their accessory function in T-cell proliferation assays. Nonadherent PBLs were further separated by rosetting with AET-treated sheep red blood cells (SRBCs) [23]. The E^+ cells (T cells) were further purified by a direct complement lysis of HLA class II expressing cells, using the anti-HLA class II monoclonal antibody 9B5 generously provided by Dr. R.S. Mittler (Bristol Myers, CT). The E^- cells (B cells) were exposed to a second round of T-cell depletion by rosetting with SRBC and irradiated prior to examination of their accessory function.

Proliferation assays. PBL or purified T cells were adjusted to 2 to 4 × 105 cells/ml and aliquots of 100 μl were plated into individual wells of flat-bottomed 96-well plates (Costar, Cambridge, Ma) in RPMI 1640 (Gibco), and heat inactivated human serum (Whitaker, Walkersville, MD). PBL were stimulated with 1 μg/ml PHA (Sigma, St Louis, MO). Purified T cells were stimulated for 72 hr at 37°C with 3 μg/ml Concanavalin A (Con A) (Sigma) in the presence of 1×10^4 allogeneic or autologous accessory B cells or accessory adherent cells (monocyte/macrophages). To assess T-cell proliferation, T-cell DNA synthesis was measured by the addition of 1 μCi/ml ^{3}H-TdR (DuPont, Boston, Ma) 4 hr prior totermination of the cell culture. The content of individual wells was harvested on filter paper, and the thymidine incorporation assessed in a β-counter.

Fig. 2. Pre-CFU assays of 4-HC^{resistant}/CD34$^+$ normal bone marrow (A) and bone marrow obtained from the CID/CN patient (B) at 6 months of age. The 1° CFU-GM value is the number of CFU-GM per 10^5 cells using GM-CSF (1000 U/ml) as the growth factor. The 2° CFU-GM value is the number of CFU-GM per 10^5 cells inoculated into the suspension culture phase of the assay. C: Antibody inhibition of 2° CFU-GM. Marrow from the CID/CN patient was incubated with 10% MO-CM in the suspension phase of the assay with saturating concentrations of the indicated antibody. Cells were then washed and 2° CFU-GM values determined. Values are the percentage of 2° CFU-GM following antibody treatment relative to an untreated control.

RESULTS

CFU-GM Assays

Figure 1 demonstrates the effects of a variety of cytokines, at doses optimal for normal controls, alone and in combination, on CFU-GM colony formation from normal bone marrow and from marrow from the CID/CN patient. Of all the cytokines assayed, only conditioned media from the human T-cell line MO (MO-CM) which contains multiple cytokines was capable of generating normal numbers of CFU-GM colonies from the CID/CN marrow. Increasing the dosage of rh-IL3 to 50-fold higher than normal and increasing the dose of M-CSF to 10-fold higher than normal partially, but not fully, restored CFU-GM colony numbers (data not shown). Increasing the dose of rh-G-CSF and rh-GM-CSF had no effect. In contrast to the suboptimal numbers of myeloid progenitors generated by single and double cytokine treatment, erythroid progenitor number as measured by the BFU-E colony assay was three- to fourfold elevated compared to a normal control (data not shown).

Hematopoietic Precursor Cell Assays (Pre-CFU Assays)

CID/CN marrow was compared using the Pre-CFU assay to normal marrow which had been depleted of primary CFU-GM forming progenitors (4-hydroperoxy-cyclophospamide (4-HC)^{resistant}/CD34^{+} marrow) [18]. As we reported previously, 4-HC^{resistant}/CD34^{+} marrow failed to form colonies in primary CFU-GM assays, while incubation in suspension cultures with the combination of rh-IL-1 and rh-IL-3, and less effectively, rh-IL-3 alone, preferentially generated secondary CFU-GM colonies compared to other growth factor combinations [18] (Fig. 2A). Similarly, while unfractionated marrow from the CID/CN patient failed to generate colonies in primary CFU/GM assays, secondary CFU/GM colony formation was optimal following incubation in suspension cultures with rh-IL-1 combined with rh-IL-3, and less effectively with rh-IL-3, compared to other cytokine combinations (Fig. 2B). In contrast to normal bone marrow however, a high number secondary CFU-GM were also observed following incubation of CID/CN marrow in suspension phase with rh-G-CSF (Fig. 2B).

When both 4-HC^{resistant}/CD34^{+} normal marrow and CID/CN marrow were incubated with 10% MO-conditioned medium in the suspension phase of the pre-CFU assay, substantially greater numbers of secondary CFU-GM were generated compared to single cytokines and double cytokine combinations. MO-CM in suspension phase resulted in 290 secondary CFU-GM per 10^5 input cells from normal marrow, and 278 secondary CFU-GM per 10^5 input cells from CID/CN marrow (cf. Fig. 2A,B). In an effort to identify the cytokines(s) present in MO-CM which were responsible for this effect on CID/CN marrow, antibody neutralization studies were carried out in the suspension phase of the pre-CFU assay. Incubating CID/CN marrow with 10% MO-CM plus saturating amounts of anti-IL1-a and β, anti-GM-CSF, anti-CSF-1, and anti-G-CSF partially, but not completely, abolished the ability of MO-CM to restore normal response to GM-CSF in secondary CFU-GM assays (Fig. 2C).

Baseline Cytokine Expression Assays

Enzyme-linked immunosorbent assays (ELISA) for h-G-CSF were performed on samples of normal and CID/CN serum, and from CID/CN and normal fibroblast-conditioned medium. All samples from the CID/CN patient were obtained prior to the treatment course of GM-CSF. No significant differences were observed in serum G-CSF concentrations between normal control samples and CID/CN samples by ELISA (30 pg/ml and 50 pg/ml respectively). No significant differences were observed in G-CSF production as measured by ELISA from marrow fibroblasts derived from normal control samples and from CID/CN marrow, following stimulation with h-IL-1 or h-TNF. Normal fibroblast conditioned media samples yielded 860U G-CSF/ml (IL-1 stimulated) and 20U G-CSF/ml (TNF stimulated) compared to CID/CN fibroblast conditioned media samples which yielded 680 U G-CSF/ml (IL-1 stimulated) and 60 U G-CSF/ml (TNF stimulated). No significant differences in basal, IL-1 stimulated, and TNF stimulated bioactivity in fibroblast conditioned media samples were observed in the NFS-60 bioassay. Normal samples yielded 280 cpm (basal), 7694 cpm (IL-1 stimulated), and 2314 cpm (TNF stimulated) compared to CID/CN samples that yielded 517 cpm (basal), 8236 cpm (IL-1 stimulated), and 1963 cpm (TNF stimulated). RNA blot analysis was performed to assess IL-1, M-CSF, G-CSF, and GM-CSF mRNA expression in unstimulated and IL-1/TNF stimulated fibroblasts derived from the CID/CN and normal control marrow. No differences in cytokine mRNA expression levels or in RNA species were observed (data not shown).

Immune Function Studies

The proliferative responses to PHA of PBL which were derived from the CID/CN patient were less than 1/10 the response of normal PBL (Fig. 3A). Since this may be due to either an intrinsic T-cell defect of due to deficient accessory cell function, T cells, monocytes, and B cells were isolated and studied separately. The proliferative function of purified T cells derived from the CID/CN patient to ConA in the presence of normal allogeneic accessory B cells was not distinguishable from background activity, suggesting a deficiency in T-cell responsiveness (Fig. 3B). The proliferative response of normal purified T cells to Concanavalin A (Con A) in the presence of the CID/CN patient's B-cells was only 30% of the proliferative response on normal T cells to Con A duplicate with normal accessory B cells (Fig. 3C). This suggests that there was a deficiency in the B-cell accessory function in the CID/CN patient. Similarly, the proliferative response on normal T cells, in the presence of monocyte/macrophages derived from the CID/CN patient, was only 50% of the level of normal T-cell proliferation in the presence of normal monocyte/macrophages (Fig. 3D). These findings suggest that the monocyte/macrophages accessory functions were also deficient in the CID/CN patient. Addition of 30% conditioned media obtained from the C5MJ cell line did not restore proliferation in any of these assays (data not shown).

CFU-GM Assays Following GM-CSF Therapy

Immediately following a 2 week course of rh-GM-CSF (see Case Report), CFU-GM assays utilizing a variety of cytokine combinations were performed on a bone marrow sample obtained from the CID/CN patient. Increased

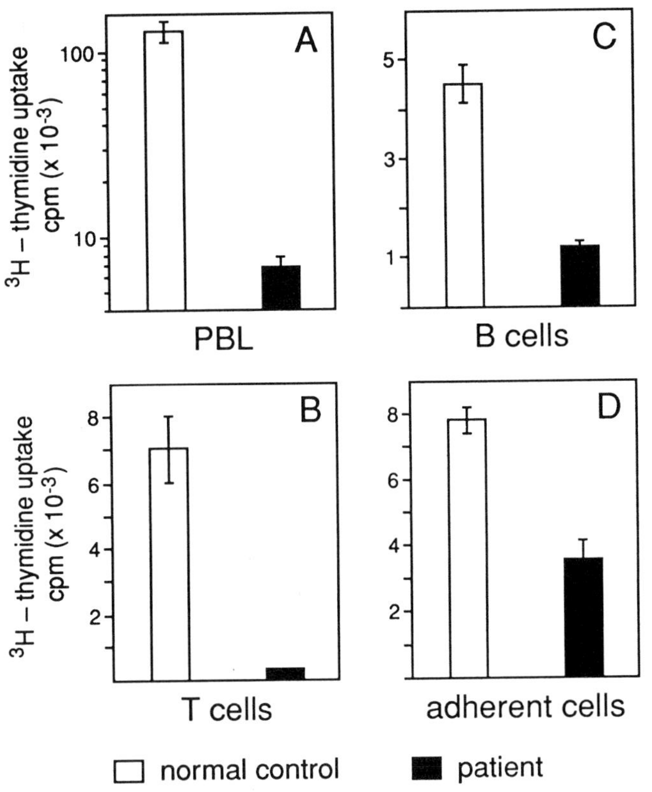

Fig. 3. Immune function assays. On the y-axes, the T-cell proliferative responses are represented. A: Proliferative response of PBL from a normal control (open bar) to PHA was compared to PBL from the CID/CN patient (closed bar). B: Proliferative response of purified T cells from a normal control (open bar) to Con A plus normal accessory B cells was compared to T cells from the CID/CN patient (closed bar). C: Proliferative response of normal T cells to Con A in the presence of normal accessory B cells (open bar) and B cells derived from the CID/CN patient (closed bar) was compared. In Figure 3D, the proliferative response of normal T cells to Con A in the presence of normal adherent cells (open bar) and adherent cells derived from the CID/CN patient (closed bar) was compared.

numbers of CFU-GM colonies were generated with rh-IL3 and rh-GM-CSF following in-vivo GM-CSF treatment (Fig. 4) compared to the previous CFU/GM assays performed prior to growth factor treatment (see Fig. 1). In addition, large numbers of CFU-GM were generated with rh-kit-ligand (stem cell factor) in combination with rh-IL3, and a variety of other cytokines. The combination of rh-IL9 + rh-IL6 + rh-IL1 + rh-GM-CSF was chosen because it represents the known cytokines present in conditioned media from the cell line C5MH, which had previously been demonstrated to have effects similar to MO-CM on CID/CN and normal marrow (data not shown). Additionally, the C5MJ combination of defined cytokines generated extremely large colonies (all typically >0.5 mm in diameter) with granulocyte/macrophage morphology, as opposed to the small colonies (50–200 cells) seen with the other defined cytokine combinations.

DISCUSSION

The form of combined immune deficiency associated with neutropenia (CID/CN) described in this report is characterized by developmental arrest in the neutrophil/monocyte lineages, B-cell developmental arrest at the CALLA$^-$CD21$^+$ stage, and deficiencies in mature T-lymphoid cell numbers and mitogen proliferative responses. No overt deficiencies in eosinophil, erythroid, and platelet number or function were observed. No improvement in hematopoietic indices or immune function occurred following treatment with steroids, androgens, IgG, or a short course of rh-GM-CSF.

The laboratory studies described in this report indicate that the block in myeloid differentiation in this disorder occurs at the level of the committed monocyte/granulocyte progenitor after the divergence of the erythro-myeloid precursor into distinct erythroid and myeloid lineages. Anemia was not present and BFU-E erythroid progenitor numbers were elevated compared to controls, possibly due to a shunt of erythro-myeloid hematopoietic precursors to the erythroid pathway. In contrast, the patient demonstrated significant neutropenia and his marrow yielded fewer colony forming progenitors in clonogenic assays (i.e., CFU-GM) than normal controls when incubated with a number of single cytokines or double cytokine combinations. Increasing the dose of single cytokines to concentrations substantially greater than optimal doses for normal marrow did not significantly overcome the myeloid developmental defect in the CID/CN marrow observed in clonogenic assays. In contrast, marrow from the CID/CN patient generated secondary CFU/GM in pre-CFU assays in a manner quantitatively and qualitatively similar to normal CFU-GM depleted marrow (CD34$^+$/4-HC^{resistent} marrow). Both marrows generated similar numbers of secondary CFU-GM following incubation in suspension cultures with MO-CM, the combination of IL-1–IL-3, and less effectively, with IL-3 alone. These findings imply that the myeloid precursors in CID/CN marrow are functionally and numerically intact. One difference between normal and CID/CN marrow was that the CID/CN marrow yielded high numbers of secondary CFU-GM following suspension culture with G-CSF, while this was not observed in normal CD34$^+$/4-HC^{resistant} marrow. Differences in accessory cell populations present in the secondary CFU assay system or intrinsic differences in stem cell biology may account for this observation.

When CID/CN marrow was incubated in CFU-GM and Pre-CFU-GM assays with conditioned media obtained

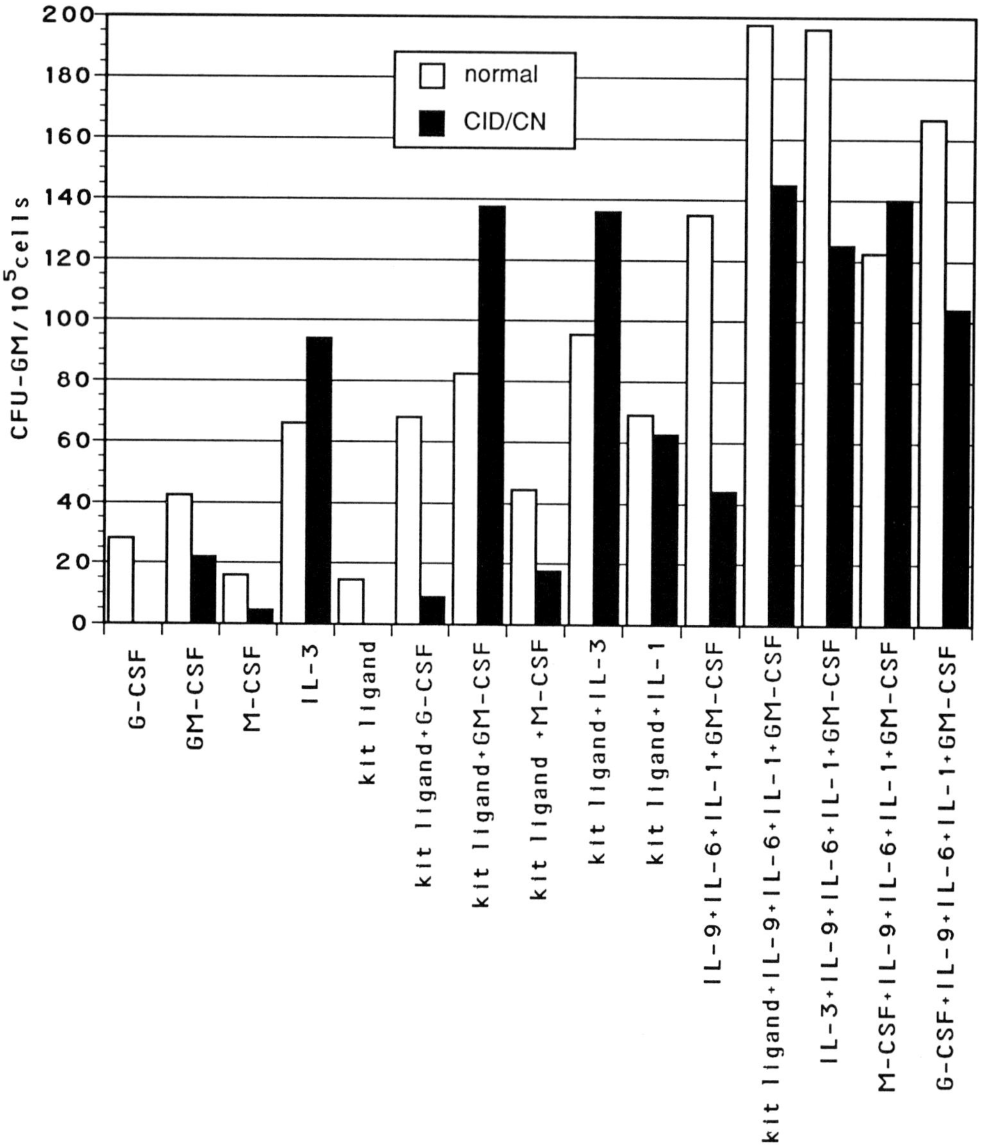

Fig. 4. CFU/GM assays following treatment of the CID/CN patient with GM-CSF. Marrow obtained from the CID/CN patient at 18 months of age following a 2-week course of GM-CSF. Cytokine concentrations at the same as in Fig. 1 with the addition of: rm-MGF (kit ligand) 20 ng/ml, rh-IL-9 30 U/ml, and rh-IL-6 10 U/ml.

from the T-cell line MO (MO-CM), normal colony number, size, and morphology was restored. MO-CM is known to contain a number of cytokines including GM-CSF, IL-1, G-CSF, CSF-1 and other unidentified growth factors [19,24]. Antibody inhibition of each of these cytokines failed to eliminate the growth supporting activity of MO-CM. These results indicate that there is either an unknown cytokine activity in MO-CM capable of supporting myelopoiesis in CID/CN marrow, or more likely, that the presence of multiple cytokines in MO-CM overcomes the defect in myelopoiesis. The observation in the pre-CFU assays that sequential exposure of CID/CN marrow to the combination of IL-1 with IL-3 then GM-CSF generated optimal numbers of secondary CFU-GM supports the contention that multiple cytokine combinations are more effective than single or double combinations in restoring normal myelopoiesis in CID/CN marrow. In an attempt to define further cytokine combinations that would correct the defect in myeloid ontogeny in CID/CN, CFU-GM assays were performed using a number of recently identified cytokines including kit ligand (MGF) [25], IL-9 [26], and IL-6 [20], which were not available during the initial evaluation of this patient at six months of age. Marrow for these experiments was obtained from the CID/CN patient at 18 months of age following a short treatment course of GM-CSF. In contrast to the results of CFU-GM assays performed on marrow obtained at 6 months of age, at 18 months of age, GM-CSF and IL-3 stimulation generated significant numbers of CFU-GM colonies from CID/CN marrow. It is unclear whether the CFU-GM response to GM-CSF and IL-3 observed at this time point was due to the in-vivo administration of GM-CSF or to evolution of the patient's disease. Even at this time however, combinations of multiple cytokines including IL-9, IL-6, IL-1, and GM-CSF with either M-CSF, IL-3, or kit ligand (MGF), generated much more numerous and larger granulocyte/macrophage colonies than single and double cytokine combinations.

Several in vitro studies were performed in an attempt to define and correct the immune dysfunction in this form of CID/CN. PBL and T cells obtained from this patient demonstrated a profound deficiency in their proliferative response to normal mitogenic stimuli. In addition, the patient's B-cells and monocyte/macrophages were deficient in their ability to support the proliferation of normal control T lymphocytes. No improvement in any of these immunologic parameters was observed when C5MJ-conditioned media containing combinations of cytokines was added to the lymphocyte proliferation assays. As opposed to the CFU-GM and pre-CFU assays, lymphocyte proliferation assays assess functional rather than developmental properties. Recently described in vitro lymphocyte culture systems [28] and murine/human lymphoid chimeras which support lymphocyte ontogeny (29) may be more useful assays for determining the effects of cytokine combinations on the lymphoid lineages in CID/CN than the functional assays described in this report.

Multiple potential explanations for the abnormalities in hematopoiesis and immune function in this form of CID/CN are possible. Several cytokines have been observed to have pleiotropic effects on both the myeloid and lymphoid lineages including, IL-1, IL-2, IL-3, IL-4, IL-6, and IL-9 [29]. In our studies, no defect in G-CSF, GM-CSF, M-CSF, or IL-1 production by accessory cells could be demonstrated by bioassay, ELISA, or Northern hybridization studies; however, defects in the production and activity of other cytokines remains a possibility. Alternatively, defects in cytokine receptors and/or signal transduction pathways, defects in the development or function of a particular accessory or hematopoietic cell critical to normal development of myeloid and lymphoid cells, overproduction of suppressing cells and/or factors [30], or intrinsic defects in myeloid/lymphoid stem cells may underlie this disorder. The observation that the erythroid and megakaryocytic lineages are intact argues against a gobal defect in totipotent hematopoietic stem cells. A recent report however, indicates that myeloid and lymphoid cells may be derived from developmentally restricted stem cells in addition to totipotent stem cells [31]. This indicates that a defect may occur in a myelolymphoid stem cell that spares stem cells of other lineages.

Regardless of the mechanism, our results indicate that combinations of cytokines, particularly those utilizing kit-ligand, IL-9, IL-6, GM-CSF, IL-1, and IL-3, may have clinical utility in correcting the neutropenia of CID/neutropenia and other congenital neutropenias not responsive to G-CSF or GM-CSF alone. It remains to be determined if cytokine combinations can correct the defect in lymphopoiesis and immune function in this disorder. In addition, these observations are based on a single case of CID/CN. It is very likely that CID/CN is the common manifestation of a spectrum of molecular abnormalities, so that the findings presented here may not be universal.

ACKNOWLEDGMENTS

C.S. is supported by NIH grant CA-09512-05. C.G. is a Fellow of the Leukemia Society of America. M.F. is supported by the Cornell University Department of Biology. D.D., A.G., and T.S. are supported by NIH grants 5PO1CA23766 and 5PO1CA33050

REFERENCES

1. Buckley R: Immunodeficiency diseases. JAMA 258:2841, 1987.
2. Proceedings: Combined immune deficiency: Its nature and treatment. Report of a Symposium Sponsored by the Fogarty International Center, National Institutes of Health, Bethesda, Maryland Clin Immunol Immunopathol 6:115, 1976.
3. Pollara B, Moore JJ, Pickering RJ, Gabrielsen AE, Meuwissen HJ: Combined immunodeficiency disease: An inborn error of purine metabolism. Birth Defects 11:120, 1975.
4. Chusid MJ, Pisciotta AV, Duquesnoy RJ, Camitta BM, Tomasulo AP: Congenital neutropenia: Studies of pathogenesis. Am J Hematol 8:315, 1980.
5. Koren A, Sela PB, Barak Y, Jammalieh J, Katzuni E: Congenital dysgranulopoietic neutropenia in two siblings: Clinical, ultrastructural, and in vitro bone marrow culture studies. Pediatr Hematol Oncol 6:293, 1989.
6. Parmley RT, Crist WM, Regab AH, Boxer LA, Malluh A, Lui VK, Darby CP: Congenital dysgranulopoietic neutropenia: Clinical, serologic, ultrastructural, and in vitro proliferative characteristics. Blood 56:465, 1980.
7. Kawaguchi Y, Kobayashi M, Tanabe A, Hara M, Nishi Y, Usui T, Nagai S, Nishibayashi Y, Nagao K, Yokoro K: Granulopoiesis in patients with congenital neutropenia. Am J Hematol 20:223, 1985.
8. Bonilla MA, Gillio AP, Ruggerio M, Kernan NA, Brochstein JA, Abboud M, Fumagalli L, Vincent M, Gabrilove JL, Welte K, Souzq L, O'Reilly RJ: Effects of recombinant human granulocyte colony-stimulating factor on neutropenia in patients with congenital agranulocytosis. N Engl J Med 320:1574, 1989.
9. Revoltella RP, Vigneti E, Cucina A, Stegagno M, Marolla L, Carapella DE: Congenital neutropenia: Sustained myeloid cell proliferation and neutrophil differentiation in vitro. Haematologica (Pavia) 73:455, 1988.

10. Espanol T, Compte J, Alvarez C, Tallada N, Laverde R, Peguero G: Reticular dysgenesis: Report of two brothers. Clin Exp Immunol 38:615, 1979.
11. Levinsky RJ, Tiedeman K: Successful bone-marrow transplantation for reticular dysgenesis. Lancet 1:671, 1983.
12. Roper M, Parmley RT, Crist WM, Kelly DR, Cooper M: Severe congenital leukopenia (reticular dysgenesis). Immunologic and morphologic characterizations of leukocytes. Am J Dis Child 139:832, 1985.
13. Ochs HD, Davis SD, Mickelson E, Lerner KG, Wedgwood RJ: Combined immunodeficiency and reticuloendotheliosis with eosinophilia. J Pediatr 85:463, 1974.
14. Ownby DR, Pizzo S, Blackmon L, Gall SA, Buckley RH: Severe combined immunodeficiency with leukopenia (reticular dysgenesis) in siblings: Immunologic and histopathologic findings. J Pediatr 89:382, 1976.
15. Shokeir MH: Short stature, absent thumbs, flat facies, anosmia and combined immune deficiency (CID). Birth Defects 14:103, 1978.
16. Wilson WG, Aylsworth AS, Folds JH, Whisnant JK: Cartilage-hair hypoplasia (metaphyseal chondrodysplasia, type McKusick) with combined immune deficiency: Variable expression and development of immunologic functions in sibs. Birth Defects 14:117, 1978.
17. Wyss M, Von Flieder V, Jacot DE, Jeannet M, Despont JP, Kapanci Y, Cox JN: A lymphoproliferative syndrome, "cutaneous dystrophy" and combined immune deficiency with lack of helper T-cell factor. Clin Immunol Immunopathol 23:34, 1982.
18. Smith C, Gasparetto C, Collins N, Gillio A, Muench MO, O'Reilly RJ, Moore MAS: Purification and partial characterization of a human hematopoietic precursor population. Blood 77:2122, 1991.
19. Gasson JC, Weisbart RH, Kaufman SE, Clark SC, Hewick RM, Wong GG, Golde DW: Purified human granulocyte-macrophage colony-stimulating factor: Direct action on neutrophils. Science 226:1339, 1984.
20. Ikebuchi K, Ihle JN, Hiria Y, Wong G, Clark SC, Ogawa M: Synergistic factors for stem cell proliferation: Further studies of the target stem cells and the mechanism of stimulation by interleukin-1, interleukin-6, and granulocyte colony-stimulating factor. Blood 72:2007, 1988.
21. Lu L, Broxmeyer HE: The selective enhancing influence of hemin and products of human erythrocytes on colony formation by human multipotential (CFU-GEMM) and erythroid (BFU-E) progenitor cells In-Vitro. Exp Hematol 8:721, 1983.
22. Chomczynski P, Sacchi N: Single step method of RNA isolated by acid guanidinium thiocyanate-phenol-chloroform extraction. Analy Biochem 162:156, 1987.
23. Keever CA, Small T, Flomemberg N, Heller G, Packle K, Black P, Pecora A, Gillio A, Kernan N, O'Reilly RJ: Immune reconstitution following bone marrow transplantation: Comparison of recipients of T-cell depleted marrow with recipients of conventional marrow grafts. Blood 73:1340, 1989.
24. Gasson JC, Bersch N, Golde DW: Characterization of purified human erythroid-potentiating activity. Prog Clin Biol Res 184:95, 1985.
25. Broxmeyer HE, Cooper S, Lu L, Hangoc G, Anderson D, Cosman D, Lyman SD, Williams DE: Effect of murine mast cell growth factor (C-Kit Proto-Oncogene Ligand) on colony formation by human marrow hematopoietic progenitor cells. Blood 77:2142, 1991.
26. Holbrook ST, Ohls RK, Schibler KR, Yang YC, Christensen RD: Effect of interleukin-9 on clonogenic maturation and cell-cycle status of fetal and adult hematopoietic progenitors. Blood 77:2129, 1991.
27. Dorshkind K, Johnson A, Harrison Y, Landreth KS: A colony assay system that detects B cell progenitors in fresh and cultured bone marrow. J Immunol Methods 123:93, 1989.
28. Lubin I, Faktorowich Y, Lapidot TT, Gan Y, Eshar Z, Gazit E, Levite M, Reisner Y: Engraftment and development of human T and B cells in mice after bone marrow transplantation. Science 252:427, 1991.
29. Moore MAS: Haemopoietic growth factor interactions: In vitro and in vivo preclinical evaluation. Cancer Surv 9:7, 1990.
30. Cashman JD, Eaves AC, Raines EW, Ross R, Eaves C: Mechanisms that regulate the cell cycle status of very primitive hematopoietic cell in long term human marrow cultures. I. Stimulatory role of a variety of mesenchymal cell activators and inhibitory role of TGF-β. Blood 75:96, 1990.
31. Harrison DE, Zhong RK: The same exhaustable multilineage precursor produces both myeloid and lymphoid cells as early as 3–4 weeks after marrow transplantation. Proc Natl Acad Sci USA 89:10134, 1992.

American Journal of Hematology 45:73–78 (1994)

Clinical Studies in Hemostasis and Thrombosis at Temple University School of Medicine

Factor XI Deficiency and Hemostasis

Robert W. Colman, A. Koneti Rao, and Ronald N. Rubin, Editors
Department of Medicine and Sol Sherry Thrombosis Research Center, Temple University School of Medicine, Temple University, Philadelphia

DISCUSSANT AND PRESENTER: *Dr. Peter N. Walsh, Professor of Medicine and Biochemistry.*

The subject of today's conference is factor XI deficiency and hemostasis. First, I would like to present two patients with factor XI deficiency and discuss their evaluation and management since the problems posed by these two patients focus on the biological role of factor XI in normal hemostasis.

The first patient is a 53-year-old white female who was referred for evaluation of a prolonged activated partial thromboplastin time (APTT) discovered during presurgical screening for cosmetic surgery. Her past medical history was negative for any abnormal bleeding problems either spontaneous or post-traumatic. Specifically she had undergone tonsillectomy at the age of 6 and a cholecystectomy at age 35 without bleeding complications and without the administration of any blood products. Her medications included Prozac and Premarin. Her hemostatic evaluation showed a bleeding time of 5 min, prothrombin time of 12.3 sec (normal 11.0–14.0), and APTT of 61 sec (normal 25–40). Since she had a prolonged APTT with a normal prothrombin time, patient plasma was mixed at various ratios with normal plasma and the APTT repeated to rule out the possibility of a coagulation inhibitor including a lupus inhibitor. However, the normal plasma corrected the abnormality in patient plasma. In addition, the dilute Russell's viper venom time, although slightly prolonged, was not sufficiently abnormal to indicate a lupus inhibitor. Further, her tissue thromboplastin inhibition test, another test for lupus inhibitor, was normal. In the presence of a prolonged APTT with a normal prothrombin time, an intrinsic clotting factor deficiency was suspected and, therefore, factor assays for factor VIII, factor IX, and factor XI, and factor XII were carried out. These were normal with the exception of the factor XI level which was 0.05 U/ml (normal 0.6–1.4 U/ml). The patient underwent uneventful cosmetic surgery without excessive bleeding, having previously received sufficient immunopurified virus-inactivated factor XI to raise her factor XI level to 50% of normal.

The second patient is a 51-year-old white female who was referred for evaluation of a prolonged APTT (58 sec) discovered during presurgical evaluation for foot surgery. She gave a past medical history of abnormal bleeding after tonsillectomy in childhood and subsequently abnormal bleeding after both dental extraction and ovarian surgery during adulthood. She also noted the presence of periodic ecchymoses. Laboratory evaluation disclosed an APTT of 60 sec and a prothrombin time of 11.8 sec. Her thrombin time was normal at 22 sec and her fibrinogen level was 320 mg/dl. Because of the prolongation of APTT with a normal PT, a mixing study was done to exclude the possibility of an inhibitor either of the lupus type or directed against a specific intrinsic coagulation factor. Normal plasma corrected the defect in the patient's APTT, and the dilute Russell's viper venom time and a tissue thromboplastin inhibition test were both normal. Factor assays were carried out disclosing normal values for factor VIII, factor IX, and factor XII, whereas her factor XI level was 0.07 U/ml.

Thus, we have two middle-aged white females with moderately severe factor XI deficiency (0.05–0.07 U/ml), one of whom has a history of severe posttraumatic and postsurgical hemorrhage and the other of whom has never experienced abnormal bleeding despite multiple surgical challenges. The clinical and laboratory findings in these two patients pose the question, why do some patients with factor XI deficiency have abnormal bleeding whereas other patients appear to be hemostatically normal?

A number of years ago we carried out a study [1] aimed to address this question and to define the bleeding manifestations in patients with factor XI deficiency. Since one of the objectives of this study was to determine whether patients with bleeding problems could be distinguished

Received for publication February 21, 1993; accepted May 19, 1993.

Address reprint requests to Dr. Peter N. Walsh, Thrombosis Research Center, Temple University School of Medicine, 3400 N. Broad Street, Philadelphia, PA 19140.

from those without bleeding problems by virtue of the presence of abnormal factor XI protein in plasma, we developed a radioimmunoassay for factor XI as well as a coagulation assay. Those patients with "crossreacting-material-positive" (CRM+) factor XI deficiency would be expected to have factor XI antigen levels in excess of the coagulant activity. The correlation between the factor XI antigen and the factor XI coagulant activity was excellent and only two patients with significantly higher levels of antigen than activity were detected.

We next carried out factor XI coagulant activity measurements and factor XI antigen measurements on plasmas obtained from 78 different members of 25 factor-XI-deficient kindreds. Factor XI deficiency was defined as a factor XI level less than 0.50 U/ml, and patients meeting this criterion were prospectively classified either as bleeders (22) or nonbleeders (21) based on carefully and uniformly collected historical information.

The mean factor XI coagulant activity and factor XI antigen levels were identical in both bleeders and nonbleeders. Thus, no evidence emerged from this study that one could distinguish patients with a propensity to bleed abnormally on the basis of either factor XI coagulant activity or factor XI antigen levels.

We then examined the distribution of factor XI coagulant activity and factor XI antigen levels in bleeding and nonbleeding factor-XI-deficient patients classified as having either severe factor XI deficiency (0–0.05 U/ml) or mild to moderate factor XI deficiency (0.06–0.50 U/ml). Even among patients with severe factor XI deficiency there was no tendency for bleeders to have a lower level of factor XI than nonbleeders.

We concluded from this study that there is a strong correlation between factor XI coagulant activity and factor XI antigen in plasmas obtained from study of factor-XI-deficient kindreds. Furthermore, at least 50% of the factor-XI-deficient individuals had no history of abnormal bleeding. An interesting observation made as a part of this study was that the bleeding tendency appears to be consistent within a given factor-XI-deficient kindred. Thus, if the propositus had a bleeding history so did other factor-XI-deficient members of that family. On the other hand, a factor-XI-deficient individual without a history of bleeding had other family members who were similarly unaffected by hemostatic abnormalities.

Recent new information emerging from the seminal work of Asakai et al. [2] has focused on the genetics of factor XI deficiency. Factor XI deficiency has been observed to be a rare autosomal dominant trait with only about one affected individual per 100,000 in the population. In contrast, however, it has been shown that in Jewish people of Ashkenazi descent the frequency of the disorder is about 1 in 190 individuals. Recently it has been shown that three independent point mutations, designated types I, II, and III, account for factor XI deficiency in Ashkenazi Jews. A mutation at an intron-exon boundary that disrupts normal mRNA splicing accounts for the type I deficiency whereas premature polypeptide termination due to a nonsense mutation at position 117 accounts for type II deficiency. An amino acid substitution of phenylalanine 283 to leucine accounts for the type III mutation which apparently results in a decreased rate of protein secretion. Recently, an analysis of two of these genetic mutations (Types II and III) was carried out in 52 unrelated families utilizing the polymerase chain reaction and restriction enzyme digestion. The mean factor XI level in patients with homozygous type III deficiency was significantly higher (9.7%) than in patients with the homozygous type II deficiency (1.2%), and compound heterozygotes for type II/III defects had an intermediate factor XI level (3.3%). Furthermore, the fraction of surgical procedures complicated by bleeding in patients with severe factor XI deficiency appeared to be larger in patients with heterozygous type II deficiency than in patients with the type III deficiency, suggesting that lower plasma levels of factor XI are associated with more severe bleeding complications. These interesting and elegant studies, however, do not address the unanswered question posed by the fact that some patients with severe factor XI deficiency appear not to have defects in hemostatic function whereas others do.

Dr. Ronald N. Rubin, Professor of Medicine: Did the authors mention what these surgical procedures were?

Dr. Walsh: Yes. They were other than tonsillectomy, urological, nasal surgery, or tooth extractions. Thus they were apparently major operations.

Dr. H. James Day, Professor of Medicine: In my reading of the paper by Asaki et al. [2] there did not seem to be a clearly documented relationship between the factor XI level and the propensity to bleed.

Dr. Walsh: The patients with the type II deficiency had levels of 1.2% and were said to bleed more extensively, although I agree the numbers were small and the differences in bleeding frequencies seemed marginal. Furthermore, these data still do not answer the question of why some patients with factor XI deficiency are not bleeders. The authors also indicate that tissues in which there is a high level of fibrinolytic activity, such as dental or nasal tissue, are relatively unaffected by the level of factor XI whereas tissues where the fibrinolytic system is not quite so active are more affected. The hypothesis that I am very interested in examining is whether patients in the bleeding category have lower levels of *platelet* factor XI than those in the nonbleeding category. We are currently carrying out studies aimed at detecting factor XI mRNA in platelets using reverse transcriptase and the polymerase chain reaction. I will discuss platelet factor XI later.

Dr. Robert W. Colman, Professor of Medicine: Well, I am very attracted to that explanation for another reason. There is already an example of this phenomenon with respect to factor V. Factor V_{Quebec} patients who are bleeders have about 50% factor V in their plasma which does not cause any hemostatic defects but they have 2% factor V in their platelets. There is a single family described by Ken Mann's group. This disease is unlike classical factor V deficiency where synthesis is decreased. Factor V_{Quebec} is presumably due to biosynthetic failure of expression of factor V in megakaryocytes. However, there is a quantitative difference for factor XI. Platelet factor V is 25% of blood factor V whereas factor XI in platelets is 0.5%.

Dr. Walsh: Next, to place this problem in some perspective, I would like to review the biochemical mechanisms involved in the activation of the coagulation cascade and the clinical consequences of deficiencies of the various coagulation proteins. The proteins involved in the activation of factor XI include factor XII, prekallikrein, and high molecular weight kininogen which interact on negatively charged surfaces including those provided by platelet membranes to promote the reciprocal proteolytic activation of factor XII and prekallikrein. Factor XIIa, generated both by the action of kallikrein and also through autocatalysis with factor XIIa, then accelerates the activation of factor XI. Factor XI circulates in plasma in a noncovalent complex with high molecular weight kininogen which is required for binding of factor XI to negatively charged surfaces including activated platelets which can increase rates of factor-XI activation by factor XIIa. The factor XIa thus generated recognizes factor IX as its normal macromolecular substrate. As I have pointed out, about 50% of factor-XI-deficient patients have abnormal bleeding whereas in contrast, patients with factor XII deficiency, prekallikrein deficiency, and high molecular weight kininogen deficiency have not been reported to experience defective hemostasis.

Thus, the conundrum posed by the clinical and biochemical information concerning factor XI is as follows. The facts are, first, that about 50% of factor-XI-deficient patients have defective hemostasis; second, that factor XII, prekallikrein, and high molecular weight kininogen are essential for contact activation of factor XI in vitro; and, third, that deficiencies of factor XII, prekallikrein, and high molecular weight kininogen are not associated with defective hemostasis. Thus, the two central problems which emerge from these facts are first, how is factor XI activated in vivo? And, second, how is the requirement for factor XI obviated in some people?

There are two hypotheses that have been advanced in the past to deal with this central problem and account for the activation of factor XI in vivo. The first of these has been advanced by our laboratory and focuses on redundant or alterative platelet-mediated pathways of factor-XI activation by either factor XIIa or kallikrein [3,4]. The second of these hypotheses arises from recent elegant work by Naito and Fujikawa [5] and by Gailani and Broze [6] and focuses on the dextran sulfate-mediated factor-XI activation either by thrombin or by factor XIa.

The second of these two hypotheses [5,6] suggests that the initial event in hemostasis is the exposure of tissue factor at sites of vascular injury which results in generation of factor VIIa and the subsequent activation of factor X. The generation of factor Xa allows the tissue factor pathway inhibitor (TFPI) to inactivate factor VIIa and to prevent further factor Xa formation but not before small quantities of thrombin are formed which can initially feed back to activate factor V and factor VIII and, in addition, activate factor XI by a factor XII-independent pathway. Both Naito and Fujikawa [5] and Gailani and Broze [6] have shown that both thrombin and factor XIa can catalyze the conversion of factor XI to factor XIa, but this reaction requires the presence of dextran sulfate, a substance not normally found at sites of hemostatic plug formation. There are two serious problems with this intriguing and otherwise elegant hypothesis, one of which is that the presence of high molecular weight kininogen [5,6,7] and fibrinogen [7], both found in large molar excess in plasma in relation to concentrations of thrombin or factor XIa, both inhibit factor-XI activation by both thrombin and factor XIa. The second problem is that no physiological surface has been identified which might serve to assemble these proteins in vivo. Nonetheless, further work is required to investigate the validity of this attractive hypothesis since it does potentially explain why factor XI is required for normal hemostatsis but factor XII, prekallikrein, and high molecular weight kininogen are not.

Our laboratory has presented a series of observations focusing on the role of platelets in the activation of factor XI which indicate that activated platelets can promote factor-XI activation by factor XIIa in the presence of high molecular weight kininogen [3,4,8]. Moreover, activated platelets can promote factor-XI activation in the absence of factor XII provided kallikrein is present [4]. In addition, factor XI binds specifically to high affinity saturable receptors on activated platelets in the presence of high molecular weight kininogen and zinc ions [9]. These observations and others suggest that high molecular weight kininogen mediated factor XI binding to activated platelets can promote factor-XI activation by factor XIIa and by factor XII-independent kallikrein-dependent mechanisms. Since there is no evidence that factor XI can serve as an alternative substrate for kallikrein, the mechanism by which this alternative pathway occurs is as yet unknown.

Dr. A. Koneti Rao, Professor of Medicine: Is high molecular weight kininogen required for activation of factor XI by both these two alternative pathways?

Dr. Walsh: No. We showed that the presence of high molecular weight kininogen enhanced rates of factor-XI activation by both pathways but was not an absolute requirement. Perhaps in the absence of plasma high molecular weight kininogen, the protein secreted from platelets can suffice.

Next we have shown that factor XIa formed on the platelet surface binds specifically to high affinity saturable receptors on activated platelets in the presence of high molecular weight kininogen [10]. A careful analysis of rates of factor-IX activation by platelet-bound and unbound factor XIa indicate that these reaction rates are nearly identical. However, platelet-bound factor XIa appears to be protected from inhibition by and complex formation with α-1-protease inhibitor, the major plasma inhibitor of factor XIa [11]. In addition, activated platelets secrete two specific potent inhibitors of factor XIa from which platelet-bound factor XIa is protected. One of these inhibitors has been purified and characterized in our laboratory and is referred to as the *p*latelet *i*nhibitor of factor *XI*a (or PIXI) whereas the other is protease nexin II which is a truncated form of the transmembrane Alzheimer's amyloid β-protein precursor. The conclusion to be drawn from these observations is that the binding of factor XIa and factor IX to activated platelets may localize factor-IX activation to the platelet surface. Factor IXa then binds to a platelet receptor in the presence of factor VIIIa which is bound to a distinct site on platelet membranes with a resultant 20 million-fold acceleration of the catalytic efficiency of factor-X activation [13].

Next, I would like to discuss the second major enigma related to the biological function of factor XI. Why do half the patients with severe factor XI deficiency have no apparent defects in hemostatic function often in the face of severe traumatic or surgical challenge? About 20 years ago our laboratory discovered that careful repeated and extensive platelet washing was unable to remove factor XI activity completely and that well-washed platelet suspensions which lacked many of the other coagulation proteins still had significant quantities of factor XI [3,8]. Subsequent work from our laboratory demonstrated that this activity resided in the platelet plasma membrane [14]. To explore this curious and interesting observation further, we prepared a monospecific polyclonal antibody to factor XI and used it in immunofluorescence studies. We demonstrated that well-washed platelets incubated with antifactor XI antibody and then with fluorescein-labeled goat antirabbit IgG showed immunofluorescence reflecting the presence of factor XI antigen, whereas if the antibody was previously adsorbed with factor XI this immunofluorescence was abolished [15]. Preincubation of platelets with factor XI further enhanced this immunofluorescence. These results indicated that not only did the platelets possess factor XI activity but they also possessed a protein specifically recognized by an antifactor XI antibody. We, therefore, carried out both immunoprecipitation and partial purification studies aimed at the further characterization of platelet factor XI. An SDS gel of a radiolabeled platelet extract immunoprecipitated with antifactor XI antibody demonstrated a 220,000 da platelet protein under nonreducing conditions, whereas immunoprecipitated plasma purified factor XI migrated at a molecular weight of 160,000 da as expected. Platelet extract immunoprecipitated with control serum showed no evidence of a radioactive band. Under reducing conditions, immunoprecipitated plasma factor XI showed a radioactive band at 80,000 da as expected whereas the immunoprecipitated platelet factor XI migrated at a subunit molecular weight of 55,000. This suggests that platelet factor XI may exist as a 220,000 da tetramer consisting of four 55,000 molecular weight subunits compared with plasma factor XI which has a molecular weight of 160,000 da and consists of two identical 80,000 da subunits. Our data indicate that platelet factor XI accounts for approximately 0.5% of the total factor XI activity in blood.

Dr. Colman: Would it be worthwhile to use a factor XI probe and screen a megakaryocyte or HEL cell library to detect a cDNA for platelet factor XI? Alternatively, one could use reverse transcriptase followed by polymerase chain reaction on platelets to try to detect mRNA for platelet factor XI.

Dr. Walsh: Yes, as I mentioned previously, we are doing just that currently.

Dr. Colman: I think this situation is not unprecedented because we know from the work of Altieri and Edgington that there is a factor V-like molecule in monocytes which has different molecular properties but retains the biological activities of factor V such as binding of factor Xa. Thus, platelet factor XI is an interesting molecule that deserves a second look with the molecular biological techniques that were not available in 1985 when you did the studies in collaboration with our group.

Dr. Walsh: I agree.

Dr. Robin Pixley, Research Associate Professor: Did you detrmine whether platelet factor XI might be present as a factor XIa-antitrypsin complex on the membrane? Its molecular weight would be 220,000 da. Did you look to see if there was an antitrypsin component?

Dr. Walsh: No, but the labeled factor XIa in the putative complex would not be expected to disassociate to 55,000 da.

Dr. Pixley: However, antitrypsin has a molecular weight of 55,000 da.

Dr. Walsh: But it wasn't antitrypsin that was labeled; rather platelets were labeled. Where would the antitrypsin come from?

Dr. Colman: Platelets contain α-1-antitrypsin as we and Dr. Ralph Nachman's group showed a number of years ago.

Dr. Walsh: However, the platelets were surface-labeled and since factor XI is a membrane protein, whereas antitrypsin (α-1-protease inhibitor) is an α-granular protein, one would expect factor XI but not antitrypsin to be available for labeling in unactivated platelets.

Additional observations indicated that platelet factor XI was present in normal concentrations in the platelets of selected patients with less than 1% plasma factor XI and no evidence of abnormal bleeding despite surgical or traumatic challenge. A small number of additional selected patients with less than 1% plasma factor XI who had excessive bleeding histories showed the absence of platelet factor XI in platelets and in plasma. These observations [15] give rise to the hypothesis that platelet factor XI can substitute for plasma factor XI in some patients with severe plasma factor XI deficiency. I hasten to add that this hypothesis is currently unproven and would require the development of sensitive techniques for measuring platelet factor XI antigen and activity to be applied to the study of larger numbers of patients with and without abnormal bleeding, all of whom lack plasma factor XI.

Finally, I would like to discuss some studies done in collaboration with the laboratory of Dr. Robert Colman that focus on the evaluation of naturally occurring human antibodies against two distinct functional domains in factor XI [16]. From the sequence of a cDNA insert coding for factor XI the amino acid sequence has been deduced [17]. In addition to a typical trypsin-like serine protease catalytic domain comprising the light chain of factor XI cleaved by factor XIIa, the resultant heavy chain contains four tandem repeat sequences termed Apple domains because of the characteristic disulfide linkages mediated by six of the six or seven cysteines within each of the Apple domains. Utilizing a variety of approaches including monoclonal antibodies, molecular modeling, and synthetic peptides we have defined functions for two of these four Apple domains. The Apple 1 domain mediates the binding of factor XI to high molecular weight kininogen with which it circulates in a noncovalent complex in plasma and with which it is bound to negatively charged surfaces such as platelets [18]. We have described a monoclonal antibody which specifically interferes with the binding of factor XI to high molecular weight kininogen [19]. In addition, the Apple 2 domain contains a substrate binding site for factor IX, the normal macromolecular substrate for factor XIa [20,21]. Another monoclonal antibody developed in our laboratory competes with binding of factor IX to the Apple 2 domain of factor XIa [22]. Therefore, when two patients were referred for evaluation of antifactor XI antibodies we utilized similar techniques for assessing the effects of these antibodies both in terms of binding of factor XI to high molecular weight kininogen and the role of factor XIa in the activation of factor IX [16].

The first of these patients was a 79-year-old Jewish man referred from Baltimore with congenital factor XI deficiency and recurrent episodes of urinary bleeding for which he received fresh frozen plasma. The patient had a prior history of hematuria requiring the administration of fresh frozen plasma, and subsequently he had experienced rectal bleeding and hematuria for which he was given additional fresh frozen plasma. Mixing studies of the patient's plasma and normal plasma showed a prolongation of the APTT indicating the presence of an inhibitor. This inhibitor was purified and characterized and used in an assay which measures the binding of factor XI to high molecular weight kininogen. This antibody is a potent inhibitor of factor XI binding to high molecular weight kininogen, whereas an antibody obtained from a patient referred from Winston-Salem had no such inhibitory activity. Thus, it is interesting that although this patient certainly had significant bleeding, the development of an antibody against the high molecular weight kininogen binding domain in factor XI was associated with an increased propensity to hemorrhage that was reasonably easily controlled.

The second patient is a 28-year-old Jewish woman who had a past medical history of moderate bleeding after tonsillectomy at age 18 for which she required the administration of fresh frozen plasma after a diagnosis of factor XI deficiency was established. Subsequently, at age 25, after a normal pregnancy and delivery, she experienced abnormal uterine bleeding and received 2 U of fresh frozen plasma which corrected her APTT from 85 to 43 sec. After 24 hr of continuous uterine bleeding her hemoglobin fell to 7.7 g/dl and she required multiple transfusions with packed red cells and fresh frozen plasma. Although she received daily infusions of fresh frozen plasma for 5 days, she had to be readmitted 48 hr after discharge because of recurrent uterine hemorrhage. A factor XI antibody was diagnosed on the basis of mixing studies, and after a rather stormy course her bleeding was finally controlled with the administration of multiple units of packed red blood cells, fresh frozen plasma, and epsilon aminocaproic acid therapy. The antibody from this patient's plasma was also purified, characterized, and studied along with the antibody from the Baltimore patient in an assay which measures the activation of factor IX by factor XIa. The purified antibody from the Winston-Salem patient was a potent inhibitor of factor-XIa-catalyzed factor-IX activation whereas the antibody from the Baltimore patient had no such inhibitory effect.

Dr. Rao: What was the factor XI antigen in both these patients?

Dr. Walsh: We did not measure platelet factor XI because we require a whole unit of platelets in order to measure factor XI antigen, which is not feasible. We also did not measure plasma factor XI antigen. I assume that it would probably be low since both patients had congenital factor XI deficiency with very low levels of factor XI. Antibodies in both these patients arose on the basis of prior transfusions.

Dr. Walsh: Thus, we have two patients with antibodies with apparently limited epitope specificity [16] that are quite similar to monoclonal antibodies raised in mice and evaluated in our laboratory [19,20–23]. I find it particularly interesting that the patient who developed an antibody against the Apple 2 domain and the factor IX substrate binding site in factor XIa had particularly malignant bleeding that required rather heroic measures for control. This implies to me that the Apple 2 domain which contains the factor IX substrate binding site in factor XIa is particularly important in the biological function of factor XI. These observations [16] go a long way toward proving that factor XI is an essential coagulation protein whose deficiency or inhibition, particularly of its enzymatic activity against factor IX, can promote serious defects in hemostatic function.

In summary, a large amount of new information has focused recently on the biochemistry, genetics, and biology of factor XI which have given rise to a resurgence of interest in this fascinating and unique protein. Information I have only briefly discussed today has focused on the domain structure and the structure-function relationships of factor XI as well as its molecular and cellular interactions. In addition, elegant work on the molecular genetics of factor XI has yielded new insights into the organization of the gene and its abnormalities in patients with factor XI deficiency. Although novel pathways of activation of factor XI have been described, it is my view that we still do not have the full story about the mechanisms by which factor XI is activated in vivo either by contact phase-dependent pathways or by other factor XII-independent mechanisms. In addition, recent work on the expression and regulation of the enzymatic activity of factor XI has provided new insights about how this protein functions in normal hemostasis and about the control mechanisms involved in regulating its enzymatic activity. Finally, I have tried to focus on the physiological role of factor XI in hemostasis and to propose testable hypotheses that focus on two related questions, one of which is why some patients with factor XI deficiency bleed abnormally and the second of which is why some patients with factor XI deficiency do not bleed abnormally.

REFERENCES

1. Ragni MV, Sinha D, Seaman F, Lewis JH, Spero JA, Walsh PN: Comparison of bleeding tendency, factor XI coagulant activity and factor XI antigen in twenty-five factor XI deficient kindreds. Blood 65:719–724, 1985.
2. Asakai R, Chung DW, Davie EW, Seligsohn U: Factor XI deficiency in Ashkenazi Jews in Israel. New Engl J Med 325:153–158, 1991.
3. Walsh PN. The effects of collagen and kaolin on the intrinsic coagulant activity of platelets. Evidence for an alternative pathway in intrinsic coagulation not requiring factor XII. Br J Haematol 22:393–405, 1972.
4. Walsh PN, Griffin JH: Contributions of human platelets to the proteolytic activation of blood coagulation factors XII and XI. Blood 57:106–118, 1981.
5. Naito K, Fujikawa K: Activation of human blood coagulation factor XI independent of factor XII. Factor XI is activated by thrombin and factor XIa in the presence of negatively charged surfaces. J Biol Chem 266:7353–7358, 1991.
6. Gailani D, Broze GJ Jr: Factor XI activation in a revised model of blood coagulation. Science 253:909–912, 1991.
7. Scott CF, Colman RW: Fibrinogen blocks the autoactivation and thrombin-mediated activation of factor XI on dextran sulfate. Proc Natl Acad Sci USA 89:11189–11193, 1992.
8. Walsh PN: The role of platelets in the contact phase of blood coagulation. Br J Haematol 22:237–254, 1972.
9. Greengard JS, Heeb MJ, Ersdal E, Walsh PN, Griffin JH: Binding of blood coagulation factor XI to human platelets. Biochemistry 25:3884–3890, 1986.
10. Sinha D, Seaman FS, Koshy A, Knight LC, Walsh PN: Blood coagulation factor XIa binds specifically to a site on activated human platelets distinct from that for factor XI. J Clin Invest 73:1550–1556, 1984.
11. Walsh PN, Sinha D, Keuppers F, Blankstein KB, Seaman FS: Regulation of factor XIa activity by platelets and alpha-1-protease inhibitor. J Clin Invest 80:1578–1586, 1987.
12. Cronlund AL, Walsh PN: A low molecular weight platelet inhibitor of factor XIa (PIXI): Purification, characterization and possible role in blood coagulation. Biochemistry 31:1685–1694, 1992.
13. Rawala-Sheikh R, Ahmad SS, Ashby B, Walsh PN: Kinetics of coagulation factor X activation by platelet-bound factor IXa. Biochemistry 29:2606–2611, 1990.
14. Lipscomb MS, Walsh PN: Human platelets and factor XI. Localization in platelet membranes of factor-XI-like activity and its functional distinction from plasma factor XI. J Clin Invest 63:1006–1014, 1979.
15. Tuszynski GP, Bevacqua SJ, Schmaier AH, Colman RW, Walsh PN: Factor XI antigen and activity in human platelets. Blood 59:1148–1156, 1982.
16. De La Cadena RA, Baglia FA, Johnson CA, Wenk RE, Amernick R, Walsh PN, Colman RW: Naturally occurring human antibodies against two distinct functional domains in the heavy chain of FXI/FXIa. Blood 72:1748–1754, 1988.
17. Fujikawa K, Chung DW, Hendrickson LE, et al.: Amino acid sequence of human factor XI, a blood coagulation factor with four tandem repeats that are highly homologous with plasma prekallikrein. Biochemistry 25:2417–2424, 1986.
18. Baglia FA, Jameson BA, Walsh PN: Fine mapping of the high molecular weight kininogen binding site on blood coagulation factor XI through the use of rationally designed synthetic analogs. J Biol Chem 267:4247–4252, 1992.
19. Sinha D, Koshy A, Seaman FS, Walsh PN: Functional characterization of human blood coagulation factor XIa using hybridoma antibodies. J Biol Chem 260:10714–10719, 1985.
20. Sinha D, Seaman FS, Walsh PN: Role of calcium ions and the heavy chain of factor XIa in the activation of human coagulation factor IX. Biochemistry 26:3768–3775, 1987.
21. Baglia FA, Jameson BA, Walsh PN: Identification and chemical synthesis of a substrate-binding site for factor IX on coagulation factor XIa. J Biol Chem 266:24190–24197, 1991.
22. Akiyama H, Sinha D, Seaman FS, Kirby EP, Walsh PN: Mechanism of activation of coagulation factor XI by factor XIIa studied with monoclonal antibodies. J Clin Invest 78:1631–1637, 1986.
23. Baglia FA, Sinha D, Walsh PN: Functional domains in the heavy chain region of factor XI: A high molecular weight kininogen-binding site and a substrate-binding site for factor IX. Blood 74:244–251, 1989.

American Journal of Hematology 45:79–80 (1994)

Autoimmune-Thrombocytopenia and SLE in a Patient With 5q-Anomaly and Deletion of the c-fms Oncogene

Ulrich Jaeger, Simon Panzer, Claus Bartram, Oskar Haas, Beatrix Volc-Platzer, Wolfgang Graninger, Klaus Geissler, Thaddaeusz Radaszkiewicz, and Klaus Lechner

Divisions of Haematology (U.J., S.P., K.G., K.L.), Dermatology (B.V.-P.), Chemotherapy (W.G.), and Pathology (T.R.), University of Vienna, St. Anna Children's Hospital (O.H.), Vienna, Austria; Department of Pediatrics II, Ulm, Germany (C.B.)

Autoimmune-thrombocytopenia was the striking feature in a patient with typical clinical symptoms of systemic lupus erythematosus (SLE), complement C_4 deficiency, and positive lupus serology. However, myelodysplasia was found in the bone marrow and chromosome analysis revealed a deletion of the long arm of chromosome 5 (5q− anomaly), which was confirmed by a hemizygosity for the c-fms oncogene (CSF-1-receptor) on Southern blot. Autoimmune phenomena reported in conjunction with myelodysplastic syndromes (MDS), e.g., an elevation of antinuclear antibodies, are usually regarded as nonspecific. This case report suggests that SLE can occur in patients with MDS and that a concomitant autoimmune-thrombocytopenia may mask the typical signs of the 5q− syndrome.

Key words: myelodysplastic syndrome, immunologic phenomena, SLE

INTRODUCTION

Chromosomal deletion of the long arm of chromosome 5 results in a specific form of the myelodysplastic syndrome (MDS) associated with normal or high platelet counts, the 5q− syndrome [1–3]. On the DNA level it is associated with a deletion of the c-fms oncogene (CSF-1-receptor) [4,5], which has been implicated in the pathogenesis of the syndrome, but can also serve as a molecular marker for the allelic loss. Although various serological autoimmune phenomena (e.g., the elevation of antinuclear factors, ANF) have been reported in patients with MDS, these findings are regarded to be nonspecific manifestations appearing during the course of the neoplastic disease [6]. Here we report on a patient with a 5q− anomaly in whom frank systemic lupus erythematosus (SLE) and an associated autoimmune-thrombopenia have initially obscured the typical features of the 5q− syndrome.

CASE REPORT

A 35-year-old woman with a 6-month history of joint pain, recurrent headaches, visual disturbances, hair loss, and Raynaud's phenomenon was admitted because of severe menorrhagia. The patient had never received cytostatic treatment or irradiation and had no medication at the time of admission. On physical examination she appeared well. There was no evidence of lymphadenopathy or hepatosplenomegaly.

Peripheral blood tests showed severe thrombocytopenia (platelets 29 × 10^9/L), as well as an anemia (hemoglobin 11,9 g/dl) and leukocytopenia (WBC 2.0 × 10^9/L with 41% neutrophils, 7% eosinophils, 2% basophils, 40% lymphocytes, and 10% monocytes).

Tests for antinuclear antibodies (titer 1:800), anti-double-stranded DNA (780 IU/ml), as well as anti-Ro (SS-A) were positive. The direct Coomb's test was positive and the haptoglobin was less than 45 mg/dl. The total hemolytic complement (CH_{50}) was 103 IU/l, C_3 was 62.2 mg/dl, and C_4 was decreased to less than 8 mg/dl. The diagnosis of SLE was confirmed by direct immunofluorescent staining of a skin biopsy from a non-sun-exposed area which showed deposits of IgM and C_3 within blood vessels of the papillary dermis.

In addition, the thrombocytopenia was diagnosed to be of autoimmune origin, since the platelet-associated IgG

Received for publication January 17, 1993; accepted February 18, 1993.

Address reprint requests to Dr. Ulrich Jaeger, Klinik fuer Innere Medizin I, Abteilung Haematologie, Waehringer Guertel 18-20, A-1090 Vienna, Austria.

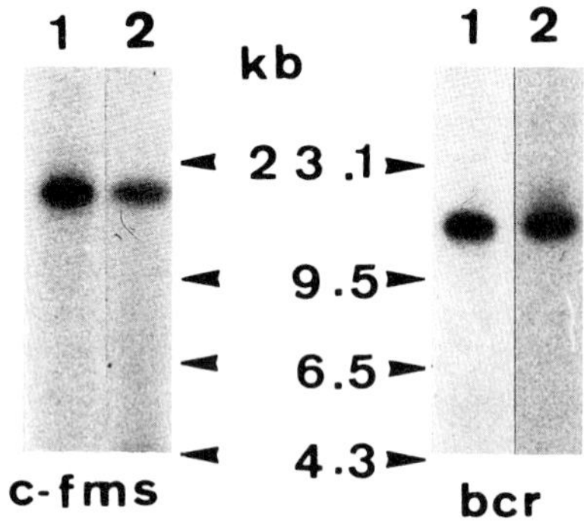

Fig. 1. Southern blot analysis of bone marrow DNA hybridized to c-fms sequences. Left: The patient's sample (lane 2) shows a normal-sized band which has only half the intensity of a normal control (lane 1). Right: Rehybridization of the same filter to sequences of the human bcr gene (from chromosome 22) shows equal intensity of control and patient samples. The data confirm a hemizygosity of the c-fms oncogene typical for a 5q− syndrome.

was 3.9% (normally less than 2.5%) and the autologous[111] Indium labeled platelet survival was only 2 days.

While the above features were indicative of an autoimmune disease, an additional bone marrow biopsy was performed because of the pancytopenia. Surprisingly, the histologic examination showed the classical signs of myelodysplasia like dyserythropoiesis and hypolobulated megacaryocytes as well as micromegacaryocytes. The blast cell count was less than 5%. Cytogenetic analysis of bone marrow cells revealed a deletion of the long arm of chromosome 5 (46 XX, 5q−) in 36% and a 5q− anomaly combined with a loss of chromosome 18 (45 XX, 5q−, −18) in 7% of the metaphases. The diagnosis was confirmed by Southern blot analysis of the patient's bone marrow DNA which showed a deletion of the c-fms oncogene (Fig. 1).

DISCUSSION

Thrombocytopenia was the diagnostic clue in this patient. The destruction of platelets due to an autoimmune mechanism in conjunction with serological and clinical features clearly established the diagnosis of SLE [7,8]. On the other hand, the patient has an underlying myelodysplastic syndrome with typical maturation defects in the bone marrow biopsy. The cytogenetic and molecular findings confirm the deletion of the long arm of chromosome 5 which is a very common finding in MDS [1,4,5]. However, the 5q− syndrome is characterized by normal or elevated platelet counts [2,3]. This typical feature was masked by the autoimmune thrombocytopenia in our case. Although, SLE and MDS are considered to be independent diseases, the occurrence of unspecific immune phenomena has been noted repeatedly in patients with MDS [6]. Increased amounts of platelet-bound immunoglobulin and circulating anti-platelet antibodies are frequently found in these patients [9]. However, frank SLE in conjunction with MDS is very rare [10] and has not been reported for a 5q− anomaly. It is noteworthy that despite the persistence of the serological signs of SLE, the thrombocyte count has spontaneously risen to more than 100×10^9/L over a period of 6 years, possibly indicating an increased 5q− activity. This case report suggests that the immunological abnormalities in MDS may not always be unspecific and that an underlying 5q− syndrome may be obscured by autoimmune-thrombocytopenia.

REFERENCES

1. List AF, Garewal HS, Sandberg AA: The myelodysplastic syndromes: Biology and implications for management. J Clin Oncol 8:1424, 1990.
2. Van den Berghe H, Vermaelen K, Mecucci C, Barbieri D, Tricot, G: The 5q− anomaly (Review article). Cancer Genet Cytogenet 17:189, 1985.
3. Wisnjewski LP, Hirschorn K: Acquired partial deletions of the long arm of chromosome 5 in hematologic disorders. Am J Hematol 15:295, 1985.
4. Kerkhofs H, Hagemaijer A, Leeksma CHW: The 5q− abnormality in haematological disorders: a collaborative study of 34 cases from the Netherlands. Br J Haematol 52:365, 1982.
5. Bartram R: Molecular genetic aspects of myelodysplastic syndromes. Haematol Oncol Clin North Am 6:557, 1992.
6. Mufti GJ, Figes A, Hamblin TJ, Oscier DG, Copplestone JA: Immunological abnormalities in myelodysplastic syndromes. Br J Haematol 63:143, 1986.
7. Anderson MJ, Peebles CL, McMillan R, Curd JG: Fluorescent antinuclear antibodies and anti-SS-A/Ro in patients with immune thrombocytopenia subsequently developing systemic lupus erythematosus. Arthritis and Rheumatism 25:1271, 1985.
8. Tan EM, Cohen AS, Fries JF, Masi AT, McShane DJ, Rothfield NF, Schaller JG, Talal N, Winchester RJ: The 1982 revised criteria for the classification of systemic lupus erythematosus. Arthritis and Rheumatism 25:1271, 1982.
9. Stadtmauer E, Cassileth P, Edelstein M: Thrombocytopenia in myelodysplasia: Response to danazol. Blood 72:299a, 1988 (suppl).
10. Ballas SK: Sideroblasic refractory anemia in a patient with systemic lupus erythematosus. Am J Med Sci 265:225, 1973.

American Journal of Hematology 45:81–84 (1994)

A Novel Mediterranean "δβ-Thalassemia" Determinant Containing the δ^+27 and $\beta^\circ 39$ Point Mutations in Cis

Lina Oggiano, Luciana Guiso, Laura Frogheri, Georgios Loudianos, Paola Pistidda, Elena Rimini, Mario Pirastu, Antonio Cao, and Maurizio Longinotti

Istituto di Ematologia ed Endocrinologia, Università degli Studi Sassari (L.O., M.L.); Istituto per lo Studio della Patologia del Sangue-CNR, Sassari (L.G., L.F., P.P., E.R.); Istituto di Clinica e Biologia dell'Età Evolutiva-Università degli Studi di Cagliari (G.L., A.C.); Istituto di Ricerca sulle Talassemie e Anemie Mediterranee CNR, Cagliari (M.P.), Italy

The term δβ-thalassemia with normal HbF has been recently proposed to define heterogenous δ and β globin gene molecular defects involving the same chromosome in cis. Here, we describe a Sardinian family in which three members showing microcytosis, border-line HbA_2 levels and normal HbF proved to be heterozygotes for δ^+27 and $\beta^\circ 39$ point mutations in cis by allele specific oligonucleotyde hybridization as well as by ECO 0 109 I endonuclease digestion and electrophoresis. As some of these β-thalassemia carriers shows normal HbA_2 levels, knowledge of the molecular basis of this novel δβ-thalassemia silent phenotype would be useful in thalassemia screening and genetic counselling.

Key words: novel δ^+27 $\beta^\circ 39$ thalassemia allele in cis

INTRODUCTION

Multiple thalassemic defects involving the δ- and β-globin genes in cis have been documented in cases of the Corfù δ (7.2 Kb del) β-thalassemia [1], δ°59-Hb Knossos [2,3], δ^+27-β^+ IVS II nt 745 [4], and δ+69-β^+IVSII nt 745 [5] alleles found in Mediterranean populations.

To define these conditions, usually characterized in heterozygotes by microcytosis, hypochromia and normal hemoglobin A_2 and HbF levels, the term "δβ-thalassemia with normal HbF level" has been proposed [4]. Since such heterozygous subjects may escape detection in HbA_2 quantitation based β-thalassemia screening, we now describe a Sardinian family in which a further "δβ-thalassemic" determinant has been detected bearing the δ^+27 (G-T) substitution and the non-sense $\beta^\circ 39$ defect in cis.

METHODS

Hematological and hemoglobin data were obtained by standard methods. DNA extraction, α-globin gene mapping, β-globin gene restriction fragment length polymorphism (RFLP), as well as the polymerase chain reaction (PCR) and dot blot analysis of amplified β and δ globin gene sequences with allele-specific oligonucleotide (ASO) hybridization were carried out as previously described [6]. The PCR based analysis of normal and mutated δ-globin genes by endonuclease digestion and agarose gel electrophoresis was as follows. Briefly, a δ-gene fragment spanning from position −297 bp upstream of CAP site to 371 bp of IVSII was amplified using direct 5′TACATTCCACTATATTAGCC3′ and reverse 5′CAGTATTCTATGCCTCTCAT3′ primers. 15 uL of the PCR product were digested by 10 U of ECO O 109 I at 37°C overnight according to the manufacturer's buffer conditions (New England Biolabs, Beverly, MA) and then subjected to TBE buffer/ethidium bromide agarose gel electrophoresis.

CASE REPORT

The family tree and the relevant hamatological and molecular data are shown in Figure 1. All members have a normal α-globin gene complement on Bam HI and Bgl II Southern blot analysis.

Received for publication April 30, 1993; accepted May 13, 1993.

Address reprint requests to Dr. Maurizio Longinotti, Istituto di Ematologia ed Endocrinologia, Università degli Studi di Sassari, viale San Pietro 12, 07100 Sassari, Italy.

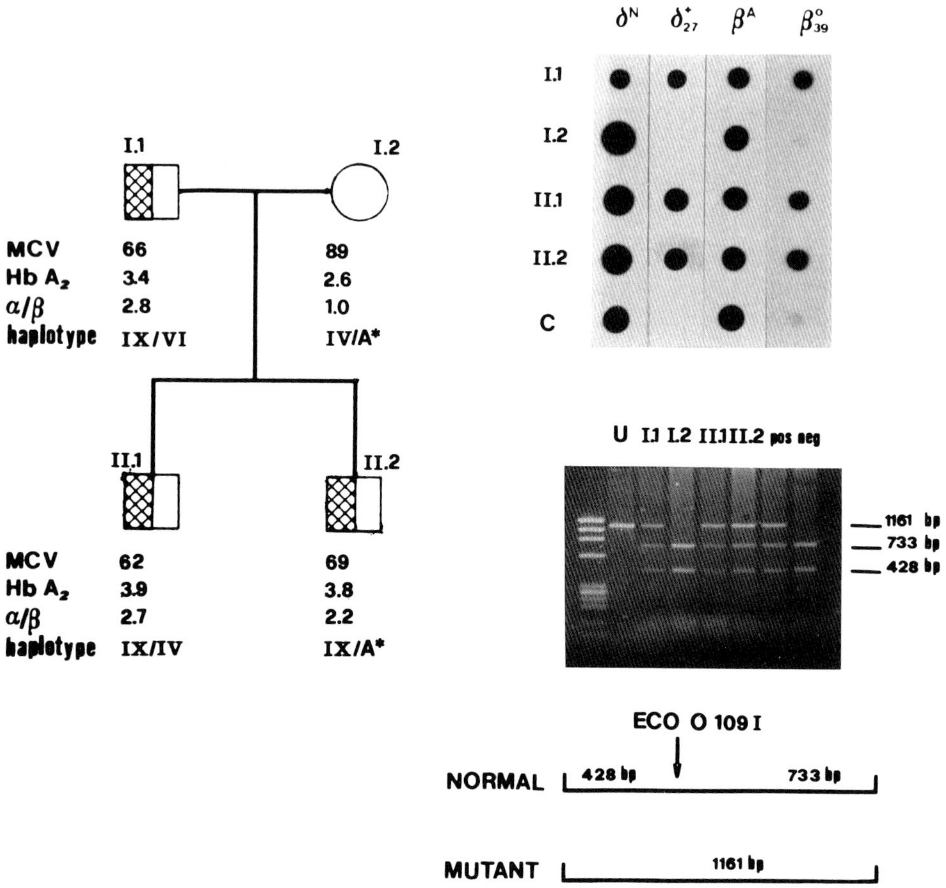

Fig. 1. Genealogical tree, hematological data, and β-globin gene haplotypes of the family studied. ⊠ indicates the chromosome carrying the $\delta^{+}27$ and the β°39 mutations in cis. A* indicates the haplotype − + + − + − + not included in Orkin's nomenclature (11). Dot blot analysis (right side, top) shows that amplified DNA of the father and sons hybridize with both normal and mutated β and δ ASO probes while that of the mother hybridizes with normal ASO probes only. C = Normal control. On the right side, bottom, detection of $\delta^{+}27$ (G-T) mutation has been performed by ECO O 109 I cleavage of a PCR amplified δ-globin gene fragment. The father (I,1) and the sons (II,1 and II,2) showing the 1161 bp fragment of the mutated allele as well as the restricted 733-bp and 428-bp bands of the normal allele are heterozygotes for the defect while the mother (I,2) is unaffected. Amplified undigested DNA (U) and known positive (pos) and negative (neg) controls are shown.

The father (I,1) as well as the sons II,1 and II,2 with typical thalassemic red cell indices, normal HbF levels and severe deficiency of β-globin chain synthesis, proved to be heterozygotes for the β°39 mutation on dot blot analysis with an ASO probe (Fig. 1, top).

The HbA_2 levels are however border-line (I,1) or only slightly increased (II,1 and II,2) in these otherwise typical β°39 carriers. This prompted us to investigate their δ-globin genes for the presence of the $\delta^{+}27$ (G-T) substitution which, when present in cis [4] as well as in trans [7], usually normalizes the HbA_2 levels of β-thalassemia heterozygotes of Mediterranean descent.

As postulated, the father and both sons also proved to be $\delta^{+}27$ thalassemia carriers while the mother, hematologically normal, was negative for $\delta^{+}27$ and β°39 defects on dot blot analysis (Fig. 1, top).

The heterozygosity for $\delta^{+}27$ mutation in the family members I,1, II,1 and II,2 was also demonstrated by the Eco O 109 I digestion of a PCR amplified 1161 bp δ-globin gene fragment (Fig. 1, bottom), which, if mutated, loses the specific cleavage restriction site. RFLP analysis confirms that $\delta^{+}27$ and β°39 mutations in cis are contained on a determinant showing haplotype IX, for which the father and the sons resulted heterozygotes at the β-globin gene cluster.

DISCUSSION

The Sardinian family investigated was shown to carry a new δβ-thalassemia determinant. This novel $\delta^{+}27$-β°39 allele might have originated from a crossing over of two different chromosomes (Fig. 2A), the first containing

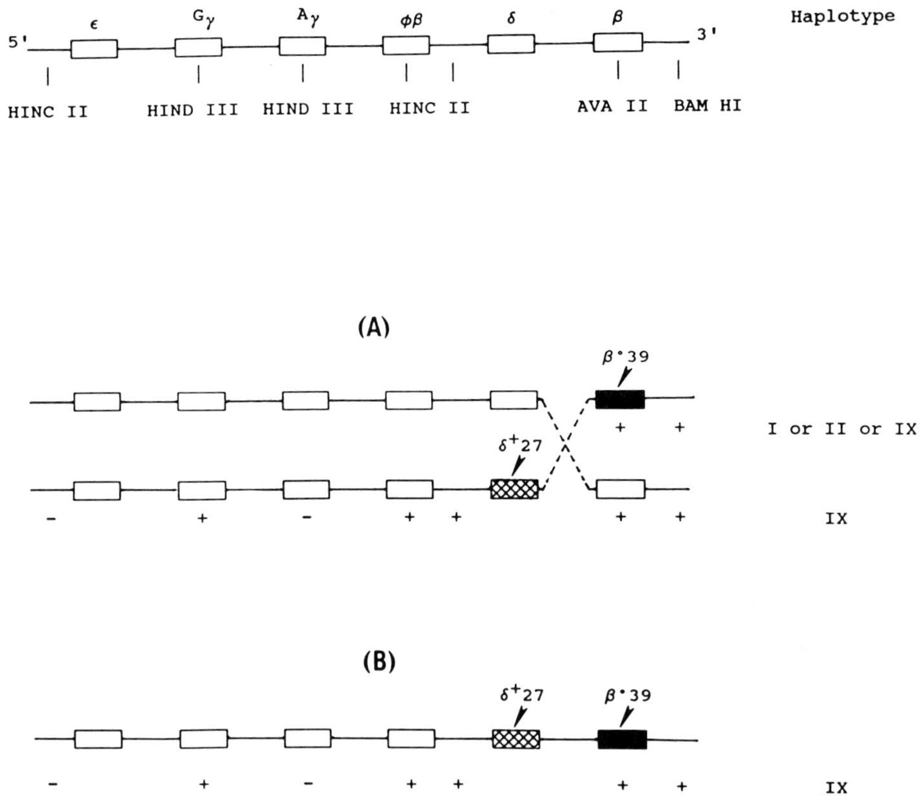

Fig. 2. Schematic illustration of the mechanisms by which the δ^+27-$\beta^\circ 39$ chromosome might have originated. Hypothesis A describes a crossing-over of two different chromosomes sharing the same 3′ AVA II and BAM HI restriction sites (+ +) on the β-globin gene cluster. In hypothesis B, the two thalassemic point mutations have occurred on the same chromosome showing haplotype IX. Haplotypes of the β-globin gene cluster, according to Orkin et al. [11], are shown at the top.

the $\beta^\circ 39$ mutation linked to the β globin gene cluster haplotypes I or II or IX, which share the same 3′ end subhaplotype (+ +); and the second containing the δ^+27 defect linked to haplotype IX (− + − + +/+ +), which has so far been described to characterize the isolated δ^+27 in both Sardinians [8] and Greeks [4].

As in Sardinians the $\beta^\circ 39$ is associated with haplotype IX in 4% of cases [9], it cannot be excluded that in this family an additional mutation may have occurred on a single chromosome bearing the $\beta^\circ 39$ or, viceversa, the δ^+27 thalassemia clearly linked to haplotype IX (Fig. 2B).

Finally, the absolute HbA_2 levels remain border-line or even slightly increased in these three δ^+27-$\beta^\circ 39$ heterozygotes (HbA_2 ranging from 0.66 pg/cell to 0.76 pg/cell) whereas they are constantly within the normal range (mean HbA_2 0.58 ± 0.08 pg/cell, range 0.45–0.68 pg/cell) in six subjects in whom such mutations were detected in trans (unpublished results).

Since the elevated HbA_2 levels in heterozygous β-thalassemia are determined by overexpression of both δ-chain loci [10], if these data were confirmed in a large series, they would suggest that δ^+27 thalassemia diversely affects δ chain synthesis in cis or in trans to $\beta^\circ 39$ mutation, perhaps by a different transcriptional activity of the corresponding normal δ-globin gene.

ACKNOWLEDGMENTS

We thank Mrs. Jenny Martin for editorial assistance. Supported by grants from CNR-MISM Progetto Strategico and MPI 60% to M.L.

REFERENCES

1. Kulozik AE, Yarwood N, Jones RW: The Corfù δβ°-thalassemia: A small deletion acts at a distance to selectively abolish β-globin gene expression. Blood 71:457, 1988.
2. Olds RJ, Sura T, Jackson B, Wonke B, Hoffbrand AV, Thein SL: A novel δ° mutation in cis with Hb Knossos: A study of different genetic interactions in three Egyptian families. Br J Haematol 78:430, 1991.
3. Loudianos G, Cao A, Pirastu M, Vassilopoulos G, Kollia P, Loukopoulos D: Molecular basis of the δ thalassemia in cis to hemoglobin Knossos variant. Blood 77:2087, 1991.
4. Loudianos G, Cao A, Ristaldi MS, Pirastu M, Tzeti M, Kannavakis E, Kattamis C: Molecular basis of δβ-thalassemia with normal fetal hemoglobin level. Blood 75:526, 1990.
5. Moi P, Loudianos G, Lavinha J, Murru S, Cossu P, Casu R, Oggiano L, Longinotti M, Cao A, Pirastu M: δ-Thalassemia due to a mutation

in an erythroid-specific binding protein sequence 3′ to the δ-globin gene. Blood 79:1, 1992.

6. Oggiano L, Rimini E, Frogheri L, Guiso L, Pistidda P, Longinotti M: Haematological phenotypes in a family with triplicated α-globin gene, β°_{39} and δ^{+}_{27} thalassaemia mutations. Clin Lab Haematol 14:289–292, 1992.
7. Moi P, Paglietti E, Sanna A, Brancati C, Tagarelli A, Galanello R, Cao A, Pirastu M: Delineation of the molecular basis of δ- and normal HbA_2 β-thalassemia. Blood 72:530, 1988.
8. Pirastu M, Galanello R, Melis MA, Brancati C, Tagarelli A, Cao A, Kan YW: δ^{+}-thalassemia in Sardinia. Blood 62:341, 1983.
9. Pirastu M, Galanello R, Doherty MA, Tuveri, P, Cao A, Kan YW: The same β-globin gene mutation is present on nine different β-thalassemia chromosomes in Sardinian population. Proc Natl Acad Sci USA 84:2882, 1987.
10. Weatherall DJ, Clegg JB: "The Thalassemia Syndromes." 3rd Ed. Oxford: Blackwell, 1981.
11. Orkin S, Kazazian HH Jr, Antonarakis SE, Goff SC, Boehm CD, Sexton JP, Waber PG, Giardina PJV: Linkage of β-thalassaemia mutations and β-globin gene polymorphism with DNA polymorphism in human β-globin gene cluster. Nature 296:627–631, 1982.

American Journal of Hematology 45:85–87 (1994)

Laboratory Monitoring of Warfarin Therapy in Utah

Susan B. Garr and George M. Rodgers
Departments of Pathology (S.B.G., G.M.R.) and Medicine (G.M.R.), University of Utah Medical Center, Veterans Affairs Medical Center, Associated Regional and University Pathologists, Salt Lake City, Utah

Accurate laboratory monitoring of oral anticoagulation has been emphasized as an important factor in providing safe and effective therapy for patients with thromboembolism. However, recent reports indicate that coagulation laboratories may not be providing optimal clinical information to clinicians who treat these patients. We surveyed all hospital coagulation laboratories in Utah to determine their format for reporting prothrombin time results in patients receiving oral anticoagulants. We found that less than 50% of laboratories used the reliable reporting format, i.e., the International Normalized Ratio (INR), and that many of the laboratories using the INR format may be reporting incorrect values. Our survey also found a significant lack of interest by physicians in requesting that their laboratories adopt reliable reporting methods. These results indicate a substantial lack of understanding by laboratories and clinicians of the importance of using reliable methods to monitor oral anticoagulation. Significant educational efforts will be required to correct this problem.

Key words: anticoagulation, prothrombin time, thromboplastin

INTRODUCTION

Laboratory monitoring of oral anticoagulation has been a major area of interest for physicians who treat patients with thromboembolism and for pathologists responsible for monitoring laboratory anticoagulation. Recent consensus statements on recommended guidelines for anticoagulation have emphasized the importance of the INR as a format for reporting the intensity of oral anticoagulation.[1] Nevertheless, a recent survey indicates that many hospital laboratories not only do not utilize the INR format, but also that many laboratory personnel are not aware of the meaning or clinical importance of this format. For example, a recent survey of Massachusetts hospitals found that almost 70% of laboratory supervisors had minimal or no understanding of the INR concept and that only 5% of these laboratories reported their prothrombin time (PT) values as on INR.[2]

To determine the level of acceptance and attitudes of clinical laboratories in our state on this issue, we surveyed all hospital laboratories in Utah. We also inquired as to the level of interest in the INR format by physicians, as judged by laboratory personnel responsible for coagulation testing. These survey results confirm a lack of understanding and importance of the INR format by laboratory personnel as previously reported for Massachusetts laboratories.[2] Our survey also points out a failure of clinicians to appreciate the benefits of the INR format and a lack of interest in requesting that their hospital laboratories offer this format.

METHODS

A listing of all 38 Utah hospital laboratories was obtained from the University of Utah Medical Center Admitting Department. Between November 1992–January 1993, the laboratory supervisor, chief technologist, or staff technologist of each laboratory responsible for coagulation testing was contacted by telephone and asked a series of questions about monitoring of oral anticoagulation by their laboratory. Survey results were then tabulated.

RESULTS

A 100% response rate was obtained in this survey representing the 38 hospital laboratories in Utah. The hospitals ranged in size from >200 beds (8 hospitals),

Received for publication April 30, 1993; accepted May 13, 1993.

Address reprint requests to Dr. George M. Rodgers, Division of Hematology-Oncology, University of Utah Medical Center, Salt Lake City, UT 84132.

TABLE I. Format of Prothrombin Time Assay Reports of Utah Hospital Laboratories

Format	No. of laboratories	(%)
Seconds	11	30
Seconds and control	7	18
Seconds and INR	15	39
Seconds and INR and control	3	8
Seconds and PT ratio	2	5

50–200 beds (10 hospitals), and 0–49 beds (20 hospitals). Only 3 laboratories did >50 PT assays daily, while 19 laboratories did 9 or fewer PT assays daily. All hospitals used PT reagents from 5 manufacturers (Ortho, Dade, Organon-Teknika, Helena, Instrumentation Laboratory); all reagents were labeled with an International Sensitivity Index (ISI) value. Table I summarizes the PT format reported by the hospital laboratories; less than 50% of the laboratories (18 of 38) reported an INR value with a PT value. Only 37% of laboratories (14 of 38) provided clinicians with recommended therapeutic ranges for patients on oral anticoagulation. When asked whether using the INR format would be clinically useful, 57% (22 of 38) of laboratory personnel answered in the affirmative.

In terms of laboratory personnel understanding the INR format, of those hospitals that do not report an INR value but are often asked to do so, 90% (10 of 11) use the manufacturer's established ISI value and did not know the reagent/instrument combination on which the ISI value was established. When calculating an INR value, 40% (4 of 10) used the mean of the reference range, 30% (3 of 10) used the mean of the normal control value, and 20% (2 of 10) used the normal control value of that day. It should also be noted that one hospital was unaware of the derivation of any of the values because the reagent sales representative programmed the parameters in their instrument. Of those hospitals that routinely report INR values, 89% (16 of 18) used the manufacturer's established ISI, and 11% (2 of 18) established their own. 17% (3 of 18) knew the reagent/instrument combination on which the ISI was established, while 83% (15 of 18) did not. 50% (9 of 19) of these hospitals use the mean of the reference for the denominator when calculating an INR value. 33% (6 of 18) use the mean of the control range and 17% (3 of 18) use the mean of the control for that day.

With regard to clinician interest in using the INR format, only 16% (3 of 19) laboratories not using the INR format reported that clinicians had either requested the format be used or had inquired about the clinical significance of the INR format.

DISCUSSION

Recognition of variability in commercial thromboplastin reagents and their effects on the PT determination led to efforts to standardize this test for patients receiving oral anticoagulants.[3] The INR format was introduced in 1983 as a means to "normalize" the PT assay between laboratories and to permit uniform safe and effective anticoagulation. A mechanism for quantitating the variability of commercial thromboplastins led to the term ISI, which refers to the "responsiveness" of a particular thromboplastin reagent. Despite acceptance of the INR format by many academic hospitals, it appears that a substantial number of hospital laboratories have not adopted this format and do not undertstand its utility. Additionally, as suggested by our survey results, many clinicians are not aware of the importance of this format.

A Massachusetts survey provided the first evidence that the INR format was not used or correctly understood by a majority of clinical laboratories.[2] This survey covered 86% of that state's laboratories. Our survey covered all Utah clinical laboratories and represented not only academic and reference laboratories of large medical centers, but also small to intermediate-size community hospitals. The results of our survey are similar to those of the Massachusetts survey in that both indicate a lack of acceptance by laboratories to adopt the INR format. However, we did find a higher percentage of Utah laboratories using this format (47% vs. 5%). On the other hand, as noted above, many Utah hospitals that use the INR format do so in an inaccurate manner.

Previous consensus recommendations on monitoring anticoagulant therapy had suggested that the PT ratio would be a reasonable substitute for using the INR format[4]; this recommendation assumed that thromboplastin reagents used by U.S. laboratories had similar ISI values. However, as recently summarized by Bussey et al.,[5] manufacturers of thromboplastin reagents used in the United States provide reagents with widely variable ISI values (1.4–2.8). Under these circumstances, it can no longer be considered acceptable to use reporting methods other than the INR format. Equally disturbing in our survey was the finding that there appears to be a lack of knowledge and interest by clinicians in using the INR format. Since we contacted the laboratory person responsible for coagulation testing for each hospital, we believe that our survey results are representative of the level of interest in the INR in our state. This subject was not surveyed in the Massachusetts report, so we cannot state with certainty that our data can be extrapolated to U.S. physicians in general, but we believe it likely that many physicians are not fully aware of or understand the INR format.

The solution to this problem is difficult. Institution of the requirement by journals to exclusively use the INR format when reporting clinical trial data[6] will be helpful. However, a more direct approach would be to target coagulation laboratory personnel, including directors, supervisors, and technologists for extensive education in this area. Improved understanding by laboratory personnel should lead to more laboratories adopting this format. Routine reporting of anticoagulant intensity in terms of the INR should lead to more rapid acceptance by clinicians. Widespread appreciation of the INR format should lead to more effective oral anticoagulation therapy.

ACKNOWLEDGMENTS

The support of the Hemostasis/Thrombosis Laboratory of Associated Regional and University Pathologists is acknowledged. Dr. Rodgers is supported by research funds from the Department of Veterans Affairs and the Utah Affiliate, American Heart Association. The manuscript was typed by Bryan Peterson.

REFERENCES

1. Hirsh J, Dalen JE, Deykin D, Poller L: Oral anticoagulants: Mechanism of action, clinical effectiveness, and optimal therapeutic range. Chest 102(Suppl):312S–326S, 1992.
2. Ansell JE: Imprecision of prothrombin time monitoring of oral anticoagulation: A survey of hospital laboratories. Am J Clin Pathol 98:237–239, 1992.
3. Poller L, Taberner DA: Dosage and control of oral anticoagulants: An international survey. Br J Haematol 51:479–485, 1982.
4. Hirsh J, Poller L, Deykin D, et al: Optimal therapeutic range for oral anticoagulants. Chest 95:5S–11S, 1989.
5. Bussey HI, Force RW, Bianco TM, Leonard AD: Reliance in prothrombin time ratios causes significant errors in anticoagulation therapy. Arch Intern Med 152:278–282, 1992.
6. Hirsh J: Inadequate monitoring of warfarin dosage. Editorial response. Blood 80:562–563, 1992.

SURVEY QUESTIONS

1. What is your title and specialty?
   Supervisor or Chief Technologist __30__
   Medical Technologist __8__
2. How many beds does your institution have?
   0–49 __19__ 50–200 __10__ >200 __8__
3. How many PT assays do you perform daily?
   0–9 __19__ 10–29 __10__ 30–50 __6__ >50 __3__
4. What format do you use to report PT results?
   Sec __11__ Sec & Control __7__ Sec & INR __15__ Sec, INR & Control __3__ Sec & Ratio __2__
5. Does you facility provide clinicians with a recommended therapeutic range for patients on oral anticoagulants?
   Yes __14__ No __24__
6. If yes, what are your therapeutic ranges?
   1.5–2.5 × normal control __10__
   1.5–2.5 × normal control and INR __2__
   INR __2__
7. If your institution does not report an INR, are you ever asked to calculate one?
   Yes __11__ No __9__
8. When calculating an INR:
   a. Do you use the manufacturer's ISI?
      Yes __10__ No ______
   b. Do you know the instrument/reagent combination used to establish the ISI?
      Yes ______ No __10__
   c. What number do you use for the denominator when calculating the INR?
      (1) Mean of reference range __4__
      (2) Mean of normal control __3__
      (3) Normal daily control __2__
      (4) Other __1__
9. Is the reference range adjusted with each new lot of PT reagent?
   Yes __6__ No __13__
10. Have you been asked by clinicians about the significance of an INR?
    Yes __3__ No __16__
11. Have you been asked to bring the INR format into your laboratory?
    Yes __3__ No __16__
12. If your laboratory reports INR values:
    a. Do you use the manufacturer's ISI?
       Yes __17__ No __2__
    b. Do you know the instrument/reagent combination used to establish the ISI?
       Yes __3__ No __16__
    c. What number do you use for the denominator when calculating the INR?
       (1) Mean of reference range __10__
       (2) Mean of normal control __6__
       (3) Normal daily control __3__
13. Would reporting an INR be of value when monitoring oral anticoagulant therapy of hospitalized patients?
    Yes __18__ No __4__ Uncertain __15__

American Journal of Hematology 45:88–90 (1994)

Production of Parathyroid Hormone-Related Protein by Cultured Human Myeloma Cells

Akira Suzuki, Takayuki Takahashi, Yoshiaki Okuno, Reiko Tsuyuoka, Yutaka Sasaki, Manabu Fukumoto, Hideki Katakami, Kenkichi Kita, and Tsunefumi Shibuya

Second Department of Internal Medicine (A.S., T.T., Y.O., R.T., Y.S.), The First Department of Pathology (M.F.), Faculty of Medicine, Kyoto University, Kyoto, The Third Department of Internal Medicine, Miyazaki Medical College, Miyazaki (H.K.), The Second Department of Internal Medicine, Faculty of Medicine, Mie University, Mie (K.K.) and The Department of Internal Medicine, Hamanomachi General Hospital, Fukuoka, Japan (T.S.)

We examined whether or not parathyroid hormone-related protein (PTH-rP) is produced in cultured human myeloma cells. PTH-rP protein was detected in the cell extract of one (U266) of 6 myeloma cell lines examined by radioimmunoassay. Also we demonstrated the expression of PTH-rP mRNA in all of the 6 lines. These findings indicate that PTH-rP may be one of the factors responsible for the bone destruction or hypercalcemia in multiple myeloma.

Key words: multiple myeloma, hypercalcemia, PTH-rP

INTRODUCTION

Human myeloma cells have been supposed to produce bone resorbing factors that activate adjacent osteoclasts [1]. The bone resorbing activity of human myeloma cells has been attributed to tumor necrosis factor β (TNFβ) [2] or interleukin-1 β (IL-1β) [3]. In a previous study, neutralizing antibodies against TNFβ incompletely blocked the bone resorbing activity produced by human myeloma cell lines, suggesting the presence of other resorbing factors [4].

PTH-rP, a powerful stimulator for osteoclastic bone resorption and the most important factor in humoral hypercalcemia of malignancy was recently isolated and molecularly cloned. The plasma PTH-rP level has been reported to be increased in some patients with multiple myeloma associated with hypercalcemia [5], although the cellular source of PTH-rP in such patients remains to be clarified. These findings prompted us to examine whether or not PTH-rP is produced by human myeloma cells.

MATERIALS AND METHODS

Cell Lines and Measurement of PTH-rP Concentration

Six human myeloma cell lines—U266, RPMI8226, MM-S1 [6], MM-M1 [6], KMM56, 1180 (IgD-λ) (manuscript in preparation)—were studied. CHU-2, Raji, and HL60 were examined as controls for PTH-rP production.

Cells from each cell line were cultured (5×10^5 cells/ml) in RPMI1640 medium with 10% FCS for 3 days. Culture supernatants were concentrated 10-fold by ultrafiltration using a PM-10 membrane (Amicon, Tokyo, Japan). The cell extracts were prepared as described previously [7]. Concentrations of PTH-rP were measured by radioimmunoassay (RIA) for N-terminal peptide as described previously [8].

Northern Blotting

Messenger RNA (2 μg) was extracted from cells as described previously [8]. The gel-purified 320 bp of reverse transcriptase polymerase chain reaction (RT-PCR) product from mRNA of CHU-2 was cloned into pBR322, then used as the probe for PTH-rP mRNA.

Primers for Amplification

Primers used to amplify PTH-rP cDNA by PCR were as follows: GAGGGTCTCAGCCGCCGCCT, 5′ sense

Received for publication April 30, 1993, accepted May 13, 1993.

Address reprint requests to Dr. Takayuki Takahashi, Second Department of Internal Medicine, Faculty of Medicine, Kyoto University, 54 Shogoin Kawahara-cho, Sakyo-ku, Kyoto 606, Japan.

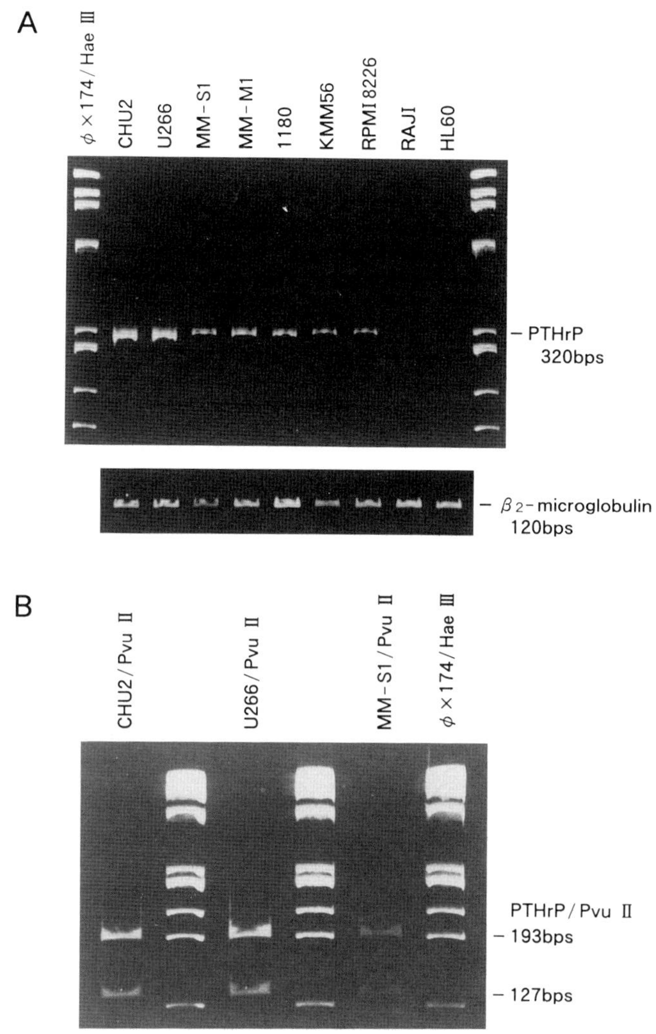

Fig. 1. A: RT-PCR products of cDNA from myeloma and control cell lines after 40-cycle amplification. B: PvuII digestion of the PTH-rP RT-PCR products from CHU-2, U266, and MM-S1 cDNA, after 40-cycle amplification.

primer (2nd exon) [9]; TTGCGTTTCCCGGGCTTGCC, 3′ antisense primer (3rd exon). The amplified product was 320 bp and was digested into 193 bp and 127 bp by PvuII. For internal control, we also prepared primers for β_2-microglobulin: ACCCCCACTGAAAAAGATGA, 5′ sense primer (2nd exon); ATCTTCAAACCTCCATGATG, 3′ antisense primer. The amplified product was 120 bp. RT-PCR was performed as described previously [7].

RESULTS

PTH-rP was not detectable (<8 pg/ml) by RIA in the ten-fold concentrated culture supernatant of any of the 6 myeloma cell lines, whereas it was detected (5 pg/10^7 cells) in the cell extract of U266 line. The lower limits of detection with the RIA for the cell extract was 4 pg/10^7 cells. The PTH-rP concentration in the concentrated culture supernatant and cell extract of CHU-2 employed as the positive control was 311 pg/ml and 75 pg/10^7 cells, respectively.

PTH-rP mRNA was detectable only in CHU-2 cells, and not in 6 myeloma cell lines by Northern blotting (data not shown). The reverse-transcribed cDNA from 6 myeloma cell lines, CHU-2, Raji and HL60 cells were amplified up to 40 cycles. As shown in Fig. 1A, all 6 myeloma cell lines expressed PTH-rP mRNA, showing the most intensive expression in U266 cells. PvuII digestion of the amplified products from U266 cells demonstrated that the band of 320 bp was a part of the PTH-rP cDNA (Fig. 1B).

DISCUSSION

In the present study, we demonstrated the PTH-rP production by all 6 human myeloma cell lines examined. Although the amount of PTH-rP produced appears to be minute, it might be sufficient to activate osteoclasts, because myeloma cells are present close to them in the bone marrow. Furthermore, Sato et al. reported that PTH-rP and IL-1α synergistically stimulate bone resorption in vitro and increase the serum calcium level in vivo [10]. Because of similar biological activities between IL-1α and IL-1β, PTH-rP and IL-1β which can be co-produced by myeloma cells, may synergistically promote bone resorption and ultimately produce hypercalcemia. Further studies are required to clarify the interaction between PTH-rP and IL-1β or TNFβ in the bone resorption and hypercalcemia in multiple myeloma.

ACKNOWLEDGMENTS

This work was supported in part by a Grant-in-Aid for Scientific Research 04671521 from the Ministry of Education, Science, and Culture of Japan, and by The Research Committee on Idiopathic Hematopoietic Disorders, Ministry of Health and Welfare, Japan.

REFERENCES

1. Mundy GR, Raisz LG, Cooper RA, Schechter GP, Salmon SE: Evidence for the secretion of an osteoclast stimulating factor in myeloma. N Engl J Med 291:1041–1046, 1974.
2. Garrett R, Durie BGM, Nedwin GE, Gillespie A, Bringman T, Sabatini M, Bertolini DR, Mundy GR: Production of lymphotoxin, a bone-resorbing cytokine, by cultured human myeloma cells. N Engl J Med 317:526–532, 1987.
3. Kawano M, Yamamoto I, Iwato K, Tanaka H, Asaoku H, Tanabe O, Ishikawa H, Nobuyoshi M, Ohmoto Y, Hirai Y, Kuramoto A: Interleukin-1 beta rather than lymphotoxin as the major bone resorbing activity in human multiple myeloma. Blood 73:1646–1649, 1989.
4. Mundy GR: Incidence and pathophysiology of hypercalcemia. Calcif Tissue Int 46(Suppl):S3–S10, 1990.

5. Budayr AM, Nissenson RA, Klein RF, Pun KK, Clark OH, Diep D, Arnaud CD, Stewler GJ: Increased serum levels of a parathyroid hormone-like protein in malignancy-associated hypercalcemia. Ann Intern Med 111:807–812, 1989.
6. Suzuki A, Takahashi T, Okuno Y, Fukumoto M, Fukui H, Koishihara Y, Ohsugi Y, Ohno Y, Imura H: Estimation of interleukin 6 production by reverse transcriptase-polymerase chain reaction in four human myeloma cell lines. Leuk Res 15:1043–1050, 1991.
7. Katakami H, Downs TR, Frohman LA: Decreased hypothalamic growth hormone-releasing hormone content and pituitary responsiveness in hypothyroidism. J Clin Invest 77:1704–1711, 1986.
8. Mune T, Katakami H, Kato Y, Yasuda K, Matsukura S, Miura K: Production and secretion of parathyroid hormone-related protein in pheochromocytoma: Participation of α-adrenergic mechanism. J Clin Endocrinol Metab, 76:757–762, 1993.
9. Yasuda T, Banville D, Hendy GN, Goltzman D: Characterization of the human parathyroid hormone-like peptide gene. J Biol Chem 264:7720–7725, 1989.
10. Sato K, Fujii Y, Kasono K, Ozawa M, Imamura H, Kanaji Y, Kurosawa H, Tsushima T, Shizume K: Parathyroid hormone–related protein and interleukin-1α synergistically stimulate bone resorption in vitro and increase the serum calcium concentration in mice in vivo. Endocrinology 124:2172–2178, 1989.

American Journal of Hematology 45:91–93 (1994)

Quantities of α^Q Chain Variants in Heterozygotes With and Without a Concomitant β-Thalassemia Trait

W.-B. Qin, E. Baysal, K.F. Wong, T.P. Molchanova, D.D. Pobedimskaya, S. Sharma, J.B. Wilson, and T.H.J. Huisman

Department of Biochemistry and Molecular Biology, Medical College of Georgia, Augusta, Georgia (W.-B.Q., E.B., T.P.M., D.D.P., S.S., J.B.W., T.H.J.H.); Institute of Pathology, Queen Elizabeth Hospital, Kowloon, Hong Kong (K.F.W.)

We have analyzed the quantities of α^X chain-containing hemoglobins ($\alpha_2{}^X\beta_2$ and $\alpha_2{}^X\delta_2$) in 14 heterozygotes for Hb Q-India [α64(E13)Asp→His] or Hb Q-Thailand [α74(EF3)Asp→His]; both amino acid replacements are the result of mutations in the α1-globin gene. Five of these persons (three with Hb Q-India and two with Hb Q-Thailand) had an additional β°-thalassemia heterozygosity. The average quantities for Hb Q + Hb Q_2 in the four groups were 17.2% ($\alpha\alpha^Q/\alpha\alpha$; β^A/β^A), 9.5% ($\alpha\alpha^Q/\alpha\alpha$; $\beta^A/\beta^{\circ Th}$), 26.8% ($-\alpha^Q/\alpha\alpha$; β^A/β^A), and 16.95% ($-\alpha^Q/\alpha\alpha$; $\beta^A/\beta^{\circ Th}$). These variations can best be explained by a posttranslational control mechanism; an imbalance in the α^A, α^Q, and β^A chain ratio will favor the $\alpha_2{}^Q\beta_2$ formation when an α-thalassemia is present and will reduce its formation in the presence of a β-thalassemia heterozygosity.

Key words: α-thalassemia, Hb Q-India, Hb Q-Thailand, globin gene

INTRODUCTION

There is considerable evidence that the level of an α chain variant in a heterozygote is lower when this person also has a β-thalassemia (β-thal) gene, although some investigators have reported that this is not the case [reviewed in 1]. It may well be that both the type of α chain variant and that of the β-thal allele (mainly β°− and β^+-) are responsible for these observations. Recently, we had the opportunity to reexamine this phenomenon for two closely related α chain variants, Hb Q-India [α64(E13) Asp→His] and Hb Q-Thailand [α74(EF3) Asp→His], in heterozygotes with and without a well-defined β°-thal allele.

MATERIALS AND METHODS

Blood samples were collected in vacutainers with EDTA as anticoagulant and shipped by fast air service to Augusta, Georgia. Hematological data were collected with an automated cell counter. Red cell lysates were examined by isoelectrofocusing [2], and quantitation of the hemoglobin (Hb) components was by cation-exchange high-performance liquid chromatography (HPLC) [3]. The amino acid replacements in the α chains were identified through protein analysis [4] and sequencing of amplified DNA segments, which includes either the α2- or the α1-globin gene [5]. The β-thal mutations were characterized by a similar procedure [6]. The possible presence of deletional α-thal determinants was evaluated with polymerase chain reaction (PCR) methodology; the method of Bowden et al. [7] was used to detect the SEA α-thal-1 deletion and that of Baysal and Huisman [8] for the detection of the smaller $-\alpha^{3.7}$ and $-\alpha^{4.2}$ α-thal-2 deletions.

RESULTS

Hb Q-India [α64(E13)Asp→His]

Eight Indian heterozygotes living in Canada, South Africa, and India participated. All had four α-globin genes (αα/αα); the Asp→His mutation was found to be located in the minor α1-globin gene. Three subjects had an additional β°-thal heterozygosity, which involved the splice junction mutant IVS-I-1 (G→T) common among Indians [9]. Table I lists the available hematological data and the quantities of Hb Q ($\alpha_2{}^Q\beta_2$), Hb Q_2 ($\alpha_2{}^Q\delta_2$), and Hb A_2; all were obtained with the same cation-exchange

Received for publication May 31, 1993; accepted June 30, 1993.

Address reprint requests to Dr. Titus H.J. Huisman, Department of Biochemistry and Molecular Biology, Medical College of Georgia, Augusta, GA 30912-2100.

TABLE I. Hematological and Hb Composition Data for Hb Q-India [α64(E13)Asp→His] and Hb Q-Thailand [α74(EF3)Asp→His] Heterozygotes With and Without a β°-Thal Trait

Subject	Sex-age (years)	Hb (g/dl)	PCV (liter/liter)	RBC (10^{12}/liter)	MCV (fl)	MCH (pg)	Hb A_2 (%)	Hb Q_2 (%)	Hb Q (%)
Hb Q-India ($\alpha\alpha^Q/\alpha\alpha$;:$\beta^A/\beta^A$)									
M.G.	F-adult	—	—	—	—	—	2.2	0.2	17.2
B.S.	M-adult	12.0	0.345	4.21	92.0	28.5	3.2	0.3	16.8
D.N.	F-adult	—	—	—	—	—	2.4	0.4	15.7
C.H.	F-adult	11.2	0.370	3.89	95.0	28.8	2.4	0.3	16.1
S.J.	F-16	15.7	0.436	4.90	89.0	32.0	2.0	0.3	18.7
						Average	2.44	0.3	16.9
Hb Q-India ($\alpha\alpha^Q/\alpha\alpha;\beta^A/\beta^{oTh}$)									
W.C.M.	M-32	—	—	—	—	—	4.4	0.5	8.0[a]
Y.J.	F-41	13.5	0.390	6.00	65.0	22.5	4.5	0.5	9.5[a]
P.K.	F-28	11.7	0.367	5.66	64.9	20.8	4.9	0.5	9.5[a]
						Average	4.6	0.5	9.0
Hb Q-Thailand [$-\alpha^Q(4.2)/\alpha\alpha;\beta^A/\beta^A$]									
D.N.	M-adult	14.7	0.525	5.42	96.0	27.1	2.3	0.6	25.9
L.F.	M-49	15.8	0.475	6.13	77.0	25.8	1.6	0.5	27.4
C.C.	M-32	14.7	0.438	5.59	78.4	26.3	1.9	0.6	24.4
N.N.	F-61	9.1	0.283	3.63	80.0	25.1	1.3	0.4	27.4
						Average	1.8	0.5	26.3
Hb Q-Thailand [$-\alpha^Q(4.2)/\alpha\alpha;\beta^A/\beta^{oTh}$]									
L.M.	F-22	12.1	0.373	5.59	66.8	21.6	5.5	1.3	14.7[b]
L.C.	M-21	12.6	0.405	6.03	67.2	20.9	4.8	1.4	16.5[b]
						Average	5.15	1.35	15.6

[a]The β-thal allele was identified as the IVS-I-1 (G→T) mutation.
[b]The β-thal allele was identified as the frameshift at CDs 41/42 (−TTCT).

HPLC procedure. The average value for the α^Q-containing Hbs in the heterozygotes was 17.2% in the absence of a β°-thal and 9.5% when a β°-thal heterozygosity was present.

Hb Q-Thailand [α74(EF3)Asp→His]

Six Chinese adults carried the Hb Q-Thailand abnormality; the mutation was in codon (CD) 74 of the α1-globin gene on a chromosome with a 4.2 kb deletion, which includes the entire α2-globin gene (data not shown). The average levels of Hb Q and Hb Q_2 in the four subjects without an additional β-thal were 26.3% and 0.5%, respectively (Table I). The two Hb Q-Thailand heterozygotes who were also heterozygous for the CDs 41/42 (−TTCT) frameshift, common among Chinese [9], were the children of a Chinese patient with Hb Q-Thailand/Hb H disease; his genotype was determined to be $-\alpha^Q/--(SEA);\beta^A/\beta^A$ (data not shown). The children apparently inherited the β-thal allele from their mother, who was not available for study. Their average Hb Q and Hb Q_2 levels were 15.6% and 1.35%, respectively.

All five patients with a β°-thal heterozygosity had the expected increase in δ chain-containing Hbs; in the three with Hb Q-India, this value was 5.1%, and, in the two with Hb Q-Thailand, it was 6.5% (Table I).

DISCUSSION

It is of interest to compare the quantitative data in all 14 subjects with a Hb Q heterozygosity. In doing so, it is assumed that the α-Q-India and α-Q-Thailand chains have an equal affinity for combining with β chains to form the $\alpha_2{}^Q\beta_2$ tetramer; both Hb Q tetramers have a normal stability as determined via several stability methods.

The level of 17.2% for an $\alpha\alpha^Q/\alpha\alpha$ heterozygote is as expected for a mutation in an α1-globin gene and is definitely lower than that observed for stable α variants with a mutation in the α2-globin gene. The presence of an additional β°-thal trait (genotype: $\alpha\alpha^Q/\alpha\alpha;\beta^A/\beta^{oTh}$) reduces the Hb Q level to 9.5%, a reduction of nearly 50%. Apparently the formation of normal Hb A ($\alpha_2\beta_2$) is preferred over that of HbQ ($\alpha_2{}^Q\beta_2$) probably because of the replacement of an acidic for a basic amino acid. The presence of an α-thal-2 trait (genotype: $-\alpha^Q/\alpha\alpha;\beta^A/\beta^A$) increases the level of α^Q-containing Hbs to 26.8%, an increase of ~50%. The additional presence of a β°-thal (genotype: $-\alpha^Q/\alpha\alpha;\beta^A/\beta^{oTh}$) reduces this level from 26.8% to 16.95%, which is the same as the 17.2% for the α^Q heterozygote (genotype: $\alpha\alpha^Q/\alpha\alpha;\beta^A/\beta^A$). Assuming that a difference in affinity between α^Q and β^A chains and between α^A and β^A chains is the major cause for this variation in the level of Hb Q in these patients, one can conclude that the synthesis ratio between α^A and α^Q chains in the $\alpha\alpha^Q/\alpha\alpha;\beta^A/\beta^A$ and the $-\alpha^Q/\alpha\alpha;\beta^A/\beta^{oTh}$ conditions is nearly identical. The loss of one normal α2-globin gene in the $-\alpha^Q/\alpha\alpha;\beta^A/\beta^A$ heterozygote greatly promotes the formation of the $\alpha_2{}^Q\beta_2$ tetramer (26.8%), while the (functional) loss of one normal β-globin gene in the $\alpha\alpha^Q/\alpha\alpha;\beta^A/\beta^{oTh}$ affects the formation of $\alpha_2{}^Q\beta_2$ to the extent that $<10\%$ of this variant is present in such persons. Indeed, the posttranslational mechanism of tetramer formation is a powerful determinant for the quantity of the α chain-containing Hbs in heterozygotes.

REFERENCES

1. Weatherall DJ, Clegg JB: "The Thalassaemia Syndromes. 3rd ed." Oxford: Blackwell Scientific Publications, 1981.
2. Righetti PG, Gianazza E, Bianchi-Bosisio A, Cossu G: Conventional isoelectric focusing and immobilized pH gradients for hemoglobin separation and identification. In Huisman THJ (ed): "The Hemoglobinopathies." Edinburgh: Churchill Livingstone, 1986, p 47.
3. Bissé E, Wieland H: High-performance liquid chromatographic separation of human haemoglobins—Simultaneous quantitation of foetal and glycated haemoglobins. J Chromatogr 434:95, 1988.
4. Wilson JB, Lam H, Pravatmuang P, Huisman THJ: Separation of tryptic peptides of normal and abnormal α, β, γ, and δ hemoglobin chains by high-performance liquid chromatography. J Chromatogr 179:271, 1979.
5. Yüregir GT, Aksoy K, Çürük MA, Dikmen, N, Fei Y-J, Baysal E, Huisman THJ: Hb H disease in a Turkish family resulting from the interaction of a deletional α-thalassaemia-1 and a newly discovered poly A mutation. Br J Haematol 80:527, 1992.
6. Divoky V, Bissé E, Wilson JB, Gu L-H, Wieland H, Heinrichs I, Prior JF, Huisman THJ: Heterozygosity for the IVS-I-5 (G→C) mutation with a G→A change at codon 18 (Val→Met; Hb Baden) in cis and a T→G mutation at codon 126 (Val→Gly; Hb Dhonburi) in trans resulting in a thalassemia intermedia. Biochim Biophys Acta 1180:173, 1992.
7. Bowden DK, Vickers MA, Higgs DR: A PCR-based strategy to detect the common severe determinants of α-thalassaemia. Br J Haematol 81:104, 1992.
8. Baysal E, Huisman THJ: PCR-based methodology for the detection of common α-thal-2 determinants. Abstract, 5th International Conference on Thalassaemias and the Haemoglobinopathies, Nicosia, Cyprus, April 1993.
9. The β- and δβ-thalassemia repository. Hemoglobin 16:237, 1992.

American Journal of Hematology 45:94–101 (1994)

LETTERS AND CORRESPONDENCE

Letters and correspondence submitted for possible publication must be identified as such. Text length must not exceed 500 words and five bibliographic references. A single concise figure or table may be included if it is essential to support the communication. Letters not typed double-spaced will not be considered for publication. Letters not meeting these specifications will not be returned to authors. Letters to the Editor *are utilized to communicate a single novel observation or finding.* Correspondence *is to be used to supplement or constructively comment on the contents of a publication in the journal and cannot exceed the restrictions for Letters to the Editor. The Editor reserves the right to shorten text, delete objectional comments and make other changes to comply with the style of the journal. Permission for publication must be appended as a postscript. Submissions must be sent to Marcel E. Conrad, M.D., Associate Editor, American Journal of Hematology, USA Cancer Center, Mobile, Alabama 36688 to permit rapid consideration for publication.*

Acute Lymphoblastic Leukemia in Fanconi's Anemia

To the Editor: Fanconi's anemia (FA) is an autosomal recessive disorder characterized by a high incidence of aplastic anemia, diverse assortment of congenital malformations, and chromosomal anomalies. Recently, the diagnosis of FA was based on chromosomal breakage in lymphocytes following treatment with a DNA cross-linking agent [1–3]. The disease has a premalignant component of leukemia, which is nearly always of the acute nonlymphoblastic type (ANLL) or solid tumors. We report a patient with FA who developed acute lymphoblastic leukemia (ALL). Only one patient has been described previously with these combined disorders [4].

A 5-year-old girl first presented in 1986 with FA at another university hospital, and she was treated with androgen 3 mg/kg and prednisolone 1 mg/kg in addition to blood transfusion. Past history revealed only paleness of the patient over the previous years. Family history revealed two healthy sisters, and healthy parents who had had three miscarriages. Physical examination revealed short stature (height 100 cm weight 15 kg head circumferences 46.5 cm), epicantic fold with two cafe-au-lait spots and two hypopigmented areas on the chest. The remainder of the physical examination was normal.

Laboratory findings were as follow: Hb 10 g/dl, WBC 6×10^9/liter, reticulocyte 4%, platelets 70×10^9/liter, erythrocytes morphology macrocytic, bone marrow aspiration was mildly hypocellular and fatty, and HbF 15%; *x*-ray findings (hands, vertebra, intravenous pyelography) were normal. Chromosomal studies were not performed. She was treated with the same therapy except that prednisolone dose was changed to 10 mg daily.

In 1991 she was transferred again to our department with the possible diagnosis of acute nonlymphoblastic leukemia (ANLL). It was learned that she had been treated during last 5 years with the androgen and prednisolone therapy intermittently and with blood transfusions at 2–3 months intervals for the last year.

Hematologic examination of the patient showed 33% blasts in the peripheral smear and 35% blasts in the bone marrow smear, with a lymphoblastic appearance. Immunohistochemical and immunophenotyping studies of blasts showed that periodic acid-Schiff stain was positive, Sudan black was negative, myeloperoxidase 6% positive, terminal deoxynucleotidyl transferase (Tdt) 34% positive. CALLA was 0%, CD2 22%, CD19 15%, CD33 6%, CD34 11%.

Cytogenetic studies of the patient were as follows. Bone marrow chromosome analysis revealed 46,XX. Peripheral blood lymphocyte cultures established normal and diepoxybutane (DEB) induction of chromosome and chromatid breaks and gaps. Chromosome analysis of 50 metaphases showed 3.20% breaks/cell.

The patient was treated with vincristine, L-asparaginase, daunorubicine, and prednisolone therapy, and she died.

Recently, in the identification of FA, the chromosome breakage test has become more specific with the addition of DNA cross-linking agents into lymphocyte culture [1–3]. In our patient, DEB positivity proved that the patient had FA. FA has a heterogeneity in clinical and cytogenetic findings [2]. The significance of marrow clonal cytogenetic abnormalities is unclear and does not necessarily indicate impending leukemia. Analysis of data from the International FA Registry revealed a high risk of leukemic transformation in between 32% and 50% of FA patients [5]. Although most leukemias observed in children are ALL, nearly all FA-associated leukemias are of myeloid origin [4]. This association suggests that FA is a preleukemic condition for AML. While the occurrence of ALL in patients with FA may be a coincidence, the possibility that FA may predispose patients to develop ALL must be considered.

Sevgi Yetgin
Murat Tuncer
Ertuğrul Güler
Feride Duru
Department of Pediatric Hematology, Faculty of Medicine, Hacettepe University, Ankara, Turkey

Mehmet Ali Kaşifoğlu
Department of Genetics, Faculty of Medicine, Hacettepe University, Ankara, Turkey

References

1. Auerbach AD, Rogatko A, Schroeder-Kurth TM: International Fanconi Anemia Registry. Relation of clinical symptoms to diepoxybutane sensitivity. Blood 73:791, 1989.
2. Alter PB: Fanconi's anemia. Current concepts. Am J Pediatr Hematol/Oncol 14:170, 1992.
3. Strathdee CA, Buchwald M: Molecular and Cellular Biology of Fanconi's anemia. Am J Pediatr Hematol/Oncol 14:177, 1992.
4. Auerbach AD: Fanconi's anemia and leukemia. Tracking the genes. Leukemia 6(Suppl 1):1, 1992.
5. Auerbach AD, Allen RG: Leukemia and preleukemia in Fanconi's anemia patients. A review of the literature and report of the International Fanconi Anemia Registry. Cancer Genet Cytogenet 51:1, 1991.

Standard Ph Chromosome, t(9;22)(q34;q11), as an Additional Change in a Patient With Acute Myelomonocytic Leukemia (M4Eo) Associated With inv(16)(p13q22)

To the Editor: A Ph translocation, t(9;22)(q34;q11), has been found mainly in chronic myelogeneous leukemia (CML) and acute lymphocytic leukemia

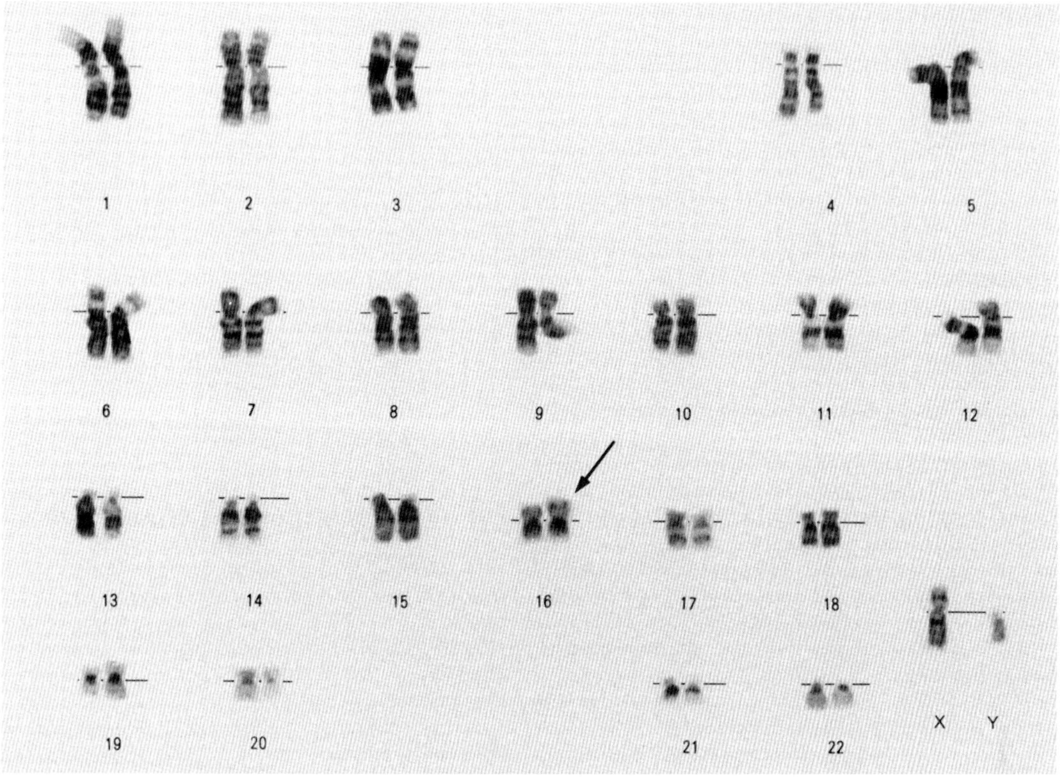

(a)

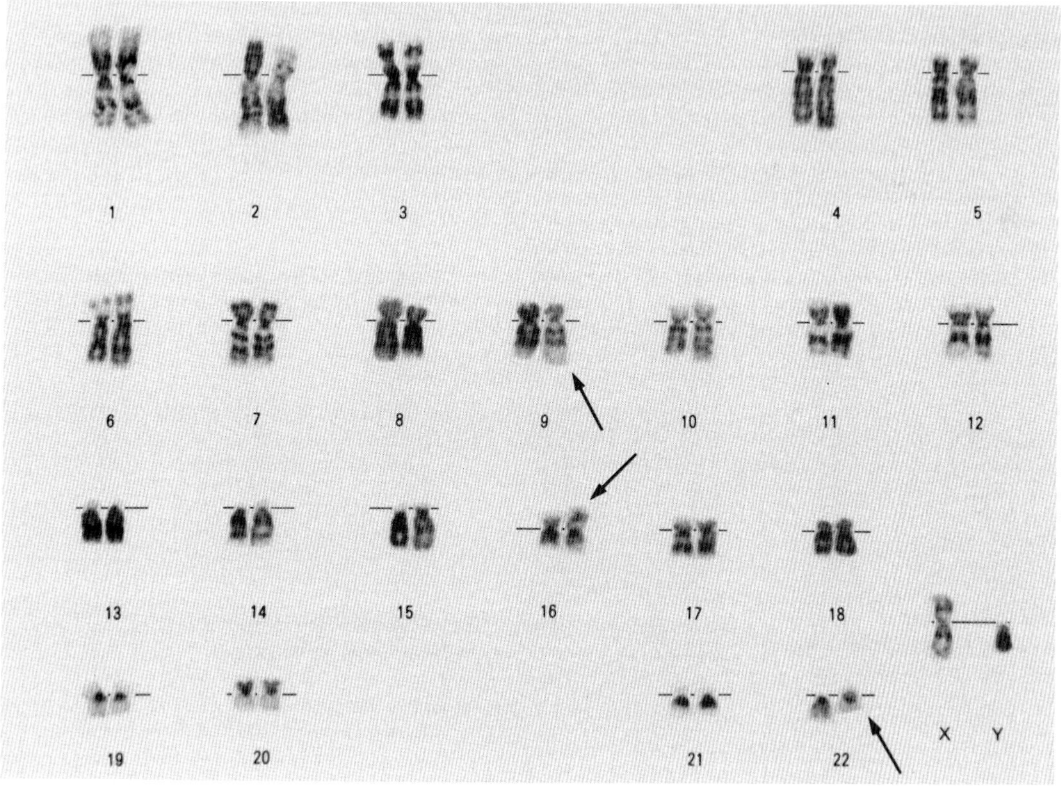

(b)

Fig. 1. **All cells had inv(16), and four of them had Ph chromosome besides this abnormality. Karyotypes showing inv(16)(p13q22) (a) and both inv(16) and t(9;22)(q34;q11) (b).**

(ALL). The presence of Ph chromosomes in acute leukemia implies an extremely poor prognosis. On the other hand, inv(16)(p13q22) is associated with acute myelomonocytic leukemia (AMMoL) with dysplastic marrow eosinophils (M4Eo; FAB classification) and suggests a favorable prognosis. Herein we describe an allografted patient with such a cytogenetic event, the combination of inv(16) and standard Ph translocation, and discuss the conflicting influences on prognosis.

A 40-year-old man was referred to our hospital because of anemia and leukocytosis in January, 1991. There was no history of leukocytosis or any other signs suggesting chronic phase of CML or myelodysplastic syndrome. Physical examination did not show hepatosplenomegaly. The Hb was 6.4 g/dl; the WBC count was 28.9 × 10^9/liter, with 59% blast cells; the platelet count was 18 × 10^9/liter. Bone marrow was hypercellular, with 36% leukemic cells and 6% eosinophils containing basophilic staining granules. The diagnosis of M4Eo was made, and the patient was treated with standard chemotherapy in Japan. After the achievement of complete remission, allogeneic bone marrow transplantation from an HLA-matched sister was undertaken on October 29, 1991. The patient has been well and free from relapse 18 months after the transplant.

Chromosome analysis showed the following (ISCN, 1991): 46,XY,inv(16)(p13q22)[17]/46,idem,t(9;22)(q34;q11)[3] (Fig. 1). No rearrangements of the major breakpoint cluster region (M-bcr) were detected with Southern blot analysis. After the achievement of complete remission, normal karyotypes were restored.

The majority of CML patients show breakpoints within the M-bcr. On the other hand, about one-half of Ph+ ALL patients have breakpoints in the minor breakpoint cluster region (m-bcr). To our knowledge, nine patients who have both Ph chromosome and inv(16) have been reported in the literature, four CML and five M4Eo patients [1–6]. Among them, four were studied by molecular biology; two CML had M-bcr breakpoints and two M4Eo had m-bcr breakpoints. Interestingly, Ph translocation detected as change additional to inv(16) has not shown M-bcr breakpoints so far. On the basis of eight patients reported in the literature and the present case, two types of combination of Ph and inv(16) are disclosed: 1) CML that has Ph chromosome, inv(16), and M-BCR+ and 2) M4Eo that has the opposite but is M-BCR−.

Regarding our patient, it is not possible to comment on the impact of these conflicting chromosomal abnormalities on prognosis. Although inv(16) carries a good prognosis in most surveys, allogeneic bone marrow transplantation from an HLA-matched sister was undertaken, because the accompanying Ph chromosome suggests a poor prognosis. All prior patients with M4Eo with inv(16) and Ph chromosome eventually relapsed. It may follow that the prognosis of M4Eo with inv(16) is hampered by the accompanying Ph chromosome.

I. Miura
H. Takatsu
A. Yamaguchi
K. Hashimoto
T. Nimura
T. Nishinari
H. Niitsu
A.B. Miura

Third Department of Internal Medicine, Akita University School of Medicine and Department of Internal Medicine, Senboku Kumiai General Hospital, Akita, Japan

References

1. Enright H, Weisdorf D, Peterson L, Rydell RE, Kaplan ME, Arthur DC: Inversion of chromosome 16 and dysplastic eosinophils in accelerated phase of chronic myeloid leukemia. Leukemia 6:381–384, 1992.
2. Heim S, Christensen BE, Fioretos T, Sorensen A-G, Pedersen NT: Acute myelomonocytic leukemia with inv(16)(p13q22) complicating Philadelphia chromosome positive chronic myeloid leukemia. Cancer Genet Cytogenet 59:35–38, 1992.
3. Secker-Walker LM, Morgan GJ, Min T, Swansburry GJ, Craig J, Yamada T, Desalvo L, Medina JW, Chowdhury V, Donahue RP, Polliack A, Catovsky D: Inversion of chromosome 16 with the Philadelphia chromosome in acute myelomonocytic leukemia with eosinophilia: report of two cases. Cancer Genet Cytogenet 58:29–34, 1992.
4. Preudhomme C, Lai JL, Plantier I, Demory JL, Zandecki M, Fenaux P: Cytogenetic and molecular remission in a case of acute myeloid leukemia (AML) with inversion of chromosome 16 [inv(16)] and Philadelphia chromosome (Ph). Br J Haematol 82:623–626, 1992.
5. Li YS, Hayhoe FGJ: Ph[1] chromosome positive acute myelomonocytic leukemia with inverted chromosome 16. Br J Haematol 69:576, 1988.
6. Evers JP, Bagg A, Himoe E, Zwiebel JA, Jacobson RJ: Temporal association of chromosome 16 in recurrent blast crises of chronic myelogeneous leukemia. Cancer Genet Cytogenet 62:134–139, 1992.

Iron Deficiency Anemia in Hemoglobinopathy

To the Editor: I have read the paper entitled "Clinical Course and Molecular Characterization of a Compound Heterozygote for Sickle Hemoglobin and Hemoglobin Kenya" by Waye et al. in the December issue of the Journal (41:289–291, 1992). The authors should be congratulated for their keen evaluation of the peripheral smear for sickling despite the finding that hemoglobin electrophoresis and PCR studies were found consistent with sickle cell anemia, as with the complaints of the patient. Because of the observation of hypochromia and microcytosis (MCV.56.fl), which could easily be explained by the presence of alpha thalassemia, the patient was treated successfully with parenteral iron administration, since her serum ferritin level was low.

Iron deficiency was observed in 22% of our patients with sickle cell anemia; most of them were children and were transfused infrequently [1]. The authors' patient was given transfusions and oral iron. I wonder how she became iron deficient despite her hemoglobinopathy? Did she have malabsorption or did she lose all the iron with hemosiderinuria or with excessive menstrual loss? Despite laborious molecular studies, I am still looking for a simple solution to the problem, for which I hope the authors will not be disturbed.

Şinasi Özsoylu

Hacettepe University Faculty of Medicine, Department of Pediatrics, Hematology Unit, Hacettepe Children's Hospital, Ankara, Turkey

Reference

1. Özsoylu Ş, Altinöz N: Sickle-cell anemia in Turkey. Evaluation of 97 cases (with parents findings). Scand J Haematol 19:85–92, 1977.

β^S-Gene-Cluster Haplotypes in Sickle Cell Anemia Patients From Two Regions of Brazil

To the Editor: The ethnic origin of the Brazilian population is heterogeneous and unevenly distributed within the country of continental dimensions. Hemoglobin S was introduced into Brazil by the slave trade and the prevalence of heterozygotes among the Black population has been estimated at 8% [1].

To our knowledge, no studies have been performed to study the frequencies of the β^S cluster haplotypes among Brazilian sickle cell anemia patients from different regions of the country. In this report we compare the frequencies of the β^S-cluster haplotypes among patients from Southeastern Brazil (São Paulo State) and Northeastern Brazil (Bahia State).

TABLE I. Haplotype Combination of Sickle Cell Anemia Patients From São Paulo and Bahia (Brazil)

Haplotypes	No. of patients (%) São Paulo	Bahia
CAR/CAR	13 (35%)	6 (16%)
CAR/Benin	19 (51%)	23 (64%)
Benin/Benin	4 (11%)	7 (20%)
Others	1 (3%)	—

Blood samples for hematological and DNA analysis were obtained from 73 nonrelated patients with homozygous sickle cell anemia (from the University Hospital of UNICAMP, Campinas, State of São Paulo, and from the University Hospital of Federal University of Bahia and of Oncology and Hematology Center "Eric Loffler," Salvador, State of Bahia). The diagnosis was based on clinical and laboratory findings [2].

High molecular weight DNA was isolated from peripheral blood leukocytes with proteinase K or urea using standard procedures [2]. The haplotype determination was carried out by PCR amplification of the region of the polimorfic site followed by digestion with appropriate enzyme. The following restriction sites were analysed: Xmn I of the position -158 of the $^{G}\gamma$ gene, Hind III in IVS2 of $^{A}\gamma$, Hind III of IVS2 of $^{G}\gamma$, Hinc II in the $\psi\beta$, Hinc II at 3' of $\psi\beta$ and Hinf I at 5' of β. The primers and conditions utilized were described by Sutton et al. [3].

Haplotype determinations in 37 samples from São Paulo and 36 samples from Bahia showed an apparently different distribution of haplotype patterns between the two groups of patients, although the difference was not significant (chi-square test). The results are shown in Table I. The samples from São Paulo exhibited 45 out of 74 (61%) chromosomes of the Central Africa Republic (CAR) type (−+−−−−), 28 (38%) of the Benin type (−−−−+−) and one of an atypical haplotype (−−−−−−). Among the samples from Bahia 35 (49%) were of CAR type and 37 (51%) were Benin type.

The data presented here suggest two distinct patterns of haplotype distribution for the two groups of patients. The most common type among patients from São Paulo State is the CAR haplotype whereas among patients from Bahia the CAR and Benin haplotypes are equally frequent. Moreover, the frequencies in both regions are different from those observed for U.S., Jamaican, and African sickle cell anemia patients [5–7].

The haplotype distribution observed in our study probably reflects the African ancestry of the patients. Brazil received slaves mainly from Angola, Congo, and Mozambique where the CAR haplotype predominates [8]. However, the State of Bahia, in contrast with the State of São Paulo, also received slaves from Nigeria and Ghana [8], regions where the Benin haplotype reaches high frequency [5]. Thus, the higher proportion of Benin haplotype in Bahia was to be expected based in the origin of the Black population. Internal migration from the less developed Northern States to the industrialized Southern States of Brazil may have contributed to the considerable proportion of the Benin haplotype in São Paulo.

Our data indicate that the pattern of β^{S}-haplotypes distribution in Brazil may be geographically heterogeneous, can be related to the origin and miscigenation of the Black population in the country and is distinct from that of the USA and Jamaica. In addition, the different proportion β^{S} of haplotypes may be a factor to explain the possible discrepancies of the clinical behaviour of the sickle cell anemia patients in different regions of Brazil.

ACKNOWLEDGMENTS

This work was supported in part by grants from FAPESP, Hemocentro-UNICAMP and CNPq, Brazil.

F.F. COSTA
V.R. ARRUDA
M.G. GONÇALVES
S.R.P. MIRANDA
M.H. CARVALHO
M.F. SONATI
S.O.T. SAAD
Department of Clinical Medicine, Hemocentro, UNICAMP, Campinas, São Paulo, Brazil
F. GESTEIRA
D. FERNANDES
M.L. NASCIMENTO
I.L. QUEIROZ
Federal University of Bahia and Hematology Center "Eric Loffler" Bahia, Brazil

REFERENCES

1. Zago MA, Costa FF: Heredity hemoglobin disorders in Brazil. Trans R Soc Trop Med Hyg 79:385–388, 1985.
2. Costa FF, Tavella MH, Zago MA: Deletion type thalassemia among Brazilian patients with sickle cell anemia. Rev Brasil Genet 12:605–611, 1989.
3. Sutton M, Bouhassira EE, Nagel RL: Polymerase chain reaction amplification applied to the determination of like globin gene cluster haplotypes. Am J Hematol 32:66–69, 1989.
4. Pagnier J, Mears JG, Dunda-Belkhodja O, Schaefer-Rego KE, Beldjord C, Nagel RL, Labie D: Evidence for the multicentric origin of the sickle cell hemoglobin gene in Africa. Proc Nat Acad Sci USA 81:1771–1773, 1984.
5. Powars DR: β^{S}-gene-cluster haplotypes in sickle cell anemia. Hematol/Oncol Clin of North Am 5:475–493, 1991.
6. Nagel RL: The origin of hemoglobin S gene: Clinical, genetic and anthropological consequences. Einstein Q J Med 2:53–62, 1984.
7. Hattori Y, Kutlar F,Kutlar A, McKie VC, Huisman THJ: Haplotypes of chromosomes among patients with sickle cell anemia from Georgia. Hemoglobin 10:623–642, 1986.
8. Saldanha PH: Mistura de raças. Mistura de genes. Ciencia Hoje 9:48–54, 1989.

Burkitt's Lymphoma Presenting as Ophthalmoplegia in an Elderly Male

To the Editor: Burkitt's lymphoma is a small noncleaved B-cell lymphoma, which was first described in 1958 as a mandibular malignancy in African children [1,2]. American Burkitt's lymphoma (AMBL) is found predominantly in older children and young adults. Although histologically identical, the American form typically presents as an intra-abdominal tumor with bone marrow involvement. Extranodal disease of the soft tissues and bones of the face occurs in less than ten percent of patients [3].

We describe a case of paranasal sinus Burkitt's lymphoma in a 70-year-old man. To our knowledge, this is the only reported case of AMBL of the nasopharynx in an older adult.

A 70-year-old man complained of nasal congestion and cephalgia and was treated empericially with cefaclor and decongestants without relief. Computed tomography of the head revealed mucosal thickening consistent with sinusitis. An antrostomy and ethmoidectomy was performed. The patient presented to our institution ten days later with complaints of bilateral ophthalmoplegia. He reported cephalgia and vertical diplopia for the preceding three days.

Examination revealed a symmetric face with a slight bilateral ptosis, no proptosis and total bilateral ophthalmoplegia. Pupils were equally reactive to light with slight anisocoria (5-mm OD and 4-mm OS). Visual acuity was without change and visual fields were intact. Fundi were normal. Neurologic examination was otherwise normal. No sinus tenderness or nasal

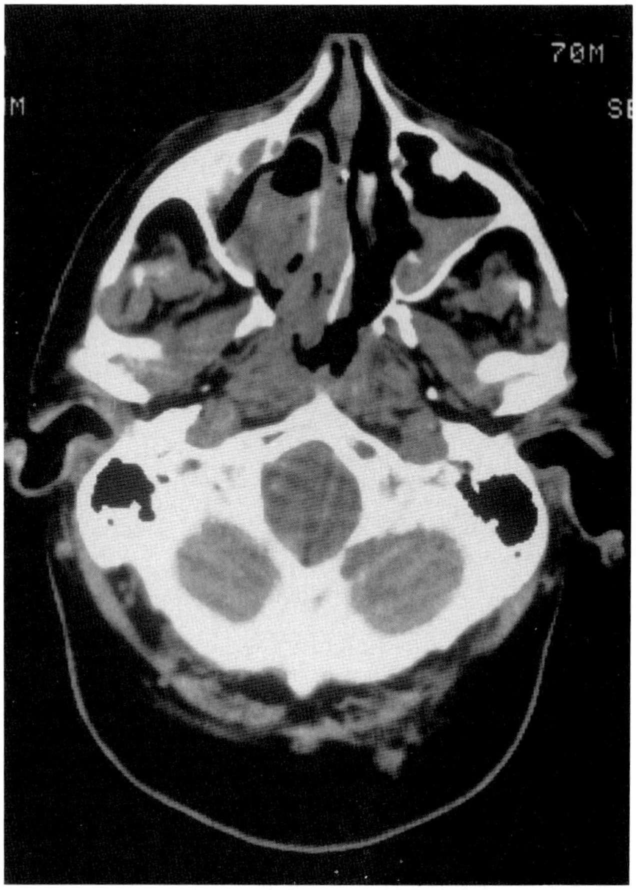

Fig. 1. Computed tomography scan of the head reveals Burkitt's lymphoma of the paranasal sinuses without extension into the orbits.

drainage was present. The cardiopulmonary exam was normal. The abdomen was soft and nontender with a palpable spleen tip, slight hepatomegaly, and a 4-cm, hard, fixed inguinal lymph node.

Laboratory studies were consistent with renal failure (BUN 94 mg/DL, creatinine 4.3 mg/dl). Electrolyte imbalances included hyponatremia (128 mmol/L), hypochloremia (94 mmol/L), hyperkalemia (5.1 mmol/L), and hyperphosphatemia (7.5 mg/dl). Biochemistry studies were otherwise normal except for an elevation of LDH (899 IU/L) and alkaline phosphatase (184 IU/L). There was a marked leukocytosis (leukocyte count 113×10^9), with lymphocytosis (81%) and anemia (hemoglobin 9 g/dl, hematocrit 31%). The peripheral smear showed mature lymphocytes with chromatin clumping. Cell marker analysis revealed an IgM/kappa population with low fluorescence intensity B-cell markers and no T-cell markers. CD5 markers were present with negative Tdt, consistent with CLL.

An aspirate of the inguinal node was obtained and revealed the presence of a high-grade lymphoma. The immunophenotype was different than that seen in the peripheral blood. Cell markers were intensely positive for IgM/kappa, CD20 (B1), CD19 (B4), and CD10 (J5 cALLa). CD5 markers were negative. Bone marrow examination revealed very few normal marrow elements with replacement by two abnormal lymphocyte populations compatible with both chronic lymphocytic leukemia and high grade lymphoma. Cerebrospinal fluid cytology was negative.

Slides of the sinus tissue were obtained from the prior ethmoidectomy. Sheets of uniform, undifferentiated small lymphocytes were noted below the respiratory epithelium. These cells had a high nucleus-to-cytoplasm ratio with numerous mitotic figures and a "starry sky" pattern formed by scattered large, pale histiocytes. The pathologic diagnosis was Burkitt's lymphoma.

In retrospect, polypoid tumors were evident on the initial CT scan of the sinuses prior to surgery (Fig. 1). A repeat study failed to reveal erosion into the orbits or brain; soft tissue densities were still present in the maxillary, ethmoid, and frontal sinuses. Magnetic resonance imaging of the head also demonstrated increased signal intensity of the lining of the sinuses without evidence of extension. CT scan of the abdomen and pelvis showed only mild hepatosplenomegaly and no mass.

The patient was treated with two cycles of cyclophosphamide, vincristine, cytarabine, methotrexate and prednisone. He developed complications of pancytopenia and pseudomonas sepsis and refused further chemotherapy. A residual palsy of right upward gaze remained for several months, followed by complete resolution of ophthalmoplegia. There has been no evidence of AMBL or CLL on restaging evaluations. The patient has had a sustained clinical remission for 2 years.

Approximately 25 new cases of AMBL are identified each year in the United States [4]. Involvement of the head and neck has never been reported in the elderly population. Only 48 cases of AMBL with extranodal involvement of the head and neck have been described in the English-language literature [3–7]. The oldest patient was a 38-year-old HIV-positive man with a palatal mass [3]. Our case is remarkable for an unusual presentation of AMBL in an elderly patient.

Sheryl A. Russ
Department of General Internal Medicine, Geisinger Medical Center, Danville, Pennsylvania

Omar H. Yumen
Department of Hematology, Geisinger Medical Center, Danville, Pennsylvania

References

1. Burkitt D: A sarcoma involving the jaws in African children. Br J Surg 46:218–223, 1958.
2. Magrath I: The pathogenesis of Burkitt's lymphoma. Adv Cancer Res 55:133–251, 1990.
3. Wang MB, Strasnick B, Zimmerman MC: Extranodal American Burkitt's lymphoma of the head and neck. Arch Otolaryngol Head Neck Surg 118:193–199, 1992.
4. Levine PH, Kamaraju LS, Connelly RR, Berard CW, Dorfman RF, Magrath I, et al: The American Burkitt's Lymphoma Registry. Cancer 49:1016–1022, 1982.
5. Pavlova Z, Parker JW, Taylor CR, Levine AM, Feinstein DI, Lukes RJ: Small noncleaved follicular center cell lymphoma: Burkitt's and non-Burkitt's variants in the United States. Cancer 59:1892–1902, 1987.
6. Patten LL, McMillan CW, Webster WP: American Burkitt's lymphoma: a 10-year review and case study. Oral Surg Med Path 69:307–316, 1990.
7. Schoem Sr, Morton AL: Paranasal sinus Burkitt's lymphoma in a human immunodeficiency virus positive male. ENT J 69:844–846, 1989.

Intracranial Hemorrhage in an Adult with Factor-VII Deficiency

To the Editor: Congenital factor-VII deficiency is a rare disorder with an autosomal recessive inheritance pattern. The gene is located on chromosome 13 [1]. Patients with severe deficiency often have clinical complications similar to those experienced by patients with hemophilia A [2]. In addition, an increased incidence of intracranial hemorrhage has been reported. It occurs most often in infants and is usually ascribed to birth trauma [3]. We report a case of an adult patient who presented with a right basal ganglia hemorrhage and was found to have a mild congenital factor-VII deficiency.

The proband is an 18-year-old white male who on the day of admission was found nearly unresponsive with a dense left hemiplegia. Prior history

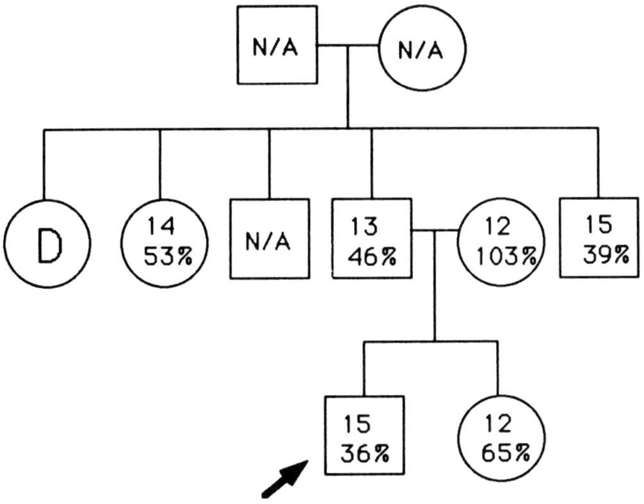

Fig. 1. Pedigree of the patient, parents and paternal relatives. The upper number in each box or circle refers to the prothrombin time in s and the lower number to factor-VII activity. The proband is marked with an arrow. N/A, not available; D, family member who died at age 9 of causes unrelated to bleeding.

included one transient episode of left sided weakness and bleeding colon ulcerations within the year prior to admission at which time the prothrombin time was elevated at 14 s. There was no family history of any bleeding abnormality. Physical examination was normal, except for somnolence and a dense left hemiplegia. Laboratory data included a prothrombin time of 15 s (reference range = 10–13) and a prothrombin time 1:1 mix with normal plasma corrected to 13 s. A factor-VII assay was 36%. Other vitamin K dependent factors, protein C at 87% and factor IX at 118% were normal. Normal studies included activated partial thromboplastin time, thrombin time, platelet count, bleeding time, fibrinogen, liver function studies, and creatinine. A head CT scan confirmed the presence of a large right basal ganglia hemorrhage. A cerebral angiogram showed a tiny 2- to 3-mm vascular anomaly in the region of the lenticulostriate arteries. Treatment was with fresh frozen plasma and vitamin K. Neurologic recovery was nearly complete.

Six family members were studied (Fig. 1). His father and paternal uncle had factor-VII levels of 46% and 39%, respectively, and prothrombin times that were at the upper limit of normal or mildly elevated. His mother, sister, and aunt were normal. This pedigree is consistent with a co-dominant gene expression for factor-VII levels and an autosomal recessive inheritance pattern with regard to clinical bleeding as would be expected from other family studies of factor-VII deficiency [4].

A 1981 review of 75 reported cases of factor-VII deficiency revealed a 16% incidence of intracranial hemorrhage [3]. Factor-VII levels ranged from <1% to 18%. The only adult in the series suffered a spontaneous subarachnoid hemorrhage [5]. Her factor-VII level was 2–3%, and she had other clinical history of significant bleeding events. No angiograms were reported on any of these patients.

The cause-effect relationship between our patient's intracranial hemorrhage and factor-VII deficiency is uncertain. Certainly, his factor level is such that significant bleeding is not expected, since spontaneous hemorrhage is rare when factor-VII levels are greater than 25% [2,4]. Although the tiny vascular abnormality demonstrated on arteriogram could cause such a hemorrhage, the incidence of bleeding from cryptic malformations in patients with factor deficiencies is unknown. It is possible that some of the patients reported by others had an undetected small cryptic vascular malformation that gave rise to the hemorrhage. However, given the described association of intracranial hemorrhage with factor-VII deficiency, the possibility must be considered that the factor-VII deficiency predisposed him to hemorrhage from the tiny vascular malformation that otherwise might have remained intact.

Barbara J. Seaborg
C. Patrick Burns
Department of Medicine, The University of Iowa College of Medicine, Iowa City, Iowa
John D. Olson
Beverly J. Pennell
Department of Pathology, The University of Iowa College of Medicine, Iowa City, Iowa
Kenneth A. Follett
Department of Neurosurgery, The University of Iowa College of Medicine, Iowa City, Iowa

References

1. Gilgenkrantz S, Briquel ME, Andre E, Alexandre P, Jalbert P, Le Marec B, Pouzol P, Pommereuil M: Structural genes of coagulation factors VII and X located on 13q34. Ann Genet 29:32–35, 1986.
2. Marder VJ, Shulman NR: Clinical aspects of congenital factor VII deficiency. Am J Med 37:182–194, 1964.
3. Ragni MV, Lewis JH, Spero JA, Hasiba U: Factor VII deficiency. Am J Hematol 10:79–88, 1981.
4. Owen CA Jr, Amundsen MA, Thompson JH Jr, Spittell JA, Jr, Bowie EJW, Stilwell GG, Hewlett JS, Mills SD, Sauer WG, Gage RP: Congenital deficiency of factor VII (hypoconvertinemia). Critical review of literature and report of three cases, with extensive pedigree study and effect of transfusions. Am J Med 37:71–91, 1964.
5. Owren PA: Prothrombin and accessory factors. Clinical Significance. Am J Med 14:201–215, 1953.

High-Dose Human Immunoglobulins in Thrombotic Thrombocytopenic Purpura

To the Editor: Thrombotic thrombocytopenic purpura (TTP) is a rare blood syndrome characterized by schistocytic and microangiopathic hemolytic anemia, thrombocytopenia, neurological symptoms, fever, and altered renal functions; its etiology is still quite unknown. Even though plasma exchange (PE) is now widely recognized as the therapy of choice in the treatment of TTP [1,2], the role is still to be defined of the various drugs which are usually combined with PE, i.e., cortisone, platelet anti-aggregating substances, and vincristine. The inhibitory effect of human immunoglobulins on platelet aggregation which was observed in vitro [3] has been considered as the rationale of their use in vivo in the treatment of TTP. However, only few reports [4,5] seem to suggest that human immunoglobulins are effective to treat TTP, at least in the rare cases not responding to more conventional therapy [5].

We briefly report on a recent case which was treated and cured by means of high-dose immunoglobulins (HDIgG) administration, after the failure of combined apheretic therapy, cortisone and platelet anti-aggregating substances. A young woman was hospitalized; she complained of bleeding gums and progressive sensorial clouding: hematochemical tests (Hb 6.8 g/dl, Ptl 19,000/mm^3, reticulocytes 18.5%, LDH 2,657 U/L, prothrombin time 12.6″, PTT 20.3″, fibrinogen 238 mg/dl, creatinine 1.1 mg/dl, bun 32 mg/dl, negative direct and indirect Coombs' test) and the observation of a peripheral blood smear (anisopoikilocytosis and schistocytes) allowed TTP to be diagnosed. The patient, after the treatment protocol suggested by the Italian Cooperative Group for TTP [2], was immediately submitted to apheretic treatment combined with i.v. acetylsalicylic acid (650 mg/day). Seven PE sessions were performed in 10 days, with the exchange of 1 plasma volume per session and the reinfusion of the same quantity of fresh frozen plasma. This combined treatment slightly improved the patient's neurological state but failed to effect so marked a change in pathologic blood variables as to allow either complete remission (CR) or partial remission (PR) (Ptl > 150,000/mm³, reticulocytes < 100,000/L, and LDH < 300 U/L for CR; Ptl < 100,000/mm³, with LDH < 300/L for PR, after Italian Cooperative Group criteria) [2]. Five more PE sessions were performed in 7 days, and i.v. cortisone (400 mg/day) was also administered from day 13 on. Once again, CR could not be achieved. Neurological symptoms increased. Therefore, HDIgG (40 g of human IgG/day) were administered. From the second day of treatment, a gradual normalization was observed in the patient's hematochemical variables; at 5 days, CR was diagnosed, with complete resolution of neurologic symptoms. The patient was discharged a week later and, 11 months after the acute episode, she remains in good health and has no signs of disease activity although receiving no consolidation treatment.

This case represents further, though certainly not conclusive, evidence of the possible efficacy of HDIgG in the treatment of the TTP forms not responding to conventional apheretic and pharmacologic (platelet anti-aggregating substances and cortisone) therapy.

Camillo Porta
Enrico Bobbio-Pallavicini

Italian Cooperative Group for TTP, Istituto di Terapia Medica, I.R.C.C.S., Policlinico "San Matteo", Università di Pavia, Pavia, Italy

References

1. Rock GA, Shumak KH, Buskard NA, Blanchette VS, Kelton JG, Nair RC, Spasoff RA: Comparison of plasma exchange with plasma infusion in the treatment of thrombotic thrombocytopenic purpura. N Engl J Med 325:393–397, 1991.
2. Bobbio-Pallavicini E, Porta C, Fornasari PM, Viarengo GL, Ascari E: Thrombotic thrombocytopenic purpura (TTP): retrospective study on 84 patients and therapeutical prospects. Transfus Sci 13:39–44, 1992.
3. Lian ECY, Mui P, Siddiqui FA, et al: Inhibition of platelet aggregating activity in thrombotic thrombocytopenic purpura plasma by normal adult immunoglobulin G. J Clin Invest 73:548–555, 1984.
4. Viero P, Cortellazzo S, Buelli M, et al: Thrombotic thrombocytopenic purpura and high dose immunoglobulin treatment. Ann Intern Med 104:282, 1986.
5. Finn NG, Wang JC, Hong KJ: High dose intravenous gamma-immunoglobulin infusion in the treatment of thrombotic thrombocytopenic purpura. Arch Intern Med 147:2165–2167, 1987.

HTLV-I Associated Adult T-Cell Leukaemia/Lymphoma in Hong Kong

To the Editor: Adult T-cell leukemia and lymphoma (ATLL) is an aggressive disease of CD4+ T-lymphocytes. The disease is endemic in the Southwestern part of Japan and the Caribbean [1]. Sporadic cases are also seen in other parts of the world [2]. Human T-cell leukemia/lymphoma virus-I (HTLV-I) has been recognised as the etiological agent of ATLL [1,2]. In Japan, 40–70% of their lymphomas are T-cell in origin and many of them are associated with HTLV-I infection [3].

Compared to the western population, a relatively high incidence of T-cell malignancies is seen in the Hong Kong Chinese [3]. About 70–80% of our cases of lymphoma are aggressive non-Hodgkin lymphoma and among them, 30% have a T-immunophenotype [3,4]. Since 1985, a total of 192 cases of T-cell lymphoma seen in our Department have been screened for HTLV-I antibody, only one of them are found to be positive.

The patient was a 42-year-old housewife presented to us in December 1992 with bilateral cervical lymphadenopathy for four weeks. She had no other symptoms. She had no history of travel except to some neighbouring cities in Southern China. There was no history of transfusion and intravenous drug abuse. Both the patient and her husband denied any extramarital sexual contact. On physical examination, there was generalised lymphadenopathy but no hepatosplenomegaly. Computerised tomography of abdo-

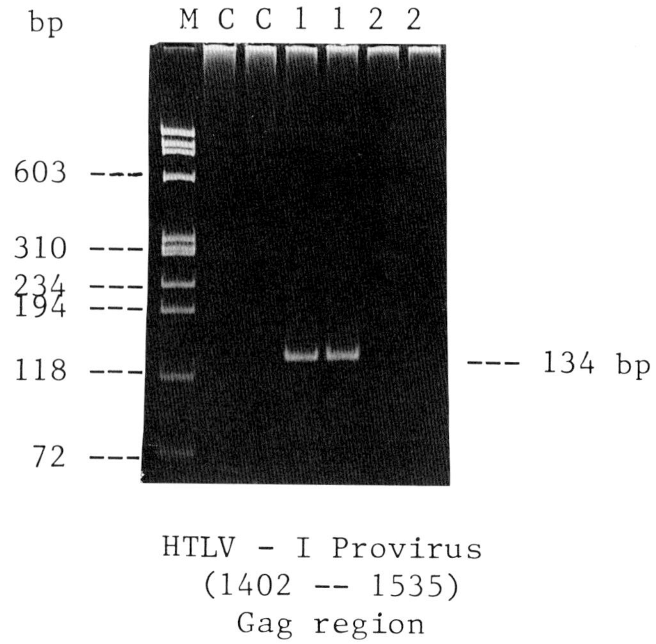

Fig. 1. Polymerase chain reaction detecting the Gag region of the HTLV-I provirus. M, markers; C, negative control; 1, peripheral blood of the ATLL patient; 2, peripheral blood of another patient with T-cell lymphoma.

men showed the presence of paraortic lymphadenopathy and a mild splenomegaly. The liver was normal. She had a hemoglobin of 10.8 g/dl, white cell 17.7 × 10⁹/L and platelet 321 × 10⁹/L. The peripheral blood showed 70% circulating abnormal lymphoid cells. There was no hypercalcemia. Lymph node biopsy revealed a pleomorphic T-cell lymphoma, and the marrow biopsy showed extensive lymphomatous infiltration. Immunophenotyping on the neoplastic cells demonstrated CD2, CD3, CD4, IL2 receptor and HLA-DR positivities. This was compatible with ATLL. She was confirmed to be seropositive for HTLV-I antibody by Western blot assay. DNA was extracted from the mononuclear cells of her peripheral blood. Using appropriate primers and conditions, polymerase chain reaction was performed for the Gag and pX regions of the HTLV-I provirus and both were positive [5] (Fig. 1).

Despite our geographic proximity to the endemic areas of HTLV-I infection in Japan, HTLV-I infection remains rare in Hong Kong. The origin of the virus of our first ATLL patient remains unknown. Although the mode of transmission of the virus is believed to be very similar to HIV, it is probably much less infectious. The relatively high incidence of T-cell malignancies in Hong Kong Chinese remains to be explained. Possibly, another retrovirus should be sought.

Raymond Liang

Department of Medicine, University of Hong Kong, Queen Mary Hospital, Hong Kong

References

1. Malik KTA, Even J, Karpas A: Molecular cloning and complete neucleotide sequence of an adult T cell leukaemia viruses/human T-cell leukaemia virus type I (ATLV/HTLV-I) isolate of Caribbean origin—relationship to other members of the ATLV/HTLV-I subgroup. J Gen Virol 69:1695–1710, 1988.
2. Sherman MP, Saksena NK, Dube DK, Yanagihara R, Poiesz BJ: Evolutionary insights on the origin of human T-cell lymphoma/leukemia virus-type I (HTLV-I) derived from sequence analysis of a new HTLV-I variant from Papua New Guinea. J Virol 66:2556–2563, 1992.

3. Ho FCS, Loke SL, Hui PK, Todd D: Immunohistological subtypes of non-Hodgkin's lymphoma in Hong Kong Chinese. Pathology 18:426–430, 1986.
4. Liang R, Loke SL, Ho FCS, Chiu E, Chan T, Todd D: Histological subtypes and survival of Chinese patients with non-Hodgkin's lymphoma. Cancer 66:1850–1855, 1990.
5. Hall WW, Liu CR, Schneewind O, Takahashi H, Kaplan MH, Roupe G, Vahlne A: Deleted HTLV-I provirus in blood and cutaneous lesions of patients with mycosis fungoides. Science 253:317–320, 1991.

AMERICAN JOURNAL OF HEMATOLOGY

INSTRUCTIONS TO AUTHORS

MANUSCRIPTS and all editorial correspondence should be sent to Ananda S. Prasad, MD, PhD, University Health Center, 5th Floor, Pod C, 4201 St. Antoine, Detroit, MI 48201, telephone and FAX (313) 577-7937. Submit the **original and three copies** of all elements arranged in the following order: title page, abstract, key words (for indexing), text, references, legends, tables, and illustrations. All **photographs** and **illustrations** must be submitted in **triplicate.**

Review of Manuscripts. All submitted articles will be reviewed by the Editor and two or more referees. **Authors may provide the Editor with a list of three to five potential reviewers.** The decision to use these reviewers remains with the Editor. Final acceptance will be based on the priority score assigned to each manuscript.

All copy must be double spaced on **8½ × 11 inch paper** and have generous margins, including the abstract, text, references, legends, and tables. Begin each part at the top of a new page. Number all pages in sequence, beginning with the title page.

Title page. This should contain the complete title of the manuscript, the names, titles, and affiliations of the authors, institution at which the work was performed, two to six indexing words as used in the Index Medicus, and the name, address, phone, telex, and fax numbers for all correspondence. Also include a shortened title, not more than 40 characters, to be used as a running head.

Abstract. This should be a factual condensation of the entire work, including a statement of its purpose, a clear description of the findings, including numbers, and finally a concise presentation of the conclusions. The abstract may not exceed 250 words.

Text. The text should follow the usual "Introduction, Materials and Methods, Results, Discussion, Conclusions" format; and it must be written in a manner that will permit the reader to easily understand what was done, the reason for it, and the conclusions drawn from the work. If the work includes data derived from human subjects, a statement that informed, written consent was obtained is mandatory. If any photographs of human subjects are to appear, a copy of the signed consent form must accompany the manuscript. Use subheadings and paragraph titles whenever possible. Define unusual abbreviations initially, e.g., chronic lymphocytic leukemia (CLL). Abbreviate measurements (cm, ml) according to The Council of Biology Editors Style Manual, 5th Edition (available from the Council of Biology Editors, Inc., One Illinois Center, Suite 200, 111 East Wacker Drive, Chicago, IL 60601-4298. Place acknowledgments as the last element of the text, before references.

References. In the text, references should be cited consecutively as numerals in parentheses. In the final bibliography, they should be in numerical order and should conform to Index Medicus style. For example:

Journal articles:

1. Awidi AS: Delivery of Infants With Glanzmann Thrombasthenia and Subsequent Blood Transfusion Requirements: A Follow-Up of 39 Patients. Am J Hematol 40:1, 1992.

Books:

2. Tunnicliff G, Raess BU, eds. GABA Mechanisms in Epilepsy. New York: Wiley-Liss, Inc., 1991.

Chapters in Books:

3. Coil WH. Platyhelminthes: Cestoidea. In Harrison FW, Bogitsh BJ, eds. Microscopic Anatomy of Invertebrates: Platyhelminthes and Nemertinea, Volume 3. New York: Wiley-Liss, Inc., 1991.

Legends. A descriptive legend completes an illustration and permits it to be useful without the necessity of referring to the text. A legend must accompany each illustration and must define all abbreviations used therein. Legends must be typed double spaced on a separate page at the end of the manuscript.

Tables. Tables must be self-explanatory and must not duplicate the text. Each must have a title and they should be numbered in order of appearance with Roman numerals.

Illustrations. 3 sets of glossy black and white photographs 5″ × 7″ or 8″ × 10″ in size are preferred. Do not submit original recordings, graphs, radiographic plates, or art work. They will be requested at a later date if needed for publication. All lettering must meet professional standards (and must be legible after reduction in size); typewritten or hand-lettering is unacceptable. All illustrations must be numbered in order of appearance with Arabic numerals. Identify each illustration on the back by affixing a gummed label on which is listed the number of the illustration, name of first author, title of manuscript, and an arrow indicating the top.

CONCISE REVIEWS. The purpose of a "Concise Review" is to provide practicing hematologists and those in training with a clear and up-to-date concept of a subject of current interest. It should be very informative, thoroughly referenced, and easily readable. The text should not exceed 3 or 4 journal pages in length. For information regarding the typing instructions and reference style, please refer to the instructions above. **Concise Reviews must be sent to Raymond Alexanian, MD, Associate Editor, American Journal of Hematology, Room AC6.005 (Box 1), MD Anderson Hospital and Tumor Institute, Texas Medical Center, 6723 Bertner Avenue, Houston, TX 77030.**

BRIEF REPORTS, LETTERS TO THE EDITOR, AND CORRESPONDENCE. These sections permit rapid publication of abbreviated communications in the field of hematology. **Brief Reports** may not exceed 750 words, 10 bibliographic references, and either one figure or concise table in the style of the Journal. **Letters to the Editor** should not exceed 500 words and five bibliographic references. A single concise figure or table may be included if it is essential to support the communication. Letters to the Editor are utilized to communicate a single novel observation or finding. Both Brief Reports and Letters may be used to communicate a laboratory observation, clinical experience, drug trial, or adverse effect. Correspondence is to be used to supplement or constructively comment on the content of a publication in the Journal and cannot exceed the restrictions for letters to the Editor. The Editor reserves the right to shorten text, delete objectionable comments, and make other changes to comply with the style of the Journal. Permission for publication must be appended as a postscript. **Brief Reports, Letters to the Editor, and Correspondence must be sent to Marcel E. Conrad, MD, Associate Editor, American Journal of Hematology, USA Cancer Center, Mobile, AL 36688, to permit rapid consideration for publication.**

All Manuscripts submitted to the American Journal of Hematology must be submitted solely to this Journal, may not have been published in any part or form in another publication of any type, professional or lay, and become the property of the publisher. Upon acceptance of a manuscript for publication, the author will be requested to sign an agreement transferring copyright to the publisher, who reserves copyright. No published material may be reproduced or published elsewhere without the written permission of the publisher and the author. The Journal will not be responsible for the loss of manuscripts at any time. All statements in, or omissions from, published manuscripts are the responsibility of the authors who will assist the editors by reviewing proofs before publication. Reprint order forms will be sent with the proofs.

Revised April 1993

American Journal of Hematology 45:103–108 (1994)

Hemophilic Pseudotumor: Multicenter Experience Over a 25-Year Period

M. Magallón , J. Monteagudo, C. Altisent, A. Ibáñez, A. Rodríguez-Pérez, J. Riba, J. Tusell, and J. Martín-Villar

Hemophilia Units, Hospital "La Paz," Madrid (M.M., A.I., A.R.-P., J.M.-V.); Hospital Clinico, Barcelona (J.M., J.R.); and Hospital "Vall d'Hebró," Barcelona (C.A., J.T.), Spain

Pseudotumor is an infrequent manifestation of bleeding diathesis seen in hemophiliacs, the management of which is still controversial. To ascertain the effectiveness of the main therapies of choice, we have reviewed 1,831 patients affected by hemophilias A (1,108) and B (172), von Willebrand's disease (329), and other miscellaneous coagulopathies (222) diagnosed between 1965 and 1990 in a multicentric, retrospective study. Pseudotumor was proven in 21 patients. Replacement therapy was given in 15 cases as the first therapeutic approach, with complete success attained in only two, whereas surgery, which was carried out in 14 patients, completely resolved the process in eight (*P* = 0.017). Patients over 40 years of age demonstrated worse prognosis than younger patients (*P* = 0.02), but no other clinical parameters were shown to have influenced the patients' evolution. Surgical management was the most effective treatment for pseudotumor, although more conservative therapies cannot be overlooked in selected cases.

Key words: **pseudocyst, hemophilia, dyshypoprothrombinemia**

INTRODUCTION

Pseudotumor is an uncommon, severe complication of bleeding diathesis occurring in a wide spectrum of bones and soft tissues in hemophiliacs; it consists of a chronically encapsulated blood collection, usually due to recurrent extraarticular hemorrhage in either bone or soft tissues. As swelling progresses, the increasing pressure within the hematoma leads to the slow destruction of adjacent structures. Although treatment of bleeding symptoms in hemophilia and other coagulopathies has progressed enormously over the last decades, at present management of bleeding-induced pseudotumors still lacks of well-established therapy rules. In addition, its relative frequency [1] further hinders the generalized elucidation of a basic treatment schedule. Several therapy approaches therefore have been used to date in managing hemophilic pseudotumors [2]. Surgery [3,4], replacement therapy [5,6], and local irradiation [5,7], alone or combined [5,6,8], as well as conservative measures [9], mainly have been described.

The choice of whether to use aggressive management as well as the influence of clinical and biological parameters on the outcome has been, to date, difficult to ascertain. In an attempt to investigate such unanswered questions, we have reviewed 1,831 individuals previously diagnosed with hemophilias A and B from 1965 to 1990 in addition to other miscellaneous coagulopathies in a multicenter, retrospective study.

PATIENTS AND METHODS

We reviewed 1,831 clinical histories of patients affected by congenital coagulopathies, diagnosed between 1965 and 1990 in three Spanish Hemophilia Centers (Units of Hemophilia from Hospitals "La Paz," Madrid, and Clinico and "Vall d'Hebró," Barcelona). The underlying coagulopathies included 1,108 patients with hemophilia A, 172 with hemophilia B, 329 with von Willebrand's disease (vWD), and 222 with other miscellaneous coagulopathies. According to the severity of the disease, 722

Received for publication April 21, 1992; accepted September 10, 1992.

Address reprint requests to M. Magallón, MD, Unidad de Hemofilia, Hospital "La Paz," P. Castellana 261, 28046 Madrid, Spain.

TABLE I. Relative Frequencies of Pseudotumor

	Patients	PTM[a]	Percent
Hemophilia A	1,108	16	1.44
Hemophilia B	172	4	2.32
Other coagulopathies	551	1	0.18
Total hemophilias	1,280	20	1.56
Severe	712	9	1.26
Moderate	252	7	2.77
Mild	316	4	1.26

[a]PTM, pseudotumor.

patients were considered severe (hemophilias A and B and vWD, with specific activities <1 U/dl), 254 moderate (between 1 and 5 U/dl), and 855 mild (>5 U/dl). Diagnosis of pseudotumor, following the clinical and radiological criteria described by several authors [2,9–12], was confirmed in 21 patients, after differential diagnosis was made with other processes, such as Ewing's tumor [9,13,14] and other sarcomas [13–17], aneurysmal bone cyst [9,16], giant cell tumor [9], malignant fibrous hystiocytoma [17], neurofibroma [17], and certain metastatic neoplasms [9,16].

The following data for patients with an established diagnosis of pseudotumor were recorded: type and the severity of the underlying disease; existence of a documented etiological antecedent; localization of the pseudotumor; and presence or absence of several clinical signs and symptoms (both induced and spontaneous local pain, signs related to the mass volume, and neurological compressive symptoms). The different treatment regimes have been classified into three major types: 1) continuous replacement therapy (as a first approach, and in the absence of any surgical procedure), in which doses ranging from 40 to 50 U/kg were transfused twice or thrice per week for a given period not less than 2 months; 2) discontinuous replacement therapy, in which the blood product was not infused following a well-established schedule; and 3) surgery. Patients have been followed by periodic examinations in the hemophilia center for 1.5–21 years.

RESULTS

Epidemiological and Clinical Data

The ages of the 21 patients, at the time of diagnosis of the pseudotumor, ranged between 8 and 61 years (median 40 years). Frequency distributions of pseudotumors according to type and severity of the coagulopathy are shown in Table I. One case was observed in a patient previously diagnosed as having abnormal prothrombin, prothrombin Barcelona [18]. The different localizations of pseudotumor are displayed in Table II. A documented relationship with an etiological antecedent was recorded in 12 patients: previous trauma in the affected zone was found in ten (47.6%), surgical procedure in one, and intramuscular injection in another. According to the localization, pseudotumor was confined to soft tissues in nine patients (42.8%), whereas in the remaining 12 (57.1%) bones were also affected (Fig. 1b). Local pain, either spontaneous or induced, was present in 17 (80.9%). Symptoms related to the great mass volume (Fig. 1a) were ascribed mainly to impaired walking in five (23.8%) cases (in whom pseudotumor was localized in the iliac, gluteus, thigh, femur, and toe). Compressive, neurological symptoms consisting of paresthesia, dysesthesia, and cubital nerve involvement were seen in three patients (14.2%). Seven patients were seropositive for HIV at the time of diagnosing pseudotumor. None had suffered, to that moment, either opportunistic infection or any other process attributable to HIV infection. The presence of a circulating factor VIII inhibitor (23 Bethesda U) was recorded in patient 18. Immunotolerance at doses of 50 U/kg/day of factor VIII during 8.5 months previous to intervention rendered the inhibitor not detectable. Follow-up determinations after surgery did not evidence inhibitory activity in plasma.

Anatomopathological Findings

Anatomopathology was recorded in 11 patients (Fig. 1c,d). Macroscopically, cysts were constituted of blood-like material in various degrees of organization. Their walls were fibrous, and intracyst tabications were occasionally seen. When bone was involved, both cortical and trabecular destruction was present, and damage or necrosis was observed in other adjacent tissues. Microscopically, cyst walls were formed mainly by connective tissue with a high content of collagen. The presence of foci of hemosiderin-loaded histyocytes was recorded in seven cases, whereas intense vascular neoformation was observed in five. Stores of hemosiderin were present in three patients and osteoid neoformation in two. Giant multinucleated cells mimicking osteoclasts were detected in one case, and foreign body-type cells in another.

Therapy, Complications, and Outcome

Continuously given replacement therapy was formerly chosen in 11 patients (Table II). Doses between 40 and 50 U/kg were transfused twice or thrice per week for periods of time ranging from 2 to 36 months (median 4 months). This regime was initially successful in three patients, but one showed a later relapse of the pseudotumor, whereas the continuous substitutive treatment did not modify the former evolution in the remaining eight (Fig. 2). Surgical treatment was subsequently carried out in five. Four patients were treated with discontinuous substitutive therapy, but in no case was such treatment demonstrated to induce noticeable improvement in the evolution of the pseudotumor (Fig. 2); amputation was indicated in two, and it was carried out in one. Surgery was employed for 14 patients (pseudotumor drainage has been considered

TABLE II. Different Therapies Given and Outcomes in Pseudotumor Patients*

Patient	Age (years)	Localization	Therapy	Outcome	Remarks
1	50	Iliopsoas	Discontinuous ST	Unchanged	Infection, fistula
2	43	Thigh	Continuous ST	Unchanged	Pathologic fracture 6 yr later
3	57	Thigh	Continuous ST	Unchanged	
4	14	Radius	Excision and ABF	Resolved	Dead, CH 12 yr later
5	35	Thigh	Discontinuous ST	Unchanged	
			Excision	Resolved	
6	17	Thigh	Continuous ST	Resolved	
7	61	Femur	Discontinuous ST	Unchanged	
			Amputation		Dead, stress ulcer
8	49	Gluteus	Continuous ST	Unchanged	
			Excision		Fistula
9	8	Toe	Discontinuous ST	Unchanged	
			Amputation		
10	32	Fibula	Continuous ST	Resolved	Relapse of PTM
			Continuous ST	Unchanged	
11	47	Thigh	Continuous ST	Unchanged	
			Excision	Resolved	Dead, HIV infection 8 mo later
12	39	Tibia	Excision	Resolved	Dead, CH 5 yr later
13	55	Ulna	Excision	Resolved	Dead, CH 11 yr later
14	42	Iliopsoas	Continuous ST	Unchanged	Infection
			Excision		Dead, postop bleeding and sepsis
15	17	Fibula	Excision and ABF	Resolved	
16	58	Iliac	Continuous ST	Unchanged	Treatment arrested by patient willing
					Dead, HIV infection
17	48	Thigh	Continuous ST	Unchanged	
			Excision	Unchanged	Local hematomata
			Re-operated	Slight improvement	Fistula
18	21	Femur	Amputation		Fistula before surg
					FVIII inhibitor
19	40	Iliac	Drainage		Fistula
			Excision		Local abscess
			Curretage	Resolved	
20	12	Radius	Continuous ST	Resolved	
21	19	Femur	Continuous ST	Unchanged	
			Excision and HBF	Improvement	Fistula, infection
			Fistulectomy	Resolved	

*ST, substitutive therapy; ABF, autologous bone filling; HBF, homologous bone filling; CH, chronic hepatopathy.

as a surgical procedure), in six as the first therapeutic approach; untractable pain, spontaneous drainage through the skin, risk of bone fracture, and a great mass had been the reasons to implement surgical management first. The remaining eight patients underwent surgery after being unsuccessfully treated with replacement therapy. Complete resolution of the process was obtained in eight (Fig. 2) of the 14 patients, in whom relapse of pseudotumor is still absent at present. Excision and curretage was performed in 11 patients, in three of whom the bone cavity was filled with either autologous (two) or homologous (one) bone tissue. Amputation was carried out in three, whereas pseudotumor was unsuccessfully punctured for evacuation in one patient.

To the present time, seven patients have died. Chronic liver disease was the immediate cause in three patients (5, 11, and 12 years after diagnosis of pseudotumor), whereas in another two death was related to complications of HIV infection several months later. Another patient died from postoperative bleeding and sepsis 1 month after surgery and the remaining case from a stress ulcer on the fourth day of the procedure. Infection of pseudotumor was seen in four patients, and fistulization appeared in six. Association of both fistula and infection was present in three patients. In all cases, either fistula or infection appeared in pseudotumors localized in the pelvis and proximally in the lower extremities. Of 14 patients with either of these localizations, seven developed infection and/or fistula; in the remaining seven cases, in whom pseudotumor appeared in other localizations, such complications were absent. In four of the seven patients with fistula or infection, pseudotumor was not resolved. Infections associated with HIV infection were not recorded in the postoperative follow-up of any patient, and no correlation was found between postsurgical infections and HIV-seropositive individuals. As miscellaneous

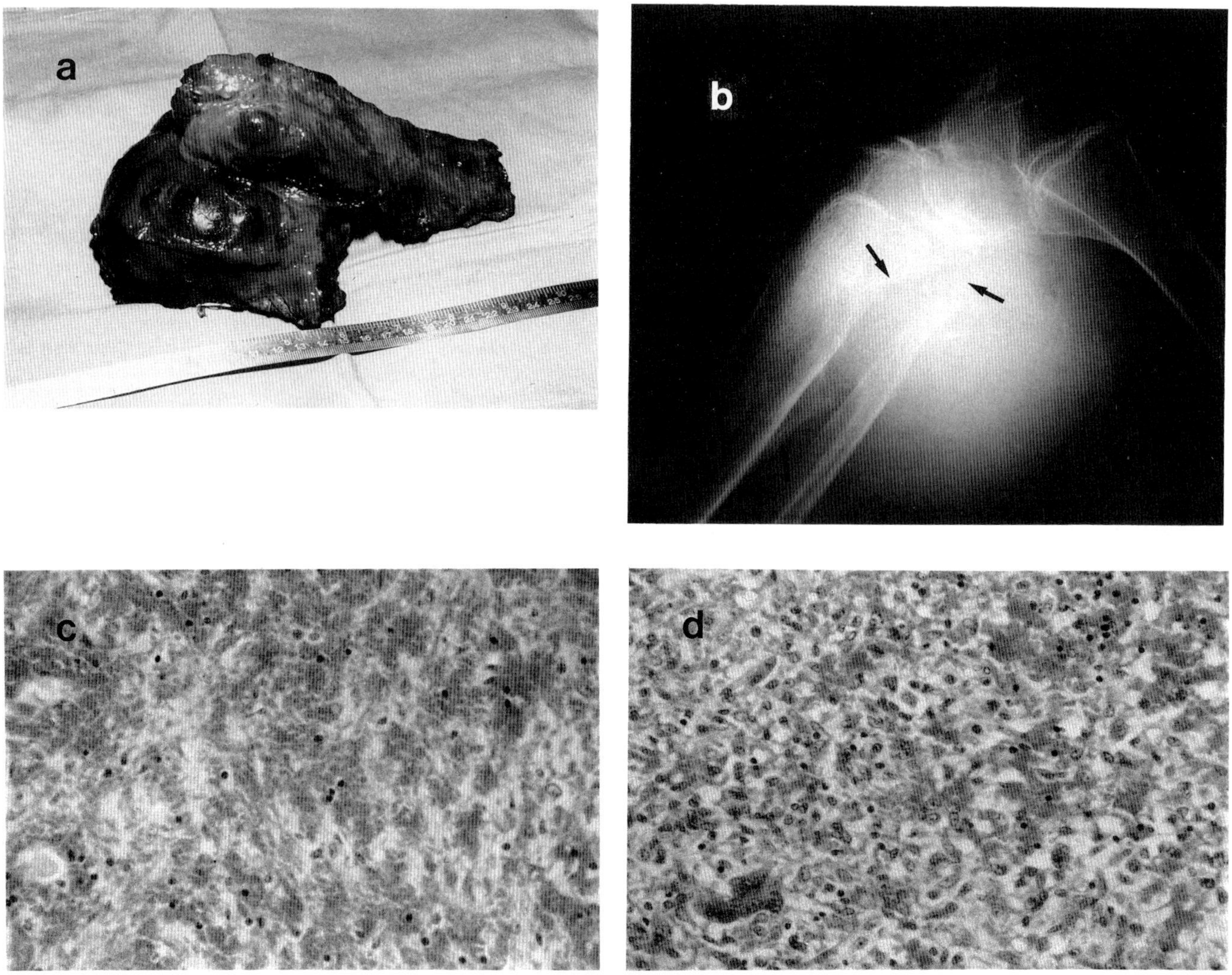

Fig. 1. Representative macroscopic, microscopic and roentegnographic examples of different pseudotumors. a: Excised pseudotumor. b: Roentgenogram showing (arrows) the complete destruction of the head of the fibula, erosion of the posterior region of the upper metaphysodiaphysiary part of the tibia, and periosteal reaction. c: Micrograph in which hemorrhagic material predominates over the presence of fibroblasts, suggesting an early stage of organization. d: Microscopic features of a more advanced degree of organization showing both larger number of fibroblastic cells and a giant multinucleated cell.

complications, a pathological fracture was observed in one patient 6 years following treatment, and another patient underwent secondary surgery for the development of local hematoma.

Patients of 40 years of age or less (n = 11) were demonstrated to have a better prognosis (resolved eight, unresolved three) than older ones (ten patients; resolved two, unresolved eight; $P = 0.02$, Fisher's exact test), whereas no differences were observed between children (18 years of age or less) and adults (over age 18 years). No correlation was found between the ages of the patients and complications or pseudocyst localization. The development of either infection or fistula was recorded only in those patients in whom pseudotumor was localized in the

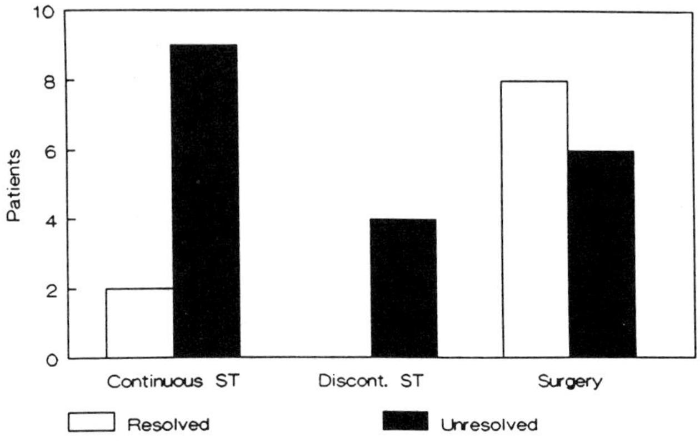

Fig. 2. Effect of the different treatment regimes on the patients' clinical evolution. ST, substitutive therapy.

pelvis or proximally. Surgery (14 patients; resolved eight, unresolved six) was found to be a safer procedure than replacement therapy alone (15 patients; resolved two, unresolved 13; $P = 0.017$, Fisher's exact test). The remaining clinical parameters did not correlate with the patients' outcome.

DISCUSSION

Hemophilic pseudotumor is a severe bleeding complication whose treatment remains difficult; as yet no specific measures have been proven to be of choice as a general approach. There is no wide agreement among authors in the management of pseudotumors [5,10,19–21], and the low numbers of previously reported patients [4,10,19,21–23] indicate that therapy is ultimately dependent on a careful case-to-case evaluation.

In our series, surgical management was related to the best results, especially in those cases when surgery was formerly chosen, whereas replacement therapy alone was successful in only two of fifteen patients. Even though this latter treatment has been the subject of great changes throughout the period studied, making comparisons difficult, the doses of either factor VIII or factor IX transfused were closely similar in terms of units/kg/day. Reported patients initially given only factor VIII transfusion have also frequently shown poor results [8,14,23–27]. Hence the choice of a conservative measure at first does not appear to be useful for most patients, as a general overview, obviously keeping in mind that an individual evaluation of each case cannot be overlooked. Furthermore, patients from our series in whom surgery was performed after replacement therapy had failed showed poorer results than those in whom surgical measures were first applied. Pseudotumor puncture is not considered a safe procedure: relapse, fistulization, and infection appear to be the usual consequences. On the other hand, HIV status did not share a well-defined relationship with postoperative infections. Even though children have not demonstrated a better evolution than adults, significant differences in the outcome observed between patients, when tailored to those younger or older than age 40 years, suggest a worse prognosis in older hemophiliacs, but their number has rendered the discrimination of the type of treatment performed impossible.

Although not statistically significant, an apparent tendency was observed in the proximal localization of pseudotumor of adults compared with the localization of pseudocysts appearing in children. The incidence of pseudotumors (1.56%) found in our study in such a large cohort of hemophiliacs confirms results of Gunning in 1966 [1]. Eleven of 20 hemophiliacs were mild to moderate, but significant differences in their outcomes, in comparison with severe patients, were not observed. Such an apparently similar incidence of pseudotumor in both types is not shown by other bleeding symptoms usually seen in hemophilia patients, and a number of mildly affected hemophiliacs have been reported in the literature [4,6,14,27–30]. A possible explanation is that the extremely frequent factor VIII transfusion needed by severe patients might partly act as a protective mechanism against the usually long lasting formation of the pseudotumor, while replacement therapy is much less frequent among mild-to-moderate hemophiliacs. Furthermore, medical consultation is more frequent for severe patients than other types, and this may be of importance in the prompt prevention of hemorrhages, which, if untreated, may progress to pseudotumor formation.

REFERENCES

1. Gunning AJ: The surgery of haemophilic cysts. In Biggs R, MacFarlane RG (eds): "Treatment of Haemophilia and Other Coagulation Disorders." Oxford: Blackwell 1966, p 262.
2. Gilbert MS: Hemophilic pseudotumor. In Brinkhous KM, Hemker HC (eds): "Handbook of Hemophilia." New York: Elsevier, 1975, p 435.
3. Rosenthal RL, Graham JJ, Selirio E: Excision of pseudotumor with repair by bone graft of pathological fracture of femur in hemophilia. J Bone Joint Surg 55A:827, 1973.
4. Post M, Telfer MC: Surgery in hemophilic patients. J Bone Joint Surg 57A:1136, 1975.
5. Hilgartner MW, Arnold WD: Hemophilic pseudotumor treated with replacement therapy and radiation. J Bone Joint Surg 57A:1145, 1975.
6. Wolff LJ, Lovrien EW: Management of fractures in hemophilia Pediatrics 70:431, 1982.
7. Lazarovits P, Griem ML: Radiotherapy of hemophilia pseudotumors. Radiology 91:1026, 1968.
8. Meyers L, Hakami N: Pseudotumor of hemophilia in the orbit: the role of radiotherapy in management. Am J Hematol 19:99, 1985.
9. Jensen PS, Putman CE: Hemophilic pseudotumor. Diagnosis, treatment, and complications. Am J Dis Child 129:717, 1975.
10. Brant EE, Jordan HH: Radiologic aspects of hemophilic pseudotumors in bone. Radiology 115:525, 1972.
11. Fernández de Valderrama JA: The haemophilic blood cysts. In Brinkhous KM, Hemker HC (eds): "Handbook of Hemophilia." New York: Elsevier, 1975, p 425.
12. Bullough PG, Bansal M: The differential diagnosis of geodes. Radiol Clin North Am 26:1165, 1988.
13. Lieberg OU, Penner JA, Bailey RW: Fibrosarcoma presenting as a pseudotumor of hemophilia. J Bone Joint Surg 57A:422, 1975.
14. Pettersson H, Ahlberg A: Computed tomography in hemophilic pseudotumor. Acta Radiol Diagn 23:453, 1982.
15. Koepke JA, Brower TW: Chondrosarcoma mimicking pseudotumor of hemophilia. Arch Pathol 80:655, 1965.
16. Sundaram M, Wolverson MK, Joist JH, Riaz MA, Rao BJ: Case report 133. Skel Radiol 6:54, 1981.
17. Hermann G, Gilbert M: Case report 471. Skel Radiol 17:152, 1988.
18. Rabiet MJ, Furie BC, Furie B: Molecular defect of prothrombin Barcelona. Substitution of cysteine for arginine at residue 273. J Biol Chem 261:15045, 1986.
19. Britten AFH, Salzman EW: Surgery in congenital disorders of blood coagulation. Surg Gynecol Obstet 123:1333, 1966.
20. Wessler S, Avioli LV: Changes in surgical management of hemophiliacs. J Am Med Assoc 206:2292, 1968.
21. Ahlberg AKM: On the natural history of hemophilic pseudotumor. J Bone Joint Surg 57A:1133, 1975.

22. Ghormley RK, Clegg RS: Bone and joint changes in hemophilia. With report of cases of so-called hemophilic pseudotumor. J Bone Joint Surg 30A:589, 1948.
23. Steel WM, Duthie RB, O'Connor BT: Haemophilic cysts. Report of five cases. J Bone Joint Surg 51B:614, 1969.
24. Coto H, Allen RC, Thomas E: CT scan diagnosis of hemophilic pseudotumor. Postgrad Med 70:82, 1981.
25. Kitchens CS: Computed tomography in two cases of hemophilic pseudotumors. Am J Hematol 12:277, 1982.
26. Marquez JL, Vinageras E, Dorantes S, Nussbaumer C, Flores A, Perez-Rolon G: Hemophilic pseudotumor of the inferior maxilla. Oral Surg 53:347, 1982.
27. Bellinazzo P, Silvello L, Caimi MT, Baudo F, de Cataldo F: Novel surgical approach to pseudotumour of ilium in haemophilia (letter). Lancet ii:1333, 1989.
28. MacFarlane RG, Mallam PC, Witts LJ, Bidwell E, Biggs R, Fraenkel GJ, Honey GE, Taylor KB: Surgery in haemophilia. The use of animal antihaemophilic globulin and human plasma in thirteen cases. Lancet ii:251, 1957.
29. Bloom AL, Enoch BA, Richards HJ: Major surgery in haemophilia. Prolonged substitution therapy for surgical treatment of haemophilic cyst and pathological fracture of the femur. Br J Surg 55:109, 1968.
30. Guilford WB, Mintz PD, Blatt PM, Staab EV: CT of hemophilic pseudotumors of the pelvis. Am J Radiol 135:167, 1980.

American Journal of Hematology 45:109–111 (1994)

Von Willebrand Factor Availability in Platelet Concentrates Stored for 5 Days

Jesús M. Cesar, Angel García-Avello, Juán Monteagudo, José I. Espinosa, José C. Lodos, Ricardo Castillo, and José L. Navarro

Servicio de Hematología, Hospital Ramón y Cajal, Madrid (J.M.C., A.G.-A., J.I.E., J.C.L., J.L.N.) and Servicio de Hemostasia y Banco de Sangre, Hospital Clinic y Provincial, Barcelona (J.M., R.C.), Spain

Von Willebrand factor (vWF) availability was assessed in platelet concentrates (PCs). After 5 days of storage, 82 ± 9% of basal levels of ristocetin cofactor activity (vWF:RCo) remained in PCs. vWF antigen (vWF:Ag) increased up to 166 ± 38% ($P < 0.05$) in the same period. Autoradiograph pattern of vW:Ag showed an increase in low molecular weight multimers, and fast migrating multimeric forms were visualized by crossed immunoelectrophoresis on day 5. Studies carried out in platelet free plasma stored as PCs showed similar changes in vWF:RCo but increments in vWF:Ag were not detected. These data indicate that PCs maintain vWF:RCo levels of clinical value even after 5 days of storage and suggest that vWF comes out from platelets to plasma during storage.

INTRODUCTION

The infusion of platelet concentrates (PCs) provides, in addition to the platelet supply, 400–600 ml of plasma [1] and therefore different proteins with potential hemostatic activities [2,3]. One of these components is the von Willebrand factor (vWF). Quantitative and qualitative deficiencies of this compound are associated with a bleeding disorder [4]. Consequently it seems useful to know the vWF availability in PCs, since changes of this protein could occur during storage. The current work studied the antigenic and ristocetin cofactor activities (vWF:Ag and vWF:RCo) in plasma of PCs stored for 5 days. Platelet influence in vWF changes was tentatively examined comparing these data with those obtained by similar studies carried out in platelet free plasma stored under the same conditions as PCs.

MATERIAL AND METHODS

Eight PCs were prepared in CLX™ bags (Cutter, Berkeley, CA) as has been previously published [5] and stored at 22 ± 0.5°C in a Hellmer agitator. Platelet free plasma (PFP) was prepared by centrifugation at 3,000g for 10 min and stored under the same conditions as PCs. On days 0, 1, 3, and 5, samples of 1 ml were removed from each container in sterile conditions and centrifuged at 1,900g for 10 min to obtain platelet poor plasma (PPP). vWF:RCo was measured using formalinized platelets as reported [6]. vWF:Ag and crossed immunoelectrophoresis were assessed according to Laurell [7]. Multimeric analyses were performed by mean of SDS-agarose gel electrophoresis [8] and autoradiographs of the electrophoretic runs were scanned in an EC 910 Transmission densitometer equipped with an EF 934 densitometer software (EC Apparatus Corporation, FL). Statistic analyses were made by the Snedecor "F" test.

RESULTS

Studies in PCs: vWF:RCo activity was arbitrarily considered as 100% on day 0 and decreased to 82 ± 9% on day 5 ($P < 0.05$, Table I). This meant a loss of 3.6%/day ($r = -0.98$). In the same period vWF:Ag increased up to 166 ± 38% ($P < 0.05$). On day 5, an increase in the fast migrating forms of vWF was detected by crossed immuno-electrophoresis (Fig. 1), and multimeric analyses showed an increase in low molecular weight bands (Fig. 2).

Studies in stored PPP:vWF:RCo decreased to 77 ± 14% on day 5 ($P < 0.05$), Table II), which was not different to the levels measured in PCs on this day. In contrast with PCs, we did not find changes in vWF:Ag.

Received for publication July 20, 1992; accepted June 30, 1993.

Address reprint requests to Dr. Jesús M Cesar, Servicio de Hematología, Hospital Ramón y Cajal, Ctera Colmenar Km 9, 28034 Madrid, Spain.

TABLE I. vWF in Plasma of PCs†

	Basal	Day 1	Day 3	Day 5
vWF:CRCo	100	92 ± 11	90 ± 17	82 ± 9*
vWF:Ag	100	128 ± 30	145 ± 37	166 ± 38*

†Figures indicate percentage ± 1 SD. Basal values were arbitrarily considered as 100%.
*$P < 0.05$.

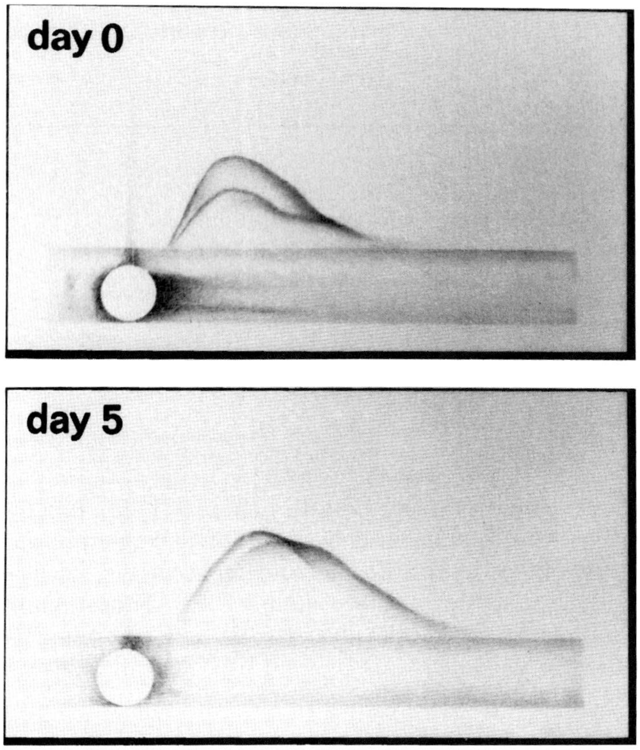

Fig. 1. Crossed immunoelectrophoresis of vWF:Ag in plasma of PCs on day 0 and on day 5 of storage. The anode is to the right in the first dimension and to the top in the second. On day 5 a wide arc resulting of a fast migrating forms of vWF can be observed.

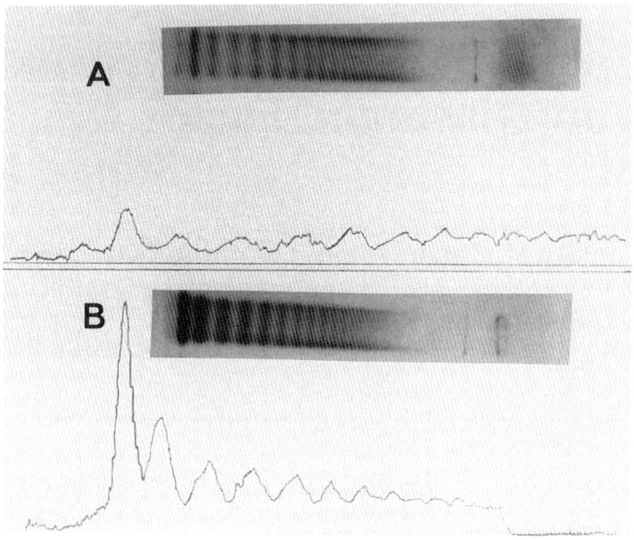

Fig. 2. Multimeric composition of vWF:Ag in plasma of PCs on day 0 (A) and on day 5 of storage (B). Autoradiograph pattern with their respective densitometer scans are showed to emphasized the increase of the most anodic bands. The arrows indicate the origin of running gel.

TABLE II. vWF in PFP Stored as PCs†

	Basal	Day 1	Day 3	Day 5
vWF:CRCo	100	96 ± 14	90 ± 17	77 ± 14*
vWF:Ag	100	98 ± 14	98 ± 15	97 ± 14

†Figures indicate percentage ± 1 SD. Basal values were arbitrarily considered as 100%.
*$P < 0.05$.

DISCUSSION

This study found that vWF:RCo activity remained with minor changes in PCs after 5 days of storage. Similar findings have been reported for most hemostatic proteins (but on, Factor V and Factor VIII) in PCs stored for 3 days [2,3]. The increase of vWF:Ag levels during PCs storage suggested the existence of a proteolytic degradation of vWF, and multimeric forms with enhanced mobility were shown by crossed immunoelectrophoresis and multimeric analyses later. This feature did not occur in PPP, which means that it was due to a platelet-mediated protease activity that has been demonstrated in these cells [9]. Despite this protein degradation, the levels of vWF:RCo in PCs on day 5 were similar to those measured on PPP, suggesting that plasma pool of vWF in PCs was replenished from some other source, probably platelets. Previous reports have shown that 10–25% of circulating vWF is confined in platelets [10,11], and the concentration of these cells is remarkably increased in PCs. The transfer from platelet vWF to plasma could occur passively or resulting of some platelet activation. This behaviour has been shown for other platelet proteins stored in granules [12,13]. Although secreted vWF is bound to membrane in activated platelets [14,15], the storage causes a reduction in platelet Gp Ib and Gp IIb-IIIa [16,17], which could impair this binding. In summary, this work demonstrated that PCs contain important levels of functionating vWF after 5 days of storage. We also suggest that platelet vWF replenish the plasmatic pool during the storage.

ACKNOWLEDGMENTS

The authors wish to thank María Teresa Urueña and Mariano Pérez for their excellent technical assistance.

REFERENCES

1. Murphy S, Kahn RA, Holme S, Phillips GL, Sherwood W, Davisson W, Buchhold DH: Improved storage of platelets for transfusion in a new container. Blood 60:194, 1982.
2. Simon TL, Henderson R: Coagulation factor activity in platelet concentrates. Transfusion 19:186, 1992.
3. Murphy S, Martinez J, Holburn R: Stability of plasma fibrinogen during storage on platelet concentrates at 22°C. Transfusion 23:480, 1983.
4. Ruggeri ZM, Zimmermann TS: von Willebrand factor and von Willebrand disease. Blood 70:895, 1987.
5. Cesar JM, Navarro JL: Arachidonic acid metabolism in platelets stored for five days. Br J Haematol 74:295, 1990.
6. Sureda A, Cesar J, García Frade LJ, Garcia Avello A, Fernández Fuertes I, Navarro JL: Hereditary hemorrhagic telangiectasia: Analysis of platelet aggregation and fibrinolytic system in seven patients. Acta Haematol 85:119, 1991.
7. Laurell CB: Quantitative estimation of proteins by electrophoresis in agarose gel containing antibodies. Analyt Biochem 15:45, 1966.
8. Monteagudo J, Pereira A, Roig S, Reverter JC, Ordinas A, Castillo R: Investigation of plasma von Willebrand factor and circulating platelet aggregating activity in mitomycin C-related hemolytic-uremic syndrome. Am J Hematol 33:46, 1990.
9. Kunicki TJ, Montgomery RR, Schulleck J: Cleavage of human von Willebrand factor by platelet calcium-activated protease. Blood 65: 352, 1985.
10. Koutts J, Walsh PN, Plow EF, Fenton JW, Bouma BN, Zimmerman TS: Active release of human platelet factor VIII-related antigen by adenosine diphosphate, collagen and thrombin. J Clin Invest 62:1 255, 1978.
11. Zucker MB, Broeckman MJ, Kaplan KL: Factor VIII-related antigen in human blood platelets. Localization and release by thrombin and collagen. J Lab Clin Med 94:675, 1979.
12. Snyder EL, Hezzey A, Katz AJ, Bock J: Occurrence of the release reaction during preparation and storage of platelet concentrates. Vox Sang 41:172, 1981.
13. Shimizu T, Ishikawa Y, Morishima Y, Fukuda T, Kato K: Platelet Factor 4 release from the platelets stored in platelet concentrates. Transfusion 25:420, 1985.
14. George JN, Onofre AR: Human platelet surface binding of endogenous secreted factor VIII-von Willebrand factor and platelet factor 4. Blood 59:194, 1982.
15. Fernández MF, Ginsberg MH, Ruggieri ZM, Batlle J, Zimmermann TS: Multimeric structure of platelet factor VIII/von Willebrand factor: The presence of larger multimers and their association with thrombin-stimulated platelets. Blood 60:1132, 1982.
16. George JN: Platelet membrane glycoproteins: Alteration during storage of human platelet concentrates. Thromb Res 8:719, 1976.
17. Bolin RB, Medina F, Cheney BA: Glycoprotein changes in fresh vs. room temperature-stored platelets and their buoyant density cohorts. J Lab Clin Med 98:500, 1981.

American Journal of Hematology 45:112–121 (1994)

Changes in Longevity and Causes of Death Among Persons With Hemophilia A

Terence L. Chorba, Robert C. Holman, Tara W. Strine, Matthew J. Clarke, and Bruce L. Evatt

National Center for Injury Prevention and Control (T.L.C.), and Division of Viral and Rickettsial Diseases (R.C.H., T.W.S., M.J.C.), and Division of HIV/AIDS (B.L.E.), National Center for Infectious Diseases, Centers for Disease Control and Prevention, Public Health Service, U.S. Department of Health and Human Services, Atlanta, Georgia

To examine recent changes in longevity and the causes of death among persons with hemophilia A, we evaluated death certificate data for persons who died in the United States from 1968 through 1989 and had hemophilia A or congenital Factor VIII disorder (ICD code 286.0) listed on the death certificate as one of the multiple causes of death. Multiple-cause-of-death mortality data for the United States from 1968 to 1989 were examined to compare death rates by year, focusing on death rates and causes of death for 1979–1981, 1983–1985, and 1987–1989. Gender, age group, race, geographic region, and median age at death of persons with hemophilia A and human immunodeficiency virus (HIV)-related disease listed as a cause of death were compared with those with hemophilia A without HIV-related disease. From 1968 through 1989, 2,792 hemophilia A deaths were reported. The death rate increased from 0.5 to 1.3 per 1,000,000 persons. From 1979–1981 through 1987–1989, mortality increased in all age groups above 9 years of age and age at death shifted markedly to lower ages. Median age at death decreased from 57 years in 1979–1981 to 40 years in 1987–1989. The percentage of deaths due to hemorrhage or diseases of the circulatory system decreased markedly as the result of the increase in deaths associated with HIV infection or infections other than HIV infection. Spread of HIV-1 infection in persons with hemophilia A has disrupted the reduction in mortality seen with factor replacement therapy, implementation of home care, and use of comprehensive hemophilia treatment centers. It is hoped that advances in the care of HIV-infected persons will improve survival in the hemophilia community.

Key words: HIV, AIDS, mortality, hemophilia

INTRODUCTION

Hemophilia A is the clinical manifestation of a congenital deficiency of procoagulant activity of the antihemophilic factor (AHF), factor VIII. In mild cases, spontaneous bleeding is rare, but exsanguinating hemorrhage can occur after injury or surgery. In severe cases, spontaneous bleeding can also be lethal because of local pressure effects. Hence, the disorder has been characterized by excess mortality and a markedly lower than normal mean age at death [1,2].

In 1937, a fraction isolated from plasma was found to correct the coagulation defect of hemophilia [3]. In 1965, it was discovered that the precipitate formed after slowly thawing frozen plasma was enriched in factor VIII coagulant activity [4], and by 1968, cryoprecipitate was widely used to treat hemorrhagic phenomena associated with hemophilia A. Purified preparations purported to be purified factor VIII were subsequently obtained from human plasma [5–9], and lyophilized factor VIII concentrates became commercially available. These are prepared either from cryoprecipitates or from preparations high in AHF that have been separated in other ways [10].

By 1982, 73% of persons with hemophilia A treated at U.S. hemophilia treatment centers received lyophilized concentrates [4], compared with 46% of persons with hemophilia A treated by U.S. physicians in 1970–1971 [2]. Also by 1982, 54% of persons with hemophilia A treated at hemophilia treatment centers received therapy almost exclusively at home [4], whereas only 10% received infusions outside of an institution in 1970–1971 [2].

Received for publication December 8, 1992; accepted June 30, 1993.

Address reprint requests to Terence L. Chorba, NCIPC, Centers for Disease Control and Prevention (K60), 4770 Buford Highway NE, Atlanta, GA 30341.

Home infusion with reconstituted factor concentrate meant that treatment of hemorrhage could begin sooner, reducing the severity of bleeding and markedly increasing longevity.

The first U.S. case of acquired immunodeficiency syndrome (AIDS) in a person with hemophilia was diagnosed retrospectively in January 1981 and reported to the Centers for Disease Control (CDC) in January 1982. By the end of 1982, considerable evidence indicated that transfused nonheat-treated factor VIII preparations that were then commercially used could potentially transmit the causative agent of AIDS, human immunodeficiency virus (HIV) [11,12].

By the end of 1992, over 253,000 persons with AIDS in the United States were reported to CDC [13]. Of these, 2,214 were persons with hemophilia A or other bleeding disorders. Most of these persons had transfusion exposure before the widespread use of heat-treated factor concentrates beginning in 1985. Because of the effect of the AIDS epidemic on the hemophilia community and the need for data for long-term planning for health care in the hemophilia community, we analyzed national mortality data from death certificates to examine recent changes in longevity and the causes of death among persons with hemophilia A.

MATERIALS AND METHODS

Multiple-cause-of-death mortality data for the United States from 1968 to 1989 were obtained from the National Center for Health Statistics (NCHS), CDC [14]. Cause-of-death classifications by NCHS from death certification data used the Eighth and Ninth Revisions of the International Classification of Diseases (ICD-9) [14–18]. For the years 1968–1978 in which the Eighth Revision was used, hemophila A deaths were defined as those in which code 286.0 [hemophilia: antihemophilic globulin deficiency, factor VIII deficiency, hemophilia (familial) (hereditary), hemophilia A] appeared in 1 of 14 record axis codes, i.e., deaths in which hemophilia A was recorded as one of the multiple causes of death. For the years 1979–1989 in which the Ninth Revision was used, hemophilia A deaths were defined as those in which code 286.0 [congenital factor VIII disorder: antihemophilic globulin deficiency, factor VIII (functional) deficiency, hemophilia, hemophilia A, classical hemophilia, familial hemophilia, hereditary hemophilia, subhemophilia] appeared in one of 20 record axis codes. The record axis coding is a method that links causes of death into categories for certification by NCHS and listed up to 14 causes of death per person for the Eighth Revision and up to 20 causes of death for the Ninth Revision. The record axis data classification is comparable to the underlying cause of death classification because it uses the same rules and category definitions. Multiple-cause-of-death data allow for mortality statistics based on a number of different causes reported on the death certificate.

Age-adjusted and unadjusted annual death rates in association with hemophilia A for the United States were calculated for the years 1968 through 1989 as the number of hemophilia A deaths per 1,000,000 persons, based on estimates of the U.S. resident population [19]. Because adjusting for age did not affect death rates for the years 1979 through 1989 by gender, race, or geographic region, we used unadjusted death rates. We calculated risk ratios (RR) with 95% confidence intervals (CI) to compare death for the periods 1979–1981 and 1987–1989 [20]. To examine age differences in death rates, we used 10-year age groups from 0 to 69 years of age and 70+. Median age at death in association with hemophilia A was determined for each 3-year period. To examine racial differences and trends, we used race categories as provided in the national mortality data: white, black, and other; the latter include American Indian, Chinese, Japanese, Hawaiian, Filipino, other Asian or Pacific Islander, and all other races. Geographic comparisons were analyzed by standard U.S. census regions: Northeast, North Central, West, and South.

To describe changes in causes of death among persons with hemophilia A, we examined the causes of death by broad disease categories, comparing the 3-year periods 1979–1981, 1983–1985, and 1987–1989. Other studies have noted considerable underreporting of HIV infection or AIDS on death certificates, possibly due to improper completion of death certificates, nonacknowledgment of HIV infection or AIDS on death certificates, causes of death unrelated to HIV infection, incomplete recognition of underlying diseases [21], or variations in terminology for certain disease categories [22]. To allow for such underreporting of HIV infection, we aggregated disease categories based on multiple causes of death listed on death certificates during 1987 through 1989, the years that specific codes for HIV infection (N042.0–N044.9) were first available for mortality coding [14,15]. These categories are presented in Table I.

To assess further the impact of HIV infection on mortality in persons with hemophilia A, we examined the characteristics of persons with hemophilia A with and without HIV-related disease listed on death certificates during 1987 through 1989. For persons with hemophilia A, gender, age, race, and region of those with HIV-related disease (including N042.0–044.9, N136.3, N279.1, N279.3, N279.9, and N795.8) listed as a cause of death were compared with those of persons with hemophilia A without HIV-related disease listed as a cause of death. The ages of persons in these groups were compared using the Wilcoxon rank-sum test [23].

RESULTS

In the 22 years from 1968 through 1989, 2,792 deaths in association with hemophilia A were reported in the multiple-cause-of-death data, 1,832 (66%) of which oc-

TABLE I. Aggregate Disease Categories Based on Multiple Cause of Death Listed on Death Certificates, 1987–1989

N001.0–139.0: Infectious and parasitic diseases other than infection with *Pneumocystis* or HIV
(excluding N042.0–044.9: HIV infection
and N136.3: Pneumocystosis)
N140.0–239.9: Neoplasms
N240.0–289.9: Endocrine, nutritional and metabolic diseases and immunity disorders, and diseases of blood and blood-forming organs, other than N286.0 (congenital factor VIII disorder)
(excluding N279.1: Deficiency of cell-mediated immunity;
N279.3: Unspecified immunity deficiency;
and N279.9: Unspecified disorder of immune mechanism)
N290.0–389.9: Mental disorders and diseases of the nervous system and sense organs
N390–459.9: Diseases of the circulatory system
(excluding N423.0: Hemopericardium;
N430–432.9: Subarachnoid, intracerebral, other than unspecified intracranial hemorrhage;
N456.0–456.2: Esophageal varices;
and N459.0: Hemorrhage, unspecified)
N460.0–519.9: Diseases of the respiratory system
N520.0–579.9: Diseases of the digestive system
(excluding N570.0–573.9: Acute and subacute necrosis of liver, chronic liver disease and cirrhosis, liver abscess and sequelae of chronic liver disease, and other disorders of liver,
and N578.0–578.9: Gastrointestinal hemorrhage)
N580.0–676.9: Diseases of the genitourinary system and complications of pregnancy, childbirth, and the puerperium
(excluding N596.7–596.8: Bladder hemorrhage
and N599.7: Hematuria)
N680.0–779.9: Diseases of the skin and subcutaneous tissue, musculoskeletal system and connective tissue, and congenital anomalies, and conditions originating in the perinatal period
(excluding N719.1: Hemarthrosis
and N767.0: Subdural hemorrhage)
N780.0–799.9: Symptoms, signs, and ill-defined conditions
(excluding N784.7–784.8: Epistaxis and hemorrhage from throat
and N795.8: Positive serological or viral culture findings for HIV)
N800.0–999.9: Injury and poisoning
(excluding N852.0–853.9: Intracranial hemorrhage following injury
and N860.2–860.5: Hemothorax and pneumothorax)
HIV-related disease: including N042.0–044.9, N136.3, N279.1, N279.3, N279.9, and N795.8, as excluded from other categories above.
Hemorrhage: including N423.0, N430–432.9, N459.0, N578.0–578.9, N596.7–596.8, N599.7, N719.1, N767.0, N784.7–784.8, N852.0–853.9, and N860.2–860.5, as excluded from other categories above.
Noncongenital, intrinsic liver disease: including N456.0–456.2 and N570.0–573.9, as excluded from other categories above.

curred in the latter 11 years (1979–1989). The death rates for hemophilia A for the United States from 1968 through 1978 decreased from 0.5 to 0.4 per 1,000,000 persons, and from 1979 through 1989 increased from 0.4 to 1.3 per 1,000,000 persons (Fig. 1). Demographic analyses of changes for the years 1979–1981, 1983–1985, and 1987–1989 are presented in Table II. The median age at death of persons with hemophilia A decreased from 57 years in 1979–1981, to 54 years in 1983–1985, and to 40 years in 1987–1989. For persons with hemophilia A listed in multiple-cause-of-death data in 1987–1989, the leading disease-specific causes of death (as categorized in Materials and Methods) were HIV-related disease (55.1%), diseases of the circulatory system (30.8%), hemorrhage (23.0%), infections other than pneumocystosis or HIV infection (16.3%), diseases of the respiratory system (15.0%), and noncongenital, intrinsic liver diseases (13.0%) (Table III).

The annual hemophilia A death rate for males was markedly higher than that for females, reflecting the inheritance pattern of congenital factor VIII deficiency and the rare occurrence of spontaneous factor VIII inhibitors in females, for example, in the postpartum period; for males, the rate significantly increased from 1979 to 1989 (Table II). Increases in death rates were seen in all racial groups. By age group, all age groups above 9 years had significant increases in mortality. The 10–19, 20–29, and 30–39 age groups had the largest relative increases in mortality; however, deaths associated with hemophilia A were most common in the 20–29, 30–39, 40–49, and 70+ age groups. Analysis by geographic regions showed significant increases in mortality in each region from

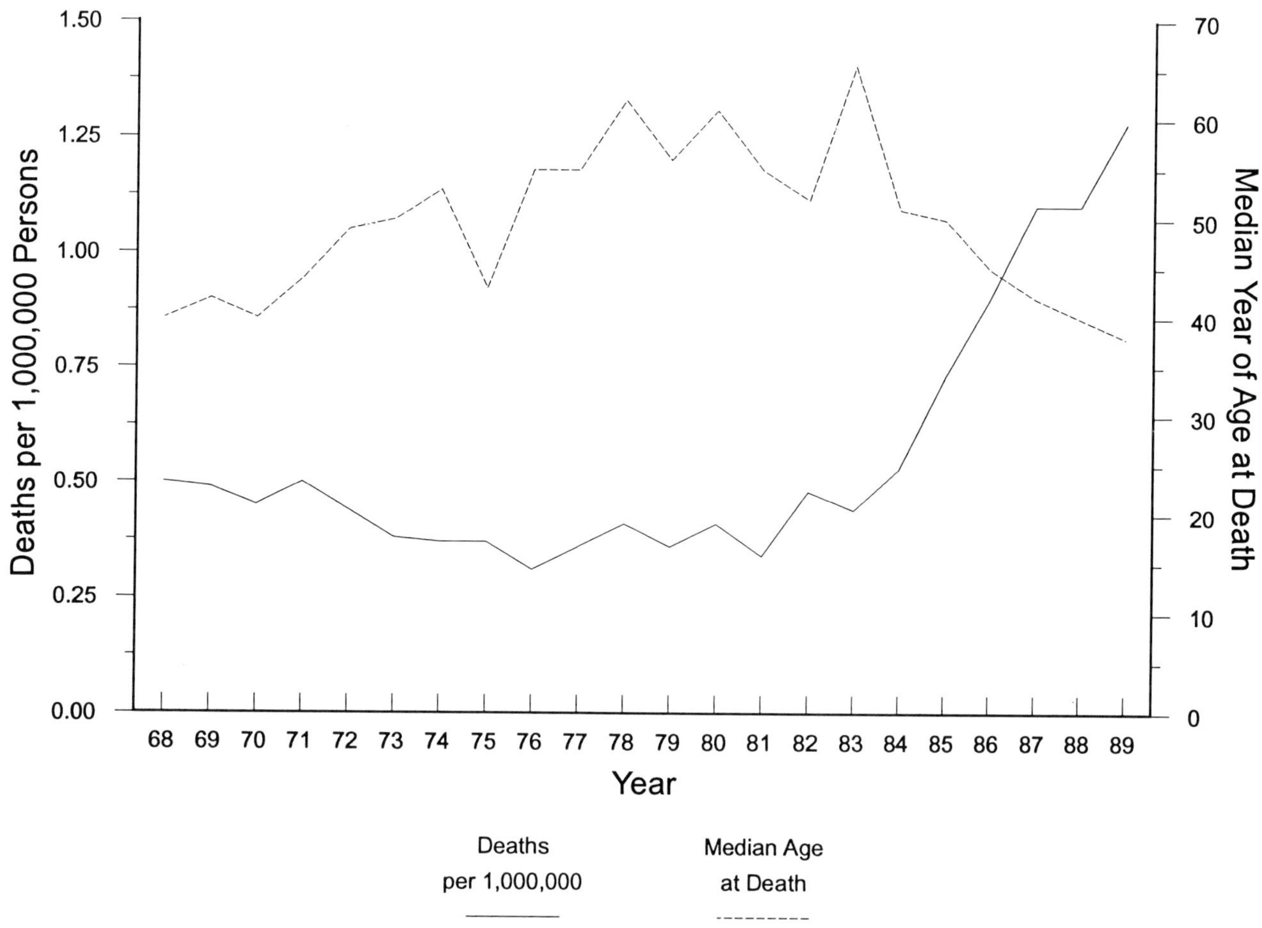

Fig. 1. Hemophilia A death rates and median age at death by year, United States, 1968–1989.

1979–1981 to 1987–1989 (Table II), with the greatest relative increases in the West. Comparisons of the age at death for 1979–1981 and 1987–1989 demonstrate the marked shift in age at death to lower ages in recent years (Fig. 2).

Deaths by disease category for the leading causes of death listed among multiple causes of death analyzed for each period (1979–1981, 1983–1985, and 1987–1989) are shown in Figure 3. Only 22 persons from 1979 through 1989 had hemophilia A listed as the sole cause of death, 9 of which were from 1987–1989. Although total number of deaths associated with hemorrhage or diseases of the circulatory system increased, the percentages of deaths associated with these causes from 1979–1981 through 1987–1989 decreased from 42.4 to 23.0% for hemorrhage and from 38.8 to 30.8% for circulatory diseases; these changes are the result of the marked increases in deaths associated with HIV or other infections (Fig. 3). For 68 persons with hemophilia A who died in 1987–1989 with infections other than pneumocystosis or HIV infection listed as a cause of death *and* without pneumocystosis or HIV infection listed in the death certificate, 41 (60%) had septicemia (streptococcal, staphylococcal, gram-negative, or unspecified), 16 (24%) had viral hepatitis, and 11 (16%) had another infection commonly associated with HIV infection: four had mycobacterial infections, two had candidiasis, two had histoplasmosis, one had blastomycosis, one had cryptococcosis, and one had an unspecified mycotic infection. By comparison, only 15 persons with hemophilia A in 1979–1981 had infections listed as a cause of death: seven had septicemia, five had viral hepatitis, one had cryptococcosis, one had listeriosis, and one had blastomycosis *and* septicemia.

Comparisons (for 1987–1989) of persons with hemophilia A for whom HIV-related disease was listed as a cause of death and persons with hemophilia A without HIV-related disease listed as a cause of death showed a marked difference in median age at death ($P < .001$): for those with HIV-related disease, median age at death was 34 years; for those without HIV-related disease, median age at death was 56 years. For persons with hemophilia A, additional comparisons by gender, age group, race,

TABLE II. Hemophilia A Annual Death Rates (per 1,000,000 Persons), United States, 1979–1981, 1983–1985, and 1987–1989

	Years							
	1979–1981		1983–1985		1987–1989		1987–1989/ 1979–1981	
	Rate	(No.)	Rate	(No.)	Rate	(No.)	Risk ratio	95% CI
Total	0.4	(250)	0.6	(403)	1.2	(853)	3.2	2.9–3.7
Gender								
Male	0.7	(228)	1.1	(368)	2.3	(815)	3.3	2.9–3.8
Female	0.1	(22)	0.1	(35)	0.1	(38)	1.6	1.0–2.7
Race								
White	0.4	(219)	0.6	(356)	1.2	(769)	3.3	2.9–3.9
Black	0.4	(29)	0.5	(42)	0.9	(79)	2.4	1.6–3.7
Other Races	0.1	(2)	0.2	(5)	0.2	(5)	1.5	0.3–7.8
Age Group								
0–9	0.2	(17)	0.2	(18)	0.2	(26)	1.4	0.8–2.6
10–19	0.1	(14)	0.2	(21)	0.8	(88)	7.1	4.0–12.4
20–29	0.2	(22)	0.3	(33)	1.1	(133)	6.0	3.8–9.4
30–39	0.2	(22)	0.5	(52)	1.4	(173)	6.2	4.0–10.0
40–49	0.4	(26)	0.7	(50)	1.5	(128)	3.9	2.5–5.9
50–59	0.5	(37)	0.8	(53)	1.2	(78)	2.3	1.5–3.3
60–69	0.9	(52)	1.1	(66)	1.6	(97)	1.7	1.2–2.4
70+	1.2	(60)	2.0	(110)	2.1	(130)	1.8	1.3–2.4
Region								
Northeast	0.5	(66)	0.6	(95)	1.3	(190)	2.8	2.1–3.7
North Central	0.4	(61)	0.5	(93)	1.2	(204)	3.3	2.5–4.4
South	0.4	(84)	0.6	(142)	1.2	(291)	3.1	2.5–4.0
West	0.3	(39)	0.5	(73)	1.1	(168)	3.7	2.6–5.2

TABLE III. Causes of Death on Death Certificates for Persons With Hemophilia A, United States, 1987–1989

Cause of death on death certificate	Number and percent[a] of persons (N = 853)
HIV-related disease	470 (55.1%)
Circulatory disease	263 (30.8%)
Hemorrhage	196 (23.0%)
Infections other than pneumocystosis or HIV	139 (16.3%)
Respiratory disease	128 (15.0%)
Noncongenital, intrinsic liver disease	111 (13.0%)
Injury or poisoning	94 (11.0%)
Endocrine, nutritional or metabolic disease	86 (10.1%)
Neoplasm	60 (7.0%)
Mental disorder or nervous system disease	60 (7.0%)
Digestive system disease	45 (5.3%)
Genitourinary disease or complication of pregnancy or childbirth	45 (5.3%)
Cutaneous, musculoskeletal, or connective tissue disease, congenital anomaly, or perinatal condition	29 (3.4%)

[a]Percent of hemophilia A deaths. Persons may have had more than one cause of death listed.

and region are presented in Table IV between those with HIV-related disease listed as a cause of death and those without HIV-related disease listed as a cause of death. More persons with hemophilia A in all age groups 10–49 years were listed with HIV-related disease than without HIV-related disease (Table IV), as reflected in the large increases in mortality in those age groups (Table II). Also, for persons with hemophilia A, the ratio of those with HIV-related disease to those without HIV-related disease was greatest in the West (Table IV), which may in part explain the greater *relative* increases in hemophilia A mortality in that region (Table II).

DISCUSSION

This study found that hemophilia A-associated death rates for the United States decreased from 1968 to 1978 but increased markedly in all age groups except the very young (0–9 year olds) from 1979–1981 to 1987–1989. These increases were most marked in association with HIV infection or HIV-related disease, with persons with HIV-related disease dying at significantly younger ages. The numbers of HIV-related deaths (Tables III and IV, and Fig. 3) represent estimates that are conservative, because possible HIV-related causes of death may be listed on the death certificate without expressly identifying HIV infection. For example, nonspecific, severe infectious processes associated with HIV infection, such as septicemia, may be listed as the cause of death. After 1979–1981, deaths due to infections other than pneumocystosis or HIV increased disproportionately to deaths associated with all other causes of death. In 1987–1989, of the 68 persons with hemophilia A with infections other than pneumocystosis or HIV infection listed as a cuase of death *and* without pneumocystosis or HIV infection

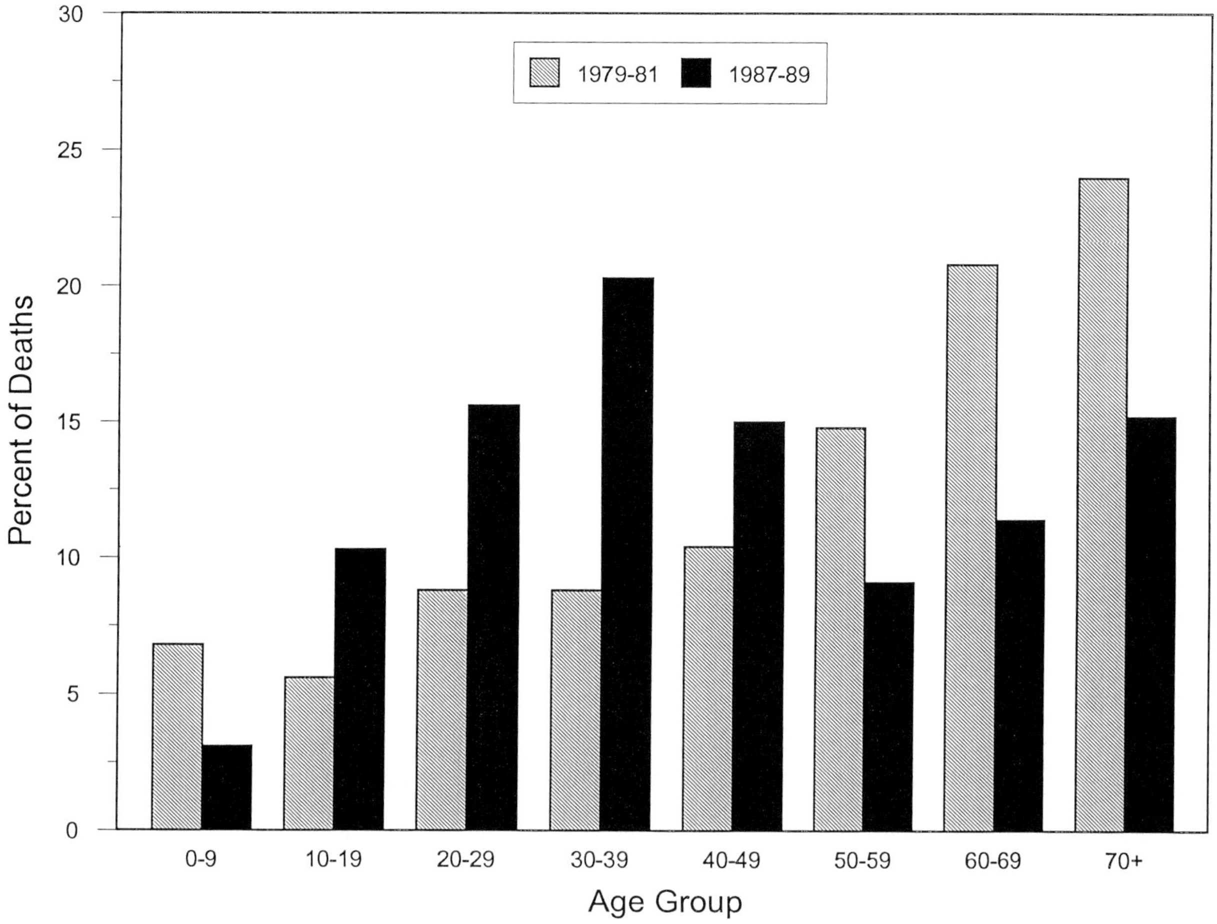

Fig. 2. Percentage of hemophilia A deaths by age group, United States, 1979–1981 and 1987–1989.

listed, 11 (16%) had mycobacterial or mycotic infections that are now commonly associated with HIV. From 1979–1981 to 1987–1989, a five-fold increase was also observed in hemophilia A deaths due to septicemia in the absence of other listed causes of death diagnostic of AIDS or HIV infection.

The spread of HIV-1 infection in persons with hemophilia A in the United States significantly disrupted the progress in mortality statistics for this population. In the 1960s and 1970s, the introduction of factor replacement therapy, the development of comprehensive hemophilia treatment centers, and the implementation of home care resulted in dramatic increases in median age at death [24] and a decrease in the number and proportion of deaths due to hemorrhage [4]. In the data presented here, these perturbations are underscored by the disparity in median age at death in 1987–1989 for persons with hemophilia A, between those with HIV-related disease (34 years) and those without HIV-related disease (56 years). Unfortunately, the adverse impact of HIV on mortality trends for persons with hemophilia A could not be fully represented in this study because death certificate data before 1968 do not differentiate hemophilia A deaths from those of other bleeding disorders. Analyses of death certificates also precluded assessment of the impact of HIV infection by severity of hemophilia A; it is likely that the greatest impact of HIV infection has been on those with severe hemophilia A, who are the predominant users of factor VIII concentrates and are more likely to be HIV-positive than are those with mild or moderate hemophilia A [25]. As in any study of death certificate data, this study also had the limitations of potential misdiagnoses or errors in death certificate preparation.

Among the very young, lack of change in the number of deaths observed here in association with hemophilia A may be explained by the widespread availability of donor-screened, heat-treated factor concentrates and implementation of blood screening programs after 1984, and by incubation period considerations, e.g., estimates of the median incubation period for transfusion-associated AIDS are as high as 11 years [26]. A low HIV-1 seroprevalence in the pediatric hemophilia population and an

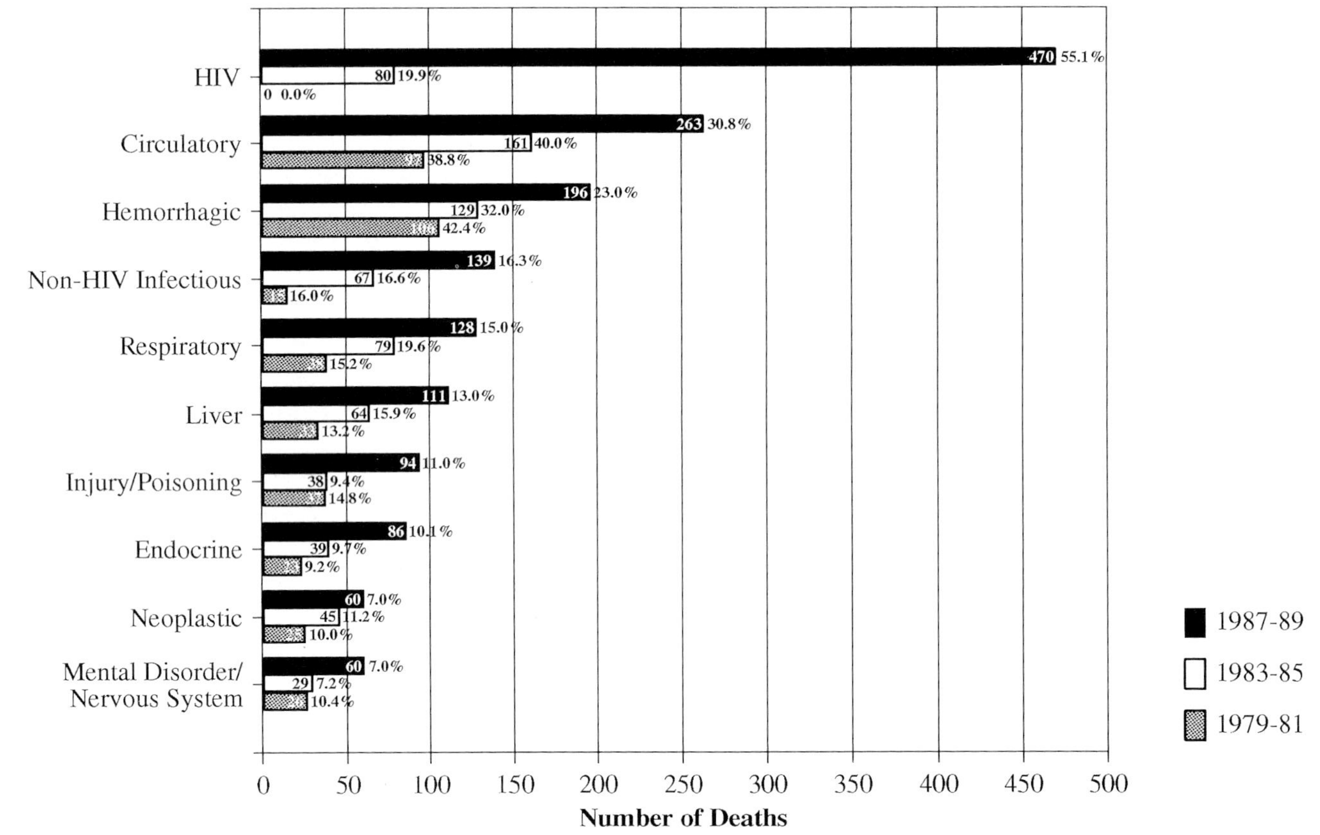

*Percent of Hemophilia A deaths in respective 3-year time frame. Persons may have more than one cause of death listed.

Fig. 3. Number and percentage* of hemophilia A deaths by cause of death listed on death certificates for leading causes of death, by period, United States, 1979–1981, 1983–1985, and 1987–1989.

increasingly greater seroprevalence among older persons with hemophilia was expected [27,28] and observed. In addition, AIDS incidence rates following HIV-1 seroconversion appear to increase with increasing age [29,30], suggesting that children and adolescents may tolerate severe immunodeficiency better than do adults [29].

Before the availability of an antibody screen for HIV, the use of alanine aminotransferase (ALT) testing to screen blood products was explored, but probably had no impact on HIV transmission through the use of concentrates: there was no clinically meaningful correlation between ALT level and evidence of HIV infection [31], and it appears that HIV infection could result from exposure to a single lot of unscreened factor concentrates that had not been heat- or solvent-treated [32]. However, it is estimated that testing for surrogate markers (such as ALT) before the introduction of anti-hepatitis C testing, reduced the rate of transfusion-associated hepatitis C from 0.45% to 0.19% per unit transfused [33].

A multifaceted approach has since reduced the risk of HIV exposure for persons with hemophilia. Pasteurization of factor concentrates is used to inactivate HIV without significantly altering the plasma recovery or plasma half-life [34,35]; dry-heat, steam treatment, and solvent detergents have also been used to inactivate HIV in preparing factor concentrates [34–36]. In January 1985, CDC recommended that all blood used for transfusion and for manufacturing of blood products be screened for HIV-1. In March 1985, the ELISA was first licensed as a screening test to be used in blood and plasma collection centers. Since May 1985, a two-phase screening procedure has been used by blood and plasma centers in the United States for all blood or blood products, to decrease the transmission of HIV through transfusion. First, potential donors are informed that if they have a risk factor for AIDS they should not donate; second, the blood or plasma accepted is screened for antibody to HIV-1, and an ELISA for HIV-2 has been licensed since April 1990 [37]. Several U.S. hemophilia treatment centers have also used cryoprecipitate from low-risk, screened donor populations. Although this approach has been very successful in preventing HIV-transmission to cryoprecipitate recipients [32], the number of hemophilia patients so treated has been small, with no apparent impact on varia-

TABLE IV. Persons With Hemophilia A With and Without HIV-Related Disease Listed as a Cause of Death on Death Certificate, United States, 1987–1989

	Number of persons with HIV-related disease (N = 470)	Number of persons without HIV-related disease (N = 383)
Gender		
Male	469 (99.8%)	346 (90.3%)
Female	1 (0.2%)	37 (9.7%)
Race		
White	433 (92.1%)	336 (87.7%)
Black	35 (7.5%)	44 (11.5%)
Other	2 (0.4%)	3 (0.8%)
Age Group		
0–9	7 (1.5%)	19 (5.0%)
10–19	71 (15.1%)	17 (4.4%)
20–29	93 (19.8%)	40 (10.4%)
30–39	134 (28.5%)	39 (10.2%)
40–49	80 (17.0%)	48 (12.5%)
50–59	37 (7.9%)	41 (10.7%)
60–69	37 (7.9%)	60 (15.7%)
70+	11 (2.3%)	119 (31.1%)
Region		
Northeast	100 (21.3%)	90 (23.5%)
North Central	110 (23.4%)	94 (24.5%)
South	157 (33.4%)	134 (35.0%)
West	103 (21.9%)	65 (17.0%)

tions in mortality in different regions of the country (Table II).

The risk of HIV exposure through blood transfusion has also been all but eliminated with application of the ELISA, in conjunction with a confirmatory assay (most commonly the Western blot [38]) for HIV-1 antibody, together with use by blood centers of self-exclusion criteria for donors at high risk, improved blood donor education, and wider HIV testing. [39,40]. The Food and Drug Administration (FDA) requires blood donors to test HIV-1 negative by Western blot as well as by ELISA to requalify for blood donation [37]. In September 1991, FDA licensed a combination HIV-1/HIV-2 test and recommended that blood centers start screening for HIV-2 by June 1992 [37]. Every donation of whole blood in the United States is now screened for HIV-1, HIV-2, human T-lymphotropic virus type I (HTLV-I), HTLV-II, the viruses of hepatitis B (HBV) and hepatitis C (HCV), syphilis and, in special pediatric units, cytomegalovirus [41]. However, new cases of transfusion-associated AIDS will probably continue to appear for two reasons: 1) since estimates of the median incubation period for transfusion-associated AIDS vary from 6.5 to more than 11 years [26,42,43], clinical manifestations, including AIDS, may develop in persons infected with HIV-1 before ELISA became available; and 2) blood from seronegative persons with recent HIV infection can transmit HIV: transmission has been reported from fully screened donors later found to have been exposed to HIV at the time of donation [44–48].

The spread of HIV-1 infection has diverted the attention of clinicians from another pair of sequelae of the treatment of hemophilia with blood and blood products, i.e., chronic hepatitis and progressive liver disease [49]. Most recipients of nonheat-treated factor concentrates have been infected with HBV [50] and HCV [51]. At least 50% of those infected with HCV get chronic hepatitis, and many eventually get cirrhosis [52]. Concentrates dry-heated at 60°C for 72 hr transmit non-A, non-B hepatitis agents to most recipients [53], although viral inactivation procedures effective against HIV and HBV do appear to reduce the risk of transmission of HCV from factor VIII concentrates [54,55]. A three-fold increase was observed when comparing 3-year periods 1979–1981 and 1987–1989 for total number of persons with hemophilia A with viral hepatitis listed as a cause of death *and* without pneumocystosis or HIV infection listed. A more than three-fold increase was also observed when comparing 3-year periods 1979–1981 and 1987–1989 for total number of deaths from hemophilia A in association with noncongenital, intrinsic liver disease, which may in part reflect the sequelae of exposures to HBV and HCV, as well as other non-A, non-B hepatitis agents [56,57].

Increases in deaths among persons with hemophilia A may continue [58], given the high prevalence of HIV-1, HBV, and HCV infection among persons who received unscreened, nonheat-treated blood products from 1978 to 1985 [29,57,59,60]. Attempts at modeling when increases in hemophilia-associated AIDS-related deaths will peak [29,59] may or may not be much affected by advances in treatment of HIV-infected persons. Continuous treatment with zidovudine [Retrovir, formerly azidothymidine (AZT)] appears to hinder the progression of disease to AIDS for HIV-1-infected persons with hemophilia [61–63]. Early treatment with zidovudine [64,65] and prophylaxis against *Pneumocystis carinii* pneumonia [62] appear to prolong survival in addition to prolonging the time until AIDS develops. However, numerous other antivirals for treating HIV infection are in development [66], some of which may have additional positive impact on the survival of HIV-infected persons with hemophilia.

ACKNOWLEDGMENTS

The authors thank Marilyn Kirk and John Hamilton for assistance with graphics.

REFERENCES

1. Larsson SA, Wiechel B: Deaths in Swedish hemophiliacs, 1957–80. Acta Med Scand 214:199–206, 1983.
2. National Heart, Lung, and Blood Institute. Pilot Study of Hemophilia Treatment in the United States. National Blood Resource Program.

DHEW Pub. No. (NIH) 73-417. Public Health Service, Washington, D.C.: U.S. Government Printing Office, 1972.

3. Pool JG, Hershgold EJ, Pappenhagen AR: HIgh-potency antihaemophilic factor concentrate prepared from cryoglobulin precipitate. Nature 203:312, 1964.
4. Johnson RE, Lawrence DN, Evatt BL, Bregman DJ, Zyla LD, Curran JW, Aledort LM, Eyster ME, Brownstein AP, Carman CJ: Acquired immunodeficiency syndrome among patients attending hemophilia treatment centers and mortality experience of hemophiliacs in the United States. Am J Epidemiol 121:797–810, 1985.
5. van Mourik JA, Mochtar IA: Purification of human antihemophilic factor (factor VIII) by gel chromatography. Biochem Biophys Acta 221:667–9, 1970.
6. Hershgold EJ, Davidson AM, Jansen ME: Isolation and some chemical properties of human factor VIII (antihemophilic factor). J Lab Clin Med 77:185–205, 1971.
7. Marchesi SL, Shulman NR, Gralnick HR: Studies on the purification and characterization of human factor VIII. J Clin Invest 51:2151–61, 1972.
8. Legaz ME, Schmer G, Counts RB, Davie EW: Isolation and characterization of human factor VIII (antihemophilic factor). J Biol Chem 248:3946–55, 1973.
9. Shapiro GA, Andersen JC, Pizzo SV, McKee PA: The subunit structure of normal and hemophilic factor VIII. J Clin Invest 52:2198–2210, 1973.
10. Brinkhous KM, Shanbrom E, Roberts HR, Webster WP, Fekate L, Wagner RH: A new high-potency glycine-precipitated antihemophilic factor (AHF) concentrate. JAMA 205:613–7, 1968.
11. Centers for Disease Control: *Pneumocystis carinii* pneumonia among persons with hemophilia A. MMWR 31:365–7, 1982.
12. Jason J, McDougal JS, Holman RC, Stein SF, Lawrence DN, Nicholson JKA, Dixon G, Doxey M, Evatt BL, and the Hemophilia/AIDS Collaborative Study Group: Human T-lymphotropic retrovirus type III/lymphadenopathy-associated virus antibody: Association with hemophiliacs' immune status and blood component usage. JAMA 253: 3409–15, 1985.
13. Centers for Disease Control and Prevention: "HIV/AIDS Surveillance Report," February pp 1–23, 1993.
14. Department of Health and Human Services, Centers for Disease Control and Prevention, National Center for Health Statistics. "Vital Statistics Mortality Data, Multiple Cause Detail, 1969–1989, Public Use Data Tape Contents and Documentation Package." Hyattsville, MD: U.S. Department of Health and Human Services, 1992.
15. National Center for Health Statistics: "Vital Statistics of the United States, 1988, Vol. II, Mortality, Part A." DHHS Pub. No. (PHS) 91-1101. Public Health Service, Washington, DC: U.S. Government Printing Office, 1991.
16. World Health Organization: "Manual of the International Statistical Classicification of Diseases, Injuries, and Causes of Death." Based on recommendations of the ninth revision conference, 1975, and adopted by the Twenty-Ninth World Health Assembly." Geneva, Switzerland: World Health Organization, 1977.
17. National Center for Health Statistics, Chamblee RF, Evans MC: TRANSAX, the NCHS system for producing multiple cause-of-death statistics, 1968–78. Vital and Health Statistics Series 1, No. 20, DHHS Pub. No. (PHS) 86-1322. Public Health Service. Washington, DC: U.S. Government Printing Office, June 1986.
18. Israel RA, Rosenberg HM, Curtin LR: Analytical potential for multiple cause-of-death data. Am J. Epidemiol 124:161–79, 1986.
19. Bureau of Census. "Intercensal Estimates of the Population of Counties by Age, Sex and Race: 1970–1990." Prepared by U.S. Bureau of Census. Washington, DC: U.S. Bureau of Census, 1992.
20. Rothman KJ. "Modern Epidemiology." Boston: Little, Brown and Co., 1986.
21. Hessol NA, Buchbinder SP, Colbert D, Scheer S, Underwood R, Barnhart JL, O'Malley PM, Doll LS, Lifson AR: Impact of HIV infection on mortality and accuracy of AIDS reporting on death certificates. Am J Public Health 82:561–4, 1992.
22. Sorlie PD, Gold EB: The effect of physician terminology preference on coronary heart disease mortality: An artifact uncovered by the 9th revision ICD. Am J Public Health 77:148–52, 1987.
23. Lehmann EL: Nonparametrics: Statistical Methods Based on Ranks. San Francisco, CA: Holden-Day, Inc., 1975, pp 5–13.
24. Aronson DL: Cause of death in hemophilia A patients in the United States from 1968 to 1979. Am J Hematol 27:7–12, 1988.
25. Fricke W, Augustiniak L, Lawrence D, Brownstein A, Kramer A, Evatt B: Human immunodeficiency virus infection due to clotting factor concentrates: Results of the Seroconverion Surveillance Project. Transfusion 32:707–709, 1992.
26. Lee CA, Phillips AN, Elford J, et al.: Progression of HIV disease in a haemophilic cohort followed for 11 years and the effect of treatment. Br Med J 303:1093–6, 1991.
27. Holman RC, Gomperts ED, Jason JM, Abildgaard CF, Zelasky MT, Evatt BL: Age and human immunodeficiency virus infection in persons with hemophilia in California. Am J Public Health 80:967–9, 1990.
28. Eyster ME, Gail MH, Ballerd JO, Al-Monhiry H, Goedert JJ: Natural history of human immunodeficiency virus infection in hemophiliacs: Effects of T-cell subsets, platelet counts, and age. Ann Intern Med 107:1–6, 1987.
29. Goedert JJ, Kessler CM, Aledort LM, Biggar RJ, Andes WA, White GC 2d, Drummond JE, Vaidya K, Mann DL, Eyster ME, et al.: A prospective study of human immunodeficiency virus type 1 infection and the development of AIDS in subjects with hemophilia. N Engl J Med 321:1141–8, 1989.
30. Brookmeyer R, Goedert JJ: Censoring in an epidemic with an application to hemophilia-associated AIDS. Biometrics 45:325–35, 1989.
31. Gjerset GF, Martin PJ, Counts RB, Fast LD, Hansen JA: Immunologic status of hemophilia patients treated with cryoprecipitate or lyophilized factor concentrate. Blood 64:715–20, 1984.
32. Gjerset GF, Clements MJ, Counts RB, Halvorsen AS, Thompson AR: Treatment type and amount influenced human immunodeficiency virus seroprevalence of patients with congenital bleeding disorders. Blood 78:1623–7, 1991.
33. Donahue JG, Munoz A, Ness PM, et al.: The declining risk of post-transfusion hepatitis C virus infection. N Engl J Med 327:369–373, 1992.
34. Heldebrant CM, Gomperts ED, Kasper CK, et al.: Evaluation of two viral inactivation methods for the preparation of safer factor VIII and factor IX concentrates. Transfusion 25:510–515, 1985.
35. Gomperts ED: Procedures for the inactivation of virus in clotting factor concentrates. Am J Hematol 23:295–305, 1986.
36. Horowitz MS, Rooks C, Horowitz B, Hilgartner MW: Virus safety of solvent/detergent-treated antihaemophilic factor concentrate. Lancet 2:186–9, 1988.
37. Sloand EM, Pitt E, Chiarella RJ, Nemo GJ: HIV testing: State of the art. JAMA 266:2861–6, 1991.
38. Centers for Disease Control: Interpretation and use of the Western blot assay for serodiagnosis of human immunodeficiency virus type 1 infections. MMWR 38:1–7, 1989.
39. Busch MP, Young MJ, Samson SM, Mosley JW, Ward JW, Perkins HA, and the Transfusion Safety Study Group: Risk of human immunodeficiency virus (HIV) transmission by blood transfusions before the implementation of HIV-1 antibody screening. Transfusion 31:4–11, 1991.
40. Cumming PD, Wallace EL, Schorr JB, Dodd RY: Exposure of patients to human immunodeficiency virus through transfusion of blood components that test antibody-negative. N Engl J Med 321:941–6, 1989.
41. Dodd RY: The risk of transfusion-transmitted infection. N Engl J Med 327:419–421, 1992.
42. Downs AM, Ancella-Park RA, Costagliolo D, Rigaut JP, Brunet JB: Transfusion-associated AIDS cases in Europe: Estimation of the incu-

bation period distribution and prediction of future cases. J Acquir Immune Defic Syndr 4:805–13, 1991.
43. Blattner WA: HIV epidemiology: Past, present, and future. Faseb J 5:2340–8, 1991.
44. Ward JW, Holmberg SD, Allen JR, Cohen DL, Critchley SE, Kleinman SH, Lenes BA, Ravenholt O, Davis JR, Quinn MG, et al.: Transmission of human immunodeficiency virus (HIV) by blood transfusions screened as negative for HIV antibody. N Engl J Med 318: 473–8, 1988.
45. Kleinman S, Secord K: Risk of human immunodeficiency virus (HIV) transmission by anti-HIV negative blood: estimates using the lookback methodology. Transfusion 28:499–501, 1988.
46. Cohen ND, Munoz A, Reitz BA, Ness PK, Frazier OH, Yawn DH, Lee H, Blattner W, Donahue JG, Nelson KE, et al.: Transmission of retroviruses by transfusion of screened blood in patients undergoing cardiac surgery. N Engl J Med 320:1172–6, 1989.
47. Donahue JG, Nelson KE, Munoz A, McAllister HA, Yawn DH, Ness PM, Cohen ND: Transmission of HIV by transfusion of screened blood. N Engl J Med 323:1709, 1990.
48. Julien A-M, Courouce A-M, Richard D, Favre M, Lefrere J-J, Habibi B. Transmission of HIV by blood from seronegative donors. Lancet 2:1248–9, 1988.
49. Hay CRM, Preston FE, Triger DR, Underwood JCE: Progressive liver disease in haemophilia: An understated problem. Lancet 1:1495–8, 1985.
50. Gerety RJ, Eyster ME, Tabor E, Drucker JA, Lusch CJ, Prager D, Rice SA, Bowman HS: Hepatitis B virus, hepatitis A virus and persistently elevated aminotransferases in hemophiliacs. J Med Virol 6:111–8, 1980.
51. Bretler DB, Alter HJ, Dienstag JL, Forsberg AD, Levine PH: The prevalence of antibody to hepatitis C in a cohort of hemophilic patients. Blood 76:254–6, 1990.
52. Alter HJ, Purcell RH, Shih JW, Melpolder JC, Houghton M, Choo QL, Kuo G: Detection of antibody to hepatitis C virus in prospectively followed transfusion recipients with acute and chronic non-A non-B hepatitis. N Engl J Med 321:1194–200, 1989.
53. Colombo M, Mannucci PM, Carnelli V, Savidge GF, Grazengel C, Schimpf K: Transmission of non-A, non-B hepatitis by heat treated factor VIII concentrate. Lancet 2:1–4, 1985.
54. Epstein JS, Fricke WA: Current safety of clotting factor concentrates. Arch Pathol Lab Med 114:335–60, 1990.
55. Fricke WA: Evaluation of the risk of hepatitis from clotting factor concentrates. In "Recent Advances in Hemophilia Care." New York: Alan R. Liss, Inc., 1990, pp 161–6.
56. Bradley DW, Maynard JE, Popper H, Cook EH, Ebert JW, McCaustland KA, Schable CA, Fields HA: Posttransfusion non-A, non-B hepatitis: physiocochemical properties of two distinct agents. J Infect Dis 148:254–65, 1983.
57. Eyster ME, Schaefer JH, Ragni MV, Gorenc TJ, Shapiro S, Cutter S, Kajani MK, Abrams J, Barron LE, Odenwelder A, et al.: Changing causes of death in Pennsylvania's hemophiliacs 1976 to 1991: Impact of liver disease and acquired immunodeficiency syndrome. Blood 79: 2494–5, 1992 (letter).
58. Jones PK, Ratnoff OD: The changing prognosis of classic hemophilia (factor VIII "deficiency"). Ann Intern Med 114:641–8, 1991.
59. McGrady GA, Jason JM, Evatt BL: The course of the epidemic of acquired immunodeficiency syndrome in the United States hemophilia population. Am J Epidemiol 126:25–30, 1987.
60. Centers for Disease Control: Human immunodeficiency virus infection in the United States: A review of current knowledge. MMWR 36:1–20, 1987.
61. Eichlinger S, Pabinger I, Hartl H, Stain C, Mayerhofer S, Schweiger C, Keir P, Shwarzinger I, Kyrle PA, Lechner K: Azidothymidine (AZT) in the treatment of symptomatic HIV-1-infected hemophiliacs. Thrombosis Haemostasis 64:108–12, 1990.
62. Merigan TC, Amato DA, Balsley J, Power M, Price WA, Benoit S, Perez-Michael A, Brownstein A, Kramer AS, Brettler D, et al.: Placebo-controlled trial to evaluate zidovudine in treatment of human immunodeficiency virus infection in asymptomatic patients. Blood 78:900–6, 1991.
63. Ragni MV, Kingsley LA, Zhou SJ: The effect of antiviral therapy on the natural history of human immunodeficiency virus infection in a cohort of hemophiliacs. J Acquir Immune Defic Syndr 5:120–6, 1992.
64. Vella S, Giuliano M, Pezzotti P, Agresti MG, Tomino C, Floridia M, Greco D, Moroni M, Visco G, Milazzo F, et al.: Survival of zidovudine-treated patients with AIDS compared with that of contemporary untreated patients. JAMA 267:1232–6, 1992.
65. Graham NHM, Zego SL, Park LP, Zenger SL, Park LP, Vermund SH, Detels R, Rinaldo CR, Phair JP: The effects on survival of early treatment of human immunodeficiency virus infection. N Engl J Med 326:1037–42, 1992.
66. Palca J: The growing anti-HIV armamentarium. Science 253:263, 1991.

American Journal of Hematology 45:122–127 (1994)

Varying Populations of CD59-Negative, Partly Positive, and Normally Positive Blood Cells in Different Cell Lineages in Peripheral Blood of Paroxysmal Nocturnal Hemoglobinuria Patients

Seitoku Fujioka and Teruo Yamada

Department of Hematology and Laboratory of Hematology, Mitsui Memorial Hospital, Tokyo, Japan

CD59-antigen expression on the surface membranes of erythrocytes, granulocytes, monocytes, lymphocytes, and platelets was determined by flow cytometry in 34 healthy controls and 17 patients with paroxysmal nocturnal hemoglobinuria (PNH). In all PNH patients, CD59-negative erythrocytes accounted for >10% of the total erythrocyte population. Two erythrocyte populations (CD59-negative and normally positive or CD59-negative and partly positive), three populations (CD59-negative, partly positive, and normally positive), and one population (CD59-negative) were demonstrated in ten, six, and one patients, respectively. However, CD59-negative granulocytes did not account for >10% of the total granulocytes in two patients, and one of them had only a CD59 normally positive granulocyte population. A particular granulocyte population extended over both CD59-negative and partly positive areas was shown in two patients. Two populations (CD59-negative and normally positive) and one population (CD59-negative) were demonstrated in monocytes and lymphocytes. CD59-negative lymphocytes accounted for >50% of the total lymphocytes in only two patients. Three patients had a CD59 normally positive lymphocyte population. Percentages of CD59-positive platelet population in normal controls were widely various. Therefore, it was usually difficult to discriminate between PNH-affected and normal platelets. Thus, the flow cytometric profiles of CD59-antigen expression varied not only between PNH patients but between cell lineages. The present results and our prior study indicate that CD59 flow cytometry using erythrocytes and granulocytes is most suitable for diagnosing PNH.

Key words: paroxysmal nocturnal hemoglobinuria, CD59 expression, flow cytometry, blood cell lineages

INTRODUCTION

Paroxysmal nocturnal hemoglobinuria (PNH) is characterized by hemoglobinuria, chronic intravascular hemolytic anemia, pancytopenia, susceptibility to infection, and venous thrombosis [1]. Complement-sensitive and -insensitive erythrocytes have been demonstrated in PNH [2]. Intravascular hemolysis is caused by the complement-sensitive erythrocytes. Membrane-bound C3b is increased about eightfold on complement-sensitive erythrocytes in PNH compared to that on normal erythrocytes [3]. A defect of decay-accelerating factor (DAF), known as a complement-regulatory protein for C3 convertases, was revealed in PNH erythrocytes in 1983 [4,5]. However, differences in the terminal steps of complement lysis of normal and PNH had been observed [6]. Complement-sensitive hemolysis of PNH erythrocytes was shown by reactive lysis [7]. CD59 (P18, MIRL, MACIF)[1] was extracted from normal erythrocyte membrane, and this contributed to protection against the complement-mediated hemolysis of normal cells [8–12]. A defect of CD59 is a major cause of the complement sensi-

Received for publication February 3, 1993; accepted June 30, 1993.

Address reprint requests to Seitoku Fujioka, MD, Director, Department of Hematology, Mitsui Memorial Hospital, 1 Kanda-Izumi-cho, Chiyoda-ku, Tokyo 101, Japan.

[1]Synonyms for CD59 include P18, protein 18 [8]; MIRL, a membrane inhibitor of reactive lysis [11]; and MACIF, a membrane attack complex-inhibitory factor [12].

tivity of erythrocytes in PNH [9]. Defective glycosylphosphatidylinositol (GPI)-anchored membrane proteins have been shown in granulocytes, monocytes, lymphocytes, platelets, and erythrocytes in peripheral blood of PNH [13–16]. In the present study, CD59-negative and -positive cells were determined in different cell lineages in peripheral blood of 17 patients with PNH. Typical patterns of CD59 flow cytometric profiles in PNH-affected cells were elucidated in each cell lineage.

MATERIALS AND METHODS

Patients

The 17 patients consisted of five males and 12 females ranging in age from 19 to 81 (mean 43) years. The patients were treated in our hospital and/or the affiliated hospitals. All of them had clinical findings consisted with PNH and showed positive acidified serum (Ham's) and/or sucrose lysis tests. Some patients received daily oral androgen treatment. However, all patients were untransfused at the time of study. Informed consent for this study was obtained from all participants. The periods after PNH diagnosis of each patient were 1–205 (median 66) months. Hematological data at the time of the study were shown as follows: red blood cell counts, 1.26–3.76 (mean 2.74) $\times 10^{12}$/liter; hemoglobin concentration, 4.8–14.2 (mean 8.9) g/dl; reticulocyte counts 53–188 (mean 121) $\times 10^9$/liter; white blood cell counts, 1.7–5.1 (mean 3.4) $\times 10^9$/liter; lymphocyte counts, 0.36–2.34 (mean 1.23) $\times 10^9$/liter; platelet counts, 8–172 (mean 86) $\times 10^9$/liter. Values of serum lactic dehydrogenase activity, total bilirubin, and plasma hemoglobin were increased. Serum haptoglobin was decreased.

Blood Cell Preparation

Whole blood from 34 healthy individuals (controls) and 17 patients with PNH was drawn via venous puncture into a tube containing EDTA or heparin. Whole blood was centrifuged at 800 rpm (16 cm radius) for 10 min. Sedimented erythrocytes were washed twice with phosphate-buffered saline (PBS, pH 7.4) and then suspended in PBS at $\sim 10^5$ cells/μl. To collect leukocytes, the sedimented cells were added to Separate-L (specific gravity 1.105; Mutoh Cehmical Co., Tokyo, Japan) and centrifuged at 1,500 rpm for 30 min. The leukocyte layer was collected and washed twice PBS, and the leukocytes were suspended at 10^3 cells/μl in PBS. Platelets in the plasma obtained by centrifugation of whole blood were washed twice with PBS containing 10 mM EDTA and were suspended in PBS at $\sim 5 \times 10^4$/μl.

Flow Cytometry

One hundred microliters of each suspension was added to 10 μl (~200 μg protein) of mouse IgG anti-CD59 monoclonal antibody (kindly supplied by Prof. M. Tomita) and incubation was done at 0°C for 30 min [12]. After washing twice with PBS, cells were resuspended in 200 μl of PBS. Then, 200 μl of diluted goat $F(ab')_2$ anti-mouse Igs (G + L) − FITC (Tago Inc., Burlingame, CA) was added, followed by incubation at 0°C for 40 min. The erythrocytes and platelets were next washed twice with PBS and prepared for flow cytometry on an Ortho Cytron (Ortho Diagnostic Co., Tokyo, Japan). Leukocytes were added to 2 ml of lysing reagent containing ammonium chloride and were let stand for 15 min. Then the leukocytes were washed twice with PBS and prepared for flow cytometry. After the gating conditions were tested with cells in different cell lineage, each blood cell population was checked on a scattergram of the Cytron. Flow cytometric profiles were drawn using the counts of CD59-negative and CD59-positive cells vs. the intensity of CD59-fluorescence on a logarithmic scale. Five to ten thousand cells were counted to draw each prolife, except in the case of monocytes. About 1,000 monocytes were counted because of their small number in the peripheral blood. The same procedure was performed omitting incubation with the anti-CD59 antibody to provide a negative control. The CD59-negative area in the flow cytometric profile was defined as the area containing 99.7% of the negative control cells.

Statistics

The significant difference of mean value between controls and PNH patients was determined by Student's t test.

RESULTS

Typical CD59 flow cytometric profiles of erythrocytes, granulocytes, monocytes, lymphocytes, and platelets from a control subject and the patients with PNH are shown in Figure 1. A CD59-negative erythrocyte population was found in all patients with PNH who were confirmed by positive Ham's test and/or sucrose hemolysis test.

The CD59-positive cells in PNH are classified into two subpopulations. Normally positive cells are those with a mean intensity of CD59-fluorescence that lay within the normal range (mean − 2 S.D. to mean + 2 S.D.) calculated from the 34 healthy controls [17]. Partly positive cells (intermediate positive cells) are shown between negative and normally positive areas. It is thought that both CD59-negative and partly positive cells are PNH affected. Percentages of CD59-negative cells and partly positive cells in each cell lineage in peripheral blood of the 17 patients with PNH are shown in Table I.

Two erythrocyte populations (CD59-negative and normally positive) and the other two populations (CD59-negative and partly positive) are demonstrated in nine patients and one patient, respectively. Three erythrocyte

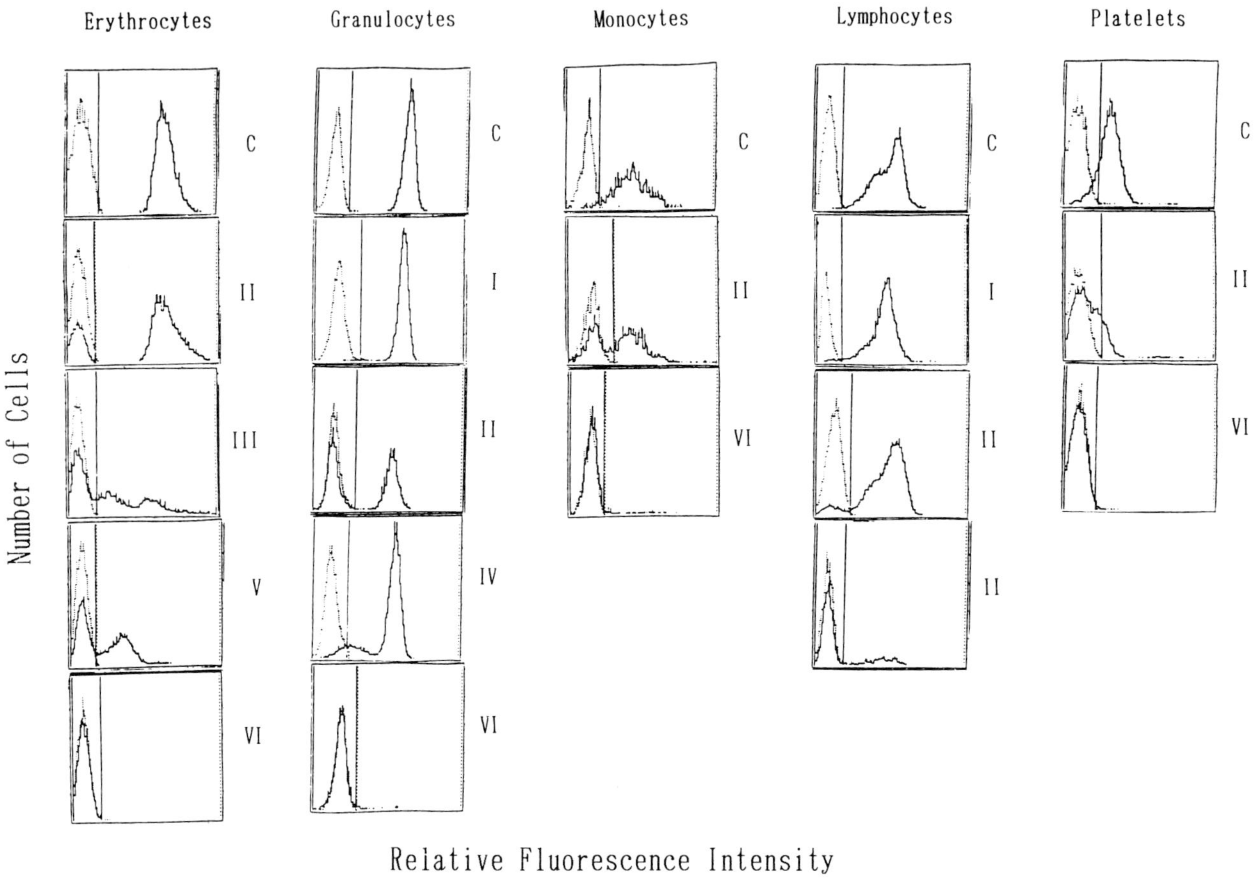

Fig. 1. Typical CD59 flow cytometric profiles of erythrocytes, granulocytes, monocytes, lymphocytes, and platelets in peripheral blood of control subjects and the 17 patients with PNH. Numbers I–VI at right indicate pattern numbers of specific combination of CD59-expressed cell populations in PNH, as shown in Table II. C indicates normal control. Dotted lines show CD59 antibody-excluded, negative-control peaks.

populations (CD59-negative, partly positive, and normally positive) are shown in six patients. In cases of two CD59-positive erythrocyte populations, the mean intensity of stronger relative fluorescence (a right peak) is always within the normal range, but that of weaker fluorescence (a left peak) is lower than the lower limit of normal (data not shown). Therefore, a right peak and a left peak in CD59-positive area consist of CD59 normally positive erythrocytes and CD59 partly positive erythrocytes, respectively, as shown in Figure 1, pattern III. In all PNH patients, CD59-negative erythrocytes accounted for >10% (i.e., 13.6–98.5%) of the total erythrocyte population. The mean percentages of CD59-positive erythrocytes (CD59 normally positive and partly positive) of the patients were significantly lower than those in control subjects.

CD59-positive granulocytes showed a single peak in all the PNH patients, except that a peak of lower mean intensity extended over both the CD59-negative and partly positive areas in two patients. Single CD59-negative and single CD59-positive granulocyte peaks were seen in two patients and one patient, respectively. The CD59-negative granulocyte peak was not detected in the latter patient. CD59-negative granulocytes also made up >10% of the total granulocyte population, except in two patients. CD59-negative monocytes were present in all the PNH patients. However, CD59-profiles of monocytes showed many notches due to a small number of cells assayed. CD59-positive lymphocytes showed a single peak in PNH, although a small shoulder was found in some patients of similar shape to that of normal controls. CD59 expression of PNH lymphocytes was considerably different from that of the other blood cells. A distinct peak of CD59-negative lymphocyte population (>50% of total lymphocytes) was demonstrated in only two patients. However, a small peak of CD59-negative lymphocytes was seen in the remainder, except for three patients who did not show a significant peak of CD59-negative lymphocytes. The mean relative fluorescence intensity of

TABLE I. Percentages of CD59-Negative Cells and Partly Positive Cells (PNH-Affected Cells) in Each Cell Lineage in Peripheral Blood of 17 Patients With PNH*

Case	Erythrocytes Neg.	Erythrocytes Partly pos.	Granulocytes Neg.	Granulocytes Partly pos.	Monocytes N	Lymphocytes N	Platelets N
1	48.9		54.6		66.1	79.8	78.0
2	79.1	16.3	94.7		82.9	13.6	97.7
3	25.5		77.2		70.7	11.8	58.2
4	98.5		96.7		95.5	2.7	97.1
5	77.0	14.5	82.0		71.6	19.5	97.0
6	55.6	44.4	96.2		90.0	66.2	98.2
7	26.3		40.5		63.0	2.9	52.1
8	32.8		8.4[a]	11.1[a]	55.5	8.3	44.2
9	17.1		11.0		66.2	7.9	81.8
10	16.2		2.2		12.7	12.0	68.6
11	16.1	71.3	84.8		89.0	14.3	42.9
12	61.3		34.4		55.2	2.5	78.8
13	54.5	36.8	86.7		90.3	6.6	97.6
14	21.6		22.5		46.5	6.6	84.5
15	58.4	21.7	80.9		83.7	14.5	97.3
16	19.5		19.5[a]	10.7[a]	41.2	8.2	71.0
17	68.6		80.2		68.2	29.5	93.7

*Other than these populations, the remainder are CD59 normally positive populations. A population <3% of the total is neglected in this study. Two, but not three, erythrocyte populations were seen in case 6.
[a]A population extended over both CD59-negative and -positive areas (see Fig. 1).

TABLE II. Specific Patterns of CD59 Flow Cytometric Profiles and Their Incidences in Each Cell Lineage in Peripheral Blood of 17 Patients With PNH*

Pattern	Combination of CD59-negative, partly positive, and normally positive cells	No. of patients E	G	M	L	P
I	Normally positive cells	0	1	0	3	0
II	Negative cells and normally positive cells	9	12	16	14	11
III	Negative cells, partly positive cells, and normally positive cells	6	0	0	0	0
IV	Cells extended over both negative and partly positive areas, and normally positive cells	0	2	0	0	0
V	Negative cells and partly positive cells	1	0	0	0	0
VI	Negative cells	1	2	1	0	6

*A cell population is defined as 3% and more of the total cells in this study. E, erythrocytes; G, granulocytes; M, monocytes; L, lymphocytes; P, platelets.

the CD59-positive lymphocyte population was within normal limits in all cases (data not shown).

CD59-relative fluorescence intensity of platelets was less than that of other blood cells in normal controls. Therefore, it was usually difficult to discriminate between PNH-affected platelets and normal platelets; although CD59-negative platelets might be present in the patients.

Specific patterns of CD59-flow cytometric profiles and their incidence in each cell lineage in peripheral blood of 17 patients with PNH are shown in Table II. Similar profiles were reproduced at different times (checked from after about 1 week to after several months) in most patients in the study.

DISCUSSION

Varying combinations and percentages of CD59-negative, partly CD59-positive, and/or normally CD59-positive cells were demonstrated in five different cell lineages (erythrocyte, granulocyte, monocyte, lymphocyte, and platelet) in the peripheral blood of the 17 patients with PNH by flow cytometry. A CD59-negative erythrocyte population was shown in all patients. However, a CD59-

negative granulocyte population was not found in any patient. This phenomenon was confirmed by a blood sample on a different day. DAF-negative granulocytes were also not detected in the sample. It has been suggested that granulocytes are most suitable to diagnose PNH by flow cytometry [15]. The present patient may be an exceptional case. However, the result indicates that two cell lineages of erythrocytes and granulocytes are best in diagnosing PNH by CD59 flow cytometry. The granulocyte population extended over both CD59-negative and partly positive areas, as shown in Figure 1; pattern IV indicates a CD59 weakly positive cell population. CD59-negative lymphocytes were not shown in three patients. The size of the CD59-negative population in each cell lineage in peripheral blood in PNH was quite variable from one patient to another. CD59-negative cells accounting for >50% of total cells of the lineage are commonly seen in granulocyte, monocyte, and platelet lineages but not in erythrocyte and lymphocyte lineages. CD59-negative erythrocytes may be decreased in number due to complement hemolysis. It has been shown that the life span of CD59-negative erythrocytes is shorter than that of CD59-positive erythrocytes [18]. Erythrocytes of intermediate sensitivity to complement lysis have been demonstrated [19,20]. CD59-negative lymphocytes accounting for >50% of the total were found in only two patients. Long periods (195 and 169 months) have passed after the PNH diagnosis in these two cases. However, it is not known whether CD59 expression in each cell lineage varies in a cell cycle or not. Percentages (mean ± 1 S.D.) of CD59-positive platelets in normal controls are 57.2% ± 21.0%. Those of erythrocytes and granulocytes are 99.9% ± 0.2% and 99.9% ± 0.1%, respectively [17]. These results indicate that platelets are not suitable in specificity for the flow cytometric diagnosis of PNH. Defects of DAF have also been observed in several cell lineages [13,14]. The combination of CD59-negative cells and CD59 normally positive cells (pattern II) is most common in each cell lineage, as shown in Table II.

It has been shown that CD59 protects erythrocytes from hemolysis by complement and that the CD59-negative erythrocytes of PNH patients therefore are complement sensitive [11]. However, peripheral blood cell counts in each lineage and reticulocyte counts were not significantly different between the patients with varying combinations of CD59-negative, partly positive, and normally positive erythrocytes (data not shown). Severe anemia was shown not only in patients with >50% CD59-negative erythrocytes but also in patients with <50%. Anemia may result from the bone marrow hypoplasia in some patients as well as the increased hemolysis. Clonal proliferation of defective erythrocytes has been shown in a patient with both PNH and heterozygous glucose 6-phosphate dehydrogenase deficiency [21]. The clonal character of PNH was also demonstrated by analysis of leukocyte X chromosome methylation [22]. A clonal defect of committed hematopoietic progenitors (CFU-E, BFU-E, CFU-GM) has been found in PNH [23,24]. The present study has shown that CD59-negative cells are present among granulocytes, monocytes, lymphocytes, platelets, and erythrocytes in PNH patients, with a few exceptions. Therefore, it is thought that PNH generally affects hematopoietic pluripotent stem cells. PNH-affected pluripotent stem cells will proliferate and differentiate into committed progenitors of each cell lineage. Competitive clonal proliferation between PNH-affected cells and normal cells will arise at several levels of progenitors in each cell lineage with different growth advantages, and the results may be quite variable. Very recently, we reported a case of PNH secondary to aplastic anemia in which CD59-negative cells appeared first in granulocytes and monocytes and later in all types of peripheral blood cells, including erythrocytes [17]. The sucrose hemolysis test was positive at the later time. The present results and this case study indicate that CD59 flow cytometry using erythrocytes and granulocytes is most suitable in the diagnosis of PNH.

CONCLUSIONS

The flow cytometric profiles of CD59 antigen expression on the surface membranes of erythrocytes, granulocytes, monocytes, lymphocytes, and platelets in 17 patients with PNH were studied. A CD59-negative erythrocyte population was found in all patients with PNH. CD59 expression varied not only between patients but also between cell lineages. Two populations of CD59-negative cells and normally positive cells were seen mostly in each cell lineage. Three populations of CD59-negative, partly positive, and normally positive cells were shown in erythrocytes. CD59-negative granulocytes were present in all PNH patients except for one. A particular granulocyte population extended over both CD59-negative and partly positive areas was found in two patients. CD59 profiles of monocytes showed many notches due to the small number of cells assayed. CD59-negative lymphocytes accounted for >50% of the total lymphocytes in only two patients. A single population of CD59 normally positive lymphocytes was shown in three patients. Percentages of CD59-positive platelet population in normal controls were widely various. The present results and our prior study indicate that two cell lineages of erythrocytes and granulocytes are best used in PNH diagnosis by flow cytometry.

ACKNOWLEDGMENTS

We are grateful to Prof. M. Tomita, Department of Pharmaceutical Sciences, Showa University, for supplying the mouse IgG anti-CD59 monoclonal antibody. This study was supported by a Research Grant for Intractable Disease from the Ministry of Health and Welfare, Japan, and was partially supported by the Iida Foundation.

REFERENCES

1. Dacie JV, Lewis SM: Paroxysmal nocturnal haemoglobinuria: Clinical manifestations, haematology and nature of the disease. Ser Haematol 5:3, 1972.
2. Rosse WF, Dacie JV: Immune lysis of normal human and paroxysmal nocturnal hemoglobinuria (PNH) red blood cells. I. The sensitivity of PNH red blood cells to lysis by complement and specific antibody. J Clin Invest 45:736, 1966.
3. Rosse WF, Adams JP, Thorpe AML: The population of cells in paroxysmal nocturnal haemoglobinuria of intermediate sensitivity to complement lysis: Significance and mechanism of increased immune lysis. Br J Haematol 28:181, 1974.
4. Nicholson-Weller A, March JP, Rosenfeld ST, Austen KF: Affected erythrocytes of patients with paroxysmal nocturnal hemoglobinuria are deficient in the complement regulatory protein, decay-accelerating factor. Proc Natl Acad Sci USA 80:5066, 1983.
5. Pangburn MK, Schreiber RD, Muller-Eberhard HJ: Deficiency of an erythrocyte membrane protein with complement regulatory activity in paroxysmal nocturnal hemoglobinuria. Proc Natl Acad Sci USA 80: 5430, 1983.
6. Rouault TA, Rosse WF, Bell S, Shelburne J: Differences in the terminal steps of complement lysis of normal and paroxysmal nocturnal hemoglobinuria red cells. Blood 51:325, 1978.
7. Parker CJ, Wiedmer T, Sims PJ, Rosse WF: Characterization of the complement sensitivity of paroxysmal nocturnal hemoglobinuria erythrocytes. J Clin Invest 75:2074, 1985.
8. Sugita Y, Nakano Y, Tomita M: Isolation from human erythrocytes of a new membrane protein which inhibits the formation of complement transmembrane channels. J Biochem (Tokyo) 104:633, 1988.
9. Holguin MH, Fredrick LR, Bernshaw NJ, Wilcox LA, Parker CJ: Isolation and characterization of a membrane protein from normal human erythrocytes that inhibits reactive lysis of the erythrocytes of paroxysmal nocturnal hemoglobinuria. J Clin Invest 84:7, 1989.
10. Davies A, Simmons DL, Hale G, Waldmann H: CD59, an Ly-6-like protein expressed in human lymphoid cells, regulates the action of the complement membrane attack complex on homologous cells. J Exp Med 170:634, 1989.
11. Holguin MH, Wilcox LA, Bernshaw NJ, Rosse WF, Parker CJ: Relationship between the membrane inhibitor of reactive lysis and the erythrocyte phenotypes of paroxysmal nocturnal hemoglobinuria. J Clin Invest 84:1387, 1989.
12. Sugita Y, Tabe T, Oda E, Tomita M, Yasukawa K, Yamaji N, Takemoto T, Furuichi K, Takayama M, Yano S: Molecular cloning and characterization of MACIF, an inhibitor of membrane channel formation of complement. J Biochem 106:555, 1989.
13. Nicholson-Weller A, Spicer DB, Austen KF: Deficiency of the complement regulatory protein, "decay-accelerating factor," on membranes of granulocytes, monocytes, and platelets in paroxysmal nocturnal hemoglobinuria. N Engl J Med 312:1091, 1985.
14. Kinoshita T, Medof ME, Silber R, Nussenzweig V: Distribution of decay-accelerating factor in the peripheral blood of normal individuals and patients with paroxysmal nocturnal hemoglobinuria. J Exp Med 162:75, 1985.
15. Van der Schoot E, Huizinga TWJ, Van't Veer-Korthof ET, Wijmans R, Pinkster J, Von dem Borne AEGK: Deficiency of glycosyl-phosphatidylinositol-linked membrane glycoproteins of leukocytes in paroxysmal nocturnal hemoglobinuria. Description of a new diagnostic cytofluorometric assay. Blood 76:1853, 1990.
16. Schubert J, Alvarado M, Uciechowski P, Zielinska-Sknowronek M, Freeund M, Vogt H, Schmidt RE: Diagnosis of paroxysmal nocturnal haemoglobinuria using immunophenotyping of peripheral blood cells. Br J Haematol 79:487, 1991.
17. Fujioka S, Yamada T: Decay-accelerating factor and CD59 expression in peripheral blood cells in aplastic anaemia and report of a case of paroxysmal nocturnal haemoglobinuria secondary to aplastic anaemia. Br J Haematol 83:660, 1993.
18. Fujioka S, Yamada T: Longer in vivo survival of CD59- and decay-accelerating factor-almost normal positive and partly positive erythrocytes in paroxysmal nocturnal hemoglobinuria as compared with negative erythrocytes: A demonstration by differential centrifugation and flow cytometry. Blood 79:1842, 1992.
19. Rosse WF, Hoffman S, Campbell M, Borowitz M, Moore JO, Parker CJ: The erythrocytes in paroxysmal nocturnal haemoglobinuria of intermediate sensitivity to complement lysis. Br J Haematol 79:99, 1991.
20. Shichishima T, Terasawa T, Hashimoto C, Ohto H, Uchida T, Maruyama Y: Heterogenous expression of decay accelerating factor and CD59/membrane attack complex inhibition factor on paroxysmal nocturnal haemoglobinuria (PNH) erythrocytes. Br J Haematol 78: 545, 1991.
21. Oni SB, Osunkoya BO, Luvvatto L: Paroxysmal nocturnal hemoglobinuria: Evidence for monoclonal origin of abnormal red cells. Blood 36:145, 1970.
22. Josten KM, Tooze JA, Borthwick-Clarke C, Gordon-Smith EC, Rutherford TR: Acquired aplastic anemia and paroxysmal nocturnal hemoglobinuria: Studies on clonality. Blood 78:3162, 1991.
23. Rotoli B, Robledo R, Scarpato N, Luzzatto L: Two populations of erythroid cell progenitors in paroxysmal nocturnal hemoglobinuria. Blood 64:847, 1984.
24. Kanamaru A, Okuda K, Ueda E, Kitani T, Kinoshita T, Nagai K: Different distribution of decay-accelerating factor on hematopoietic progenitors from normal individuals and patients with paroxysmal nocturnal hemoglobinuria. Blood 72:507, 1988.

American Journal of Hematology 45:128–135 (1994)

Topical Thrombin and Acquired Coagulation Factor Inhibitors: Clinical Spectrum and Laboratory Diagnosis

Thomas L. Ortel, Linda A. Charles, Frank G. Keller, P. Kelly Marcom, H. Newland Oldham, Jr., William H. Kane, and B. Gail Macik

Division of Hematology/Oncology, Department of Medicine (T.L.O., P.K.M., W.H.K., B.G.M.), and the Departments of Pathology (L.A.C.), Pediatrics (F.G.K.), and Surgery (H.N.O.), Duke University Medical Center, Durham, North Carolina

Topical bovine thrombin preparations are used extensively in cardiovascular, neurosurgical, and otolaryngologic procedures. Patients who are treated with these topical thrombin preparations may develop antibodies to bovine coagulation factors that may cross-react with the endogenous human clotting proteins. We have identified four patients with acquired factor inhibitors following exposure to topical thrombin at Duke University Medical Center and summarize these cases in addition to 13 patients previously reported in the literature. In most cases, the inhibitor developed following a second (or subsequent) exposure to topical thrombin. The clinical course was extremely variable, ranging from totally asymptomatic to life-threatening hemorrhage. The most consistent laboratory abnormality was a prolonged bovine thrombin clotting time, which corrected, at least partially, when human thrombin was substituted for bovine thrombin. Some of these patients also developed factor V inhibitors with prolonged prothrombin and activated partial thromboplastin times. Although these patients have prolonged clotting times, they should not be considered "autoanticoagulated," since thromboembolic complications can still occur. Therapeutic intervention is largely empirical and depends on the clinical manifestations of the individual patient.

Key words: factor V, clotting, bovine thrombin

INTRODUCTION

Bovine thrombin was first used as a topical hemostatic agent by Tidrick and coworkers in 1943 [1]. They reported on 225 patients who received "Thrombin Topical" (Parke, Davis & Co.) for control of bleeding from donor skin graft sites, cancellous or cortical bone surfaces, operative sites, and various other bleeding surfaces, including "brain tissue" [1]. It was quickly recognized that mixing purified thrombin with fibrinogen would produce a fibrin "seal," but early attempts were of limited success due to inadequate fibrinogen concentrations [2]. However, with the development of methods to produce a highly concentrated fibrinogen in the 1960s, the use of "fibrin glue" for repair of peripheral nerves, wound closure, and skin grafting spread rapidly. Currently, topical thrombin and fibrin sealants are used extensively, especially in cardiovascular surgery, otolaryngologic surgery, and neurosurgery [2,3]. For example, over 6,000 vials of topical bovine thrombin (5,000 unit and 20,000 unit vials) were used at Duke University Medical Center during 1991 (Edward H. Bailey, Administrative Manager, Department of Pharmacy, personal communication).

Until recently, the only adverse reactions associated with the use of these topical thrombin preparations were allergic responses [4,5]. In 1988, however, Stricker et al. [6] described three patients who developed antithrombin antibodies following prosthetic cardiac valve surgery. An association with topical bovine thrombin was subsequently recognized, since all three patients had been exposed to bovine thrombin during their surgical procedures [7,8]. Subsequently, Flaherty et al. [9] and Diez-Martin et al. [10] reported an additional six patients who developed prolonged thrombin clotting times after exposure to topical bovine thrombin. Although several of

Received for publication February 9, 1993; accepted June 30, 1993.

Address reprint requests to Thomas L. Ortel, MD, PhD, Division of Hematology/Oncology, Department of Medicine, Duke University Medical Center, Box 3422, Durham, NC 27710.

TABLE I. Clinical Summary of Patients With Acquired Factor Inhibitors Following Exposure to Topical Thrombin*

Patient	Age (years)	Procedure with current thrombin exposure	Prior thrombin exposure	Outcome	Reference
1	64	AVR/MVR (second)	?	Bleeding duodenal ulcer when heparin initiated; died with SBE and CNS thromboembolism	a
2	13	Multiple surgical procedures for tetralogy of Fallot	?	Minimal oozing from poorly healing mediastinal wound	a
3	62	CABG	?	Prolonged oozing from tracheostomy site	a
4	49	Left hip disarticulation	?	Intermittent oozing from left hip stump	a
5	39	MVR (second)	?	Intraperitoneal hemorrhage; died due to "multisystem failure"	8
6	43	AVR (second)	?	Expired with defect in homograft suture line and large pericardial hematoma	8
7	62	Intraventricular hematoma drained	Prior MVR	Expired following prolonged comatose state; no bleeding complications	8
8	91	CABG and AVR	No	No bleeding complications; died secondary to respiratory failure	11
9	23	Craniotomy	No	No bleeding complications	11
10	17	Multiple surgical procedures for tetralogy of Fallot	Yes	No bleeding complications	11
11	68	Revascularization procedure for ischemic lower extremities	Yes	No bleeding complications	11
12	14	Evacuation of cerebral hematoma	?	Recurrent cerebral hematoma nine months later	12
13	14	Evacuation of cerebral hematoma	Prior AVR	Subsequent cardiac surgery without complications	12
14	68	MVR (third)	Yes	Epistaxis post-operatively; subsequent uneventful cholecystectomy	18
15	65	MVR (second)	?	Hemothorax and soft tissue hemorrhage; plasmapheresis necessary for therapy	13
16	82	Open reduction and internal fixation	?	No bleeding complications	14
17	59	AVR/MVR (second)	?	Nasopharyngeal bleeding	14

*Abbreviations: MVR, mitral valve replacement; AVR, aortic valve replacement; SBE, subacute bacterial endocarditis; CNS, central nervous system; CABG, coronary artery bypass grafting.
[a]These patients are described in this paper.

these patients did have various hemorrhagic complications, it was generally thought that the antithrombin antibodies were of little clinical significance (see Table I). Zehnder and Leung [11], however, described a patient who developed a significant bleeding diathesis in association with antibodies to both bovine thrombin and factor V following exposure to topical thrombin. The authors showed that the topical thrombin preparation also contained bovine factor V, which presumably served as the immunogen [11]. Finally Rapaport et al. [12] described two patients with antibodies to bovine thrombin and factor V and showed by crossed immunoelectrophoresis that these patients possessed antibodies to multiple bovine antigens, suggesting immunization by additional proteins in the bovine thrombin preparation.

In this report, we present four additional cases of acquired coagulation factor inhibitors developing after exposure to bovine thrombin and review the literature. The purpose of this report is to summarize the clinical spectrum of these antibodies, which may range from totally asymptomatic to life-threatening hemorrhage, and the difficulties that can confound their identification in the clinical laboratory.

MATERIALS AND METHODS

Laboratory Studies

The prothrombin times (PT) were determined with Simplastin Auto (Organon Teknika, Durham, NC) and the activated partial thromboplastin times (aPTT) with

Auto aPTT reagent (Organon Teknika). The PT, aPTT, factor assays, and inhibitor titers were determined on the Coag-a-mate coagulation analyzer (Organon Teknika). All other clotting assays were performed on the ST4 coagulation analyzer (American Bioproducts Co., Parsippany, NJ). Fibrinogens were performed using bovine thrombin (80 NIH units/ml) by the method of Clauss [13]. Thrombin clotting times (TCT) were determined with bovine thrombin (Parke, Davis & Co.) or human thrombin (kindly provided by Dr. Frank Church, Chapel Hill, NC). Thrombin was diluted to give a clotting time of 20–25 sec on 100 μl normal pooled plasma (NPP), which was approximately 2 NIH units/ml. A patient TCT was considered prolonged if it was >3 sec longer than the NPP control. All assays were performed at 37°C on plasma collected in 3.2% sodium citrate.

Factor V and factor II assays were performed using PT reagent and immunodepleted factor-deficient substrates (American Bioproducts Co.). Inhibitor titers were determined according to the Bethesda method [14], mixing twofold serially diluted patient plasma with an equal volume of NPP and incubating for 2 hr at 37°C. An equal volume of factor-deficient substrate was added to the mixed plasma prior to measuring the clotting times. A calibration curve using NPP and factor-deficient substrate was used to calculate the residual factor activities. Inhibitor units were calculated as described for the Bethesda procedure [14].

Dilute Russell viper venom times (dRVVT) were determined using DVVTest (American Diagnostica, Inc., Greenwich, CT). Patient clotting times were compared to those of NPP, with a ratio ⩾ 1.2 indicative of a positive test. The presence of inhibitor(s) was confirmed by repeating the dRVVT with a 1:1 incubated mix of patient plasma and NPP with 0 and 60 min incubations. Lupus anticoagulant activity was determined by the DVV Confirm assay (American Diagnostica, Inc.). A ratio of the clotting times in the DVVTest to the DVV Confirm of ⩾ 1.2 indicated the presence of a lupus anticoagulant.

Tissue thromboplastin inhibition times (TTIT) were also determined to evaluate for lupus anticoagulants using the PT reagent diluted 1:500. The clotting times of patient plasma were compared to NPP, with a ratio ⩾ 1.3 indicative of a lupus anticoagulant.

Reptilase times were determined using Atroxin (Sigma Diagnostics, St. Louis, MO) diluted to give a clotting time of 20–25 sec (normal, within 3 sec of NPP). D-dimers were determined by latex agglutination using Dimer-Bead reagent (Baxter-Dade, Miami, FL).

Literature Review

All English-language reports of acquired factor inhibitors following exposure to topical thrombin and/or fibrin glue were identified through MEDLINE and a manual review of the literature. Only those reports that demonstrated an exposure to bovine thrombin and documented that the inhibitory effect was more prominent with bovine than with human thrombin were included in this summary.

CASE REPORTS

Patient 1

RS was a 64-year-old male who underwent placement of a Carpentier-Edwards mitral valve for rheumatic valve disease in 1982. He subsequently did well until February, 1992, when he developed shortness of breath and a cough. He was found to have a flail mitral valve as well as aortic valve insufficiency, and he underwent both mitral and aortic valve replacement with St. Jude's valves. Preoperatively, the PT was 9.1 sec (normal 9.1–10.3 sec), the aPTT was 26 sec (normal 24–35 sec), and the platelet count was 133,000/ml. The procedure was performed without complications, and bovine topical thrombin was used intraoperatively. Coumadin was started on postoperative day 4. On day 6, the PT was 40.6 sec and the aPTT was 146 sec, and further coumadin was held. Neither fresh frozen plasma (FFP) nor vitamin K had any effect on the prolonged clotting times. Additional laboratory studies revealed that the fibrinogen was 468 mg/dl (normal 152–344 mg/dl), D-dimer <2 μg/ml (normal <2 μg/ml), and the platelet count was ~496,000/ml, but the TCT was mildly prolonged at 39.1 sec (control 23.1 sec). Mixing studies did not correct the PT nor the aPTT. Factor assays revealed a factor V inhibitor with a titer of 11 inhibitor units. On day 9, the patient developed acute abdominal pain due to a perforated duodenal ulcer. A laparotomy was performed with primary closure of the ulcer with an omental patch. He received platelets during the procedure, but there was only relatively minimal bleeding. He also received intravenous IgG (1 g/kg) in an attempt to decrease the titer of his inhibitor. Because of the lack of spontaneous bleeding, as well as minimal bleeding with central line placements, intravenous heparin was slowly started (500 U/hr) to provide anticoagulation for his prosthetic valves. Within 24 hr, he developed severe gastrointestinal bleeding, and the heparin was discontinued. Arteriography confirmed that the bleeding was localized to the duodenum, but embolization of two pancreaticoduodenal arteries only briefly controlled the bleeding. A repeat laparotomy was performed, with oversewing of the duodenal ulcer and pyloroplasty. At this time, the PT was 33.7 sec, the aPTT was >150 sec, the fibrinogen was 353 mg/dl, the D-dimers were <2 μg/ml, and the factor V inhibitor titer was 3.2 units. His subsequent course was punctuated by fevers and intermittent episodes of gastrointestinal bleeding with only minimal bleeding elsewhere. A second course of intravenous IgG had little effect on the clotting times. On postoperative day 30, the patient sustained a nonhemorrhagic cerebrovascular accident with a dense hemiplegia. A target lesion was identified on the atrial surface of the prosthetic mitral valve by echocardiography. Antibiotics were started for bacterial endocarditis (blood cultures positive for *Staphylococcus epidermidis*), and heparin was slowly restarted despite continued guaiac-positive stool and melena. The patient's condition worsened 2 days later, and repeat head CT scan revealed increased herniation but no hemorrhage. He died later that day.

Patient 2

MJ is a 13-year-old male who was diagnosed shortly after birth with severe tetralogy of Fallot with pulmonic valve atresia. At 5 years of age, a right ventricle-to-pulmonary artery Hancock Dacron/porcine valve conduit was placed, with closure of the ventricular and atrial septal defects. Revision of the conduit was performed for obstruction of the conduit with elevated right ventricular pressures in June, 1992, and topical thrombin was used during the procedure. Preoperative PT and aPTT were normal. The patient's postoperative course was uncomplicated, and he was discharged on postoperative day 6. On postoperative day 8, he developed fever, chest and abdominal pain, and fatigue, and a sanguinous drainage was noted at the sternotomy site. A diagnosis of postpericardiotomy syndrome was made, and he was begun on methylprednisolone (4 mg/kg/day). The PT was 37.2 sec, the aPTT 105 sec, and the fibrinogen 444 mg/dl. The TCT using bovine thrombin was >120 sec, but the TCT using human thrombin was normal (see Table II). Mixing studies revealed that neither the PT nor the aPTT were corrected completely with a 1:1 mix. Specific factor assays revealed a factor V activity of 2% and a prothrombin activity of 26%, both with inhibitory patterns, and a factor X activity of 108%. The factor V inhibitor titer was 2.2 units. Over the next several days, his symptoms improved, and the oozing from his sternotomy site stopped. On postoperative day 14, his PT was 18.6 sec and aPTT 53 sec. Steroids were gradually withdrawn over a 10 day period. On postoperative day 24, the PT was 11.5 sec, the aPTT was 40 sec, but the TCT remained >120 sec.

Patient 3

TR is a 62-year-old man who underwent coronary artery bypass grafting in 1985. He developed recurrent ischemia in 1992, and coronary catherization revealed three-vessel disease with occlusion of the previous grafts and stenosis of the left main coronary artery. Because of continued angina refractory to medical management, a repeat bypass grafting procedure was performed. Admission laboratories included a PT of 9.7 sec, an aPTT of 119 sec (the patient was on heparin), and a platelet count of 255,000/ml. The patient tolerated surgery well with some oozing which was treated with topical thrombin. Postoperatively, the PT was 10.3 sec, the aPTT 34 sec, the fibrinogen 302 mg/dl, and the platelet count 143,000/ml. Because of difficulties in weaning the patient from the ventilator, a tracheostomy was performed on postoperative day 7. Pretracheostomy, the PT was 11.4 sec, the aPTT was 45 sec, and the platelet count was 168,000/ml. Blood continuously oozed from the tracheostomy site, and, on day 9, the PT was 13.7 sec and the aPTT was 64 sec, despite the administration of FFP. Vitamin K (10 mg) was administered. The platelet count climbed to 337,000/ml, and the fibrinogen was 448 mg/dl. On day 10, the patient developed melena, and the tracheostomy site bled profusely despite attempts to cauterize the area. The platelet count and fibrinogen remained stable, but the PT was further prolonged to 14.8 sec and the aPTT to 82 sec despite an additional dose of vitamin K.

Mixing studies did not correct the PT nor the aPTT. Factor V level was 17% with a linear curve; factors VIII, X, and VII had minimal inhibitory patterns but were within normal range; and prothrombin showed a marked inhibitory pattern. The bovine TCT was 27.8 sec. The dRVVT was prolonged, did not correct with a 1:1 mix with NPP, and did not correct with preincubation with phospholipids (DVV Confirm), indicating that the inhibitor was most likely not a lupus anticoagulant. The patient was diagnosed with a thrombin and/or factor V antibody, and, starting on day 11, he was treated with steroids, an intravenous IgG infusion, amicar, and platelet transfusions. By day 13, the PT had fallen to 11.7 sec and the aPTT to 49 sec, and the factor V had risen to 95%, but the incubated mix still was not corrected and the prothrombin remained low and inhibitory. The patient's management was further complicated by a rising creatinine and prolongation of the bleeding time to 13 min. On day 14, he was given another dose of intravenous IgG and cryoprecipitate, because he continued to require 4–6 units of packed red blood cells per day. Surgical exploration of the tracheostomy identified a single soft tissue bleeding site that was sutured, with resolution of the bleeding. Additional complications included small bowel necrosis requiring resection and mediastinitis requiring debridement and pectoral muscle flap. Both procedures were performed successfully without extensive bleeding.

Patient 4

JH was a 49-year-old female with systemic lupus erythematosus diagnosed in 1982. Her medical history was significant for transient ischemic attacks, coronary artery disease with an anterior wall myocardial infarction in 1983 and a three-vessel coronary artery bypass graft in 1986, a lupus anticoagulant, and aseptic necrosis of both femoral heads with a left total hip replacement in 1987. She was admitted for incision and drainage of a septic left hip and intravenous antibiotics. Admission laboratory studies revealed a PT of 10 sec, an aPTT of 69 sec, a bovine TCT of 20.9 sec, a TTIT ratio of 1.4, a fibrinogen

TABLE II. Summary of Diagnostic Laboratory Studies*

Patient	Postoperative day	PT (sec)	aPTT (sec)	Bovine TCT (sec)	Human TCT (sec)	Reptilase (sec)	Fibrinogen (mg/dl)	Prothrombin (%)	Factor V (%)	Inhibitor studies	Reference
1	6	40.6	146	39.1	—	—	468	Inhibitor effect	<3.2	Factor V inhibitor titer	[c]
				63.9	23.1					11 Units	
2	8	37.2	105	>120	—	29.3	444	26	2	Factor V inhibitor titer	[c]
				<120	20.7					2.2 units	
3	10	14.8	82	27.8	—	—	448	Inhibitor effect	17	—	[c]
				36.1	29.7						
4	—	10.9	82[a]	71.9	—	31.9	315	109	—	TCT did not correct with mix	[c]
				42	14.2						
5	7	33.5	73.5	>120	40.3	14.6	391	Inhibitor effect	—	Factor V inhibitor by Western blot;	8
	30	12.3	30	>120						TCT did not correct with mix	
6	36	15	44.5	>120	>120	10.9	546	Inhibitor effect	—	TCT partially corrected with mix	8
7	4	30	113	>120	35.2	11.9	346	Inhibitor effect	—	TCT partially corrected with mix	8
	~35	"Normal"	"Normal"	68.2							
8	—	"Long"	"Long"	>300	17	—	—	—	—	Elevated IgM to bovine thrombin	11
9	—	—	—	>300	20	—	—	—	—	—	11
10	—	"Normal"	"Normal"	>300	21	—	—	—	—	Protein A partially clears inhibitor	11
11	—	"Normal"	"Normal"	>300	28	—	—	—	—	Protein A partially clears inhibitor	11
12	—	18	31	>600	15	16	342	—	—	Inhibitor purified by protein A	12
13	—	18	31	>600	15	16	342	—	—	Inhibitor purified by protein A	12
14	—	17	34	>150	35	23	465	—	—	Antithrombin antibody purified	18
15	12	43.8	99.7	>100	—	12.7	383	108	1	Factor V inhibitor demonstrated by	13
	41	37.3	116.8	>100	32.7	13.7	311			ELISA	
16	—	45.4	127	>240	28	—	—	100 (human plasma)	3	—	14
17	21								27	—	
	40	17.6[b]	37.0[b]	>240	36	12.5	—	—	49	—	14

*Abbreviations: PT, prothrombin time; aPTT, activated partial thromboplastin time; TCT, thrombin clotting time; ELISA, enzyme-linked immunosorbent assay.

[a]Patient 4 had a lupus anticoagulant with a prolonged aPTT prior to exposure to topical thrombin.

[b]Patient 17 was on coumadin when the PT and aPTT were determined.

[c]These patients are described in this paper.

of 660 mg/dl, and a prothrombin level of 105%. Because of the anticipated prolonged immobilization during treatment of her hip, the patient was started on prophylactic coumadin anticoagulation. This was stopped after 4 days due to the development of epistaxis (PT 13.9 sec). Because of persistent fevers, the Bateman hemiarthroplasty was removed on hospital day 17. Her subsequent hospital course was characterized by multiple bleeding episodes, a left leg deep venous thrombosis, and a complex multifactorial coagulopathy. The left hip wound continued to bleed profusely despite multiple therapeutic interventions including topical thrombin and repeated packings. She eventually underwent left hip disarticulation on day 49, due to our inability to treat the local infection adequately or to control the bleeding. Her subsequent hospital course was characterized by a prolonged, gradual recovery and intermittent oozing from the left hip stump. Laboratory studies on day 126, when she was no longer bleeding, revealed the PT to be 10.9 sec, the aPTT to be 63 sec, the TTIT ratio to be 1.7, and the fibrinogen to be 315 mg/dl. Her bovine TCT was now prolonged, however, at 71.9 sec, with a prothrombin level of 104% with an inhibitory pattern. The reptilase time was 31.9 sec (control 22.4 sec). A repeat bovine TCT determination was 42 sec (control 20.4 sec), and this was corrected incompletely with a 1:1 mix (29.4 sec). With human thrombin, her TCT was 14.2 sec, with a control TCT of 9.9 sec.

DISCUSSION

Coagulation factor inhibitors are antibodies that bind to specific coagulation factors and either neutralize their procoagulant activity or result in their clearance from the circulation [15]. Factor inhibitors may develop as alloantibodies in patients with congenital deficiencies who receive replacement therapy or, more rarely, as autoantibodies in patients with no known prior factor deficiency. Most inhibitors are directed against factor VIII, although patients with antibodies directed against factor VII, von Willebrand factor, factor IX, factor V, and thrombin have been reported [15]. Inhibitors to coagulation factor V are relatively rare and have been described most frequently in the postsurgical setting and/or in association with aminoglycoside antibiotics [16]. Many of these patients have a low-titer inhibitor, with minimal, if any, hemorrhagic complications [16]. A subset of patients with factor V inhibitors develop a severe hemorrhagic diathesis, however, and may die in spite of aggressive therapeutic intervention [17]. Acquired inhibitors to thrombin are also relatively rare, and, as with factor V inhibitors, carry a variable clinical presentation [18–20]. One type of autoantibody to prothrombin that does occur with slightly more frequency, however, is the clearing antiprothrombin antibody that is seen in association with the lupus anticoagulant [21,22]. This antibody does *not* neutralize the procoagulant activity of thrombin but does result in a decreased level of prothrombin due to in vivo clearance [21,22].

Recently, there have been several reports of patients developing coagulation factor inhibitors following exposure to heterologous procoagulant proteins [6,9–12,18]. Including the four patients described here, there have been a total of 17 patients who developed coagulation factor inhibitors following exposure to topical bovine thrombin (Table I). An additional 19 patients have been reported in abstract form [23–25]. Because individual patient information is not available, these patients are not included in this summary. Most of the patients were treated with topical thrombin during a cardiovascular or neurosurgical procedure, with the remainder associated with orthopedic procedures (Table I). In addition, most of the patients had also been exposed to topical thrombin during a *preceding* surgical procedure or had previously undergone a procedure in which topical thrombin is frequently used. For example, of the 17 patients summarized in Table I, ten had previously undergone either aortic and/or mitral valve replacement or other open cardiac surgery. Prior exposure is clearly not required, however, since at least two of the patients had never been treated previously with topical thrombin.

The clinical course is markedly variable, with some patients having absolutely no bleeding complications, whereas others have life-threatening hemorrhagic episodes. Of the 17 patients summarized here, five (patients 8–11 and 16) had no bleeding complications associated with the acquired inhibitor(s). The remainder experienced some degree of bleeding, ranging from minimal (patients 2, 10, and 17) to life-threatening (patient 15). Of those patients developing clinical bleeding, most did not demonstrate spontaneous hemorrhage but bled more readily from structural lesions (patients 1–4, 6, and 12). In contrast, four of these patients (patients 1, 3, 13, and 14) underwent major surgical procedures with minimal, if any, bleeding. In general, spontaneous hemorrhagic events appear to be relatively uncommon, similar to most patients with spontaneously acquired inhibitors to factor V or thrombin. Similar clinical outcomes were observed for the 19 patients described in abstract form only, with the majority experiencing no clinical bleeding. Two of these patients did die, however, one death being associated with significant "bleeding complications" [24].

Similar to the case with the clinical course, there is also considerable variation in the laboratory abnormalities that these patients develop (Table II). The most consistently observed laboratory abnormality is a marked prolongation of the TCT. In most clinical laboratories, bovine thrombin is used in this test; therefore, it will be the most sensitive to the development of antibovine thrombin antibodies. Typically, substitution of human thrombin for bovine thrombin results in a marked decrease in the inhibitory effect (Table II), although this does not occur in all cases (patient 6). Lawson and coworkers [18] demonstrated that the antithrombin antibody from their patient (patient 14) reacted with greater affinity to bovine thrombin than human thrombin in an enzyme-linked immunosorbent assay. They interpreted this result as being consistent with the development of antibovine antibodies that cross-reacted with a lesser affinity to the human protein [18]. This variability in cross-reactivity to human thrombin is also seen in determinations of prothrombin levels, which can vary from decreased levels (patient 2 and 3) to normal levels (patients 4, 13, and 14). As with the TCT, this test can also yield variable results depending on whether the test plasma is from a bovine or a human source [12]. Interestingly, bovine thrombin is also frequently used to determine functional fibrinogen levels. The amount of thrombin added is considerably greater, however, and is presumably in excess of the antibody titer, since fibrinogen levels are consistently within the normal range (Table II).

In addition to antithrombin antibodies, a significant number of these patients have also developed cross-reacting antibodies to factor V (patients 1–3, 5, and 15–17). Zehnder and Leung [11] demonstrated that bovine factor V was present in two commercial thrombin preparations. Thrombostat (Parke-Davis) and Thrombinar (Armour Pharmaceutical Company), and this was presumably serving as the immunogen. As with the antithrombin antibodies, the antifactor V antibodies from two patients (patients 16 and 17) were shown to react more strongly with bovine factor V than with human factor V, consistent with a heterologous antigenic exposure rather than spontaneous development of an autoantibody [12]. Although it was initially proposed that the antifactor V antibodies were more likely to be associated with significant clinical bleeding, this has not been consistently observed. Of the seven patients described who clearly had antifactor V antibodies, four developed significant hemorrhagic complications (patients 1, 3, 5, and 15), with patient 1 bleeding only when heparin was started for his prosthetic valves. The other three patients (patients 2, 16, and 17) experienced essentially no bleeding. Similarly, 16 of the 19 patients described in abstract form developed factor V inhibitors, but only five of these patients developed clinically significant bleeding.

Because they are frequently asymptomatic, many of these inhibitors are not detected until weeks to months following the surgical procedure. In those patients identified early, however, the clotting times begin to be prolonged within 1–2 weeks after exposure, consistent with the timing of the antigenic exposure (Table II). Interestingly, in three of the patients (patients 2, 5, and 7), the PT, aPTT, and TCT were all initially prolonged. Within several weeks, however, only the TCT remained significantly prolonged. In contrast, two of our patients (patients 1 and 3) developed inhibitors that prolonged predominantly the PT and aPTT, with little if any prolongation of the TCT. This spectrum of laboratory findings was also observed in eight of 11 patients reported in one abstract [23]. These patients appear to have a predominantly antifactor V effect, with minimal antithrombin activity. Finally, neither of our patients nor any of the patients described in the literature developed acquired factor inhibitors against any of the other coagulation proteins. In one abstract, however, all 11 patients with factor V inhibitors also developed factor XI inhibitors [23].

Treatment, *when required,* is similar to the treatment for spontaneously acquired coagulation factor inhibitors and has included transfusion therapy, steroids, cytotoxic therapy, intravenous IgG, and plasmapheresis if necessary [15,16]. However, if the patient develops no hemorrhagic complications, no specific treatment is indicated. Nevertheless, all patients who develop antibovine thrombin antibodies should be evaluated for the presence of antifactor V antibodies, because these patients may benefit from platelet transfusions in the setting of acute hemorrhage [26]. Platelets contain ~20% of the circulating factor V and therefore may serve as a "protected" source of this essential cofactor [16]. Conversely, although these patients may develop markedly prolonged clotting times, they should not be considered "autoanticoagulated." For example, one of our patients (patient 1) died from a septic thromboembolism originating on a prosthetic mitral valve despite markedly prolonged clotting times. Attempts to anticoagulate him with heparin were hindered by recurrent bleeding from his ulcer and by his baseline prolonged aPTT, which significantly complicated therapeutic monitoring. Indeed, management of anticoagulant therapy in these patients may be one of the most difficult aspects of their care, due to the abnormally prolonged clotting times and the need for specialized laboratory monitoring. Finally, we recommend minimizing the use of topical thrombin preparations in patients with known prior exposure, since these patients appear to be at greatest risk for developing factor inhibitors. The actual frequency of inhibitor development in this patient population remains to be determined.

In summary, acquired coagulation factor inhibitors developing after exposure to heterologous procoagulant proteins are probably more common than is currently appreciated, especially given the extent of topical thrombin use. They should be suspected in any patient developing abnormally prolonged clotting times (PT, aPTT, and/or TCT) within 1–2 weeks of a surgical procedure in which topical thrombin or fibrin glue is frequently used. Although frequently clinically benign, these inhibitors may be associated with life-threatening hemorrhage. If required, treatment is the same as for spontaneously acquired inhibitors to factor V or thrombin.

ACKNOWLEDGMENTS

We thank Julie Leumas, MT (ASCP), for determining the human and bovine thrombin clotting times and the Duke University Coagulation Laboratory for expeditiously performing the multiple studies required to diagnose these complex patients. This work was performed during the tenure of a Clinician Scientist Award (91-419) from the American Heart Association and Genentech (T.L.O.) and an Established Investigatorship Award (91-181) from the American Heart Association and Smithkline Beecham (W.H.K.).

REFERENCES

1. Tidrick RT, Seegers WH, Warner ED: Clinical experience with thrombin as an hemostatic agent. Surgery 14:191, 1943.
2. Brennan M: Fibrin glue, Blood Rev 5:240, 1991.
3. Matras H: Fibrin seal: the state of the art. J Oral Maxillofac Surg 43:605, 1985.
4. "Physicians Desk Reference, 46th ed." Oradell, NJ: Medical Economics Data, 1992, pp 1765–1766.
5. Tadokoro K, Ohtoshi T, Takafuji S, Nakajima K, Suzuki S, Yamamoto K, Ito K, Miyamoto T, Muranaka M: Topical thrombin-induced IgE-mediated anaphylaxis: RAST analysis and skin test studies. J Allerg Clin Immunol 88:620, 1991.
6. Stricker RB, Lane PK, Leffert JD, Rodgers GM, Shuman MA, Corash L: Development of antithrombin antibodies following surgery in patients with prosthetic cardiac valves. Blood 72:1375, 1988.
7. Flaherty MJ, Wener MH: Antibodies to thrombin in postsurgical patients. Blood 73:1386, 1989.
8. Stricker RB, Corash L: Antibodies to thrombin in postsurgical patients. Response. Blood 73:1386, 1989.
9. Flaherty MJ, Henderson R, Wener MH: Iatrogenic immunization with bovine thrombin: A mechanism for prolonged thrombin times after surgery. Ann Intern Med 111:631, 1989.
10. Diez-Martin J, Sikkink RA, Gilchrist GS, Bowie EJW, Fass DN: Development of anti-bovine thrombion antibodies following neurosurgical procedures. Br J Haematol 74:369, 1990.
11. Zehnder JL, Leung LLK: Development of antibodies to thrombin and factor V with recurrent bleeding in a patient exposed to topical bovine thrombin. Blood 76:2011, 1990.
12. Rapaport SI, Zivelin A, Minow RA, Hunter CS, Donnelly K: Clinical significance of antibodies to bovine and human thrombin and factor V after surgical use of bovine thrombin. Am J Clin Pathol 97:84, 1992.
13. Clauss A: Gerinnungsphysiologische schneliomethode zur bestimmung des fibrinogens. Acta Haematol 17:237, 1957.
14. Kasper CK, Aledort LM, Counts RB, Edson JR, Fratantoni J, Green D, Hampton JW, Hilgartner MW, Lazerson J, Levine PH, McMillan CW, Pool JG, Shapiro SS, Shulman NR, van Eyes J: A more uniform measurement of factor VIII inhibitors. Thromb Diath Haemorrh 34:869, 1975.
15. Feinstein DI: Acquired inhibitors of blood coagulation. In Hoffman R, Benz EJ, Shattil SJ, Furie B, Cohen, HJ (eds): "Hematology: Basic Principles and Practice." New York: Churchill Livinstone, 1991, pp 1380–1394.
16. Nesheim ME, Nichols WL, Cole TL, Houston JG, Schenk RB, Mann KG, Bowie EJ: Isolation and study of an acquired inhibitor of human coagulation factor V. J Clin Invest 77:405, 1986.
17. Coots MC, Muhleman AF, Glueck HI: Hemorrhagic death associated with a high titer factor V inhibitor. Am J Hematol 4:193, 1978.
18. Lawson JH, Pennell BJ, Olson JD, Mann KG: Isolation and characterization of an acquired antithrombin antibody. Blood 76:2249, 1990.
19. Costa JM, Fiessinger JN, Capron L, Aiach M: Partial characterization of an autoantibody recognizing the secondary binding site(s) of thrombin in a patient with recurrent spontaneous arterial thrombosis. Thromb Hemost 67:193, 1992.
20. Sié P, Bezeaud A, Dupouy D, Archipoff G, Freyssinet J-M, Dugoujon J-M, Serre G, Guillin M-C, Boneu B: An acquired antithrombion autoantibody directed toward the catalytic center of the enzyme. J Clin Invest 88:290, 1991.
21. Bajaj SP, Rapaport SI, Fierer DS, Herbst KD, Schwartz DB: A mechanism for the hypoprothrombinemia of the acquired hypoprothrombinemia-lupus anticoagulant syndrome. Blood 61:684, 1983.
22. Fleck RA, Rapaport SI, Rao LVM: Anti-prothrombin antibodies and the lupus anticoagulant. Blood 72:512, 1988.
23. Spero JA, Triplett DA, Cmolik BL, Reid C, Clark RE: A family of clotting factor inhibitors primarily involving FV and FXI occurring after cardiovascular and neurosurgical procedures. Blood 78 (Suppl): 63a, 1991 (abstract).
24. Nichols WL, Daniels TM, Fisher PK, Owen WG, Figueroa PI, Pineda AA: Inhibitors of coagulation factor V and thrombion associated with surgical use of topical bovine thrombin or fibrin glue. Blood 78 (Suppl):63a, 1991 (abstract).
25. Tsang PWK, Naiman SC: Development of antibodies to bovine thrombin and to other coagulation factors in three patients after cardiac surgery. Blood 78(Suppl):65a, 1991 (abstract).
26. Chediak J, Ashenhurst JB, Garlick I, Desser RK: Successful management of bleeding in a patient with factor V inhibitor by platelet transfusions. Blood 56:835, 1980.

ADDENDUM

While this manuscript was in review, three additional publications have appeared describing acquired thrombin and/or factor V inhibitors developing after exposure to topical bovine thrombin [27,28,29]. As with the cases summarized here, clinical and laboratory manifestations were variable.

27. Berruyer M, Amiral J. Ffrench P. Belleville J, Bastien O, Clerc J, Kassir A, Estanove S, Dechavanne M: Immunization by bovine thrombin used with fibrin glue during cardiovascular operations. Development of thrombin and factor V inhibitors. J Thorac Cardiovasc Surg 105:892, 1993
28. Cmolik BL, Spero JA, Magovern GJ, Clark RE, Reid C: Redo cardiac surgery: Late bleeding complications from topical thrombin-induced factor V deficiency. J Thorac Cardiovasc Surg 105:222, 1993.
29. Spero JA: Bovine thrombin-induced inhibitor of factor V and bleeding risk in postoperative neurosurgical patients. Report of three cases. J Neurosurg 78:817, 1993.

American Journal of Hematology 45:136–141 (1994)

Transgenic Mouse Model of Pharmacologic Induction of Fetal Hemoglobin: Studies Using a New Ribonucleotide Reductase Inhibitor, Didox

B.S. Pace, H.L. Elford, and G. Stamatoyannopoulos

Division of Medical Genetics, Department of Medicine, University of Washington, Seattle, Washington; (B.S.P., G.S.) Molecules For Health, Inc., Richmond, Virginia (H.L.E.)

Evaluation of pharmacologic agents that stimulate fetal hemoglobin production has been done mainly in baboons and macaques. We investigated whether results in transgenic mice can predict the stimulation of fetal hemoglobin in primates, by testing γ globin induction in response to a new ribonucleotide reductase inhibitor, Didox. A transgenic mouse line carrying the human Aγ gene linked to a locus control region cassette was used. Treatment of transgenic mice with Didox resulted in induction of γ gene expression as documented by an increase in F reticulocytes and F cells and an elevation of γ/γ + β biosynthetic ratio. Similarly, administration of Didox to a baboon in the nonanemic and chronically anemic state resulted in induction of γ gene expression as shown by increases in F reticulocytes, F cells, and Hb F. These results suggest that the μLCR-Aγ transgenic mice can be used to screen new pharmacologic compounds for γ globin inducibility.

Key words: globin, γ globin, Aγ gene, F reticulocytes, anemia

INTRODUCTION

Stimulation of fetal hemoglobin synthesis has been achieved in primates and patients with hemoglobin S disease with various cell cycle specific compounds and hemopoietins, such as 5-azacytidine [1,2], hydroxyurea [3–5], erythropoietin [6], and normal metabolites such as butyric acid [7–10]. The induction of fetal hemoglobin by these compounds was discovered with studies in baboons or macaques. Recently, it has been shown that a transgenic mouse line carrying a 2.5 kb cassette containing four DNaseI hypersensitive sites of the locus control region (LCR) linked to a 3.3 kb HindIII fragment of the human Aγ gene (μLCR-Aγ) expresses the γ gene in the embryonic and fetal stages of development and, at a lower level, in the adult [11]. Fetal hemoglobin was induced when these mice were treated with known Hb F inducers [12] suggesting that μLCR-Aγ transgenic mice can be used to screen new pharmacologic agents for their ability to induce fetal hemoglobin in vivo.

Hydroxyurea presumably augments fetal hemoglobin (Hb F) synthesis by perturbing erythroid progenitor cell kinetics secondary to cytoreduction; it has been suggested that the sudden regeneration that follows the cytoreduction by hydroxyurea treatment may result in recruitment of immature progenitors having an active γ gene expressing program [5,13]. Newer, more potent ribonucleotide reductase inhibitors are available for evaluation of their potential to induce Hb F and their toxic side effects. Didox (N,3,4-trihydroxybenzamide) has been tested in vivo and in vitro and shown to be tenfold more potent than hydroxyurea as an inhibitor of ribonucleotide reductase [14]. This compound was more effect in prolonging the life span of L1210 leukemic mice at one-third the dosage of hydroxyurea [15,16]. In view of the in vivo activity of Didox and the ability of hydroxyurea to induce Hb F production, it was desirable to investigate the effectiveness of this compound as an inducer of γ gene expression. This was initially accomplished by testing the effect of Didox on γ globin expression in μLCR-Aγ transgenic mice and subsequently examining whether the results in transgenic mice would be reproduced in baboons.

Received for publication February 10, 1993; accepted June 30, 1993.

Address reprint requests to B. Pace, MD, RG-25, Health Sciences Building, University of Washington Medical Center, Seattle, WA 98195.

MATERIALS AND METHODS

Animals

Transgenic mice that are progeny of the 1279 line carrying the construct μLCR-Aγ, containing four hypersensitive sites from the 5′ region of the β globin locus within a 2.5 kb fragment [11], linked to a 3.3 kb Hind III fragment containing a copy of the human Aγ globin gene were used in these experiments. The 5′ end of the Aγ gene extends to −1350, and hence this line is defined as μLCR (−1350) Aγ. One female juvenile baboon *(Papio cynocephalus)* housed and cared for at the Regional Primate Center, University of Washington, was also used in the study.

Drugs

Transgenic mice received human recombinant erythropoietin (rhuEpo; Genetic Institute, Cambridge, MA) and hydroxyurea (Sigma, St. Louis, MO) intraperitoneally in doses and schedules as described below. Didox (Molecules for Health, Inc., Richmond, VA) was given both intraperitoneally and intravenously to transgenic mice and a juvenile baboon respectively.

Hematologic Studies

Approximately twenty microliters of blood was drawn from the mouse for the following analyses. Blood smears were prepared and counted for reticulocytes, calculated by counting 1,500 cells. The proportion of red blood cells containing Hb F (F cells) was determined as previously described [17–19]. Reticulocytes containing hemoglobin F (F reticulocytes) were prepared by incubating the blood with 1% brilliant cresyl blue (1% BCB) to precipitate the reticulum; smears prepared and fixed with methanol, labeled with anti-γ-chain monoclonal antibody and anti-mouse F(ab′)2-FITC in the presence of .001% acridine orange [19]. The preparations were viewed on a Zeiss Universal Fluorescent microscope (Zeiss Inc., New York, NY) equipped with epillumination and a 200 mercury/150 zenon power source. From the baboon, approximately 1 ml of blood was drawn before treatment and at designated intervals throughout the study. The hematocrit and white blood cell and platelet counts were determined using standard methods.

Globin Chain Analysis

Blood aliquots were incubated in the presence of [^{3}H]leucine (specific activity 40 Ci/mmol), in leucine free Iscove's modified Dulbecco's medium (IMDM) for 12–16 hr at 37°C. After incubation, the samples were washed three times in Na, K, Mg (NKM) saline and stored at −70°C or analyzed immediately. Cell lysates were prepared and globin chain isoelectric focusing followed by flurography was performed as previously described [20]. From the flurogram obtained, automated densitometry (Gelman Automatic Computing Densitometer, Ann Arbor, MI) was used to determine the relative proportions of various synthesized globin chains.

Hemoglobin F Measurement

Aliquots of packed red blood cells were lysed by the addition of an equal volume of distilled water and subjected to hemoglobin F determination by the standard method of alkaline denaturation [21]. Hemoglobin levels were measured on the Beckman Spectrophometer at 540λ wavelength with a visual light source.

RNA Analysis

Packed red blood cells were used for slot blot cytoplasmic hybridization of globin mRNA analysis as follows. The sample was washed three times in NKM saline, after which 5 μl aliquots were resuspended in cold Tris-EDTA (RE) buffer (10 mMol/liter Tris, 0.1 mMol/liter EDTA) with 20 U RNase inhibitor (RNasin; Promega, Madison, WI). The cells were lysed with 5% Nonidet-40 (NP40) solution and centrifuged, and the supernatant was combined with 20× SSC (0.15 Mol/liter NaCl, 0.015 mol/liter trisodium citrate) and 37% formaldehyde final. The samples were denatured at 65°C for 15 min and stored at −70°C for later analysis. The slot blot technique was performed using the Schleicher & Schell (Kuene, NH) Minifold II apparatus, as previously described [22]. In brief, the samples were diluted to a final volume of 300 μl with 15× SSC and loaded on prewet nitrocellulose paper under vacuum. The nitrocellulose was dried, then baked at 80°C for 45 min. The membrane was prehybridized for 3–4 hr at 65°C in a water bath, then hybridized with 50 ng of in vitro transcribed radioactive (α-^{32}P-UTP) RNA probe. Mouse 3′β major globin RNA probe was used to detect mouse globin [23]. Human γ globin mRNA was detected with a 0.6 kb EcoRI/HindIII fragment from the 3′ end of the human Gγ globin gene. The filter was hybridized for 16 hours in a 65°C water bath, followed by extensive washing under stringent conditions [2× SSC with 0.1% sodium dodecyl sulfate (SDS) at room temperature twice, 1× SSC with 0.1% SDS at 65°C for one wash, then 0.7× SSC with 0.1% SDS at 65°C for two final washes]. The blots were analyzed by phosphorimaging.

RESULTS

μLCR (−1350)Aγ transgenic mice were the offspring of a founder containing three copies of the human Aγ globin gene. Heterozygote adult animals having 30–38% γ-positive cells were used for these studies. In control experiments adult μLCR (−1350)Aγ mice were treated with erythropoietin by intraperitoneal bolus injection of 3,000 units/kg body weight every 12 hr for 3 days. Erythropoietin induced a sharp rise in reticulocytes from 5.5%

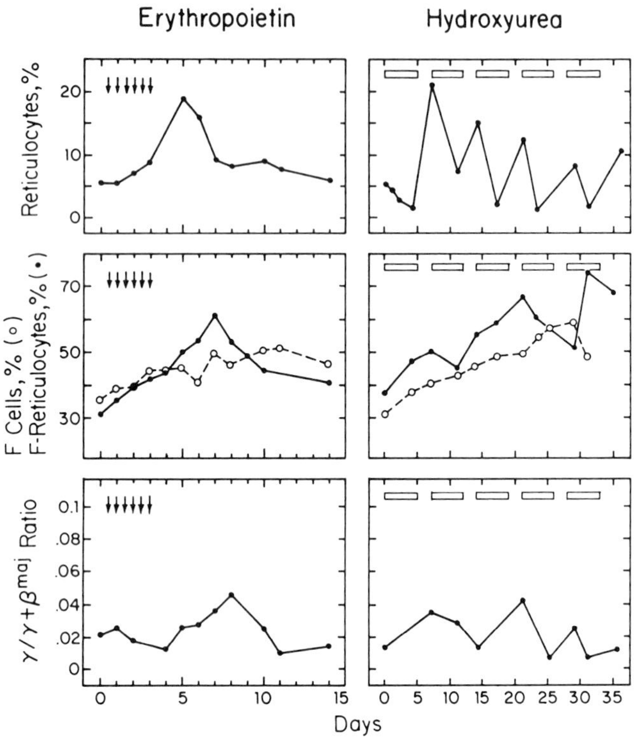

Fig. 1. Treatment of μLCR (−1350)Aγ transgenic mice with erythropoietin and hydroxyurea. The mice were injected with erythropoietin (3000 U/kg body weight) every 12 hr for 3 days of hydroxyurea (200 mg/kg body weight) for 5 days per week for a total of 5 weeks. Treatment days are indicated by the arrows (erythropoietin) or boxes (hydroxyurea).

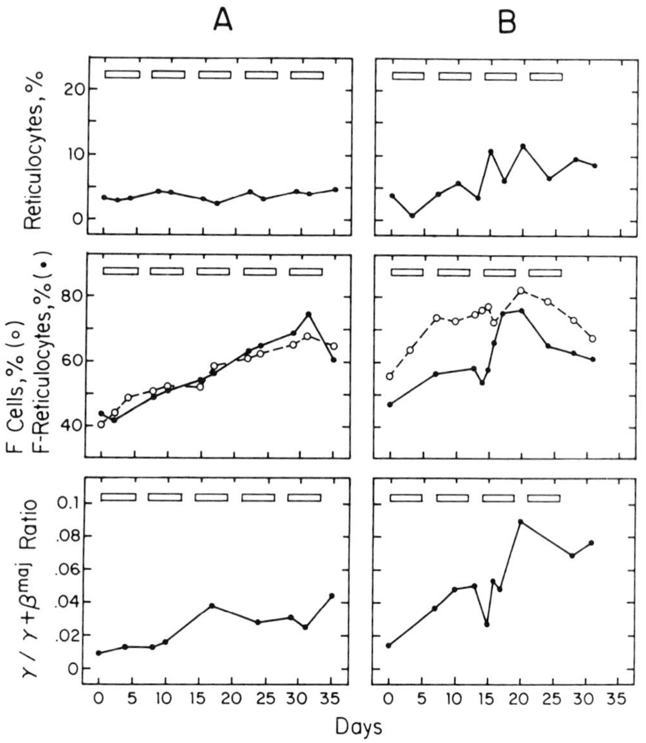

Fig. 2. Induction of γ globin produced in μLCR (−1350)Aγ transgenic mice treated with Didox. Mice were treated with Didox 100 mg/kg (A) or with 450 mg/kg (B) 5 days per week for 5 and 4 weeks, respectively. Treatment days are indicated by boxes.

to 19.2%, and, concurrently, it induced γ gene expression as indicated by the increase in F reticulocytes (from 32.1% to 60.7%), F cells (from 34.5% to 50%), and γ chain biosynthesis (Fig. 1). Hydroxyurea was administered intraperitoneally at a dose of 200 mg/kg body weight for 5 days each week for a total of 5 weeks. The treatment resulted in sharp changes in reticulocyte production consistent with sequential cycles of cytoreduction and erythroid regeneration; in parallel there was a gradual increase in F-reticulocytes from 38% to 72% (Fig. 1).

μLCR (−1350)Aγ mice were subsequently treated with one of two schedules of Didox based on the maximum tolerated dose established in human trials [24]. Didox was administered by intraperitoneal bolus injections of 100 or 450 mg/kg body weight daily 5 days per week for a total of 4 weeks with 450 mg/kg and 5 weeks with 100 mg/kg. As is shown in Figure 2A, the 100 mg/kg dose produced minimal bone marrow suppression (as indicated by a stable reticulocyte count). Nevertheless, induction of γ globin expression was observed, as shown by an increase in F reticulocytes from 41% to 75% and a transient increase in the γ/γ + β major ratio by globin chain biosynthesis. Didox at a dose of 450 mg/kg body weight produced changes in the reticulocyte production similar to hydroxyurea (Fig. 2B). In parallel, there was an increase in F reticulocytes from 47% to 76% and in F cells from 54% to 68% and a five fold increase in the γ/γ + β major globin chain ratio from 0.017 to 0.085.

To examine whether Didox can induce Hb F in a primate, a nonanemic baboon was treated with Didox 150 mg/kg/day for 3 days; this protocol failed to induce production of F cells or F reticulocytes. The same dose was given 5 days per week for 3 weeks followed by escalating doses of 250 mg/kg/day for 3 weeks and a further escalation to 350 mg/kg on the same treatment schedule. The animal was also given supplemental iron (iron dextran, 100 mg) and folic acid (5 mg) weekly. Treatment at 350 mg/kg was discontinued in the second week when clinical toxicity was noted. During the second week of Didox treatment at 250 mg/kg, there was an increase of F reticulocytes and F cells, reaching a peak in the third week (Fig. 3). The increase from baseline values to peak was 1.1% to 6.2% for F reticulocytes and 2.1% to 5.1% for F cells. The same animal was used to test whether Didox can increase fetal hemoglobin in a chronically anemic state. Daily phlebotomies were begun at 50 mls (10% of blood volume) for 3 days, followed by ~30 ml for the duration of the study. During the treatment period, the

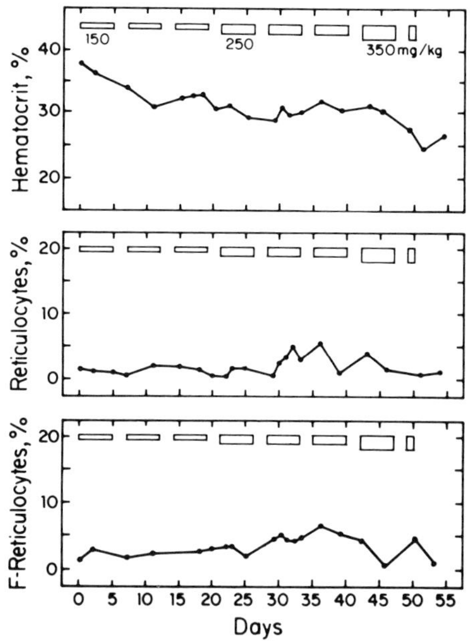

Fig. 3. Treatment of a nonanemic baboon with escalating doses of Didox. Doses of 150 and 250 mg/kg were each given intravenously for 3 weeks followed by 350 mg/kg for 7 days. Days of treatment are shown by the boxes. The hematocrit decreased initially but thereafter remained stable at 28–30%. Fluctuations in the reticulocyte count appeared by the second week of treatment at 250 mg/kg. At higher doses, bone marrow toxicity ensued without recovery of reticulocytes.

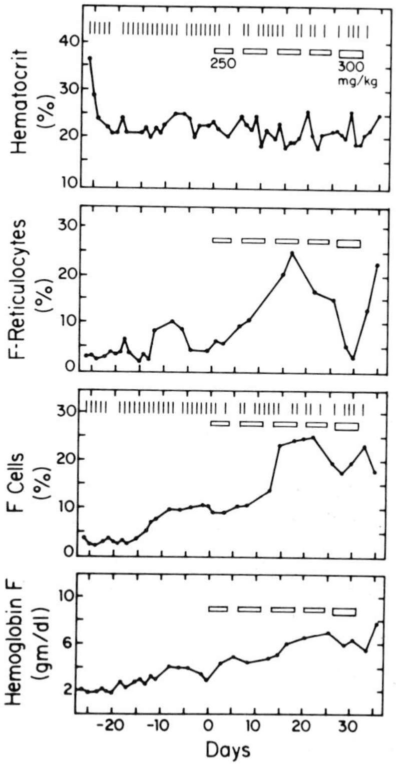

Fig. 4. Treatment of an anemic baboon with Didox. Vertical lines indicate days of bleeding. Boxes indicate days of administration of Didox. Note the increase in F reticulocytes, F cells, and Hb F in response to chronic anemia and the additional induction of Hb F production following administration of Didox.

hematocrit was maintained in a range of 20–25% (Fig. 4). When the F cells and F reticulocytes were stable at ~10% and ~4%, respectively, Didox, 250 mg/kg, was administered 5 days per week for 4 weeks followed by an increased dose of 300 mg/kg for 1 week.

In response to anemia, F cells rose from a baseline of 2.5% to 10% and F reticulocytes from 2.9% to 9.2% (Fig. 4). Administration of Didox, 250 mg/kg/day, resulted in a further increase of F reticulocytes to a peak value of 24.7% and F cells to 25.7% (Figs. 4, 5). The $\gamma/\gamma + \beta$ major biosynthetic ratio changed from a baseline value of 0.014 to 0.024 in response to bleeding alone, and to a peak value of 0.135 (a five fold increase) in response to treatment with Didox. The chemically determined hemoglobin F increased from a baseline value of 1.7% to 4% in response to bleeding and to 7% following 4 weeks of treatment with Didox.

Certain side effects of Didox treatment were also observed. Hematological toxicity (anemia, thrombocytopenia, and leukopenia) appeared during treatment of the nonanemic animal with 350 mg/kg Didox. The animal also developed clinical signs of toxicity (vomiting, abnormal behavior) and laboratory findings of hepatic toxicity (as indicated by the SGOT changing from 58 to 191 U/liter and SGPT from 47 to 163 U/liter). Both clinical and laboratory findings of toxicity resolved after discontinuation of Didox. There were no significant signs of toxicity at the dose of 250 mg/kg. Hepatic toxicity (indicated by an increase in SGPT from 63 to 125 U/liter) became apparent by day 6 during treatment of the anemic animal. Subsequently, the enzyme abnormalities began to resolve despite continued administration of Didox (SGPT decreased to 92 U/liter by day 22). In the anemic baboon, no nausea or behavior abnormalities were observed at 300 mg/kg, the highest dose tested.

DISCUSSION

Following the observation that 5-azacytidine can stimulate Hb F production in vivo [1,2], several investigations were performed with the aim of identifying pharmacologic agents that can induce fetal hemoglobin in the adult. In spite of the availability of in vitro erythroid cell culture systems for testing the effects of drugs on Hb F production [25], all studies that have identified inducers of fetal hemoglobin were done using animal models. Thus the first evidence for induction of an embryonic globin gene by butyrate was obtained in studies of anemic

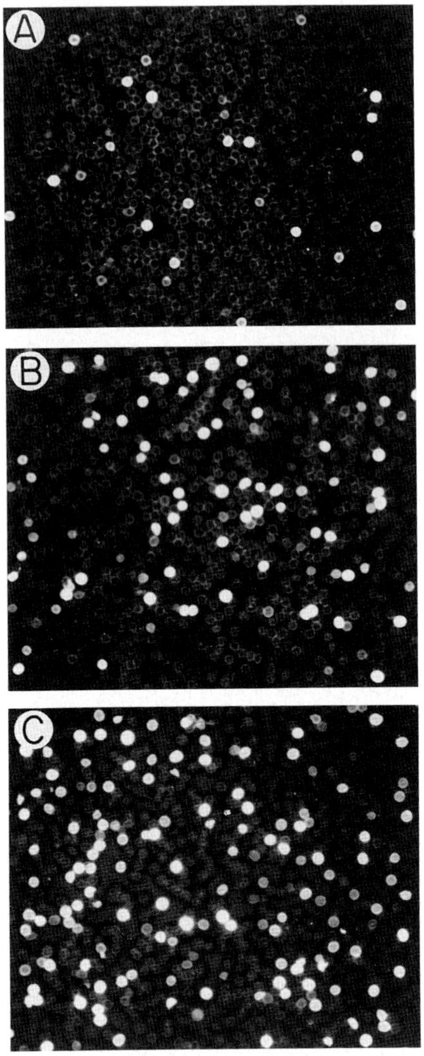

Fig. 5. Staining of baboon red cells with anti-γ globin-fluorescent antibodies before treatment (A), after bleeding (B) and during treatment with Didox (C). Note the increase in F-positive cells as the study progresses.

chickens [26], while the effect of this compound on fetal hemoglobin production was discovered with studies in sheep [27] and baboons [7,8]. Similarly, the induction of Hb F by hydroxyurea [3], erythropoietin [6], and AraC [28] was first observed in studies using baboons or macaques.

The majority of animal species display only one hemoglobin switch from embryonic to adult. Only certain primates, goats, sheep, and cattle display γ globin expression in the fetal stage of development. Goats and sheep have three developmental switches: from embryonic to fetal globin expression, from fetal to the neonatal hemoglobin C, and from Hb C to adult globin formation. When genetically AA sheep are subjected to severe hypoxia, they respond with induction of Hb C [29]. Genetically, BB sheep lack the Hb C gene, however, in this animal, fetal hemoglobin is not induced even when the sheep are subjected to very severe perturbations of erythropoiesis (Wood, personal communication). Globin gene switching in macaques is very similar to that in humans; however, most adult macaques have very low fetal globin production and rare F cells. In such animals, Hb F cannot be induced upon treatment with AraC or erythropoietin (unpublished observations). The most useful animal model for studying Hb F induction is the baboon. Although there exists a genetically defined variation in the level of Hb F production [30,31], this animal model consistently responds with Hb F induction when treated with cell cycle-specific drugs or erythropoietin [1,6,28]. The low level of F cells produced in response to chronic anemia indicates that the baboon used in our study is a low responder. Nevertheless, in this baboon the degree of F cell, F reticulocyte, and Hb F induction in response to Didox treatment was at least as high if not higher than that seen with hydroxyurea in previous studies.

The μLCR (−1350)Aγ transgenic mouse line we used in our study expresses γ globin in the embryonic, fetal, and adult stages of development. γ Globin expression in the fetus (per copy of transgene) is 20–25% of the endogenous murine α globin. γ Globin expression in the adult is about one-third to one-fifth of that in fetus [11,32]. Approximately 30–40% of the red cells of these animals contain human Hb F. To test whether induction of fetal hemoglobin in this transgenic line by a pharmacologic agent can predict Hb F induction in a primate, we first treated transgenic mice and subsequently baboons with a new ribonucleotide reductase inhibitor, Didox, which has not been evaluated before for Hb F inducibility. Didox induced Hb F production in the μLCR (−1350)Aγ transgenic mice, and a similar result was obtained when the compound was tested in a nonanemic and anemic baboon. This result adds to the evidence that the μLCR (−1350)Aγ transgenic line can be used as a convenient small animal model for screening pharmacologic agents for their potential to induce Hb F. Use of transgenic mice will facilitate the in vivo assessment of interesting compounds without the limitations and the cost of experimentation with large animals.

Clinical trials are currently in progress to test the usefulness of hydroxyurea in the treatment of patients with sickle cell disease. The major limiting factor of this treatment is bone marrow suppression. Induction of γ globin was achieved in mice by administration of 250 mg/kg Didox without significant bone marrow suppression. At doses higher than 300 mg/kg, reversible bone marrow toxicity and reversible hepatoxicity appeared. The potential usefulness of Didox as an Hb F inducer cannot be inferred from these results, since only one baboon was treated, and this animal was a low Hb F responder. More information about the in vivo toxicity of Didox from ongoing studies in humans will be required to justify studies assessing whether this compound represents a more effective agent than hydroxyurea for treatment of patients with sickle cell disease.

ACKNOWLEDGMENTS

This study was supported by NIH grant HL20899 and a Robert Woods Johnson grant (17585) to B.S.P.

REFERENCES

1. DeSimone J, Heller P, Hall L, Zwiers D: 5-Azacytidine stimulates fetal hemoglobin synthesis in anemic baboons. Proc Natl Acad Sci USA 79:4428, 1982.
2. Ley TJ, DeSimone J, Anagnou NP, Keller GH, Humphries RK, Turner P, Young NS, Heller P, Nienhuis AW: 5-Azacytidine selectively increases γ globin synthesis in patients with β^+-thalassemia. N Engl J Med 307:1469, 1982.
3. Levtin NL, Linch DC, Beardsley GP, McIntyre KW, Nathan D: Augmentation of fetal hemoglobin production in anemic monkeys by hydroxyurea. N Engl J Med 310:869, 1984.
4. Platt OS, Orlan SH, Dover G, Beardsley GP, Meller B, Nathan DG: Hydroxyurea enhances fetal hemoglobin production in sickle cell anemia. J Clin Invest 74:652, 1984.
5. Veith R, Galanello R, Papayannopoulou T, Stamatoyannopoulos G: Stimulation of F cell production in patients with sickle cell anemia treated with cytarabine or hydroxyurea. N Engl J Med 313:1571, 1985.
6. Al-Khatti A, Veith RW, Papayannopoulou T, Fritsch EF, Goldwasser E, Stamatoyannopoulos G: Stimulation of fetal hemoglobin synthesis by erythropoietin in baboons. N Engl J Med 317:415, 1987.
7. Constantoulakis P, Papayannopoulou T, Stamatoyannopoulos G: α-Amino-N-butyric acid stimulates fetal hemoglobin in the adult. Blood 72:1961, 1988.
8. Constantoulakis P, Knitter G, Stamatoyannopoulos G: On the induction of fetal hemoglobin by butyrates: In vivo and in vitro studies with sodium butyrate and comparison of combination treatments with 5-AzaC and AraC. Blood 74:1963, 1989.
9. Dover GJ, Brusilow S, Samid D: Increased fetal hemoglobin in patients receiving sodium 4-phenylbutyrate. N Engl J Med 327:569, 1992.
10. Perrine SP, Ginder GD, Faller DV, Dover GH, Ikuta T, Witkowska E, Shi-Ping C, Vichinsky EP, Olivieri NF: A short-term trial of butyrate to stimulate fetal-globin-gene expression in the β globin disorders. N Engl J Med 328:81, 1993.
11. Enver T, Ebens A, Forrester W, Stamatoyannopoulos G: The human β globin locus activation region alters the developmental fate of a human fetal globin gene in transgenic mice. Proc Natl Acad Sci USA 86:7033, 1989.
12. Constantoulakis P, Josephson B, Mangahas L, Papayannopoulou T, Enver T, Constantini F, Stamatoyannopoulos G: Locus control region Aγ transgenic mice: A new model for studying the induction of fetal hemoglobin in the adult. Blood 77:1326, 1991.
13. Stamatoyannopoulos G, Veith R, Galanello R, Papayannopoulou T: Hb F production in stressed erythropoiesis: observations and kinetic models. Ann NY Acad Sci 445:188, 1985.
14. Elford HL, Wampler GL, van't Riet B: New ribonucleotide reductase inhibitor with antineoplastic activity. Cancer Res 39:844, 1979.
15. Elford HL, van't Riet B: Inhibitors of ribonucleoside diphosphate reductase activity. In: Cory J, Cory A, (eds). "International Encyclopedia of Pharmacology and Therapeutics." Elmsford, NY: Pergamon Press, 1989, p 217.
16. van't Riet B, Wampler GL, Elford HL: Synthesis of hydroxy- and amino-substituted benzohydroxamic acids: inhibition of ribonucleotide reductase and antitumor activity. J Med Chem 22:589, 1979.
17. Wood WG, Stamatoyannopoulos G, Lim G, Nute PE: F cells in the adult: Normal values and levels in individuals with hereditary and acquired elevations of HbF. Blood 46:671, 1975.
18. Stamatoyannopoulos G, Farquhar M, Lindsley D, Brice M, Papayannopoulou T, Nute P: Monoclonal antibodies specific for globin chains. Blood 61:530, 1983.
19. Papayannopoulou T, Vichinsky E, Stamatoyannopoulos G: Fetal Hb production during acute erythroid expansion. Br J Hematol 44:535, 1980.
20. Papayannopoulou T, Kurachi S, Brice M, Nakamoto B, Stamatoyannopoulos G: Asynchronous synthesis of Hb F and Hb A during erythroblast maturation II. Studies of Gγ, Aγ and γ chain synthesis in individual erythroid clones from neonatal and adult BFUe cultures. Blood 57:531, 1981.
21. Betke D, Marti HR, Schlicht I: Estimation of small percentage of Hb F. Nature 184:1877, 1959.
22. Kafatos F, Jones W, Efstratiadis A: Determination of nucleic acid homologies and relative concentrations by dot hybridization procedure. Nucleic Acids Res 7:1541, 1979.
23. Magram J, Chada K, Constantini F: Developmental regulation of a cloned adult beta-globin gene in transgenic mice. Nature 315:338, 1985.
24. Veale D, Carmichael J, Cantwell BMJ, Elford HL, Blackie R, Kerr DJ, Kaye SB, Harris AL: Phase I and pharmacokinetic study of Didox: A ribonucleotide reductase inhibitor. Br J Cancer 58:70, 1988.
25. Galanello R, Stamatoyannopoulos G, Papayannopoulou T: Mechanism of Hb F stimulation by S-stage compounds in vitro studies with bone marrow cells exposed to 5-azacytidine, AraC or hydroxyurea. J Clin Invest 81:1209, 1988.
26. Ginder GD, Matthew WJ, Pohlman JK: Activation of a chicken embryonic globin gene in adult erythroid cells by 5-azacytidine and sodium butyrate. Proc Natl Acad Sci USA 81:3954, 1984.
27. Perrine SP, Rudolph A, Faller DV Roman C, Cohen RA, Chen S, Kan YW: Butyrate infusions in the bovine fetus delay the biologic clock for globin gene switching. Proc Natl Acad Sci USA 85:8540, 1988.
28. Papayannopoulou T, Torrealba de Ron A, Veith R, Knitter G, Stamatoyannopoulos G: Arabinosylcytosine induces fetal hemoglobin in baboons by perturbing erythroid cell differentiation kinetics. Science 224:617, 1984.
29. Barker JE, Pierce JE, Nienhuis AW: Hemoglobin switching in sheep. In Stamatoyannopoulos G, Nienhuis AW (eds): "Hemoglobins in Development and Differentiation." New York: Alan R. Liss, Inc., 1981, p 321.
30. DeSimone J, Heller P, Amsel J, Usman M: Magnitude of the fetal hemoglobin response to acute hemolytic anemia in baboons is controlled by genetic factors. J Clin Invest 65:224, 1980.
31. DeSimone J, Heller P, Biel M, Zwiers D: Genetic relationship between fetal Hb levels in normal and erythropoietically stressed baboons. Br J Haematol 49:175, 1981.
32. Enver T, Raich N, Ebens AJ, Papayannopoulou T, Constantini E, Stamatoyannopoulos G: Developmental regulation of human fetal-to-adult globin gene switching in transgenic mice. Nature 344:309, 1990.

American Journal of Hematology 45:142–145 (1994)

Continuous Infusion of Monoclonal Antibody-Purified Factor VIII: Rational Approach to Serious Hemorrhage In Patients With Allo-/Autoantibodies to Factor VIII

Erlinda M. Gordon, Fatma Al-Batniji, and Jonathan C. Goldsmith

Divisions of Hematology/Oncology (E.M.G., J.C.G.) and Medical Genetics (E.M.G.), Childrens Hospital of Los Angeles and University of Southern California School of Medicine, Los Angeles, California; Riaydh Military Hospital, Riaydh, Saudi Arabia (F.A.-B.)

Hemorrhage in a patient with factor VIII inhibitor is associated with increased morbidity and mortality. Treatment with factor IX complex concentrates or recombinant factor VIIa (rVIIa) may not control bleeding and may induce thrombosis. In this study, continuous infusion of a monoclonal antibody-purified factor VII concentrate (Monoclate-P) was used successfully in two hemophilic patients with factor VIII alloantibodies and one nonhemophilic patient with a factor VIII autoantibody. In two patients, hemorrhage was life-threatening, and, in one, bleeding did not stop with repeated infusions of activated factor IX complex concentrates. The patients' ages ranged from 4 to 15 years, and the inhibitor levels from 6 to 300 Bethesda units/ml. Clinical hemostasis was excellent, and in vivo recovery of infused factor VIII was achieved. When an excess of monoclonal factor VIII was added to the inhibitor plasma in vitro, a stable level of residual factor VIII activity was noted after an initial rapid loss. This second-order reaction occurs in plasmas of patients with type I factor VIII inhibitors. In one patient, we showed that the saturation dose of the factor VIII inhibitor predicted in vivo recovery of factor VIII:C. These data emphasize the importance of characterizing the kinetic reactions of the factor VIII inhibitor. Furthermore, we confirm previous reports that continuous infusion of monoclonal factor VIII is a safe and effective treatment of patients with factor VIII inhibitors in whom hemorrhage is either life-threatening or refractory to standard treatment.

Key words: MoAb FVIII, Monoclate-P, bleeding, clotting, hemophilia

INTRODUCTION

The treatment of acute hemorrhage in a person with a factor VIII inhibitor can be challenging. In a hemophilic person without an inhibitor, therapeutic efficacy is measured by control of bleeding and by in vivo recovery of infused factor VIII. If a person with a factor VIII inhibitor could be infused with sufficient factor VIII to overcome the inhibitor, this approach would be preferred, since both clinical hemostasis and factor VIII levels could be assessed. In such patients, treatment with factor IX complex concentrates or recombinant factor VIIa (rVIIa) may control bleeding, but plasma levels of factor VIII coagulant activity (factor VIII:C) cannot be used to evaluate therapy [1]. Furthermore, factor IX complex concentrates and rVIIa can induce life-threatening and fatal thrombosis [2,3].

In this study, we assessed the therapeutic efficacy of continuous infusion of monoclonal factor VIII (MoAb factor VIII) in patients with low- and high-titer inhibitors, and characterized the inhibitors' kinetic reactions. In one patient, we tested whether in vitro kinetic reactions of the factor VIII inhibitor could predict in vivo response to therapy.

MATERIALS AND METHODS

A monoclonal antibody-purified factor VIII preparation (Monoclate P; Armour Pharmaceutical Company, Collegeville, PA) was used. This preparation retains its potency at room temperature, making it suitable for continuous infusion [4]. It has no known contaminating coagulant proteins, making it suitable for administration of

Received for Publication March 8, 1993; accepted June 9, 1993.

Address reprint requests to Erlinda M. Gordon, MD, Childrens Hospital Los Angeles, Mailstop #57, 4650 Sunset Boulevard, Los Angeles, CA 90027.

TABLE I. Clinical Characteristics of the Three Patients

Patient	Age (years)	Diagnosis	Clinical manifestation
1	4	Hemophilia A	Subarachnoid hemorrhage
2	4	Hemophilia A	Lingual hemorrhage
3	15	Autoimmune ds	Knee hemarthrosis refractory to activated factor IX concentrates

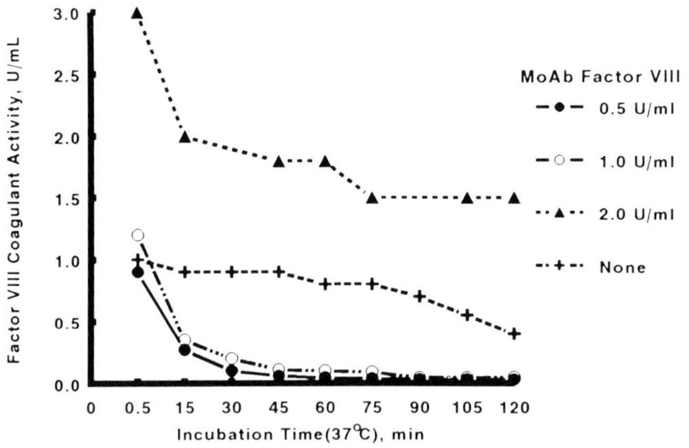

Fig. 1. Time course of inactivation of factor VIII:C in normal plasma (None, no added MoAb factor VIII), and in mixtures of patient 1's plasma (6 B.U./ml) and monoclonal antibody-purified factor VIII (MoAb factor VIII). Factor VIII coagulant activity (factor VIII:C), measured by clotting assay, is plotted on the vertical axis, and incubation time (min) is plotted on the horizontal axis.

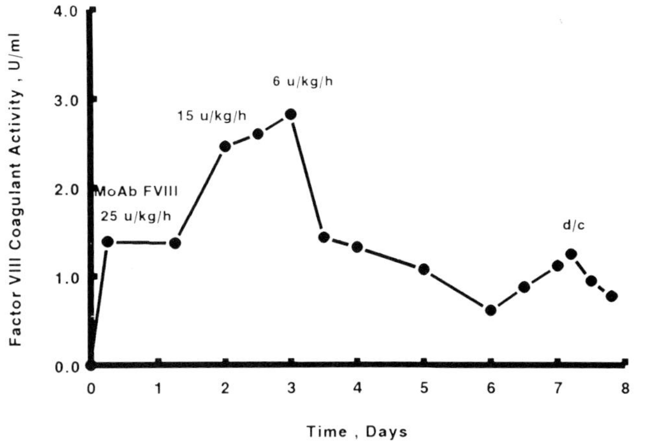

Fig. 2. Effect of continuous infusion of monoclonal factor VIII (Monoclate-P) on in vivo recovery of factor VIII:C in patient 1 (inhibitor level 6 B.U./ml). A loading dose of 100 U MoAb factor VIII/kg was given before continuous infusion of MoAb factor VIII. Factor VIII:C, measured by clotting assay, is plotted on the vertical axis, while infusion time, (days) is plotted on the horizontal axis. The dose of infused factor VIII was adjusted to maintain the desired factor VIII:C level (1.0 U/ml).

large doses [5]. Factor VIII coagulant activity [6] and factor VIII inhibitor [7] assays were performed by established techniques.

The kinetics of factor VIII:C inactivation were studied in mixtures of patient's inhibitor plasma and various doses of monoclonal factor VIII (MoAb FVIII) [8,9]. Factor VIII:C was measured in factor VIII-treated inhibitor plasmas at serial intervals during incubation at 37°C for 2 hr. The in vitro saturation dose of the factor VIII inhibitor was defined as the amount of added MoAb factor VIII that induced a stable residual factor VIII:C level >0.5 U/ml during a 2 hr incubation period. Table I shows the clinical characteristics of the three patients studied.

RESULTS

Patient 1, a 4-year-old white boy, was admitted to Childrens Hospital Los Angeles for management of subarachnoid hemorrhage. He had been on immune tolerance induction with daily injections of MoAb factor VIII for 4 weeks. A factor VIII inhibitor titer, obtained 1 week before admission, was 6 B.U./ml. Figure 1 represents the in vitro kinetic reactions of patient 1's inhibitor. A sharp decline in factor VIII:C was noted in mixtures of patient plasma and MoAb factor VIII, at doses of 0.5 and 1 U factor VIII/ml. In contrast, at 2 U factor VIII/ml, a stable level of residual factor VIII:C was noted after an initial sharp decline. The induction of stable levels of factor VIII:C indicated that the inhibitor had been saturated. Hence, the in vitro saturation dose of the factor VIII inhibitor of this patient was determined to be 2 U/ml.

The therapeutic loading dose of MoAb factor VIII was then calculated by considering the in vitro saturation dose of the patient's inhibitor. Thus a loading dose (100 U MoAb factor VIII/kg) was given that would raise the factor VIII:C level of a hemophilic person without an inhibitor to 2 U/ml. In vivo recovery of infused factor VIII, obtained 15 min after injection, was 1.4 U/ml (Fig. 2). The factor VIII:C level recovered in vivo correlated with that recovered in vitro (Fig. 1) 15 min after addition of a dose of MoAb factor VIII (2 U/ml) that saturated the factor VIII inhibitor.

Figure 2 further shows in vivo recovery of infused MoAb factor VIII in patient 1. After a loading dose of 100 U/kg, the dose of MoAb factor VIII for continuous infusion was adjusted to maintain a factor VIII:C level >1.0 U/ml. Clinical hemostasis was excellent, without untoward side effects. The patient received a total dose of 1,636 U MoAb factor VIII/kg. He was discharged on his immune tolerance regimen of 100 U MoAb factor VIII/kg/day. One week later, his factor VIII inhibitor level was <1B.U./ml, and, 4 months later, it was still <1B.U./ml. Thus immune tolerance was induced within 7 days by continuous infusion of monoclonal factor VIII.

Patient 2 had a type I inhibitor with second-order kinetic reactions on in vitro testing. This 4-year-old black boy, with severe hemophilia A and a factor VIII inhibitor level of 100 B.U./ml, was admitted for profuse lingual hemorrhage and hypotension [9]. As was reported previously [9], the inhibitor's in vitro saturation dose was 200 U MoAb factor VIII/ml. Therefore, a loading dose of 10,000 U MoAb factor VIII/kg would be required to obtain in vivo factor VIII:C recovery. Since clinical hemostasis could be evaluated by visualization of the bleeding site, the dose of MoAb factor VIII was adjusted until bleeding ceased at 75 U factor VIII/kg/hr. On the third day, in vivo factor VIII:C recovery was achieved, after a total dose of only 6,400 U/kg had been given. On the fifth day, the factor VIII:C level was >3.0U/ml, at which time a cumulative dose of 9,000 U factor VIII/kg had been given. This dose approximates the predicted dose of 10,000 U/kg at which in vivo factor VIII:C recovery could be expected. The patient was then discharged on 100 U factor VIII/kg/day. One week later, his inhibitor titer was 120 B.U./ml. Thus immune tolerance was not achieved by continuous infusion of monoclonal factor VIII, although anamnesis did not occur. Subsequently, immune tolerance induction was discontinued due to recurrent central line infections. Minor bleeding episodes were treated with activated prothrombin complex concentrates. Nine months later, the inhibitor level was 32 B.U./ml.

Patient 3 had a type I inhibitor with second-order kinetic reactions on in vivo testing. This 15-year-old white boy with an autoimmune disorder characterized by a factor VIII autoantibody (300 B.U./ml), nephrotic syndrome, and insulin-dependent diabetes mellitus presented with right knee hemarthrosis. He was treated for 1 week with twice daily injections of activated factor IX concentrates, without improvement. The in vitro saturation dose of the factor VIII inhibitor was 200 U MoAb factor VIII/ml. Thus a loading dose of 10,000 U MoAb factor VIII/kg would be required to obtain a measurable in vivo factor VIII level. Because patient 3 did not have a life-threatening bleed, an empiric loading dose of 100 U/kg was given, followed by continuous infusion of factor VIII that was adjusted to gain control of bleeding. Clinical hemostasis was excellent, with no untoward reactions. Low levels of factor VIII:C (0.02–0.04 U/ml) were detected in vivo during continuous infusion of 25 U MoAb factor VIII/kg/hr. He was discharged on the sixth hospital day after receiving a total dose of 3,900U factor VIII/kg. No further attempt at immune tolerance induction was made. Hence, his inhibitor level ranged from 250 to 500 B.U./ml during a 12 month follow-up.

In vitro kinetic reactions of the factor VIII inhibitors in ten inhibitor plasmas were then evaluated. As expected, the saturation dose of factor VIII inhibitor was directly related to the respective factor VIII inhibitor level

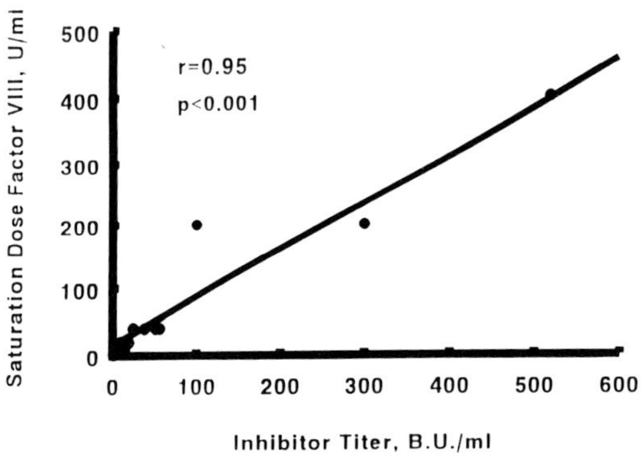

Fig. 3. Saturation dose of the factor VIII inhibitor in 10 inhibitor plasmas. The saturation dose of MoAb factor VIII, defined as the amount of factor VIII required to saturate the inhibitor and to induce a stable residual factor VIII:C level >0.5 U/ml, is plotted on the vertical axis, while the factor VIII inhibitor titer (B.U./ml) is plotted on the horizontal axis.

($r = 0.95$, $P < .001$; Fig. 3). These data indicate that the in vitro saturation dose of the factor VIII inhibitor may be used as a guide in calculating the loading dose of MoAb factor VIII for treatment of patients with factor VIII inhibitors, before hemorrhage occurs.

DISCUSSION

Hemorrhage in persons with allo- or autoantibodies to factor VIII can be life or limb threatening [1]. Common therapies include repeated bolus infusions of large doses of factor VIII in patients with low-titer inhibitors, infusion of factor VIII bypassing agents [10–12] or porcine factor VIII [13] for those with moderately high-titer inhibitors, and combined modality therapy with or without plasma exchange, and use of immunosuppressive agents and intravenous immunoglobulins for those with high-titer inhibitors [1,14]. Experimental use of recombinant factor VIIa is available for selected patients who do not respond to standard therapy [3]. In most cases, therapeutic efficacy cannot be evaluated by measuring factor VIII:C levels, and clinical hemostasis may not be adequate. Furthermore, use of factor VIII bypassing agents can induce coagulopathy and disseminated intravascular coagulation (DIC) and organ damage [2,15,16]. In this study, continuous infusion of MoAb factor VIII was used successfully in two hemophilic patients with factor VIII alloantibodies and in one nonhemophilic patient with a factor VIII autoantibody. In two patients, hemorrhage was life-threatening, and, in one, bleeding did not stop with repeated infusions of activated factor IX complex concentrates. Clinical hemostasis was excellent, in vivo recovery of infused factor VIII was achieved, and anamnesis did not occur. In vitro testing of the plasmas showed that all three patients had type I inhibitors exhibiting second-order kinetic reactions. The in vitro saturation dose of the factor VIII inhibitor was used as a guide for determining the therapeutic loading dose of MoAb factor VIII in one patient. Furthermore, immune tolerance was induced in this patient by continuous infusion of factor VIII for 7 days.

In conclusion, we confirm that continuous infusion of monoclonal antibody-purified factor VIII is a safe and effective treatment of patients with factor VIII inhibitors in whom hemorrhage is life threatening or is refractory to standard treatment. Studies are in progress to determine whether in vitro kinetic reactions of the factor VIII inhibitor could be used to predict a patient's in vivo response to therapy, before hemorrhage occurs. If so, serial assessments of in vitro kinetic reactions of the factor VIII inhibitor may be required, since inhibitor levels tend to fluctuate over time, particularly during immune tolerance induction. Finally, in patients with low-titer inhibitors, continuous infusion of factor VIII may be used in a cost-effective manner to induce immune tolerance. When the amount of MoAb factor VIII required to control bleeding can be anticipated, the cost of such therapy can then be negotiated with the manufacturer, the federal government, and/or the third-party payor.

ACKNOWLEDGMENT

The authors are grateful to Armour Pharmaceutical Company (Collegeville, PA) for providing the monoclonal antibody-purified factor VIII (Monoclate P) used in determining the kinetic reactions of the factor VIII inhibitor in vitro.

REFERENCES

1. Kasper CK: Treatment of factor VIII inhibitors. Progr Hemostas Thromb 9:57–86, 1989.
2. Lusher JM: Thrombogenicity associated with factor IX complex concentrates. Semin Hematol 28(Suppl 6):3–5, 1991.
3. Hender U: Experiences with recombinant factor VIIa in haemophiliacs. Curr Stud Hematol Blood Transfus 58:63–68, 1991.
4. Weinstein RE, Bona RD, Rickles FR: Continuous infusion of monoclonal antibody-purified factor VIII. Am J Hematol 36:211–212, 1991.
5. Schreiber AB: The preclinical characterization of Monoclate factor VIII:C antihemophilic factor human. Semin Hematol 25:27–32, 1988.
6. Nilsson IM, Kirkwood TBL, Barrowcliffe TW: In vivo recovery of factor VIII: A comparison of one-stage and two-stage assay methods. Thromb Haemostas 42:1230–1239, 1979.
7. Kasper CK, Aledort LM, Counts RB: A more uniform measurement of factor VIII inhibitors. Thromb Diath Haemorrh 34:875–876, 1975.
8. Allain JP, Frommel D: Antibodies to factor VIII: Specificity and kinetics of iso- and hetero-antibodies in hemophilia A. Blood 44:313–322, 1974.
9. Gordon EM, Mungo R, Goldsmith JC: Lingual hemorrhage in a patient with a high factor VIII inhibitor titer: Management by continuous infusion of monoclonal antibody-purified factor VIII. Am J Pediatr Hematol Oncol 15:107–110, 1993.
10. Lusher JM, Shapiro SS, Palascak JE, Rao AV, Levine PH, Blatt PM, and the Hemophilia Study Group: Efficacy of prothrombin-complex concentrates in hemophiliacs with antibodies to factor VIII: A multicenter therapeutic trial. N Engl J Med 303:421–425, 1980.
11. Sjamsoedin LJM, Heijnen L, Mauser-Bunshoten EP: The effect of activated prothrombin complex concentrate (FEIBA) on joint and muscle bleeding in patients with hemophilia A and antibodies to factor VIII: A double-blind clinical trial. N Engl J Med 305:717–721, 1981.
12. Lusher JM, Blatt PM, Penner JA: Autoplex versus Proplex: A controlled, double-blind study of effectiveness in hemophiliacs with inhibitors to factor VIII. Blood 62:1135–1138, 1983.
13. Hay CR: Innovative use of porcine factor VIII:C for immune tolerance induction. Am J Med 91:27–29, 1991.
14. Nilsson IM, Berntorp E, Zettervall O: Induction of immune tolerance in patients with hemophilia and antibodies to factor VIII by combined treatment with intravenous IgG, cyclophosphamide and factor VIII. N Engl J Med 318:947–980, 1988.
15. Rodeghiero F, Castronovo S, Dini E: Disseminated intravascular coagulation after infusion of FEIBA (factor VIII inhibitor by-passing activity) in a patient with acquired hemophilia. Thromb Haemostas 48:339–340, 1982
16. Gruppo RA, Vove KE, Donaldson VH: Fatal myocardial necrosis associated with prothrombin-complex-concentrate therapy in hemophilia A. N Engl J Med 309:242–243, 1983.

American Journal of Hematology 45:146–149 (1994)

Prevalence of Abnormal Iron Studies in Heterozygotes for Hereditary Hemochromatosis: An Analysis of 255 Heterozygotes

Paul C. Adams

Department of Medicine, University Hospital, University of Western Ontario, London, Ontario, Canada

Iron studies were compared in 434 patients from 80 hemochromatosis families classified as putative homozygotes, heterozygotes, and normal by HLA typing. There were 28 of 255 (11%) heterozygotes with an elevated serum ferritin and 22 of 255 (8.6%) with an elevated transferrin saturation. Serum ferritin (140 ± 10.2 μg/liter; mean ± standard error) was greater in heterozygotes than in normal subjects (87 ± 8.5 μg/liter; *P* < .05, Mann Whitney test). Transferrin saturation was greater in heterozygotes (38% ± 0.88%) than in normal patients (29% ± 1.1%; *P* < .0001). Mean hepatic iron concentration was 54 ± 6 μmol/g (n = 17), and the hepatic iron index was <2 in these patients. Most heterozygotes for hemochromatosis have a normal serum ferritin and transferrin saturation. Heterozygotes with minor elevations in serum ferritin or transferrin saturation do not have significant iron overload as assessed by hepatic iron concentration.

Key words: ferritin, transferrin saturation, iron absorption, hepatic iron

INTRODUCTION

Hemochromatosis is a genetic disease with an autosomal recessive inheritance pattern. Because of the close linkage between the hemochromatosis gene on chromosome 6 and the HLA-A complex, patients can be "genotyped" into putative homozygotes, heterozygotes, and normals by using conventional HLA-A and -B tissue typing [1–3]. Most homozygotes will show phenotypic expression of the disease with iron overload of parenchymal organs such as the liver, pancreas, heart and endocrine glands [4,5]. Heterozygotes have not been shown to develop the symptom complex associated with hemochromatosis, although some heterozygotes have biochemical and histological evidence of iron overload [6–9]. To assess the iron status of heterozygotes, biochemical and histological iron studies were carried out in 434 subjects from 80 families.

MATERIALS AND METHODS

The diagnosis of hemochromatosis was established in the proband cases by the demonstration of parenchymal iron overload on liver biopsy, elevated hepatic iron concentration and hepatic iron index (hepatic iron/age [10–13] and the absence of other conditions associated with iron overload, such as alcoholism, iron-loading anemias, multiple transfusions, and porphyria cutanea tarda. All available family members were investigated with serum ferritin, transferrin saturation, and HLA-A and -B typing. Siblings who shared two HLA haplotypes with the proband were considered to be putative homozygotes, those who shared one haplotype putative heterozygotes, and those who shared no haplotypes putative normal. Children of homozygotes were considered to be putative heterozygotes. Serum ferritin was measured using a commercial radioimmunoassay (Biorad), and transferrin saturation was measured using a commercial colorimetric assay (Roche). The reference ranges for serum ferritin were established at this center and were 30–350 μg/liter for men and 15–200 μg/liter for women. The reference ranges for serum ferritin were established from a random sample of 13,689 persons who participated in a Nutrition Canada national survey. Upper limits of the reference range were based on the 90th percentile and were 350 μg/liter in men at age 50 years or older and 200 μg/liter in

Received for publication April 2, 1993; accepted June 30, 1993.

Address reprint requests to Dr. Paul C. Adams, Department of Medicine, University Hospital, P.O. Box 5339, 339 Windermere Rd., London, Ontario, Canada N6A 5A5.

TABLE I. Iron Studies in 434 Patients From 80 Hemochromatosis Families†

Patients	n	Ferritin	% Tf saturation	Hepatic iron
Normal	81	87 ± 8.5	29 ± 1.1	17 ± 4.1[a]
Heterozygotes	255	140 ± 10.2*	38 ± .88*	54 ± 6.0 (n = 17)
Homozygotes	98	1,784 ± 191	74 ± 1.7	348 ± 13

†Reference ranges: serum ferritin, males 30–350 μg/liter, females 15–200 μg/liter, transferrin saturation 20–55%, hepatic iron concentration 10–40 μmol/g dry weight.
[a]Hepatic iron concentration in normal controls was established in 30 patients with normal liver at autopsy or resection [10]. Data are expressed as the mean ± standard error.
*The mean serum ferritin and transferrin saturation was significantly greater in heterozygotes than in the normal subjects ($P < .05$, Mann Whitney test).

women at age 70 years and older [14]. The reference range for transferrin saturation was 20–55%. Samples were collected during routine clinic visits and at random times throughout the day. HLA-A and -B locus antigens were assayed using standard microlymphocytotoxicity tests in Terasaki plates [15]. Mean serum ferritin and transferrin saturations between heterozygotes and normals were compared by the Mann Whitney test. Liver biopsy was performed (after informed consent was obtained) in selected putative heterozygotes in whom there was an elevated serum ferritin or transferrin saturation to rule out the possibility of a homozygote being misclassified as a heterozygote as a result of a genetic recombination or an unsuspected homozygote-heterozygote mating in the parents. Since most of the heterozygotes had a normal serum ferritin and transferrin saturation, liver biopsy was uncommon in the heterozygote group, although the cohort of 17 patients represents one of the largest reported series of hepatic iron determinations in heterozygotes. Hepatic iron concentration was measured in liver tissue dried to constant weight by atomic absorption spectrophotometry as previously described [10]. The normal range for hepatic iron concentration was considered to be 10–40 μmol/g dry weight. Hepatic iron index was the hepatic iron concentration (μmol/g) divided by the age of the patient (normal <2) [10–12].

RESULTS

Iron studies were compared in 434 patients classified as homozygotes, heterozygotes, and normal by HLA typing from 80 families. There were 98 homozygotes, 255 heterozygotes, and 81 normal patients. The clinical characteristics of the homozygotes have been described previously [5,15,16]. There were 28 of 255 (11%) heterozygotes with an elevated serum ferritin and 22 of 255 (8.6%) with an elevated transferrin saturation. The mean serum ferritin, transferrin saturation, and hepatic iron concentration in the homozygotes, heterozygotes, and normals are shown in Table I. Mean serum ferritin and transferrin saturation was within the normal range in male and female heterozygotes. Biochemical abnormalities were more common in siblings of probands [5] than in children of probands, but this may be related to the older age of the sibling group. There was only one normal patient with an abnormal serum ferritin or transferrin saturation (a 55-year-old male; serum ferritin 366 μg/liter). Heterozygotes who underwent liver biopsy had a mean serum ferritin of 303 ± 61 μg/liter (range 53–775) and a mean transferrin saturation of 57% ± 3.2% (range 29–75%). Mean hepatic iron concentration in 17 heterozygotes (54 ± 6 μmol/g) was significantly greater than in a normal control population (17 ± 4.4 μmol/g) [10,11]. All heterozygotes had a hepatic iron index <2 (range 0.45–1.77). The range of serum ferritin and transferrin saturation in the male and female homozygotes, heterozygotes and normal patients is shown in Figures 1 and 2.

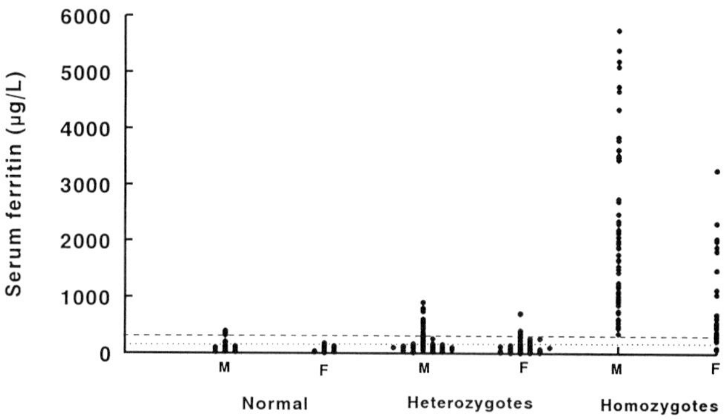

Fig. 1. Serum ferritin in normal patients, putative heterozygotes, and putative homozygotes for hemochromatosis. M, male; F, female. The reference range was 15–200 μg/liter for females and 30–350 μg/liter for males [13]. The lines represented the upper limit of normal in males (dashed lines) and females (dotted lines).

Several genetic recombinations were observed in these patients. In two putative heterozygotes in two families, there were recombinations in the "nonhemochromatosis" haplotype as assessedby HLA-A and -B typing. Both these patients had a normal serum ferritin and transferrin

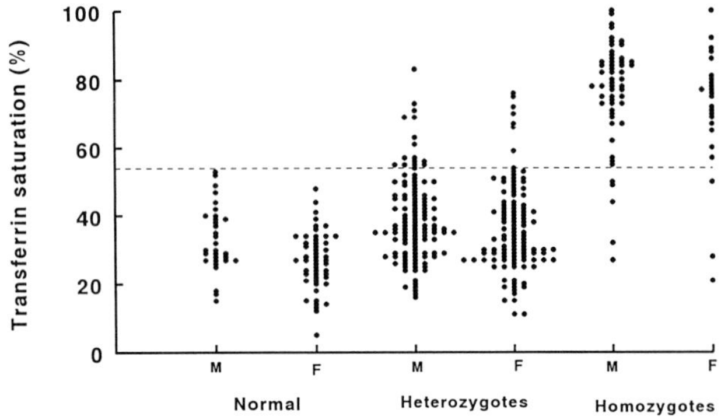

Fig. 2. Transferrin saturation (%) in normal patients, putative heterozygotes, and putative homozygotes for hemochromatosis. M, male; F, female. The reference range was 20–55%. The dashed line represents the upper limit of the reference range.

saturation. In one phenotypic homozygote (serum ferritin 948 μg/liter, transferrin saturation 84%) there was a recombination at the B locus so that this patient shared three of four HLA antigens with his proband sibling. There were six putative homozygotes in three families who were HLA identical to a proband with a normal serum ferritin and transferrin saturation as previously described [5]. There was one putative heterozygote (son of a proband) who was initially classified as a heterozygote by HLA typing, but because of a significantly elevated ferritin and transferrin saturation (ferritin 648 μg/liter, transferrin saturation 57%) he underwent liver biopsy. Liver biopsy showed marked parenchymal iron overload, with a hepatic iron concentration of 110 μmol/g and hepatic iron index of 3.05. He underwent 30 weekly venesections, after which his serum ferritin had decreased to 152 μg/liter. Three years later, without venesections, his serum ferritin had risen to 680 μg/liter and transferrin saturation to 79%, and venesections were restarted. This case illustrates the value of a percutaneous liver biopsy with hepatic iron determination in a putative heterozygote. It is likely that the parents of this man were a homozygote married to a heterozygote [16].

DISCUSSION

Hemochromatosis is a common genetic disease among whites, with an autosomal recessive inheritance. The prevalence of the heterozygous state has been estimated to be as high as 1 in 10 members of the general population in studies from Australia, Utah, France, Sweden, and Canada [3]. Most homozygotes will have phenotypic expression of the disease, with iron overload as assessed by biochemical and histological iron studies and, in the late stages of the disease, clinical symptoms related to end-organ damage. Previous studies have demonstrated evidence of iron overload in patients who are putative heterozygotes for the disease, and the occasional homozygote may be misclassified as a heterozygote because of a homozygous-heterozygous mating in the parents or a genetic recombination [6–8,16,17]. The partial expression of an autosomal recessive defect in patients who are heterozygotes has been suggested for other autosomal recessive liver diseases such as α_1-antitrypsin deficiency and Wilson's disease [18,19].

In this study, heterozygotes had a significantly greater mean serum ferritin and transferrin saturation than normal control patients, although in most cases it was still within the normal range. The use of putative normal patients from within hemochromatosis families is preferable to using controls from the general population, which would include a significant number of undetected heterozygotes. Biochemical evidence of iron overload in ~10% of our patients was less common than in previous studies. Simon et al. [8] described an elevated serum ferritin or serum iron in 53 of 247 heterozygotes (21.5%) using an upper limit for serum ferritin of 180 μg/liter in women and 300 μg/liter in men. Cartwright et al. [7] described a transferrin saturation >50% in 45 of 145 heterozygotes (31%) and no clinical symptoms in any of the heterozygotes. Milman [9] described an elevation in transferrin saturation (>50%) in 12% of heterozygotes (n = 84). Bassett et al. [6] found biochemical abnormalities in serum ferritin and transferrin saturation in ~25% in a survey of 98 heterozygotes. In their study the normal range for serum ferritin (<150 μg/liter females, <200 μg/liter males) and transferrin saturation were lower (<50%), and 44 heterozygotes followed for a mean of 6.7 years did not develop any clinical evidence of hemochromatosis [6]. If this range had been applied to our patient cohort, the percentage of heterozygotes with biochemical abnormalities would have increased to 14–21%. The mean hepatic iron concentration of 54 μmol/g is similar to the mean of 55 μmol/g reported for ten patients by Bassett et al. [6] and is much less than the range seen in homozygotes [10–13,17]. This also is likely an overestimation of the hepatic iron stores of the entire heterozygote cohort, because only selected patients with biochemical abnormalities underwent liver biopsy.

The mechanism for the mild iron overload seen in a minority of heterozygotes is as elusive as the fundamental pathophysiological defect in hemochromatosis. Homozygotes usually have an increased intestinal absorption of iron relative to body iron stores [20–22]. Recently a high-affinity iron binding protein has been demonstrated on intestinal and hepatic membranes in hemochromatosis homozygotes [23], but the expression of this protein in heterozygotes has not been described. The role of this protein in the pathogenesis of hemochromatosis will require further study. We have previously studied intestinal iron absorption in 19 of the heterozygotes in this study and could not demonstrate a hyperabsorption of intestinal iron relative to body iron stores, although a small increase in intestinal iron absorption would be difficult to demonstrate given the variability in this methodology [21].

Previously, authors have suggested the need for follow-up of heterozygotes [3] because of the possibility of a genetic recombination or an unsuspected homozygous-heterozygous mating in the parents. The incidence of genetic recombination has been estimated to be <1% [24]. In the present study, there were no known genetic recombinations that resulted in a homozygote being misclassified as a heterozygote. In one case, a homozygote was misclassified as a heterozygote probably as a result of a homozygous-heterozygous mating between his parents, but further investigations (liver biopsy, hepatic iron index) led to him being classified as a homozygote, and venesection therapy was initiated. If there are abnormalities in the serum ferritin and transferrin saturation at the time of initial assessment that appear to be consistent with the levels seen in homozygotes [17], a percutaneous liver biopsy with hepatic iron concentration should be performed. Hepatic iron concentration in heterozygotes is much less than in homozygotes of a comparable age. The hepatic iron index has been demonstrated in several studies to be useful in distinguishing between homozygotes and heterozygotes [11,12]. A morphological iron index has also been shown to be useful in the differentiation of heterozygotes from homozygotes [25].

Heterozygotes should be reassured that they are not at risk of developing the clinical manifestations of hemochromatosis. However, because of the high prevalence of heterozygotes among the general population, children of heterozygotes within known hemochromatosis families should be screened as young adults for the disease with a serum ferritin and transferrin saturation. Heterozygotes were not treated with venesections, although, if further studies confirm a preliminary report suggesting an association between serum ferritin and coronary artery disease, this may require reassessment [26].

ACKNOWLEDGMENTS

The author acknowledges the advice and assistance of Dr. L.S. Valberg and A.E. Kertesz and is a Career Scientist of the Ministry of Health of Ontario.

REFERENCES

1. Simon M, Bourel M, Genetet B, et al: Idiopathic hemochromatosis: Demonstration of recessive transmission and early detection by family HLA typing. N Engl J Med 297:1017–1021, 1977.
2. Dadone MM, Kushner JP, Edwards CQ, et al: Hereditary hemochromatosis; analysis of laboratory expression of the disease by genotype in 18 pedigrees. Am J Clin Pathol 78:196–207, 1982.
3. Adams PC, Halliday JW, Powell LW: Early diagnosis and screening for hemochromatosis. Adv Intern Med 34:111–126, 1989.
4. Powell LW, Summers KM, Board PG, et al: Expression of hemochromatosis in homozygous subjects. Implications for early diagnosis and prevention. Gastroenterology 98:1625–1632, 1990.
5. Adams PC, Kertesz AE: Human leucocyte antigen typing of siblings in hereditary hemochromatosis: A cost approach. Hepatology 15:263–268, 1992.
6. Bassett ML, Halliday JW, Powell LW: HLA typing in idiopathic hemochromatosis: distinction between homozygotes and heterozygotes with biochemical expression. Hepatology 1:120–126, 1981.
7. Cartwright GE, Edwards CQ, Kravitz K, et al: Hereditary hemochromatosis. Phenotypic expression of the disease. N Engl J Med 301:175–179, 1979.
8. Simon M, Fauchet R, Hespel JP, et al: Idiopathic hemochromatosis: A study of biochemical expression in 247 heterozygous members of 63 families. Evidence for a single major HLA-linked gene. Gastroenterology 78:703–708, 1980.
9. Milman N: Iron status markers in hereditary haemochromatosis: distinction between individuals being homozygous and heterozygous for the haemochromatosis allele. Eur J Haematol 47:292–298, 1991.
10. Bassett ML, Halliday JW, Powell LW: Value of hepatic iron measurements in early hemochromatosis and determination of the critical iron level associated with fibrosis. Hepatology 6:24–29, 1986.
11. Summers K, Halliday JW, Powell LW: Identification of homozygous hemochromatosis subjects by measurement of hepatic iron index. Hepatology 12:20–25, 1990.
12. Adams PC: Hepatic iron in hemochromatosis. Dig Dis Sci 35:690–692, 1990.
13. Bonkovsky H, Slaker DP, Billes E, et al: Usefulness and limitations of laboratory and hepatic imaging studies in iron storage disease. Gastroenterology 99:1079–1091, 1990.
14. Valberg LS, Sorbie J, Ludwig J, et al: Serum ferritin and the iron status of Canadians. Can Med Assoc J 114:417–421, 1976.
15. Terasaki P, Bernoco D, Park M, et al: Microdroplet testing for HLA A, B, C and D antigens. Am J Clin Pathol 69:103–120, 1978.
16. Bassett ML, Doran TJ, Halliday JW, et al: Idiopathic hemochromatosis: demonstration of homozygous-heterozygous mating by HLA-typing in families. Hum Genet 60:352–356, 1982.
17. Adams PC, Kertesz AE, Valberg LS: Clinical presentation of hemochromatosis: A changing scene. Am J Med 90:445–449, 1991.
18. Hodges J, Millward-Sadler G, Barbatis C, et al: Heterozygous MZ Alpha-1-antitrypsin deficiency in adults with chronic active hepatitis and cryptogenic cirrhosis. N Engl J Med 304:557–560, 1981.
19. Scheinberg IH, Sternlieb I: Wilson's disease. In Smith LH (ed): "Major Problems in Internal Medicine, Vol XXIII." Philadelphia: W.B. Saunders, 1984, p 13.
20. Adams PC, Frei JV, Bradley C, et al: Hepatic iron and iron absorption in hemochromatosis. Clin Invest Med 13:256–259, 1990.
21. Borwein ST, Ghent CN, Flanagan PR, et al: Genetic and phenotypic expression of hemochromatosis in Canadians. Clin Invest Med 6:171–179, 1983.
22. Valberg LS, Lloyd DA, Ghent CN, et al: Clinical and biochemical expression of the genetic abnormality in idiopathic hemochromatosis. Gastroenterology 79:884–892, 1980.
23. Stremmel W, Teichmann R, Arweiler D, et al: In primary hemochromatosis the membrane iron binding protein is highly enriched in duodenum and liver. Gastroenterology 100:A254, 1991.
24. Lalouel J, Jorde L: Idiopathic hemchromatosis: Significance and implications of linkage to HLA. Ann NY Acad Sci 526:34–46, 1988.
25. Deugnier Y, Halliday JW, Summers KM, et al: Differentiation between heterozygotes and homozygotes in genetic hemochromatosis by means of a morphological iron index: A study of 192 cases. Hepatology 17:30–34, 1993.
26. Salonen JT, Nyyssonen K, Korpela H, et al: High stored iron levels are associated with excess risk of myocardial infarction in eastern Finnish men. Circulation 86:803–811, 1992.

American Journal of Hematology 45:150–155 (1994)

CD21 Antigen in T-Lineage Neoplastic Lymphoid Cells: Characteristic Expression at Thymic Stage

Eiji Tatsumi, Noriko Yoneda, Seiji Kawano, and Nobuo Yamaguchi
Department of Laboratory Medicine, Kobe University School of Medicine, Kobe, Japan

The expression of CD21 antigen, a receptor for the C3d fragment of complement and Epstein-Barr virus (EBV), was investigated in a total of 85 cases of neoplastic lymphoid cells including 39 cases of T-lineage acute lymphoblastic leukemia (ALL)/lymphoblastic lymphoma (LBL), although CD21 antigen is usually regarded as a pan-B antigen. The CD21 antigen was expressed by one of the eight cases of neoplastic lymphoid cells expressing the CD7 antigen as a sole pan-T antigen, by three of the 20 cases of pro- or early thymic stage (CD7+ CD5+ CD2−, CD7+ CD5− CD2+, or CD7+ CD5+ CD2+), and ten of 11 cases of thymic stage (CD3± CD4+ CD8+), but not by one case of late thymic stage (CD3+ CD4+ CD8−) T-ALL/LBL cells. The CD21 antigen was not expressed by any of the 11 cases of adult T-cell leukemia (ATL) or two cases of chronic T-lineage leukemia. At most 4% of the normal thymocytes obtained from seven infants or children expressed the CD21 antigen. While only a very limited population of normal thymocytes expresses CD21 antigen, T-ALL/LBL cells at the thymic stage characteristically express CD21 antigen in contrast to pro- or early thymic ALL/LBL or peripheral-stage neoplastic T cells. The estimation of the expression of CD21 antigen is useful for delineating stages of differentiation in T-ALL/LBL. Furthermore, these observation are notable, considering the possibility that the reported EBV-carrying T-cell lymphomas result from the penetration of EBV into EBV-negative neoplastic T cells.

Key words: CD21 antigen, Epstein-Barr virus, T-lineage neoplasms, thymic stage

INTRODUCTION

The receptor for Epstein-Barr virus (EBV-R) was formerly studied by virus adsorption onto the cell surface [1]. While the distribution of EBV-R was, then, regarded to be confined to B-lineage (B) cells, a T-lineage acute lymphoblastic leukemia (T-ALL) cell line, MOLT4, was found to express EBV-R by Menezes et al. [2]. Tatsumi et al. [3] also showed that MOLT4 was not exceptional by detecting EBV-R on a few other T-ALL cell lines with fluorescein isothiocyanate (FITC)-conjugated EBV. The EBV-R expressed by the T-ALL cell lines apparently did not mediate EBV penetration, suggesting that the receptor was functionally inert. On the other hand, the physical association between the receptor for C3d component of complement (C3d-R) and EBV-R was first found by Klein and colleagues [4,5]. Thereafter, some monoclonal antibodies that had been developed for detecting B-lineage-specific antigen turned out to bind specifically with the C3d-R (CD21 antigen [6–9]. Studies using mainly these monoclonal antibodies confirmed that the C3d-R/CD21 antigen is an EBV-R. However, the distribution of the expression of CD21 antigen has not been fully determined in human non-B-lymphoid neoplasms. In addition to this situation, recent observations indicating that some non-B-lymphoid neoplasms can carry EBV [10–13], prompted us to estimate the distribution of the CD21 antigen in T-lymphoid neoplastic cells. The findings showed that T-ALL/LBL at the thymic stage characteristically express the CD21 antigen, while the implications of the expression of CD21 antigen in this stage of human T-cell differentiation remain unknown.

MATERIALS AND METHODS

Samples and Patients

All neoplastic cells were negative for cytochemical myeloperoxidase (MPO). Cases studied included eight

Received for publication March 4, 1993; accepted August 18, 1993.

Address reprint requests to Eiji Tatsumi, MD, Department of Laboratory Medicine, Kobe University School of Medicine, Kusunoki-Cho, Chuo-Ku, Kobe, 650 Japan.

TABLE I. Antigen Expression (%) and TdT in CD7+ CD5− CD2− Cases*

Case	Age/sex[a]	CD21[b]	CD7	CD5	CD2	CD10	CD11b	CD13	CD33	HLA-DR	CD34	TdT
1	54/M PB	1 (1)	98	2	2	1	3	3 (3, 6)[d]	66	80	48	−
2	42/M PB	1 (0)	63	1	1	0	9	97	77	48	89	−
3	40/F PB	1 (0)	60	1	0	1	4	2 (1, 6)	12	4	NT[e]	−
4	53/M LN	42 (38)	94	18[c]	3	28	3	8 (6, 58)	77	21	NT	+
5	30/M PB	2	83	3	4	1	2	6 (18, 28)	4	78	NT	NT
6	35/M PB	1	79	8	9	1	4	2 (1, 1)	38	11	58	NT
7	15/F PB	1	94	1	2	0	4	72 (58, 82)	19	43	20	+
8	16/M PB	2	94	3	2	1	91	19 (28, 63)	93	1	95	NT

*In all cases, the positive percentages for CD1, CD3, CD4, or CD8 were below 3% except for case 4.
[a]Source of material: PB, peripheral blood; LN, lymph node.
[b]Only case 4 is positive for CD21 antigen among the CD7+ CD5+ CD2− group. The percentage in parentheses is for the B2 antibody.
[c]In case 4, CD1+ cells were 1%; CD3+, 12%; CD4+, 7%; and CD8+, 4%. Therefore, the 18% for CD5 was interpreted to be negative.
[d]Expression (%) of CD13 antigen of blasts cultured for 2 days in the absence and presence of TPA 2 (ng/ml) is shown in parentheses.
[e]NT, not tested.

TABLE II. Antigen Expression (%) and TdT in CD7+ CD5+ CD2−/CD7+ CD5− CD2+ T-ALL/LBL Cases*

Case	Age/sex[a]	CD21[b]	CD7	CD5	CD2	CD10	CD11b	CD13	CD33	DR	CD34	TdT
9	32/M PE	2 (1)	90	73	15	6	47	8 (10, 42)[c]	10	13	NT[d]	−
10	14/M BM	38 (35)	90	69	7	5	12	10 (35, 56)	12	11	NT	+
11	10/F PB	2 (1)	93	81	10	1	18	2 (2, 23)	17	33	NT	+
12	36/M PB	1	98	27	5	0	1	6 (45, 61)	4	1	9	−
13	57/M LN	55 (48)	93	30	2	0	77	21 (55, 73)	61	8	1	+
14	27/F BM	1	95	19	1	0	89	14 (30, 74)	70	1	84	+
15	30/M BM	1	94	42	1	0	2	2	21	1	6	−
16	35/M PE	3	87	4	67	3	13	16 (21, 39)	40	1	NT	−

*In all cases, the positive percentages for CD1, CD3, CD4, or CD8 were below 3%. Only case 16 is CD7+ CD5− CD2+.
[a]Source of material: PB, peripheral blood; PE, pleural effusion; BM, bone marrow; LN, lymph node.
[b]Cases 10 and 13 were positive. The percentage in parentheses is for the B2 antibody.
[c]Expression (%) of CD13 antigen of blasts cultured for 2 days in the absence and presence of TPA (2 ng/ml) is shown in parentheses.
[d]NT, not tested.

TABLE III. Antigen Expression (%) and TdT in CD7+ CD5+ CD2+ T-ALL/LBL Cases*

Case	Age/sex[a]	CD21[b]	CD7	CD5	CD2	CD10	CD11b	CD13	CD33	DR	CD34	TdT
17	21/F PB	1 (1)	96	85	80	1	NT[c]	12 (15, 61)[d]	NT	2	48	+
18	17/M PB	2 (1)	96	88	90	1	23	3 (21, 40)	1	1	NT	+
19	14/M PB	1 (1)	91	60	56	1	52	15 (22, 50)	25	8	38	+
20	15/F LN	3	96	75	23	3	14	2 (9, 8)	4	22	42	+
21	18/F PB	3	38	73	23	1	21	4 (11, 16)	22	3	NT	−
22	75/M PB	46 (43)	96	19	35	1	44	21 (18, 71)	33	46	19	+

*In all cases, the positive percentages for CD1, CD3, CD4, or CD8 were below 3%.
[a]Source of material: PB, peripheral blood; LN, lymph node.
[b]Only case 21 was positive for CD21 antigen in this group. The percentage in parentheses is for the B2 antibody.
[c]NT, not tested.
[d]Expression (%) of CD13 antigen of blasts cultured for 2 days in the absence and presence of TPA (2 ng/ml) is shown in parentheses.

cases of neoplastic lymphoid (negative for cytochemical myeloperoxidase) cells expressing the CD7 antigen as the sole pan-T antigen, 26 cases of T-ALL/LBL, two cases of chronic T-lineage leukemia, and 11 cases of adult T-cell leukemia (ATL). In addition to these T-lineage neoplastic cases, 22 cases of pre-B ALL negative for cell-surface Ig (S-Ig), two cases of B-cell (S-Ig$^+$) ALL, four cases of CLL, and six cases of B-cell lymphoma were investigated.

The diagnosis of ATL was made from the clinical features, including the appearance of characteristic leukemia cells with lobulated nucleus, positive anti-HTLV-1 antibody, and derivation from the southern part of Japan [14]. Neoplastic lymphoid cells were derived from the peripheral blood, bone marrow, lymph nodes, or pleural effusion. The neoplastic cells were isolated by discontinuous gradient centrifugation [15] from the peripheral blood or from pleural effusion. Lymph nodes were

TABLE IV. Antigen Expression (%) and TdT in Thymic (CD3± CD4+ CD8+) and Late Thymic (CD3+ CD4+ CD8−) T-ALL/LBL Cases*

Case	Age/sex[a]	CD21[b]	CD1	CD3	CD4	CD8	CD7	CD5	CD2	CD10	TdT
23	12/F PB	58 (53)	60	3	61	91	89	89	84	13	+
24	16/M PB	51 (46)	45	6	67	70	75	51	78	3	+
25	9/M BM	80 (79)	71	2	89	75	96	29	96	17	+
26	28/M PB	84	85	6	50	81	88	85	93	0	+
27	3/M PB	44	33	10	76	57	82	61	80	11	+
28	14/M PB	3	5	3	41	63	23	84	93	1	−
29	33/M PE	58 (53)	8	64	78	79	61	86	75	3	+
30	16/M PB	54 (50)	54	88	80	49	84	36	88	7	+
31	9/M PB	33 (31)	17	58	25	50	76	64	83	0	+
32	15/M PE	98	99	82	96	99	91	76	93	39	+
33	9/M PE	30	83	82	77	82	69	86	54	2	+
34*	28/M PB	2	4	56	80	5	76	75	9	72	+

*In all cases, the blasts were negative (below 5%) for CD11b, CD13, CD33, or HLA-DR antigen. CD13 antigen was not induced in vitro above 8%. Cases 29–33 were positive for TCR-1, but negative for TCRδ 1. Case 34 was negative for TCR-1 but positive for TCRδ 1. Only case 34 (CD2− CD3+ CD4+ CD8−) is late thymic.
[a]Source of material: PB, peripheral blood; PE, pleural effusion; BM, bone marrow.
[b]Cases 28 and 34 were negative for CD21 antigen in this group. The percentage in parentheses is for the B2 antibody.

TABLE V. Antigen Expression (%) in ATL and Chronic T-Lineage Leukemia*

Case	Age/sex[a]	CD21[b]	CD3	CD4	CD8	CD2	CD5	CD7	CD25	CD28	DR
35	54/M PB	3 (1)	86	84	2	85	91	7	61	81	3
36	57/M PB	4 (2)	57	65	23	46	62	36	30	48	16
37	42/F PB	4 (1)	78	85	2	75	83	4	10	81	5
38	59/M PB	3 (1)	58	75	2	71	88	1	42	81	23
39	48/F PB	3	96	95	2	98	96	4	84	84	6
40	53/M PB	4	6	97	2	12	92	4	46	86	23
41	67/F PB	3	90	94	2	95	96	3	69	92	6
42	56/M PB	4	50	87	3	92	91	8	17	85	6
43	83/F PB	4	96	97	4	2	96	7	82	94	93
44	72/M LN	6	89	99	4	1	97	17	79	95	4
45	54/F PB	4	89	90	3	90	72	10	5	NT[c]	6
46	65/M PB	3	94	92	2	63	67	55	3	68	3
47	81/M PB	1	1	92	1	98	99	88	10	85	1

*In all cases, the blasts were negative (below 4%) for CD10, CD11b, CD19, CD20, CD13, or CD33. ATL, cases 35–45; chronic T-lineage leukemia, cases 46 and 47.
[a]Source of material: PB, peripheral blood; LN, lymph node.
[b]No case was positive for CD21 antigen. The percentage in parentheses is for the B2 antibody.
[c]NT, not tested.

minced, and a free cell suspension was made after sedimentation of cell debris or aggregates. Cell separation was performed within 10 hr after venipuncture, bone marrow tap, or pleural tap.

Cell Surface Antigen Analysis

Cell-surface immunofluorescence analysis for cell-surface antigen was performed using a total of 18 monoclonal antibodies [16]. NUT2 (CD1b), NUT-ER (CD2), NUT3 (CD3), NUTH/I (CD4), NUT-PAN (CD5), NUT-S/C (CD8), NU-B2 (CD20), MCS-2 (CD13), and NU-IA (HLA-DR) were purchased from Nichirei (Tokyo, Japan); BA-1 (CD24) was from Boeringer Manheim (Manheim, Germany); Leu9 (CD7), Leu12 (CD19), and CR2 (CD21) were from Becton-Dickinson (Mountainview,

TABLE VI. Expression of CD21 Antigen in T-Lineage Neoplastic Cells

Disease type	No. cases analyzed
Undifferentiated[a] CD7+ CD5− CD2−	1/8
T-ALL/LBL CD7+ CD5+ CD2−	2/7
T-ALL/LBL CD7+ CD5− CD2+	0/1
T-ALL/LBL CD7+ CD5+ CD2+	1/6
T-ALL/LBL CD3± CD4+ CD8+	8/10
T-ALL/LBL CD3+ CD4+ CD8−	0/1
Adult T-cell leukemia	0/11
T-lineage chronic leukemia	0/2

[a]Cases that express CD7 antigen as a sole pan-T antigen.

CA); and Mol (CD11b), B2 (CD21), and My9 (CD33) were from Coulter (Hialeah, FL). TAC (CD25) antibody was a generous gift from Dr. T. Uchiyama (Virus Research Institute, Kyoto University). Fluorescein isothiocyanate (FITC)-conjugated Fab fragment of goat antimouse IgG and IgM (Dako, Munksgard, Denmark) were used for indirect immunofluorescence. To block Fc receptors, heat-aggregated (56°C, 30 min) human IgG (50 mg/ml) (Venilon; Fujisawa, Osaka, Japan) was added to each specimen 10 min prior to each incubation, which was for 30 min at 4°C.

The FITC-conjugated Fab fragment of goat antihuman IgG, IgM, IgA, κ, λ, or human immunoglobulins (Tago, Burlingame, CA) was used for detecting S-Ig. In the detection of cell-surface immunoglobulin, heat-aggregated (56°C, 30 min) calf γ-globulin was added 10 min prior to each incubation to block Fc receptors. The stained cells were assayed with an Epics-C flow cytometer (Coulter).

Short-Term In Vitro Culture for Induction of CD13 Antigen Expression

The CD13 antigen has previously been reported to be induced frequently in vitro in immature T-lineage neoplastic cells [17]. The induction was examined in the T-lymphoid cases tested here. Cells were suspended in RPMI1640 supplemented with 10% fetal calf serum (FCS; Hi-Clone, Logan, UT) at a cell concentration of 2×10^6/ml in a round-bottom tube (2058; Falcon, Oxnard, CA), and cultured in both the absence and the presence of 12-O-tetradecanoyl phorbol-13-acetate (TPA; 2.0 ng/ml; Sigma, St. Louis, MO) in a CO_2 incubator (Tabai, Tokyo, Japan) in an atmosphere of 95% air and 5% CO_2 at 100% humidity for 24 hr. Harvested cells were tested for the expression of CD13 antigen.

Terminal Deoxynucleotidyl Transferase (TdT)

Terminal deoxynucleotidyl transferase (TdT) was tested by indirect immunofluorescence with a fixed smear using rabbit anti-TdT antibody (Bethesda Research Laboratory, Bethesda, MD).

RESULTS

Table I shows the expression of CD21 antigen in the group of blasts expressing the CD7 antigen as the sole pan-T antigen. Only one of eight cases expressed the CD21 antigen. Table II shows the results of seven cases of CD7+ CD5+ CD2− and one CD7+ CD5− CD2+ immature T-ALL/LBL. Two of the eight cases were positive for the CD21 antigen. One of the six CD7+ CD5+ CD2+ CD3− CD4− CD8− cases expressed the CD21 antigen, as shown in Table III. In contrast to these immature T-lineage neoplastic cells at pro- or early thymic stage [18], nine of the ten cases of thymic (CD3± CD4+ CD8+) stage [18] T-ALL/LBL cells expressed the CD21 antigen (Table IV). However, one case of late thymic (CD3+ CD4+ CD8−) stage [18] T-ALL/LBL cells did not.

TABLE VII. Antigen Expression (%) of Thymus Cells

Age[a]/sex	CD21[b]	CD1	CD2	CD3	CD4	CD5	CD7	CD8
4m/M	0 (1)	76	84	22	55	32	2	60
1y/M	2 (1)	89	98	31	71	NT	45	90
1y9m/M	2 (1)	88	99	41	93	97	54	92
1y11m/M	1	90	98	23	49	65	23	91
2y/F	1	67	94	33	80	64	48	74
4y/M	0	92	95	20	83	40	5	91
6y/M	4	79	99	22	89	73	41	91

[a]Y, years; M, months.
[b]The percentages in parentheses are for the B2 antibody.

In most of the group expressing the CD7 antigen as the sole pan-T antigen or pro- or early thymic stage (CD7+ CD5+ CD2−, CD7+ CD5− CD2−, CD7+ CD5+ CD2+, or CD3− CD4− CD8−) neoplastic T cells, the fresh blasts expressed the CD13 antigen or were induced to express it in the presence of TPA, as previously reported [17].

Eleven cases of ATL were investigated for the expression of CD21 antigen as well as other antigens, as shown in Table V. None of the ATL cases was positive for the CD21 antigen. The CD21 antigen was also negative in two chronic T-lineage leukemia cases.

Table VI shows the overall results of CD21 antigen expression in the CD7+ CD5− CD2− and T-lineage neoplasms. Obviously, the T-ALL/LBL cells at the thymic stage characteristically express the CD21 antigen. Normal thymus cells were interpreted to express it to a very limited degree or to be negative for CD21 antigen, as shown in Table VII.

Table VIII shows the results for CD21 antigen expression in various types of B-lineage neoplastic cells. Only three of the 26 pre-B (negative for S-Ig) cases expressed the CD21 antigen. By contrast, the CD21 antigen was expressed by the neoplastic cells from all CLL and B-lymphoma cases. Evidently, the CD21 antigen is expressed by mature S-Ig-positive neoplastic cells in the B lineage, but mostly not in the (S-Ig-negative) pre-B ALL stage. The findings obtained with B2 antibody were in accordance with those obtained with CR2 antibody in the cases tested.

DISCUSSION

The findings for the CD7+ CD5− CD2− and T-ALL/LBL cases showed that the CD21 antigen is characteristically expressed by the T-ALL/LBL cells at the thymic stage (Tables I–IV, VI), but only very rarely by the CD7+ CD5− CD2− neoplastic lymphoid cells (Table I) or pro- or early thymic (CD7+ CD5+ CD2−, CD7+ CD5− CD2+, CD7+ CD5+ CD2+, or CD3− CD4−

TABLE VIII. Expression of CD21 Antigen B-Lineage Neoplastic Cells

	CD21[a]	CD19	CD10	CD20	CD24	CD5	SIg
Pre-B ALL	0/3	+	−	−	+	−	−
Pre-B ALL	2/21 (9%, 14%)	+	+	−	+	−	−
Pre-B ALL	1/2 (18%)	+	+	+	+	−	−
B ALL[b]	1/2 (14%)	+	±[c]	+	+	−	+
CLL[b]	4/4 (38–68%)	+	−	+	+	+	+
B lymphoma[b]	6/6 (32–62%)	+	−	+	+	−	+

[a]Case number, positive/total; percentages for positive blasts are shown in parentheses.
[b]SIg, B ALL, IgMκ and IgMκ; CLL, IgMκ, IgMκ, IgMκ, and IgMλ; B lymphoma, IgMκ, IgMκ, IgGκ, and IgGλ.
[c]One case was positive, but the other negative.

CD8−) neoplastic T-lineage cells (Tables II, III). None of the 13 cases of peripheral type neoplastic T cells, including 11 cases of ATL, expressed the CD21 antigen (Table V). Therefore, the CD21 antigen can be a marker delineating a stage of T-lymphoid differentiation. CD21 antigen has usually been regarded as a mature stage of pan-B antigen [7]. This was also confirmed by the present findings (Table VIII), showing that the CD21 antigen was expressed in only three of the 26 cases of pre-B ALL cells lacking the S-Ig by definition but was expressed by the S-Ig-positive leukemia/lymphoma B cells. Thus, if CD21 antigen is expressed at a high percentage by a given case of ALL without S-Ig, the ALL cells are most likely to be T-ALL at the thymic stage. This seems to be paradoxical, since the CD21 antigen is generally regarded as a pan-B antigen.

Only a very small population was found to express the CD21 antigen in the thymus cells, as shown in Table VII. However, Tsuokas et al. [19] reported a slightly higher percentage (4–28%) for CD21+ cells in normal thymus cells. The reason why thymic stage T-ALL/LBL cells usually express CD21 antigen despite the very low frequency of CD21+ normal thymocytes remains unknown. The function carried out by the CD21 molecule in the thymus is also a subject for further research.

Several T lymphomas [20–22] have recently been reported to carry the EBV DNA subsequent to the initially reported forms of EBV-carrying non-B lymphoproliferative disorders [10–13]. While children are very often afflicted, the cell-surface antigen profile of these reported T-lymphoma cells is a peripheral/activated type, such as the phenotype of CD3+ CD4+ CD8− or CD3+ CD4− CD8+ and the expression of HLA-DR antigen. These EBV-positive neoplasms may develop in a de novo manner as a result of EBV infection, on the one hand. However, on the other hand, EBV may have infected ready-made T-ALL/LBL, resulting in a peripheral/activated type. The present findings, indicating that T-ALL/LBL cells at the thymic stage express the CD21 antigen, cannot exclude such a possibility. Watry et al. [23] reported that some normal thymocytes could be infected with EBV. It seems necessary to repeat testing the infectivity in T-ALL/LBL cells by EBV under more sophisticated experimental conditions.

In our study, the number of cases investigated at the non-ATL peripheral stage of neoplastic T cells was limited. If a larger number of cases were investigated, some peripheral stage of neoplastic T cells may be found to express the CD21 antigen, and it may be a more conceivable ready-made target neoplasm that can be infected by EBV. While all fresh ATL cells lacked the CD21 antigen in our study, Koizumi et al. [24] reported that the HTLV-1-positive cell line MT2, which is of nonneoplastic origin, had the CD21 antigen and was infected by EBV.

The reported EBV-positive T-cell neoplasms [10,20–22] have not been investigated regarding the expression or absence of the CD21 antigen. As examples of EBV-positive non-B neoplastic lymphoid cells, both the fresh natural killer (NK)-type large granular lymphocytes (LGL), [12] and the NK cell line of neoplastic origin, YT [25], are known to be negative for the CD21 antigen. The absence of the CD21 antigen in these neoplastic NK cells is very unexpected, since all EBV-positive neoplastic or nonneoplastic B cells have the CD21 antigen. This is based on the fact that a high percentage of nonproducer-type EBV-positive B cells express CD21, but only a low percentage of producer-type EBV-positive B cells express it [3]. Some non-B or NK lymphoid cells may have a different type of EBV-R, undetectable with the CD21 antibody. This possibility seems to require further study in addition to the questions regarding the expression of CD21 antigen by T-ALL/LBL cells.

Not much attention has been paid to the expression of CD21 antigen by fresh T-ALL/LBL cells. The present study is the first to investigate a sufficient number of cases to estimate the distribution of CD21 antigen in T-lineage neoplastic cells. The present findings suggest the role of CD21 antigen in T-cell differentiation at the thymic stage and the possibility of EBV infection of T-ALL/LBL cells at the thymic stage. The discrepancy between normal thymocytes and thymic-stage T-ALL/LBL regarding the frequency of CD21+ cells also awaits further study.

REFERENCES

1. Jondal M, Klein G: Surface markers on human B and T lymphocytes. J Exp Med 138:1365, 1973.
2. Menezes J, Siegneurin JM, Patel P, Bourkas A, Lenoir G: Presence of Epstein-Barr virus receptors, but absence of virus penetration in cells of an Epstein-Barr virus genome-negative human lymphoblastoid T line (Molt 4). J Virol 22:816, 1977.
3. Tatsumi E, Harada S, Bechtoid T, Davis J, Volsky D, Lipscomb H, Purtilo DT: Catalogue of hematopoietic cell line with or without Epstein-Barr virus receptor expression. Leukemia Res 9:231, 1985.
4. Jondal M, Klein G, Oldstone M, Bokish V, Yefenof E: Surface markers on human T and B lymphocytes. VII. Association between complement and Epstein-Barr virus receptors on human lymphoid cells. Scand J Immunol 5:401, 1976.
5. Klein G, Yefenof E, Falk K, Westman A: Relationship between Epstein-Barr virus (EBV)-production and the loss of the EBV receptor/complement receptor complex in a series of sublines derived from the same original Burkitt's lymphoma. Int J Cancer 21:552, 1978.
6. Fingeroth JD, Weis JJ, Tedder TF, Strominger JL, Biro PA, Fearon DT: Epstein-Barr virus receptor of human B lymphocytes is the C3d receptor CR2. Proc Natl Acad Sci 81:4510, 1984.
7. Tedder TF, Clement LT, Cooper MD: Expression of C3d receptors during human B cell differentiation: Immunofluorescence analysis with the HB-5 monoclonal antibody. J Immunol 133:678, 1984.
8. Nemerow GR, McNaughton, Cooper NR: Binding of monoclonal antibody to the Epstein-Barr virus (EBV) CR2 receptor induces activation and differentiation of human B lymphocytes. J Immunol 135: 3068, 1985.
9. Nemerow GR, Wolfert R, McNaughton ME, Cooper NR: Identification and characterization of the Epstein-Barr virus receptor on human B lymphocytes and its relationship to the C3d complement receptor (CR2). J Virol 55:347, 1985.
10. JonesJF, Shurin S, Abramowsky C, Tubbs RR, Sciotto CG, Wahl R, Sands J, Gottman D, Katz BZ, Sklar J: T-cell lymphomas containing Epstein-Barr viral DNA in patients with chronic Epstein-Barr virus infections. N Engl J Med 318:733, 1988.
11. Kikuta H, Taguchi Y, Tomizawa K, Kojima K, Kawamura N, Ishizaka A, Sakiyama Y, Matsumoto S, Imai S, Kinoshita T, Koizumi S, Osato T, Kobayashi I, Hamada I, Hirai K: Epstein-Barr virus genome-positive T lymphocytes in a boy with chronic active EBV infection associated with Kawasaki-like disease. Nature 333:455, 1988.
12. Kawa-Ha K, Ishihara S, Ninomiya T, Yumura-Yagi K, Hara J, Murayama F, Tawa A, Hirai K: CD3-negative lymphoproliferative disease of granular lymphocytes containing Epstein-Barr viral DNA. J Clin Invest 84:51, 1989.
13. Yoneda N, Tatsumi E, Teshigawara K, Kawanishi M, Yamaguchi N: Detection of Epstein-Barr virus (EBV) genome in benign polyclonal T cells of a young male patient. Blood 76:172, 1990.
14. Uchiyama T, Yodoi J, Sagawa K, Takatsuki K, Uchino H: Adult T-cell Leukemia: Clinical hematologic features of 16 cases. Blood 50:481, 1977.
15. Böym A: Separation of leucocytes from blood and bone marrow. Scand J Clin Invest 21(Suppl 97):77, 1968.
16. McMichael AJ (ed): "Leucocyte Typing III, White Cell Differentiation Antigens." Oxford: Oxford University Press, 1987.
17. Arita Y, Kita K, Nasu K, Doi S, Fukuhara S, Nishikori M, Miwa H, Tatsumi E, Nosaka T, Hatanaka M, Uchino H: Frequent expression of myeloid antigen (CD13) on immature T cells in culture. Acta Hematol Jpn 53:21, 1990.
18. Reinhertz EL, Kung PC, Goldstein G, Levery RH, Schlossman SF: Discrete stages of human intrathymic differentiation: Analysis of normal thymocytes and leukemic lymphoblasts of T-cell lineage. Proc Natl Acad Sci USA 77:1588, 1980.
19. Tsoukas CD, Lambris JD: Expression of CR2/EBV receptors on human thymocytes detected by monoclonal antibodies. Eur J Immunol 18:1299, 1988.
20. Su I-J, Hsie H-C, Lin K-H, Uen W-C, Kao C-L, Chen C-J, Cheng A-L, Kadin ME, Chen JY: Aggressive peripheral T-cell lymphomas containing Epstein-Barr viral DNA: A clinicopathologic and molecular analysis. Blood 77:799, 1991.
21. Herbst H, Dallenbach F, Hummel M, Niedbitek G, Finn T, Young LS, Rowe M, Müller-Lantzsch N, Stein H: Epstein-Barr Virus DNA and latent gene products in K-i(CD30)-positive anaplastic large cell lymphoma. Blood 78:2666, 1991.
22. Lee S-H, Su I-J, Chen R-L, Lin K-S, Lin D-T, Chuu W-M, Lin K-S: A pathologic study of childhood lymphoma in Taiwan with special reference to peripheral T-cell lymphoma and the association with Epstein-Barr viral infection. Cancer 68:1954, 1991.
23. Watry D, Hedrick JA, Siervo S, Rhodes G, Lamberti JJ, Lambris JD, Tsuokas CD: Infection of human thymocytes by Epstein-Barr virus. J Exp Med 173:971, 1991.
24. Koizumi S, Zhang X-K, Imai S, Sugiura M, Usui N, Osato T: Infection of HYLV-1-harbouring T-lymphoblastoid line MT-2 by Epstein-Barr virus. Virology 188:859, 1992.
25. Yoneda N, Tatsumi E, Kawano S, Teshigawara K, Oka T, Fukuda M, Yamaguchi N: Detection of Epstein-Barr virus genome in natural-kiler-like cell line, YT. Leukemia 6:136, 1992.

American Journal of Hematology 45:156–166 (1994)

Hypofibrinolysis: A Common, Major Cause of Osteonecrosis

Charles J. Glueck, Richard Freiberg, Helen I. Glueck, Clyde Henderson, Michael Welch, Trent Tracy, Davis Stroop, Tracey Hamer, Felix Sosa, and Mark Levy

Cholesterol Center (C.J.G., T.T., T.H., F.S., M.L.) and Department of Orthopedics (R.F., C.H.), Jewish Hospital; Christ Hospital (M.W.); and Departments of Pathology and Laboratory Medicine, University of Cincinnati College of Medicine (H.I.G., D.S.), Cincinnati, Ohio

In 30 patients with osteonecrosis of the hip (12 idiopathic, 18 secondary), we assessed the role of hypofibrinolysis mediated by high levels of plasminogen activator inhibitor (PAI). We evaluated hypofibrinolysis as a common, potentially reversible, pathophysiologic cause of idiopathic osteonecrosis. In all 18 patients with secondary osteonecrosis, PAI was normal, as was the ability to activate fibrinolysis. Nine of the 12 patients with idiopathic osteonecrosis had exceptionally high PAI levels and could not normally elevate tissue plasminogen activator (tPA-Fx), the major stimulator of fibrinolysis, after 10 min of venous occlusion at 100 mm Hg. The group of 12 patients with idiopathic osteonecrosis, compared to the 18 with secondary osteonecrosis, had low mean stimulated tPA-Fx (1.92 vs. 7.6 IU/ml, $P \leqslant .001$) and very high stimulated PAI-Fx (70 vs. 7.6 U/ml, $P \leqslant .01$). Three of the 12 patients with idiopathic osteonecrosis had both normal PAI and normal stimulated tPA-Fx. These three patients and 14 of the 18 with secondary osteonecrosis had high lipoprotein (a) [Lp(a)] (>20 mg/dl). Mean Lp(a) was much higher (60 mg/dl) in the patients with secondary osteonecrosis than Lp(a) (16 mg/dl, $P \leqslant .001$) in the 12 patients with idiopathic osteonecrosis. These findings suggest that hypofibrinolysis mediated by high PAI is a common cause of idiopathic osteonecrosis, whereas high Lp(a) may play an etiologic role in secondary osteonecrosis. Prospective studies of patients with high PAI and/or high Lp(a) should be carried out to assess further their apparently causal roles in osteonecrosis.

Key words: hypofibrinolysis, plasminogen activator inhibitor, tissue plasminogen activator, osteonecrosis, Lp(a)

INTRODUCTION

Idiopathic osteonecrosis of the femoral head is characterized pathoanatomically and pathophysiologically by venous hypertension and impaired venous circulation [1–5], perhaps caused by thrombotic venous occlusion, which compromises venous drainage. Osteonecrosis is also often "secondary," with known predisposing factors such as alcoholism, sickle cell disease, hyperbaric exposure, excessive corticosteroid usage, systemic lupus erythematosus, and hip trauma [1–5]. Recently we described familial, autosomal dominant hypofibrinolysis in a 29-year-old white man with idiopathic osteonecrosis involving both hips and a shoulder [6,7]. He had very high levels of endogenous plasminogen activator inhibitor (PAI-Fx), with subsequent inability to stimulate fibrinolysis [6,7]. We postulated that the depressed fibrinolysis resulted in inadequate lysis of venous thrombi in bone, impaired bone venous circulation, and venous hypertension of bone (1–6). In 1961, Nilsson et al. [8] described a 28-year-old man who, from age 10 years, had massive, very widely disseminated venous thrombosis, obliteration of the inferior vena cava, ". . . a very high fibrinogen level, absence of fibrinolytic activity, and a high content of serum components inhibiting the activation of plasminogen by streptokinase as well as urokinase." On autopsy at age 28 years ". . . the left acetabulum was partly destroyed and the femoral head on the left side was displaced. There was a pathologic fracture of the femoral neck" [8]. Bone and hip pain were not a predominant feature of this patient's clinical course [8], and the osteonecrosis appeared to be a minor feature admidst his systemic, recurrent thromboses. His mother and sister,

Received for publication May 13, 1993; accepted August 18, 1993.

Address reprint requests to C.J. Glueck, MD, Medical Director of the Cholesterol Center, Jewish Hospital, 3200 Burnet Ave., Cincinnati, OH 45229.

both free of thrombotic disease, had high levels of plasminogen inhibitor [8]. In our kindred [6,7], with very high levels of PAI available to bind tissue plasminogen activator (tPA-Fx), the major stimulator of fibrinolysis [6,7], stimulated tPA-Fx [9] presumably could not rise. The nature of the hypofibrinolysis in our original kindred [6,7] was similar to that in the five other previously reported kindreds with familial high PAI and hypofibrinolysis but without osteonecrotic manifestations of thrombosis [10–14].

High levels of PAI as a cause of familial hypofibrinolysis are apparently rare, having been previously reported in only seven kindreds, with the high PAI inherited as an autosomal dominant trait [6–8,10–14]. Affected family members with high PAI and familial hypofibrinolysis have a very wide variety of pathophysiology, ranging from no symptoms to recurrent thrombotic events [6–8,10–14]; idiopathic osteonecrosis as the sole manifestation of familial hypofibrinolysis has been described only in our kindred [6,7]. The patient of Nilsson et al. [8] had had profound venous thrombosis for 18 years prior to diagnosis of femoral head necrosis.

In contrast to the heritable, primary elevations of PAI [6,7,10–14], high PAI levels may be secondary to varous malignancies [15], may accompany severe hypertriglyceridemia [9], and are found in some patients with premature atherosclerosis, possibly associated with hyperinsulinemia [16]. Hypofibrinolysis is most often caused by high PAI [9–17], resulting in defective activation of plasminogen, since the interplay between PAI and tPA-Fx is central to regulation of fibrinolysis. In 30 patients with osteonecrosis of the hip (12 idiopathic, 18 secondary), our specific aim was to examine basal and stimulated fibrinolytic activity to determine whether hypofibrinolysis, mediated by high PAI, was pathophysiologically related to osteonecrosis.

MATERIALS AND METHODS

Study Protocol

The study was approved by our Institutional Research Committee and was carried out with signed informed consent. Thirty patients with osteonecrosis were referred for prospective study from the clinical practices of orthopedic surgeons from the Department of Orthopedic Surgery, Jewish and Christ Hospitals, Cincinnati. The single exception to this mode of referral was idiopathic osteonecrosis patient 1, a 29-year-old white man with well documented familial hypertriglyceridemia, who initially had been referred to our Cholesterol Center for diagnosis and therapy of hypertriglyceridemia with a concurrent history of (idiopathic) osteonecrosis of both hips and a shoulder [6,7].

The patients were studied by Cholesterol Center personnel who were blinded regarding clinical, pathoanatomical, laboratory, and x-ray findings used to establish the diagnosis of osteonecrosis [1–5] and who had differentiated osteonecrosis into secondary or "idiopathic." Similarly, laboratory personnel measuring fasting lipids, lipoprotein cholesterols, apolipoproteins [18–24], and fibrinolytic regulators [6,9] were also blinded regarding the patients' diagnoses.

In each patient, a systematic personal and family history was obtained, which focused on arterial and/or venous thrombosis, trauma, alcohol intake, sickle cell disease, lupus, corticosteroid use, bone and joint disease, any other acute or chronic disease state (including infection or inflammation), endocrine status, and pregnancy. The date of any hip surgery was also recorded.

Measurement of Lipids, Lipoprotein Cholesterols, and Apolipoproteins

Fasting lipids and lipoprotein cholesterols were quantitated in our Lipid Research Clinic's standardized laboratory [18] using enzymatic methods [19–21] with calculation of LDL cholesterol when triglyceride was <400 mg/dl [22]. Serum apolipoproteins A1 and B were measured by rate nephelometry [23]. Lp(a) was measured by enzyme immunoassay with a Terumo-macra Lp(a) sequential monoclonal-polyclonal sandwich method [24]. Normal ranges are provided in Table I.

Measurement of Fibrinolytic Regulators and D-Dimer in the Basal and Stimulated States

Basal and stimulated determinants of fibrinolysis and D-dimer were quantitated as previously reported [6,9]. After a 12 hr fast, blood was obtained between 8 and 9 AM to minimize the influence of time of day on regulators of basal and stimulated fibrinolytic activity [9]. Patients were seated for approximately 10 min while their history was taken, and then, still seated, had their basal blood drawn immediately after application of a tourniquet. With the patients remaining seated, after a standard stimulus (10 min of venous occlusion at 100 mm Hg with a blood pressure cuff) [6,9–11], a second blood sample was obtained for measurement of stimulated fibrinolysis. Although we obtained measures of fibrinogen, plasminogen, and α2-antiplasmin before and after venous occlusion (in addition to tPA, PAI, and D-dimer), we did not display the postocclusion values for fibrinogen, plasminogen, and α2-antiplasmin, since they are affected primarily by hemoconcentration and are not released from the endothelium in response to increased vascular transmural pressure. Normal ranges (10th–90th percentiles) [6] are given in Table II and Figures 1–4.

Tissue plasminogen activator (tPA), the major fibrinolytic activity stimulator, was measured in two forms, the antigen form (tPA-Ag) by ELISA (Imubind total tPA; American Diagnostica, Greenwich, CT) and the active form (tPA-Fx) by chromogenic techniques [Biopool

TABLE I. Lipids, Lipoproteins, Apolipoproteins (mg/dl), Causes of Osteonecrosis, Years From Hip Surgery, and Thrombophlebitis (TP) in 30 Patients, 18 With Secondary Osteonecrosis, 12 With Idiopathic Osteonecrosis*

Causes of secondary osteonecrosis	Patient	Age (years)	Sex	Race	TC	TG	HDLC	LDLC	Apo A1	Apo B	Lp (a)	Years from surg	TP
				Normal:	<200 [41]	<250 [42]	>35 [41]	<160 [41]	96–176 [23]	43–128 [23]	<20 [9]		
Trauma—hip fracture	1	60	F	W	212	112	81	109	187	115	72	1	No
Corticosteroids	2	39	F	B	160	34	53	100	138	98	147	.1	No
Alcoholism	3	59	F	B	241	134	80	134	169	125	133	1	No
Trauma—hip fracture	4	91	M	W	188	75	59	114	161	112	31	NS	No
Trauma—hip fracture	5	82	F	W	255	262	41	162	112	184	39	1	No
Trauma—hip fracture	6	64	F	W	233	192	50	145	151	162	50	2	No
Corticosteroids	7	67	M	W	183	112	40	121	111	137	19	NS	No
Trauma—hip fracture	8	51	F	W	172	121	52	96	153	100	6	NS	No
Lupus, corticosteroids	9	30	F	B	186	30	55	125	128	112	68	2	Yes
Trauma—hip fracture	10	55	M	B	180	68	59	107	145	97	57	2	No
Trauma—hip fracture	11	66	F	W	194	75	72	107	159	106	31	1	No
Alcoholism	12	62	F	B	256	101	89	147	209	152	129	2	No
Trauma—hip fracture	13	76	F	W	221	149	46	145	109	129	45	3	No
Sickle cell disease	14	38	F	B	129	65	36	80	126	89	28	1	Yes
Lupus, corticosteroids	15	38	F	B	258	119	65	169	133	151	134	2	No
Sickle cell disease	16	33	F	B	146	77	32	99	123	99	71	NS	No
Sickle cell disease	17	36	F	B	148	118	61	63	165	77	1	9	Yes
Trauma—hip fracture	18	74	F	W	187	241	44	95	137	145	18	7	No
Idiopathic osteonecrosis													
	1	29	M	W	254	301	28	166	86	189	7	NS	No
	2	46	M	W	244	137	53	164	153	181	16	NS	No
	3	50	M	W	267	224	52	170	140	170	1	NS	No
	4	58	M	W	212	197	45	128	141	145	1	1	No
	5	62	M	W	195	201	41	114	144	139	46	1	Yes
	6	40	F	W	187	87	45	125	123	123	9	NS	No
	7	42	M	B	241	205	48	152	156	185	31	NS	No
	8	47	M	W	164	181	32	96	108	112	1	NS	No
	9	66	F	B	166	115	38	105	114	114	37	NS	No
	10	49	M	W	225	217	33	149	118	174	1	6	No
	11	51	M	W	278	428	37	155	125	213	1	7	No
	12	54	F	W	157	82	37	104	136	117	43	NS	No

*TC, total cholesterol; TG, triglyceride; HDLC, high-density lipoprotein cholesterol; LDLC, low-density lipoprotein cholesterol; Apo A1, apolipoprotein A1; Apo B, apolipoprotein B; Lp(a), lipoprotein (a), NS, no surgery.

Spectrolyse (fibrin); American Diagnostica] [6,9]. Mean and normal range [10th–90th percentile (6)] basal and stimulated tPA-Fx in normal individuals were 0.81 (0.11–1.94) and 6.34 (2.28–11.3) IU/ml and for tPA-Ag, 7.3 (3.7–13.7) and 17.4 (8.4–31.4) ng/ml.

PAI-Fx, a major inhibitor of fibrinolysis, was measured with synthetic substrates [Biopool Spectrolyse (pL); American Diagnostica] [6,9]. This assay measures only the functionally active PAI. PAI-Ag was quantitated using monoclonal antibodies and ELISA (Imubind PAI-1; American Diagnostica) [6,9]. PAI-Ag measures total activity, i.e., both latent (bound to tPA) and active PAI (free). Mean and normal range (10th–90th percentile) basal and stimulated PAI-Fx in normals were 14.9 (3.5–26.9) and 12.8 (3.6–23.9) U/ml and for PAI-Ag 25 (3.2–37.1) and 48 (11.7–95.6) ng/ml.

Additional measures of fibrinolytic regulators included α2-antiplasmin (a fibrinolytic inhibitor; S-2251; KabiVitrum, Franklin, OH), plasminogen (Spectrozyme PL; American Diagnostica), and fibrinogen (Dade Thormbin; Baxter Healthcare Corp., Miami, FL) [6,9]. Mean and normal range (10th–90th percentile) basal α2-antiplasmin was 109% (77–129%), with basal fibrinogen 341 (150–400) mg/dl and basal plasminogen 106% (75–133%).

D-dimers, split products from cross-linked fibrin, a measure of in vivo fibrinolysis [6,9], were determined by ELISA (dimertest; American Diagnostica) using monoclonal antibodies against D-dimer. Mean basal D-dimer in normals was 0.12 μg/dl, normal basal levels being <0.25 μg/dl; mean and normal ranges (10th–90th percentile) for stimulated D-dimer were 0.20 (0.085–0.257) μg/dl. Protein C was measured by ELISA [25]. The normal range for protein C is 55–145%.

Statistical Analyses

The group data were normally distributed by the Shapiro-Wilk test [26]. Parametric paired and unpaired t tests

TABLE II. Measures of Basal (B) and Stimulated (S) Fibrinolysis in 18 Patients With Secondary Osteonecrosis and in 12 Patients With Idiopathic Osteonecrosis*

	tPA-Fx (IU/ml)		tPA-Ag (ng/ml)		PAI-Fx (U/ml)		PAI-Ag (ng/ml)		D-dimer (μg/dl)		α2-Ap (% normal) (basal)	Plasminogen (% normal) (basal)	Fibrinogen (mg/dl) (basal)
	B	S	B	S	B	S	B	S	B	S			
Normal range [6]													
Basal	0.11–1.94		3.7–13.7		3.5–26.9		3.2–37.1		<0.25		77–129	75–133	150–400
Stimulated	2.28–11.3		8.4–31.4		3.6–23.9		11.7–95.6		0.085–0.257				
Secondary													
1	0.76	6.03	10.2	28.1	7.4	8.8	14.4	21.0	0.109	0.124	100	112	283
2	1.28	16.18	9.8	49.6	6.7	5.1	6.7	11.4	0.094	0.166	102	108	252
3	1.18	5.02	9.6	12.0	7.2	8.2	19.8	21.0	1.365	1.829	102	118	331
4	1.00	2.49	5.5	6.2	4.4	4.8	7.0	7.6	0.470	0.504	86	80	199
5	0.46	9.56	11.2	31.0	10.6	7.1	19.6	26.5	0.124	0.128	116	100	347
6	0.36	4.83	11.8	32.4	14.9	14.0	23.8	39.0	0.106	0.122	112	97	261
7	0.70	4.00	18.8	34.0	11.2	8.6	40.2	47.7	0.536	0.902	120	116	381
8	0.56	6.75	3.6	17.8	6.6	3.4	12.8	22.2	0.096	0.167	102	85	202
9	0.36	2.58	10.8	23.8	10.7	9.6	13.0	15.2	0.127	0.150	100	108	294
10	1.18	5.44	13.9	33.2	7.8	5.6	18.6	19.5	0.096	0.106	98	94	244
11	2.22	25.12	9.8	269.1	0.2	0.01	9.0	8.5	0.189	0.222	96	96	382
12	0.48	6.37	19.4	87.4	18.6	16.2	27.6	32.4	0.136	0.142	106	142	385
13	0.50	5.29	24.9	48.0	18.5	17.8	41.0	55.2	0.204	0.336	108	120	382
14	1.14	4.17	16.3	23.7	8.7	9.0	35.2	42.6	0.152	0.201	112	89	237
15	3.84	13.23	16.2	49.8	11.8	12.2	8.6	13.6	0.706	0.936	99	92	481
16	0.90	5.47	13.6	31.6	7.6	4.2	14.6	15.4	0.162	0.178	102	91	271
17	1.91	3.16	18.9	26.6	2.8	3.0	19.0	17.0	0.122	0.142	89	79	204
18	2.03	11.70	9.6	32.6	2.8	0.2	5.2	8.6	0.126	0.134	103	126	401
Idiopathic													
1	0.05	0.10	6.8	16.9	108.8	134.1	191.0	223.0	0.080	0.084	118	137	330
2	0.20	0.46	10.4	28.1	46.6	55.8	83.9	105.7	0.142	0.198	103	118	273
3	0.12	0.27	17.6	24.0	122.5	139.5	143.5	155.0	0.095	0.103	114	120	261
4	0.49	2.19	33.5	159.5	44.1	45.0	61.7	75.5	0.126	0.130	106	115	385
5	0.29	3.82	6.0	16.6	12.1	11.3	19.0	22.8	0.185	0.240	108	106	349
6	0.08	0.18	21.0	28.8	96.0	112.0	148.0	159.0	0.092	0.098	116	122	292
7	0.19	1.75	15.8	41.4	84.7	94.6	82.9	129.6	0.102	0.128	102	108	246
8	0.32	1.84	19.5	37.4	22.6	23.3	67.9	82.6	0.084	0.086	102	110	198
9	0.25	5.52	9.2	28.4	24.8	21.6	35.4	42.6	0.181	0.215	106	110	294
10	0.18	1.09	16.0	23.5	39.8	35.7	57.6	54.8	0.104	0.100	90	108	306
11	0.51	0.23	20.2	28.6	153.5	155.0	250.0	268.5	0.104	0.112	99	104	263
12	0.31	5.57	11.8	27.1	14.0	13.8	24.6	31.0	0.110	0.123	108	112	283

*tPA-Fx, tissue plasminogen activator activity; tPA-Ag, tissue plasminogen activator activity antigen; PAI-Fx, plasminogen activator inhibitor activity; PAI-Ag, plasminogen activator inhibitor antigen; α2-Ap, α2-antiplasmin.

[27] were used to compare basal and stimulated fibrinolytic activities within groups and to compare variables between patients with idiopathic osteonecrosis and secondary osteonecrosis. Since up to 30 paired and unpaired group comparisons were made, to reduce the likelihood that some comparisons would be significant by chance alone, only P values $\leqslant .01$, $\leqslant .001$, and $\leqslant .0001$ are presented. Pearson correlations were calculated [27], and χ^2 analyses were employed [27]. General linear models with least square means were used to compare fibrinolytic measurements between groups after first covariance adjusting for group (idiopathic vs. secondary osteonecrosis) differences in lipids, lipoproteins, and apolipoproteins [27]. Stepwise regression was also used [27], with absolute change from basal to stimulated tPA-Fx values as the dependent variable and absolute change from basal to stimulated levels in PAI-Fx and PAI-Ag, time of day when venous occlusion was done, and postocclusion Lp(a) as explanatory variables.

RESULTS

Patients' Secondary and Idiopathic Osteonecrosis

The 30 patients were differentiated into secondary or idiopathic groups by reviewing their clinical orthopedic, historical, radiographic, and (when available) postsurgical pathoanatomic and microscopic data [1–5]. Twelve patients (nine men, three women; ten whites, two blacks) had idiopathic ostonecrosis, 18 (three men, 15 women; nine whites, nine blacks) had secondary osteonecrosis (Tables I–III, Figs. 1–4).

TABLE III. Mean (SD) Plasma Cholesterol, Triglyceride, High-Density Lipoprotein Cholesterol (HDLC), Low-Density Lipoprotein Cholesterol (LDLC), Apolipoprotein A1 (APO A1), Apolipoprotein B (APO B), and Lipoprotein (a) [LP(a)] (mg/dl)

Normal		Secondary osteonecrosis (n = 18)	Idiopathic osteonecrosis (n = 12)
<200 [41]	Total cholesterol	197 (40)	216 (42)
<250 [42]	Triglyceride	116 (63)	198* (96)
>35 [41]	HDLC	56 (16)	41* (8)
<160 [41]	LDLC	118 (28)	136 (27)
96–176 [23]	Apo A1	145 (27)	129 (20)
43–128 [23]	Apo B	122 (29)	155* (34)
<20 [9]	Lp(a)	60 (47)	16** (18)

*$P \leq .01$, **$P \leq .001$ (t test), idiopathic vs. secondary.

None of the 12 patients with idiopathic osteonecrosis had trauma, systemic lupus, sickle cell disease, corticosteroid usage, hyperbaric exposure or chronic alcoholism that could be implicated in the etiology of the osteonecrosis [1–5]. Two of the patients with idiopathic osteonecrosis (Nos. 10 and 11; Tables I, II) were brothers.

Of the 18 patients with secondary osteonecrosis, nine had subcapital fractures of the femur, four took long-term corticosteroids (two of these four had systemic lupus erythematosus), two had been chronic alcoholics, and three had sickle cell disease (Tables I, II). None of the 18 patients with secondary osteonecrosis was related.

Thrombosis, Thrombophlebitis, and Clinical and Surgical Factors That Might Affect Fibrinolysis

Three of the 18 patients with secondary osteonecrosis had previously sustained thrombophlebitis, No. 9 (who had lupus) and Nos. 14 and 17 (both with sickle cell disease; Table I). One of the 12 patients with idiopathic osteonecrosis had previously sustained thrombophlebitis (No. 5; Table I). None of the 30 patients had documented evidence of pulmonary emboli, mesenteric, or cerebrovascular thrombosis.

Of the 18 patients with secondary osteonecrosis, 14 had undergone hip replacement surgery prior to our study, 13 of these 14 having had the surgery 1 or more years prior to our study (Table I). Four of the 12 patients with idiopathic osteonecrosis had had hip replacement surgery one or more years prior to our study (Table I).

None of the patients was pregnant when studied (which might elevate PAI-2). Since high basal PAI-Fx and PAI-Ag were characteristic of the patients with idiopathic osteonecrosis [present in nine of the 12 (Table II, Fig. 2)], the patients were carefully studied for factors that might elevate PAI levels. There were no malignancies, no very severe hypertriglyceridemia (>500 mg/dl), no severe premature atherosclerosis, no chronic infection, and no clinical evidence for chronic inflammatory processes. Of the nine patients with idiopathic osteonecrosis and very high basal PAI-Fx and/or PAI-Ag, patient 1 had familial elevations of PAI [6], and patients 10 and 11 were brothers from a kindred with three-generation vertical and horizontal transmission of high PAI. For the remaining six patients with idiopathic osteonecrosis and high PAI, we suspect that the high PAI was primary/familial.

Basal and Stimulated Fibrinolytic Activites in Patients With Idiopathic and Secondary Osteonecrosis

After 10 min of venous occlusion at 100 mm Hg, stimulated tPA-Fx was normal (above the 10th percentile in controls; 2.28 IU/ml) in all 18 patients with secondary osteonecrosis (Table II, Fig. 1). Stimulated tPA-Ag was low in one of these patients, normal in seven, and high in ten (Table II, Fig. 1). Overall, in the 18 patients with secondary osteonecrosis, 10 min of venous occlusion led to substantial, normal increments in tPA-Fx and tPA-Ag (Fig. 1). None of the 18 patients with secondary osteonecrosis had high (top decile) basal or stimulated PAI-Fx (Table II). As displayed in Figure 2, patients with secondary osteonecrosis had markedly lower basal and stimulated PAI-Fx and PAI-Ag than patients with idiopathic osteonecrosis.

In nine of the 12 patients with idiopathic osteonecrosis, after 10 min of venous occlusion at 100 mm Hg, stimulated tPA-Fx failed to rise into the normal range (remaining below the 10th percentile for controls; Table II, Fig. 1). Conversely, stimulated tPA-Ag was normal in six of these nine patients and high (>90th percentile for controls) in three (Table II, Fig. 1). In these nine patients, basal PAI-Fx and/or basal PAI-Ag were very high (Table II, Fig. 2). In the remaining three patients with idiopathic osteonecrosis (Nos. 5, 9, and 12), however, stimulated tPA-Fx was in the normal range, as was stimulated tPA-Ag (Table II, Fig. 1). These three patients (Nos. 5, 9, 12; Table I) were further sharply differentiated from the other nine with idiopathic osteonecrosis by having high Lp(a) (46, 37, and 43 mg/dl, respectively), normal basal PAI-Fx, and normal basal PAI-Ag (Table II, Fig. 2).

Mean basal tPA-Fx levels (0.25 IU/ml) in the 12 patients with idiopathic osteonecrosis were more than four times lower ($P \leq .001$) than in the 18 patients with secondary osteonecrosis (1.16 IU/ml; Fig. 3). Mean basal PAI-Fx levels were much higher (64 U/ml) in the 12 patients with idiopathic osteonecrosis than in the 18 patients with secondary osteonecrosis (8.8 U/ml; $P \leq .01$; Fig. 3). Similarly, mean basal PAI-Ag levels (97 ng/ml) were exceptionally high in the 12 patients with idiopathic osteonecrosis (2.6 times the upper normal limit) and 5.1 times higher than in the 18 patients with secondary osteonecrosis (18.7 ng/ml; $P \leq .01$; Fig. 3).

The patients with idiopathic osteonecrosis did not differ from those with secondary osteonecrosis in regards to

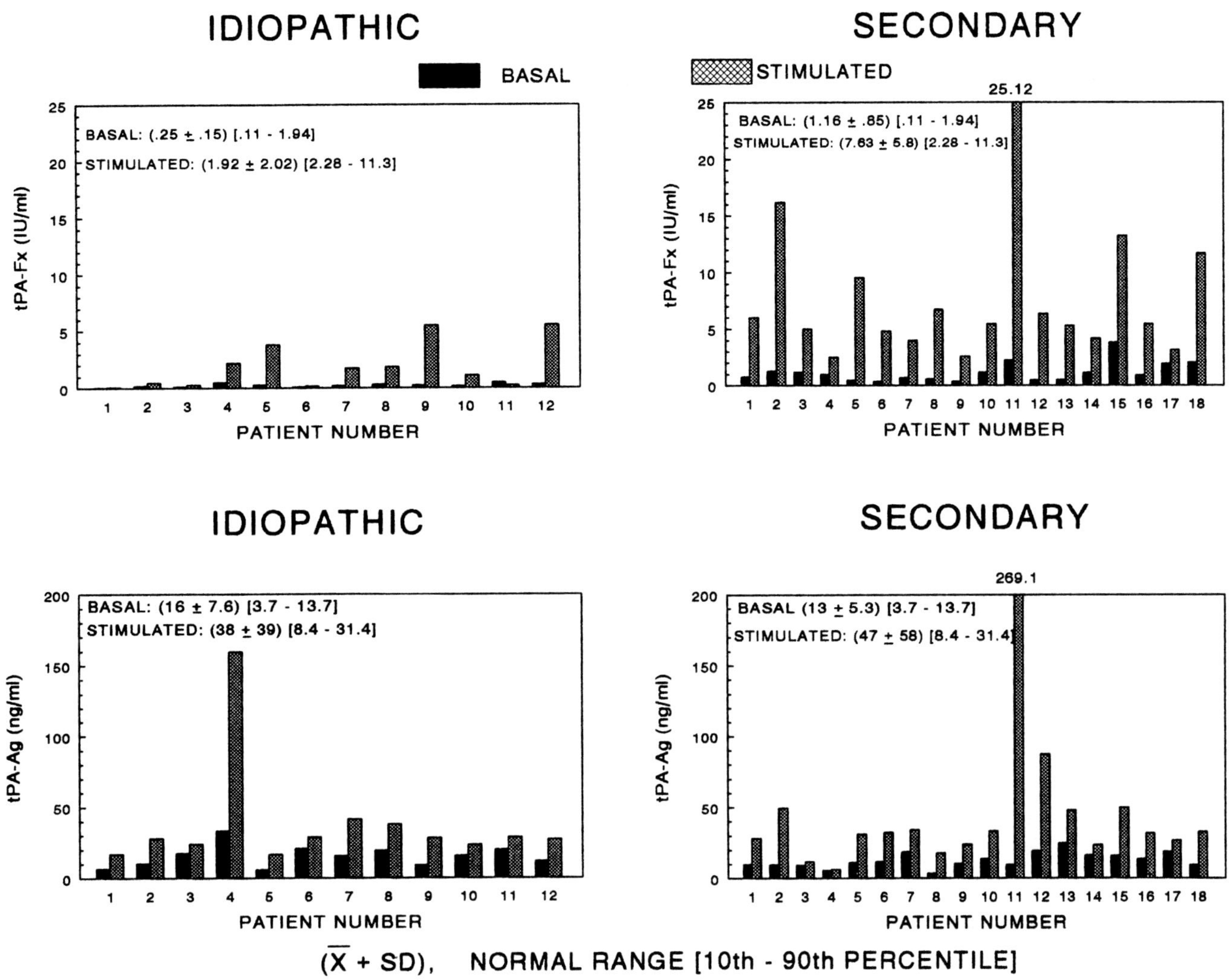

Fig. 1. Basal and stimulated tissue plasminogen activator activity (tPA-Fx) and antigen (tPA-Ag) in 12 patients with idiopathic osteonecrosis and in 18 patients with secondary osteonecrosis. Basal and stimulated group means are displayed, along with the 10th–90th percentile normal range [6].

basal tPA-Ag, α2-antiplasmin, plasminogen, fibrinogen, or D-dimer (Fig. 4).

In the 18 patients with secondary osteonecrosis vs. the 12 with idiopathic osteonecrosis, mean stimulated tPA-Fx was much higher, 7.63 vs. 1.92 IU/ml ($P \leqslant .001$; Fig. 3). The reasons for this disparity between the secondary and idiopathic cases (activation vs. nonactivation of tPA-Fx in response to venous occlusion) were seen in the striking differences in stimulated PAI-Fx and PAI-Ag when comparing idiopathic and secondary osteonecrosis (Figs. 2, 3). Stimulated PAI-Fx and PAI-Ag were markedly higher in the 12 patients with idiopathic osteonecrosis than in the 18 with secondary osteonecrosis [70 vs. 7.6 U/ml (PAI-Fx); $P \leqslant .01$], 113 vs. 24 ng/ml (PAI-Ag; $P \leqslant .01$; Fig. 3).

After covariance adjusting for triglycerides, HDLC, apo B, and Lp(a), the adjusted differences in basal and stimulated PAI-Fx and PAI-Ag in idiopathic vs. secondary osteonecrosis groups were comparable to the unadjusted differences. Thus the differences in basal and stimulated PAI-Fx and PAI-Ag between the 18 patients with secondary osteonecrosis and the 12 with idiopathic osteonecrosis (Fig. 3) could not be attributed to group differences (Table III) in triglyceride, HDLC, apo B, or Lp(a). Whereas D-dimer levels rose after venous occlusion in the 18 patients with secondary osteonecrosis from 0.27 to 0.36 μg/dl ($P \leqslant .01$; Fig. 4), they did not rise significantly in the 12 patients with idiopathic osteonecrosis.

Patients' Lipids, Lp(a), and Protein C

Mean triglycerides (198 mg/dl) were higher ($P \leqslant .01$) in the 12 patients with idiopathic osteonecrosis than in the 18 with secondary osteonecrosis (116 mg/dl; Table III).

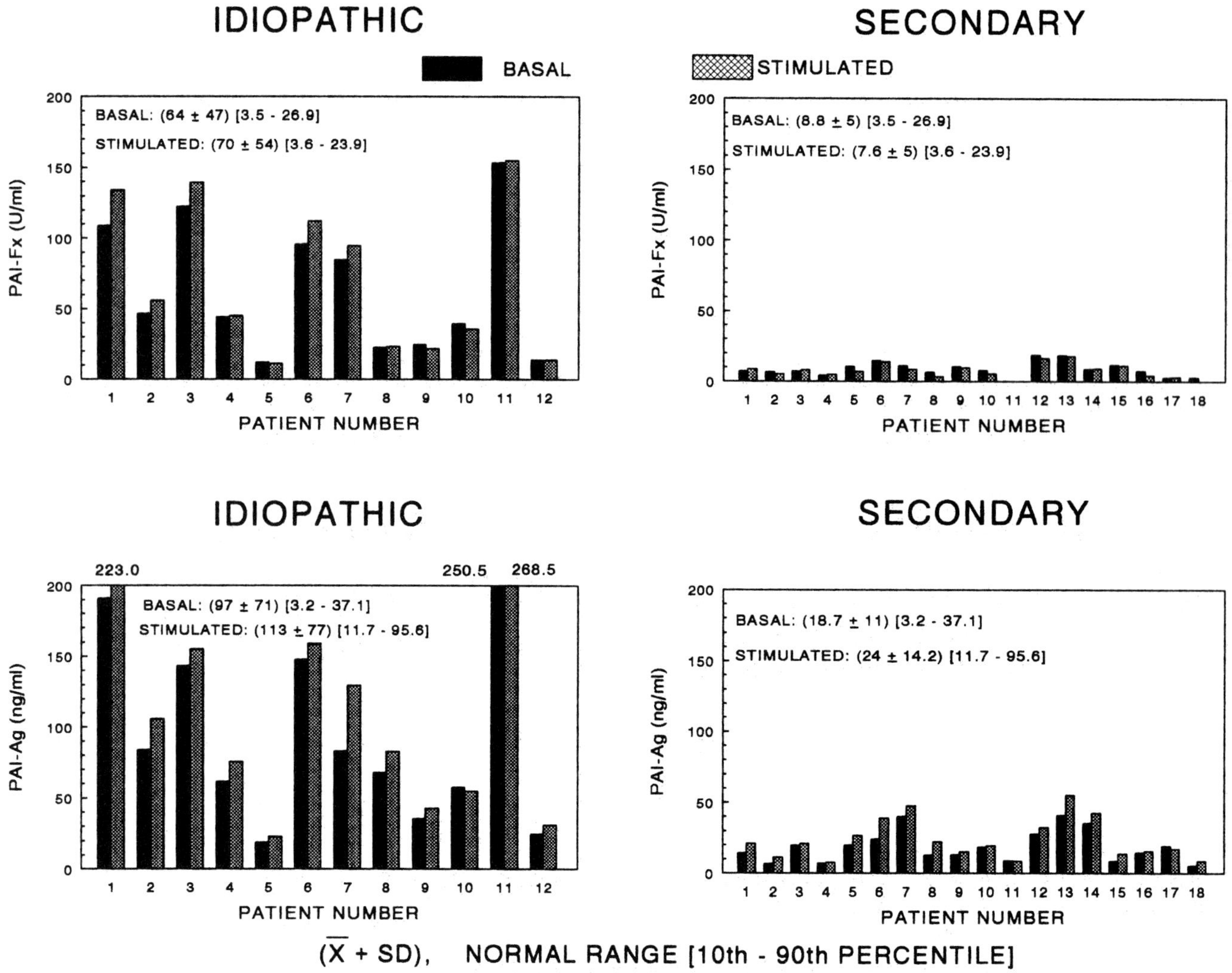

Fig. 2. Basal and stimulated plasminogen activator inhibitor activity (PAI-Fx) and antigen (PAI-Ag) in 12 patients with idiopathic osteonecrosis and in 18 patients with secondary osteonecrosis. Basal and stimulated group means are displayed, along with the 10th–90th percentile normal range [6].

Mean Lp(a) levels (16 mg/dl) were much lower in the 12 patients with idiopathic osteonecrosis than in the 18 with secondary osteonecrosis (60 mg/dl; $P \leq .001$; Table III). When we used an arbitrary cutoff of 20 mg/dl to identify high Lp(a) [9], 14 of the 18 patients with secondary osteonecrosis had high Lp(a) vs. only four of the 12 patients with idiopathic osteonecrosis (Table I; $\chi^2 = 5.9$; $P = .02$). Of the 12 patients with idiopathic osteonecrosis, only three had normal stimulated tPA-Fx (Nos. 5, 9, and 12; Table II, Fig. 1), all of whom had high Lp(a) (46, 37, and 43 mg/dl; Table I). Of the other nine patients with idiopathic osteonecrosis who uniformly failed to activate tPA-Fx after venous occlusion, only one (No. 7) had high Lp(a) (31 mg/dl; Table I).

When othe predisposing factors associated with thrombosis were analyzed in the four patients with secondary osteonecrosis who had normal Lp(a) (Table I), one patient (No. 17) had previously undiagnosed low protein C [25] (48%; normal 55–145%). Low protein C is a defect commonly associated with thrombosing disorders [28]. Protein C levels were normal in the other 29 patients.

Correlations Between PAI-Fx, PAI-Ag, and tPA-Fx in the Basal and Stimulated States in Patients With Secondary and Idiopathic Osteonecrosis

In the 12 patients with idiopathic osteonecrosis, stimulated PAI-Fx ($r = -.75$; $P = .005$) and PAI-Ag ($r = .75$; $P = .005$) were inversely correlated with stim-

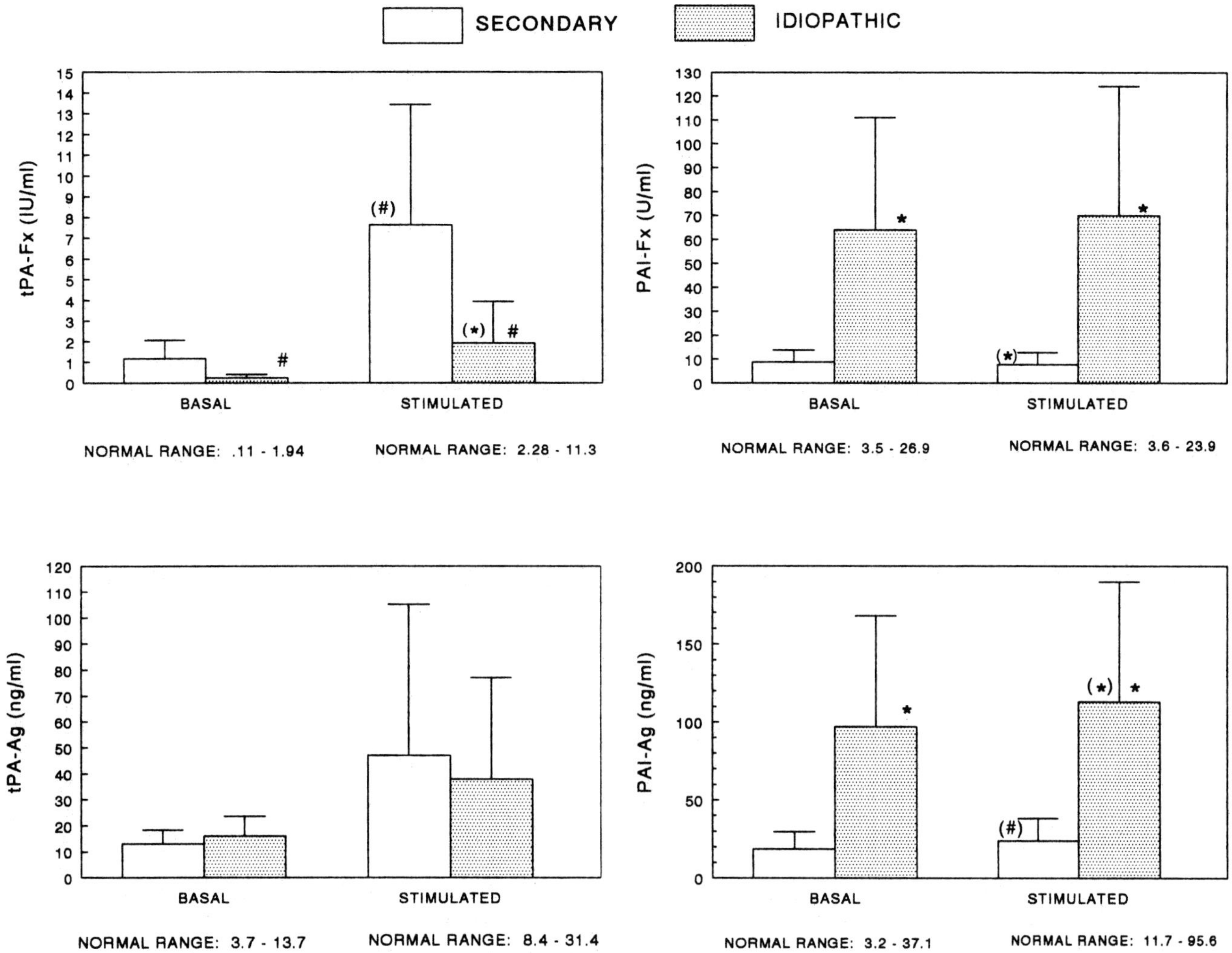

Fig. 3. Mean (SD) basal and stimulated tissue plasminogen activator activity (tPA-Fx) and antigen (tPA-Ag), and basal and stimulated plasminogen activator inhibitor activity (PAI-Fx) and antigen (PAI-Ag), in 12 patients with idiopathic osteonecrosis and in 18 patients with secondary osteonecrosis. t test, secondary vs. idiopathic. *$P \leq .01$, #$P \leq .001$. In parentheses, paired t test basal vs. stimulated, within group. (*)$P \leq .01$ (#)$P \leq .001$. The 10–90th percentile normal range [6] is also displayed.

ulated tPA-Fx. However, these correlations were not significant in the 18 patients with secondary osteonecrosis ($r = -.39$; $p = .11$; and $r = -.41$; $P = .09$).

In the 12 patients with idiopathic osteonecrosis, by stepwise regression, 78% of the change ($P = .001$) from basal to stimulated tPA-Fx levels could be accounted for by change in PAI-Ag (standardized partial regression coefficient = −0.43; $P = .02$) and by Lp(a) (standardized partial regression coefficient = .81, $P = .0006$). The greater the increment in PAI-Ag on venous occlusion, the smaller was the increment in tPA-Fx. The higher the Lp(a), the greater was the change in tPA-Fx after venous occlusion. Change in PAI-Ag was not a significant predictor ($P < 0.15$) of change in tPA-Fx in the 18 patients with secondary osteonecrosis.

Correlations Between Lp(a) and Measures of Fibrinolysis

Since 14 of the 18 patients with secondary osteonecrosis had high Lp(a) without hypofibrinolysis, we examined correlations between Lp(a) and all measures of basal and stimulated fibrinolysis. In the 18 patients with secondary osteonecrosis, there were no significant correlations between Lp(a) before or after venous occlusion with basal and stimulated measures of fibrinolysis. In the 12 patients with idiopathic osteonecrosis, the only signifi-

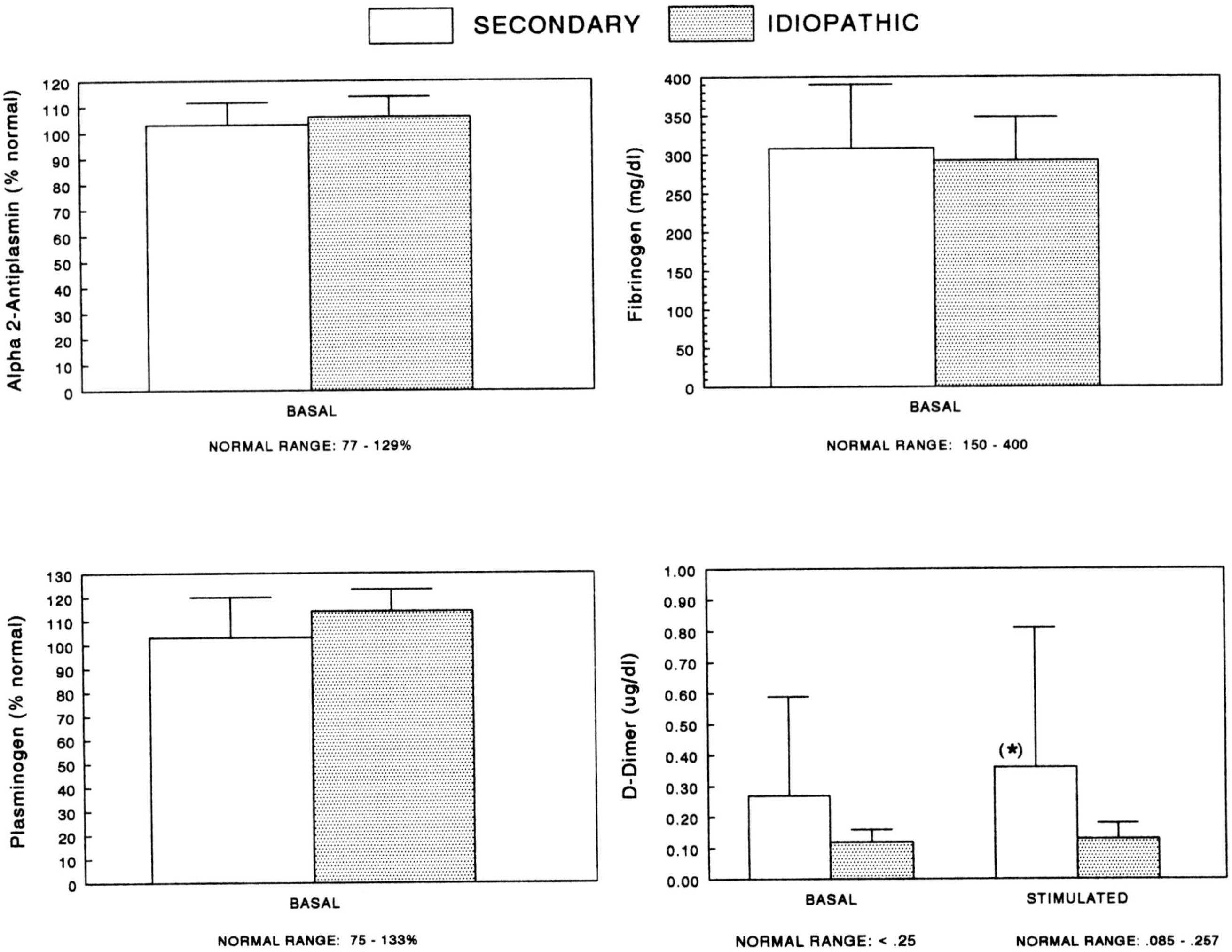

Fig. 4. Mean (SD) basal alpha 2-antiplasmin, fibrinogen, and plasminogen, and mean (SD) basal and stimulated D-dimer in 12 patients with idiopathic osteonecrosis and in 18 patients with secondary osteonecrosis. t test, secondary vs. idiopathic, *$P \leq .01$, #$P \leq .001$. In parentheses, paired t test basal vs. stimulated, within group. (*)$P \leq .01$, (#)$P \leq .001$. The 10th–90th percentile normal range [6] is also displayed.

cant correlation was between Lp(a) and stimulated tPA-Fx (r = .75; P = .01).

DISCUSSION

Central to the regulation of fibrinolysis is the interplay between the major fibrinolysis inhibitor, PAI, and its major stimulator, tPA-Fx [6–17]. Previously we reported a single patient with idiopathic osteonecrosis (patient 1 in the current study) who had familial elevations of PAI-Fx and PAI-Ag and failed to increase tPA-Fx normally and initiate fibrinolysis after venous occlusion [6,7]. We speculated that hypofibrinolysis could cause inadequate lysis of venous thrombi in bone, obstruction of bone venous drainage, and venous hypertension of bone leading to osteonecrosis [1–6].

Stimulated by our initial single case observation [6,7], we studied 30 patients with idiopathic and acquired osteonecrosis in the current report to determine how frequently primary elevations of PAI with subsequent hypofibrinolysis might cause idiopathic osteonecrosis of the hip. Nine of 12 patients with idiopathic osteonecrosis of the hip (including our initial patient [6,7]) had primary/familial elevations of PAI-Fx and/or PAI-Ag, low tPA-Fx, and inability to activate fibrinolysis. There were no diseases (malignancies, severe hypertriglyceridemia, chronic infection or inflammation, etc.) or drugs that could explain the high PAI-Fx, high PAI-Ag, or low tPA-Fx in these nine patients [6,9,11,15,16]. In the 12 patients with idiopathic osteonecrosis, the higher the stimulated PAI-Ag and PAI-Fx, the lower were the stimulated tPA-Fx levels (P = .005, .005), but these close inverse correlations were not present in the 18 patients with secondary osteonecrosis (P = .11, .09). Moreover, change from basal to stimulated PAI-Ag was a significant inverse predictor of change from basal to stimulated tPA-Fx in the 12 patients with idiopathic osteonecrosis but not in the 18 patients with secondary osteonecrosis. Presumably, this reflects the marked binding of tPA-Fx by the extraordinarily high PAI in the patients with idiopathic osteonecrosis, so that, after venous occlusion, tPA-Fx was complexed with PAI and could not be released to initiate fibrinolysis.

Three of the 12 patients with idiopathic osteonecrosis had normal PAI-Fx and normally activated tPA-Fx. However, they, along with 14 of the 18 patients with secondary osteonecrosis, unexpectedly had high Lp(a). One of the four patients with secondary osteonecrosis who had normal Lp(a) was found to have a previously undiagnosed low protein C, a known thrombophilic state [28]. Mean Lp(a) was 3.75 times higher in patients with secondary than with idiopathic osteonecrosis. High Lp(a) or possibly low protein C might thus play a major pathophysiologic role in secondary osteonecrosis and in those patients with idiopathic osteonecrosis who have normal PAI and stimulated tPA-Fx. Lp(a), by virtue of its striking homology with plasminogen [29,30] plays an antifibrinolytic role in vitro by competing with plasminogen for plasminogen receptors [29–33]. In vivo, however, Lp(a) has not yet been shown to interfere with either basal or stimulated fibrinolysis [9,34,35]. We have previously reported higher Lp(a) (28 mg/dl) in patients with a history of thrombophlebitis than in patients without such a history (15 mg/dl) [9]. Although we did not find hypofibrinolysis in vivo in the 14 patients with high Lp(a) and secondary osteonecrosis, nor in the three patients with high Lp(a) and idiopathic osteonecrosis, perhaps the limited venous drainage of the femoral head facilitates the putative hypofibrinolytic effect of high Lp(a) or the prothrombotic effect of protein C deficiency [28]. Within this frame of reference, it has been suggested that pediatric osteonecrosis (Legg-Perthe's diesease) may be caused by intravascular thrombosis due to reduced fibrinolysis [36]. For eight pediatric and young adult patients with Legg-Perthe's disease, we have recently reported that three had familial protein C deficiency, one had familial protein S deficiency, and one could not elevate tPA-Fx after venous occlusion [37]. Familial thrombophilia (protein C, protein S deficiency) or hypofibrinolysis presumably facilitates thrombotic venous occlusion of the femur, with subsequent venous hypertension and bone death, which characterize Legg-Perthes disease [37].

Prospective Lp(a) and protein C measurements should be made in patients with subcapital hip fractures that are pinned, to see whether most of those who subsequently develop secondary osteonecrosis (secondary to the fracture) have high Lp(a) or low protein C, while those who remain free of subsequent osteonecrosis have predominantly normal Lp(a) and protein C. High Lp(a) or low protein C might also predict increased risk for secondary osteonecrosis in patients with other causes of secondary osteonecrosis [lupus, corticosteroids, alcoholism, sickle cell disease, etc. (1)]. High PAI may prospectively predict increased risk of idiopathic osteonecrosis.

The current study strongly suggests that hypofibrinolysis mediated by primary high PAI may cause idiopathic osteonecrosis and that high Lp(a) or low protein C [28] may play an etiologic role in secondary osteonecrosis. We postulate that high PAI or high Lp(a) leads to inadequate lysis of venous thrombi in bone, impaired bone venous circulation, venous hypertension of bone, and subsequent development of osteonecrosis [1–5].

Since PAI can be reduced and fibrinolytic activity increased by the anabolic steroid stanozolol [38,39], we speculate that, when primary osteonecrosis is diagnosed early, prior to segmental collapse of the femoral head, it may be possible to treat defective fibrinolysis and, hence, to arrest progression or induce regression of osteonecrosis of the hip [40]. In a pilot study, we have given stanozolol (6 mg/day) to three of our nine patients with primary high PAI, inability to initiate fibrinolysis, and idiopathic osteonecrosis. In two patients, after 12 weeks of therapy, PAI-Ag and PAI-Fx were normalized, and stimulated tPA-Fx became normal [40]. Unexpectedly, but encouragingly, after 12 weeks of treatment, one of these two patients, who had been able to walk painfully for only one block prior to treatment, walked 2 miles every day despite radiographic progression of osteonecrosis [40].

ACKNOWLEDGMENTS

This study was supported by Jewish Hospital Medical Research Council grants 738 and 2728.

REFERENCES

1. Mankin JH: Nontraumatic necrosis of bone (osteonecrosis). N Engl J Med 326:1473–1479, 1992.
2. Jones JP: Intravascular coagulation and osteonecrosis. Clin Orthop Rel Res 277:41–54, 1992.
3. Rutishauser E, Rhoner A, Held D: Experimentelle untersuchungen uber die wirkung der ischamie auf den knochen und das mark. Virchow Arch Pathol Anat 333:101–118, 1960.
4. Atsumi T, Kuroki Y, Yamano K: A microangiographic study of idiopathic osteonecrosis of the femoral head. Clin Orthop 246:186–194, 1989.
5. Jones JP JR: Osteonecrosis. In McCarty D (ed): "Arthritis and Allied Conditions: A Textbook of Rheumatology, 11th Ed. Philadelphia: Lea and Febiger, 1989, pp 1545–1562.
6. Glueck CJ, Glueck HI, Mieczkowski L, et al.: Familial high plasminogen activator inhibitor with hypofibrinolysis, a new pathophysiologic cause of osteonecrosis? Thromb Haemostas 69:460–465, 1993.
7. Glueck CJ, Freiberg R, Glueck HI, Stroop D, Tracy T: High plasminogen activator inhibitor activity and antigen and hypofibrinolysis, a cause of osteonecrosis? Clin Res 41:309A (abstract), 1993.

8. Nilsson IM, Krook H, Sternby H-H, Söderberg E, Söderström N: Severe thrombotic disease in a young man with bone marrow and skeletal changes and with a high content of an inhibitor in the fibrinolytic system. Acta Med Scand 169:323–337, 1961.
9. Glueck CJ, Glueck HI, Tracy T, Speirs J, McCray C, Stroop D: Relationships between lipoprotein(a), lipids, apolipoproteins, basal and stimulated fibrinolytic regulators, and D-dimer. Metabolism 42: 236–246, 1993.
10. Jorgenson M, Bonnevie-Nielsen V: Increased concentration of fast-acting plasminogen activator in plasma associated with familial venous thrombosis. Br J Haematol 65:175–180, 1987.
11. Patrassi GM, Sartori MT, Saggiorato G, Boeri G, Girolami A: Familial Thrombophilia associated with high levels of plasminogen activator inhibitor. Fibrinolysis 6:99–105, 1992.
12. Nilsson IM, Tengborn L: Impaired fibrinolysis. New evidence in relation to thrombosis. In Jespersen J, Kluft C, Korsgaard O (eds): "Clinical Aspects of Fibrinolysis and Thrombolysis." Esbjerg: South Jutland University Press, 1983, pp 273–291.
13. Pizzo SV, Fuchs HE, Doman KA, Petruska DB, Berger H: Release of tissue plasminogen activator and its fast-acting inhibitor in defective fibrinolysis. Arch Intern Med 146:188–191, 1986.
14. Engesser L, Brommer EGP, Kluft C, Briet E: Elevated plasminogen activator inhibitor (PAI), a cause of thrombophilia? A study in 203 patients with familial or sporadic venous thrombophilia. Thromb Hemostas 62:673–680, 1989.
15. Newland JR, Haire WD: Elevated plasminogen activator inhibitor levels found in patients with malignant conditions. Am J Clin Pathol 96:602–604, 1991.
16. Juhan-Vague I, Alessi MC, Vague P: Increased plasma plasminogen activator inhibitor 1 levels. A possible link between insulin resistance and atherothrombosis. Diabetologia 34:457–462, 1991.
17. Wiman B, Hamsten A: The fibrinolytic enzyme system and its role in the etiology of thrombo-embolic disease. Semin Thromb Haemostas 26:207–216, 1990.
18. Myers GL, Cooper Gr, Winn CL, Smith SJ: The Centers for Disease Control-National Heart, Lung and Blood Institute Lipid Standardization Program. An approach to accurate and precise lipid measurements. Clin Lab Med 9:105–135, 1989.
19. Allain C, Poon LS, Chan CSG, Richmond W, Fu PC: Enzymatic determination of total serum cholesterol. Clin Chem 20:470–475, 1974.
20. McGowan MW, Artiss JD, Strandbergh DR, Zak B: A peroxidase-coupled method for the colorimetric determination of serum triglycerides. Clin Chem 29:538–543, 1983.
21. Assman G, Schriewer H, Schmitz G, Hagele EO: Quantification of high density lipoprotein cholesterol by precipitation with phosphotungstic acid/$MgCl_2$. Clin Chem 29:2026–30, 1983.
22. Friedwald WT, Levy RI, Frederickson DS: Estimation of the concentration of low density lipoprotein cholesterol in plasma without use of the preparative ultra centrifuge. Clin Chem 18:499–502, 1972.
23. Glueck CJ, McCray C, Speirs J: Measurement of serum Apo A1 and Apo B: comparison of immunoturbidimetric and rate nephelometric techniques. Clin Chim Acta 197:123–132, 1991.
24. Silberman S, Armentrout M, Vella F, Saha A: Macra Lp(a) for quantitation of human lipoprotein (a) by enzymes. Clin Chem 36:961, 1990 [Macra Lp(a) Enzyme Immunoassay Kit; catalog No. D306; Terumo Medical Corp., Elkton, MD].
25. Imubind Protein C Strip-Well American Diagnostica, Inc., Greenwich, CT, 1992.
26. Shapiro SS, Wilk MB: An analysis of variance test for normality (complete samples). Biometrika 52:591–611, 1965.
27. Snedecor GW, Cochran WG: "Statistical Methods, 7th Ed." Ames Iowa, IA: State University Press, 1980.
28. Bick RC, Ucar K: Hypercoagulability and thrombosis. Hematol Oncol Clin North Am 6:1421–1431, 1992.
29. Edelberg JM, Pizzo SV: Lipoprotein (a) inhibits plasminogen activation in a template-dependent manner. Blood Coagulation Fibrinolysis 2:759–764, 1991.
30. McLean JW, Tomlinson JE, Kuang WJ, et al.: A DNA sequence of human apolipoprotein(a) is homologous to plasminogen. Nature 300: 132–137, 1987.
31. Scanu AM, Fless GM: Lipoprotein (a) heterogeneity and biologic relevance. J Clin Invest 85:1709–1715, 1990.
32. Heinrich J, Sandkamp M, Kokoh R, Schulte H, Assman G: Relationship of lipoprotein (a) to variables of coagulation and fibrinolysis in a healthy population. Clin Chem 37:1950–1954, 1991.
33. Scanu AM: Lipoprotein(a) a potential bridge between the fields of atherosclerosis and thrombosis. Arch Pathol Lab Med 112:1045–1047, 1988.
34. Garcia Frade LG, Alvarez JJ, Rayo I, et al.: Fibrinolytic parameters and lipoprotein(a) levels in plasma of patients with coronary artery disease. Thromb Res 63:407–418, 1991.
35. Alessi MC, Parra HJ, Joly P, et al.: The increased plasma Lp(a) lipoprotein particle concentration in angina pectoris is not associated with hypofibrinolysis. Clin Chim Acta 188:119–128, 1990.
36. Gregosiewicz A, Okonski M, Stoecka D, et al.: Ischemia of the femoral head in Perthe's disease: Is the cause intra- or extravascular. J Pediatr Orthop 9:160–162, 1989.
37. Glueck CJ, Greenfield D, Freiberg R, Glueck HI, Kahn A, Hamer T, Stroop D: Protein C deficiency, protein S deficiency, and hypofibrinolysis, pathophysiologic etiologies of Legg-Perthes syndrome. Clin Res 41:649A, 1993.
38. Small M, Lowe GDO, MacCuish AC, Forbes DC: The effects of oral stanozolol on fibrinolysis in type 2 diabetes mellitus. Thromb Res 44:253–259, 1986.
39. Kluft C, Preston FE, Malia RG, et al.: Stanozolol-induced changes in fibrinolysis and coagulation in healthy adults. Thromb Hemostas 51: 157–164, 1984.
40. Glueck CJ, Freiberg R, Glueck HI, Stroop D, Tracy T, Hamer T: Idiopathic osteonecrosis, hypofibrinolysis, high lipoprotein(a), and therapy with stanozolol. Clin Res 41:661A, 1993.
41. Cholesterol Adult Treatment Panel Report: Report of the National Cholesterol Education Program expert panel on detection, evaluation, and treatment of high blood cholesterol in adults. Arch Intern Med 148:36–69, 1988.
42. NIH Consensus Conference: Triglycerides, high density lipoprotein, and coronary heart disease. JAMA 269:505–510, 1993.

American Journal of Hematology 45:167–170 (1994)

Skin Manifestation of Agnogenic Myeloid Metaplasia

Gabriel Loewy, Anna Mathew, and Ariel Distenfeld
Division of Hematology, Department of Medicine, Cabrini Medical Center, New York, New York

Agnogenic myeloid metaplasia (AMN) with myelofibrosis is a clonal malignancy of the hematopoietic stem cell. The disease is characterized by increased endothelial cell and fibroblast proliferation, resulting in increased deposition of fibronectin, laminin, and collagen in the bone marrow. In advanced disease, extramedullary hematopoiesis (EMH) is invariably seen in the spleen and liver. The lymph nodes are also frequent sites of EMH, but other organs, especially the kidneys, arenals, lungs, pleura, ovaries, gastrointestinal tract, and dura, may also be involved. Skin manifestations are rare. They may present in several ways: erythematous plaques, nodules, diffuse or papular erythema, ulcers, and bullae. Histopathology of these lesions reveals cells from one or more myeloid lineage in the dermis, erythroid, or megakaryocytic series alone or in combination. In rare cases, all three cell lines are demonstrated.

Key words: extramedullary hematopoiesis, hematopoiesis, stem cell, dermis, myelofibrosis

INTRODUCTION

Agnogenic myeloid metaplasia (AMM) with myelofibrosis is a clonal malignancy of the hematopoietic stem cell [1]. The disease is characterized by increased endothelial cell and fibroblast proliferation, resulting in increased deposition of fibronectin, laminin, and collagen in the bone marrow [1]. In advanced disease, extramedullary hematopoiesis (EMH) is invariably seen in the spleen and liver [2]. The lymph nodes are also frequent sites of EMH, but other organs, especially the kidneys, adrenals, lungs, pleura, ovaries, gastrointestinal tract, and dura, may also be involved. [2]. The skin, being a participant in embryonic hematopoiesis, may retain this capacity in adults under some conditions, including myeloid metaplasia; however, a review of the literature reveals this to be rare [3,4]. The skin manifestations may present in several ways: erythematous: erythematous plaques, nodules, diffuse or papular erythema, ulcers, and bullae [5]. We present four cases of AMM and skin lesions consistent with EMH.

CASE 1

An 84-year-old white man was evaluated for anemia. His white blood cell count was 10×10^{10} cells/liter with neutrophils 35%, bands 12%, metamyelocytes 6%, myelocytes 11%, promyelocytes 3%, blasts 25%, and lymphocytes 8%. The hematocrit was 30% and the platelet count 150×10^{10}/liter. A bone marrow aspirate and biopsy were consistent with extensive myelofibrosis (Figs. 1, 2). Cytogenetic studies on marrow revealed no growth and no mitosis. DNA probe for Philadelphia chromosome was not done. On physical examination, the most striking findings were multiple skin nodules, including nodules on the extremities, pinkish to red in color and soft and nontender in consistency. The only other physical finding was the presence of splenomegaly. Since the diagnosis 3 years ago, the patient has been treated with blood transfusions every 2–3 months.

CASE 2

A 71-year-old white woman was admitted to the hospital secondary to fever. On admission, her white blood cell count was 41.6×10^{10} cells/liter, with neutrophils 38%, bands 30%, metamyelocytes 21%, myelocytes 7%, promyelocytes 7%, and blasts 1%. The hematocrit was 27.7% and the platelet count 301×10^{10}/liter. A bone marrow aspirate and biopsy were consistent with myeloid metaplasia and myelofibrosis. There was no growth on

Received for publication February 15, 1993; accepted June 30, 1993.

Address reprint requests to Ariel Distenfeld, MD, Division of Hematology and Blood Bank, Cabrini Medical Center, 227 East 19th Street, New York, NY 10003.

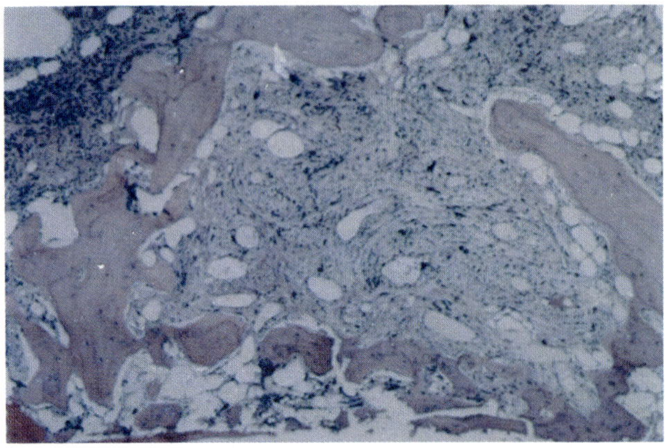

1

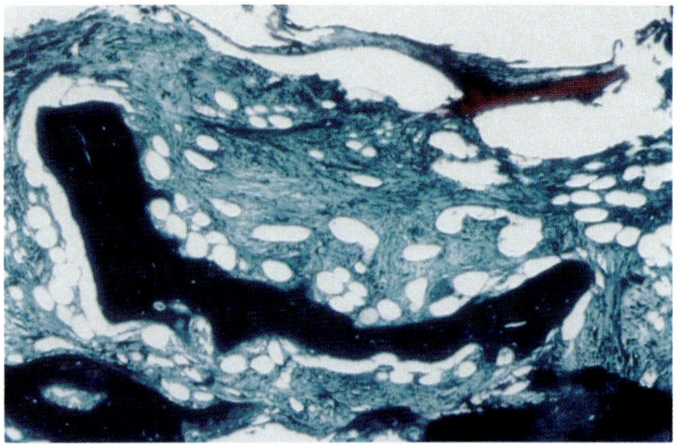

2

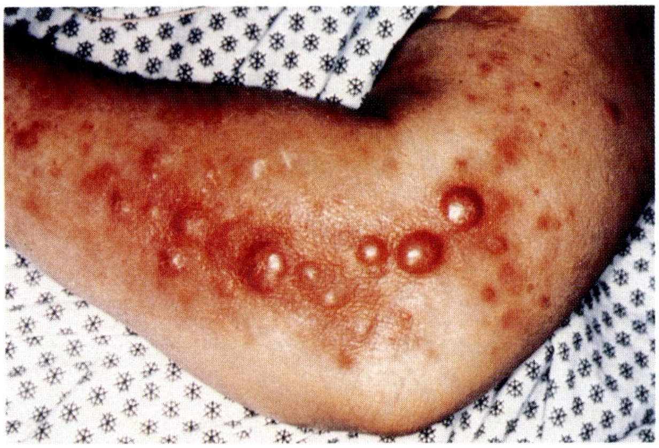

3

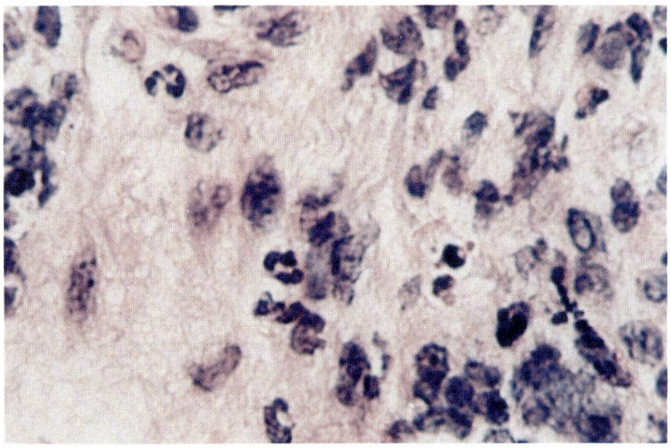

4

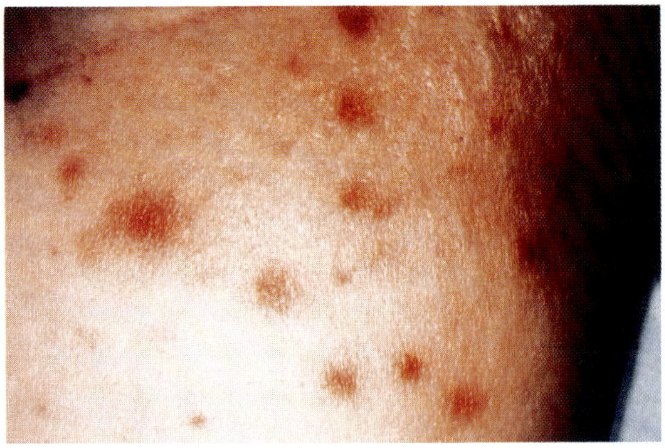

5

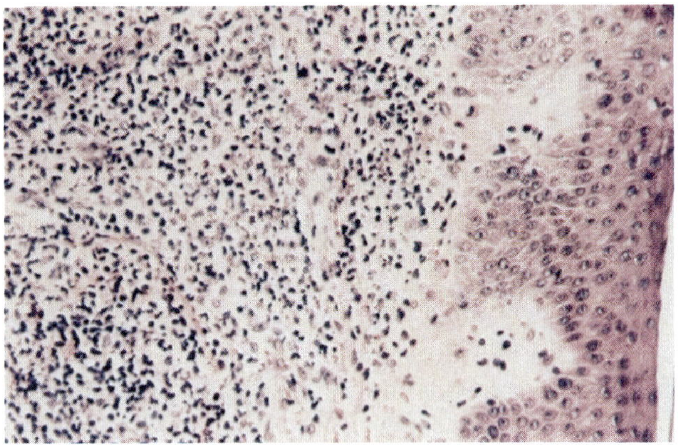

6

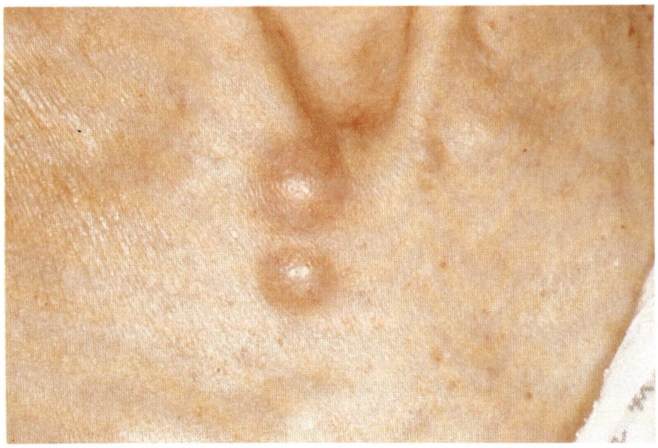

7

FIGURE GUIDE

1. Bone marrow biopsy (Hematoxylin-Eosin X400)
2. Bone marrow biopsy (Trichrome X400)
3. Skin lesions (Gross)
4. Histopathology of skin lesions (Hematoxylin-Eosin X1000)
5. Skin lesions (Gross)
6. Histopathology of skin lesions (Hematoxylin-Eosin X400)
7. Skin lesions (Gross)

culture. The Philadelphia chromosome was not found. DNA probe was not available at the time. Busulfan and Danazol were started; this therapeutic regimen over several months did not achieve improvement in the hematologic status. She was readmitted for splenectomy, necessitated by increasing splenic size and transfusion requirement.

Histopathology of the spleen revealed extramedullary hematopoiesis. Postsplenectomy, the hematologic parameters did not improve. Increasing diffuse lymphadenopathy was noted. A biopsy of one of the nodes revealed extramedullary hematopoiesis. Subsequently, due to increasing refractory anemia and thrombocytopenia, bone marrow curettage was done from the anterior iliac crest, without benefit. Shortly thereafter, red, raised, nodular-appearing nontender lesions were noted over both upper extremities (Fig. 3). Biopsy of one of the lesions was consistent with extramedullary hematopoiesis (Fig. 4). Marker and cytogenetic studies were not obtained on the skin lesion biopsy. Her condition after the appearance of the lesions rapidly deteriorated, with increasing hepatomegaly and abdominal and pelvic lymphadenopathy. She died 52 months after initial diagnosis of AMM.

CASE 3

A 68-year-old white man was evaluated for pancytopenia. The white blood cell count was 3.3×10^{10} cells/liter with neutrophils 47%, metamyelocytes 14%, myelocytes 16%, promyelocytes 10%, and lymphocytes 13%. The hematocrit was 12.7% and the platelet count 10×10^{10}/liter. Bone marrow aspirate and biopsy revealed a hypocellular marrow, with a decreased M:E ratio. Erythropoiesis was megaloblastic, and the megakaryocytes were decreased in number. Diffuse fibrosis was present and there was no growth in culture. The Philadelphia chromosome was not present. DNA probe was not available at the time. The patient required red blood cell and platelet transfusions every 2–6 weeks; a splenectomy did not improve the hematologic status. Histopathology of the spleen and a liver biopsy revealed extramedullary hematopoiesis. A subsequent bone marrow curettage from the anterior iliac crest was also performed, without benefit. Two weeks after the curettage, a generalized maculopapular rash developed, followed by red, nontender skin nodules over the trunk (Fig. 5).

Biopsy of one of the nodules was consistent with neutrophilic infiltrate (Fig. 6). Marker and cytogenetic studies were not performed on the skin biopsy. Red cell and platelet support was continued for several months, until an accidental fall was followed by confusion and right-side hemiparesis. A computed tomographic scan of the head revealed a large infarct. The patient rapidly deteriorated and died 16 months after the initial diagnosis of AMM.

Fig. 1–7. Bone marrow biopsy results and histopathology and gross appearance of skin lesions.

CASE 4

A 66-year-old white woman with an 18 month history of myeloproliferative disease was treated initially with various alklayting agents. Due to weekly platelet and red cell transfusion requirements as well as enlarging splenic size, she was admitted for splenectomy. On physical examination, a massively enlarged spleen was palpatede. Raised, purple, nontender nodules over the chest were noted (Fig. 7); clinically, these lesions were consistent with sites of EMH. Pathologic examination was unavailable. The white blood cell count was 0.8×10^{10}/liter, with neutrophils 40%, metamyelocytes 11%, myelocytes 15%, and blasts 25%. DNA probe for the break cluster region of the Philadelphia chromosome was negative. Histopathology of the spleen was consistent with EMH. Postsplenectomy, her condition rapidly deteriorated, and she died 19 months after the initial diagnosis.

DISCUSSION

The four patients reported here were seen over an 8 year span (1984–1992). During this same period, 139 patients with myelofibrosis and/or myeloproliferative disorders were seen at Cabrini Medical Center.

Marrow curettage was performed only on the two patients reported herein. Splenectomy was performed for five patients, including three described here. Other surgery was performed on eight patients.

From our own data and from reviewing the literature, it is not possible to determine the true incidence of skin involvement in myelofibrosis and myeloid metaplasia. We can state, however, that it appears to be uncommon. We were able to find 21 cases in the literature [6], excluding those with neutrophilic dermatosis (Sweet's syndrome and pyoderma gangrenosum). These include 20 cases cited by Hoss and McNutt [6] as well as their own case.

In the report by Mizoguchi et al. [5], 14 of the same cases are reviewed and information is provided regarding splenectomy. Nine of the 14 were not splenectomized, and five of the 14 were. No clear-cut relationship could be established between splenectomy and the appearance of the skin lesions. Three of our cases were splenectomized, and one was not. However, in one of them (case 4), the skin lesions preceded the splenectomy. In some cases reported in the literature, skin infiltration appeared in the splenectomy scar shortly after surgery [7]. However, many patients with myelofibrosis are splenectomized without any cutaneous complications. We were not able to find information regarding the effect of other types of surgery on extramedullary hematopoiesis and myeloid metaplasia in the skin.

It is well established that hematopoietic stem cells circulate in the peripheral blood. This fact is taken advantage of with peripheral stem cell harvesting for bone marrow transplantation. When reinfused, the stem cells home to and colonize the marrow space. The mechanism is unknown, but it may be due to attachment to stroma by adhesive integrin molecules and the effect of cytokine production by stroma cells. It is known that in myelofibrosis there is an increase in circulating hematopoietic stem cells [8,9]. These usually establish extramedullary hematopoiesis in liver and spleen. It is not known why in rare cases they produce metaplasia in the skin. This is a clonal disease, and it is possible that in some cases the clone cells have surface markers that recognize and adhere to skin collagen. The study of Kobavashi et al. [10] in which a myeloid cell line established from a patient with myelofibrosis exhibited binding to skin fibroblasts, while other myeloid cell lines did not, suggests that such a mechanism may be operative.

We were unable to obtain complete karyotypes from all patients due to marrow fibrosis. No marker or genetic studies were done on the skin biopsies. Hence we can only presume the clonality of the skin lesions.

Whereas neutrophils are known to exhibit tropism and chemotaxis to several antigens and chemicals, nothing is known about such tropism for hematopoietic stem cells. In neutrophilic dermatosis, mature neutrophils infiltrate the skin without vasculitis or infection. Our case 3 showed a pure neutrophilic infiltrate, while the other cases had true metaplasia. Other cases of neutrophilic dermatosis have been reported in association with hematological malignancies and with myelofibrosis [11]. The underlying pathophysiology may or may not be similar to myeloid metaplasia in the skin.

It is tempting to speculate that marrow curettage stimulated release of stem cells into the circulation. However, only two of our cases were treated in this way. There are no reports of curetted cases preceding skin involvement. We are not able to establish any association between marrow curettage and cutaneous myeloid metaplasia.

In summary, we report four cases of skin involvement in myeloid metaplasia. Our purpose is mainly to acquaint and to alert practicing hematologists to the presence of this complication so that it can be recognized and properly managed.

REFERENCES

1. Wolf BC, Neiman RS: Myelofibrosis with myeloid metaplasia: Pathophysiological implications of the correlation between marrow changes and progression of splenomegaly. Blood 65:803, 1985.
2. Ward HP, Block MH: The natural history of agnogenic myeloid metaplasia (AMM) and a critical evaluation of its relationship with the myeloproliferative syndrome. Medicine. 50:357–420, 1971.
3. Hocking WG, Lazar GS, Lipsett JA, Busuttil RW: Cutaneous extramedullary hematopoiesis following splenectomy for idiopathic myelofibrosis. Am J Med 76:957–959, 1984.
4. Tseng-tong K, Uhlemann J, Reinhard EH: Cutaneous extramedullary hematopoiesis. Arch Dermatol 112:1302–1303, 1976.
5. Mizoguchi M., Kawa Y, Minami T, Nakayama H, Mizoguchi H: Cutaneous extramedullary heamtopoiesis in myelofibrosis. J Am Acad Dermatol 22:351–355, 1990.
6. Hoss DM, McNutt NS: Cutaneous myelofibrosis. J Cutaneous Pathol 19:221–225, 1992.
7. Hocking WG, Lazar GS, Lipsett JA, Busuttil RW: Cutaneous extramedullary hematopoiesis following splenectomy for idiopathic myelofibrosis. Am J Med 76:956–958, 1984.
8. Chervenick PA: Increase in circulating stem cells in patients with myelofibrosis. Blood 41:67–71, 1973.
9. Chikkappa G, Carsten AL, Chanana AD, Chandra P, Crankite EP: Increased granulocytic, erythrocytic and megakaryocytic progenitors in myelofibrosis with myeloid metaplasia. Am J Hematol 4:121–131, 1978.
10. Kobavashi M, Inanura M, Soga R, Tsudd Y, Maeda S, Iwasaki H, Sugiura M, Ohizumi H, Musashi M, Morioka M, Okabe M, Sakuraada K, Kasai M, Miyazaki T: Establishment of a novel granulocytic sarcoma cell line which can adhere to dermal fibroblasts from a patient with granulocytic sarcoma in dermal tissues and myelofibrosis. Br J Hematol 82:26–31, 1992.
11. Caughman W, Stern R, Haynes H: Neutrophilic dermatosis of myeloproliferative disorders. J Am Acad Dermatol 9:751–758, 1983.

American Journal of Hematology 45:171–176 (1994)

Primary Amyloidosis Associated With a Novel Heavy-Chain Fragment (AH Amyloidosis)

Alan Solomon, Deborah T. Weiss, and Charles Murphy
Human Immunology & Cancer Program, Department of Medicine, University of Tennessee Medical Center/Graduate School of Medicine, Knoxville, Tennessee

Primary or AL amyloidosis occurs in patients with monoclonal plasma cell-related disorders and is typically associated with the systemic deposition as amyloid fibrils of the light-chain portion of the immunoglobulin molecule. Recently, the discovery that heavy chains could be involved in amyloid formation led to the designation of this type of disease process as AH amyloidosis. We have now identified a second example of heavy chain-associated amyloidosis in a patient (MAD) who had a serum IgG monoclonal gammopathy and Bence Jones proteinuria. In this case, the renal and splenic amyloid deposits consisted solely of the V_H-D-encoded portion of the heavy polypeptide chain, in contrast to the first case, where the amyloid contained an immunoglobulin component composed of the entire heavy-chain variable and third constant domains. In this respect, the chemical composition of the amyloid protein MAD differed not only from that of the first reported case of AH amyloidosis but from all other structurally abnormal components found in patients with heavy chain-associated disease. The discovery that certain forms of heavy chains, as well as light chains, can form amyloid provides further information on the chemical basis of amyloidogenicity and the diverse nature of this disease.

Key words: plasma cell, immunoglobulin molecule, IgG monoclonal gammopathy, proteinuria

INTRODUCTION

Immunoglobulin (Ig) light chains or, more commonly, light-chain variable-region (V_L) fragments constitute the protein that forms the amyloid fibrils found in patients with "primary" or multiple myeloma-associated amyloidosis, i.e., AL amyloidosis [1,2]. Recently, it has been reported that this material can instead contain the heavy-chain portion of the Ig molecule. In the first such case described, we characterized an amyloid-associated Ig (protein ART) that consisted of an internally deleted, 20 kd IgG heavy chain. This component was composed of an entire heavy-chain variable region (V_H) (including the segments encoded by the heavy-chain, V_H, diversity *(D)*, and joining *(J_H)* genes) linked directly to the third γ heavy-chain constant domain ($C_\gamma 3$); lacking were the $C_\gamma 1$, hinge, and $C_\gamma 2$ domains [3]. This Ig-related form of amyloidosis has been designated AH amyloidosis [4].

We report here a second case of AH amyloidosis in a patient with extensive renal as well as systemic amyloid deposits and a plasma-cell dyscrasia associated with a monoclonal IgGκ serum protein and a urinary κ Bence Jones protein. Chemical characterization of the amyloid protein extracted from the kidney and spleen revealed that this material was composed solely of a V_H-D heavy-chain fragment identical in sequence to that of the corresponding heavy-chain portion of the intact monoclonal IgG molecule.

CASE REPORT

Patient MAD, a 59-year-old man who presented with nephrotic syndrome, was found through kidney biopsy to have glomerular deposits of amyloid. The patient had a 5 year documented history of hypertensive cardiovascular disease and 3 months prior to the kidney biopsy became anemic and nephrotic. The pertinent laboratory findings included hemoglobin concentration, 8.2 g/100 ml; pro-

Received for publication February 22, 1993; accepted June 30, 1993.

Address reprint requests to Alan Solomon, MD, University of Tennessee Medical Center, 1924 Alcoa Highway, Knoxville, TN 37920.

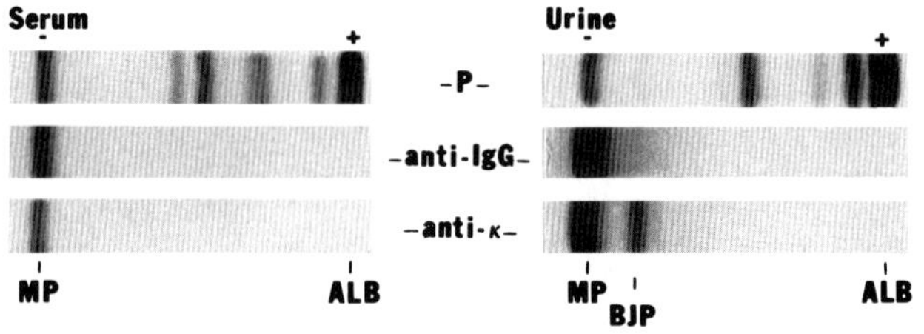

Fig. 1. Immunofixation electropherograms of serum and urine specimens from patient MAD. After electrophoresis on agarose membranes of a 1:5 dilution of serum and a 50 mg/ml solution of reconstituted, lyophilized urine, individual lanes were either chemically stained for protein (P) or were immunostained as indicated. The locations of the monoclonal IgGκ (MP), κ-type Bence Jones protein (BJP), and albumin (ALB) are indicated.

teinuria, ++++; serum albumin, 1.9 mg/100 ml; cholesterol, 326 mg/100 ml; and creatinine, 1.7 mg/100 ml. The 24 hr creatinine clearance was 100 ml/min. Serum protein electrophoresis revealed a monoclonal Ig component (0.4 g/100 ml) identified by immunofixation as an IgGκ protein (Fig. 1). The daily urine protein excretion was 20 g and consisted predominately of albumin in addition to other serum proteins, including the IgGκ component; a κ-type Bence Jones protein was also identified by immunofixation (Fig. 1). By quantitative ELISA employing a monoclonal antibody specific for free κ chains [5], 100 mg of this protein was excreted daily. The bone marrow contained ~10% plasma cells, some of which appeared binuclear and unusually large. The monoclonal nature of the atypical plasma cells was evidenced immunohistochemically using specific anti-IgG and anti-κ antisera. No osteolytic lesions were noted on skeletal X-ray survey. The renal biopsy specimen revealed extensive glomerular deposits of amyloid, but no Congophilic material was noted in the bone marrow and rectal mucosa. There was no clinical evidence of amyloid involvement of the heart, intestine, or peripheral nerves.

The patient's clinical course over the 42 months preceding his death was characterized by progressive renal insufficiency and an increase in the concentration of the serum and urinary monoclonal proteins. In an effort to reduce the synthesis of these components, the patient initially received chemotherapy consisting of alkeran and prednisone and then a combination of carmustine, cyclophosphamide, vincristine, alkeran, and prednisone. The amount and frequency of such treatments were limited due to poor bone marrow tolerance. Numerous red cell transfusions and erythropoietin injections were given for persistent anemia. In addition, recurrent deep femoral vein thrombophlebitis required continuous treatment with anticoagulants. The patient refused long-term hemodialysis and died due to sepsis and advanced uremia.

Postmortem examination revealed microscopic evidence of severe, extensive bilateral renal glomerular amyloidosis and sclerosis; minimal deposits of amyloid were found in the blood vessels of the heart, lung, thyroid, spleen, and adrenal glands. Immunohistochemical examination of the kidney using polyclonal and monoclonal anti-κ- and anti-λ-chain reagents failed to demonstrate the light-chain nature of the amyloid.

MATERIALS AND METHODS

Immunoglobulin and Amyloid Protein Isolation and Characterization

Serum specimens were stored at −70°C and 24 hr urine specimens were dialyzed extensively against distilled water and lyophilized. Agarose gel immunofixation analysis was performed using a panel of anti-γ, -α, and -μ heavy-chain and anti-κ and -λ light-chain antisera (Paragon Systems; Beckman). The monoclonal Ig components were isolated from rapidly thawed serum or water-reconstituted urine samples by zone electrophoresis on polyvinyl chloride-polyvinyl acetate blocks and further purified by gel filtration on acrylamide/agarose columns as previously described [6]. $F(ab')_2$ fragments of the monoclonal IgG protein were prepared by pepsin digestion [7]. Amyloid protein was extracted according to the method of Pras et al. [8] from 10 g portions of kidney and spleen that were obtained at autopsy and frozen in a −80°C freezer.

The purity and molecular mass of the monoclonal serum and urinary Igs, the amyloid proteins, and the pepsin-derived IgG $F(ab')_2$ fragments were determined by sodium dodecyl sulfate/polyacrylamide gel electrophoresis (SDS/PAGE) in the presence or absence of 2-mercaptoethanol. After SDS/PAGE, the proteins were transferred onto PVDF membranes, and the Ig composition was established by immunoblotting using polyclonal rabbit antisera specific for human heavy- and light-chain variable- and constant-region determinants. Included were reagents prepared in our laboratory against papain-derived Fc fragments of normal human IgG as well as κ- and λ-type Bence Jones proteins [6]. An antiserum that had been produced in rabbits against synthetic peptides encompassing the first framework region (FR1) characteristic of the V_H3 subgroup [9] was kindly furnished by Dr. Gregg J. Silverman, University of California, San Diego.

Sequence Analysis

Ten to twenty milligram samples of completely reduced and pyridylethylated amyloid and Ig proteins were cleaved chemically with cyanogen bromide and enzymatically with trypsin or a lysine-residue-specific proteinase (Endoproteinase Lys-C) as previously described [3]. Chemically and proteolytically derived peptides were separated by HPLC, and the amino acid composition of the isolated peptides was determined using an ABI 420A derivatizer and ABI 130A amino acid analyzer (Applied

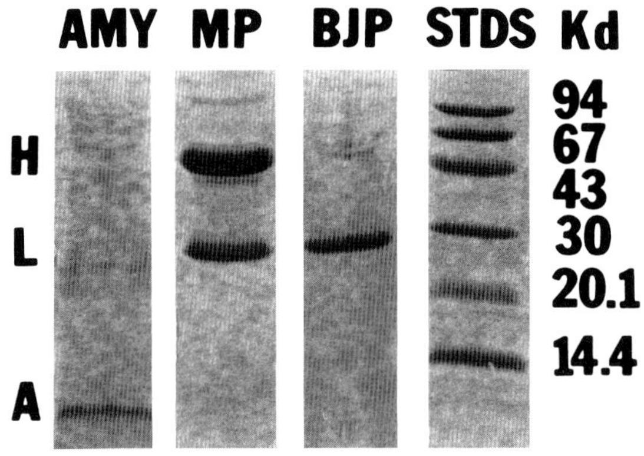

Fig. 2. Analyses by SDS/PAGE (reducing gel) of amyloid protein (AMY), monoclonal serum IgG (MP), and Bence Jones protein (BJP) from patient MAD. The location of the heavy (H) and light (L) chains and amyloid (A) component and the M_rs (kd) of the standard proteins (STDS) are indicated.

```
|---------------------------------------V_H---------------------------------------
|..............FR1...............|.......CDR1.......|.........FR2........|......CDR2......
          10        20        30        40        50        60
[ ]LVESGGGLVQPGGSLRLSCAASGFTFSNYAMSWVRQAPGKGLEWVSGITGSSGLTFY
++++++++++++++++++++++
                      <------- T1 ------><-T2><---------- T3 ---
                                              <-------- Ly1 ---

-----------------------V_H-------------------------|----D----|
..CDR2..|......................FR3......................|...CDR3...|
      70        80        90        100
ADSVKGRFTISRDNSKNTLSLHMNNLRADDTAVYYCAKALGSYN
------>                         <-- T4 ---><- T5>
---->< -- Ly2 --><-------- Ly3 ---------><-Ly4>
                         <------- CNBr ------>
```

Fig. 3. Primary structure of amyloid protein MAD. Residues marked by arrows were determined by automated amino acid sequencing of the undigested molecule. The remainder of the sequence was determined from peptides derived from enzymatic digestion with trypsin (T) or lysine-specific endoproteinase (Ly) and by cyanogen-bromide cleavage (CNBr). The absence of the three N-terminal residues is indicated by the brackets. The numbering system used is according to Kabat et al. [10], and the location of the segments encoded by the V_H and *D* genes and that of the framework and complementarity-determining regions (FR and CDR, respectively) are indicated.

Biosystems, Foster City, CA). Automated amino acid sequence analyses were performed with an ABI 477A gas-phase protein sequencer connected on line to an ABI 120A phenylthiohydantoin analyzer.

RESULTS

The material contained in the water-soluble extract of kidney as well as spleen had the characteristic tinctorial and ultrastructural features of amyloid [1]; namely, when viewed by polarizing microscopy after Congo red staining, it exhibited green birefringence; by electron microscopy, it consisted of 10 nm fibrils. The molecular mass of the amyloid extracts was determined by SDS/PAGE. Under reducing conditions (Fig. 2) and in the absence of a reducing agent (not illustrated), this material consisted of a relatively homogeneous component with a M_r of ~11 kd. The M_rs of the monoclonal IgG serum protein heavy and light chains (~55 and ~23 kd, respectively) were comparable to that of pooled normal IgG; the urinary Bence Jones protein had a M_r of ~23 kd.

That the amyloid fibrillary protein was heavy chain-related was evidenced through amino acid sequence analyses. The primary structure of amyloid protein MAD was established by automated analyses of the intact molecule and of the peptides derived from enzymatic and chemical cleavage of the completely reduced and pyridylethylated protein (Fig. 3). Amyloid protein MAD consisted of 101 residues; the first 93 were encoded by a V_H gene, while the remaining eight residues were the product of a *D* gene. That this protein consisted exclusively of a heavy chain-related component was apparent from the sequence of the first 20 amino acids. Except for the absence of three N-terminal residues, this sequence was characteristic of the first framework region (FR1) of the human Ig V_H3 subgroup [10].

The remainder of the primary structure of the 101-residue amyloid protein MAD was established though analyses of the peptides obtained from digestion with trypsin, lysine-specific endoproteinase, or cyanogen bromide. The correct ordering of these peptides was made possible by their overlapping nature and the availability of published V_H sequence data [10]. Five tryptic (T) peptides were isolated and sequenced. The first three–T1, T2, T3–included the last three FR1 residues, the first complementarity-determining region (CDR1), the entire FR2 and CDR2, and the first residue of FR3. The remaining two tryptic peptides (T4, T5) contained the last 11 FR3 and the first six CDR3 residues. From cleavage with the lysine-specific endoproteinase, four peptides were isolated—Ly1, Ly2, Ly3, Ly4; their sequences provided confirmation of the amino acids encompassing the last six residues of FR2 through the first six residues of the third CDR. The amyloid protein consisted of a single species, as demonstrated by the presence at the C-terminus of an asparagine found in peptides T5 and Ly4 as well as in the cyanogen-bromide peptide.

The structural relationship between the patient's amyloid protein and monoclonal serum IgG component was demonstrated through sequence analyses of the IgG heavy chain. One light chain- and three heavy chain-related peptides were obtained by cyanogen-bromide cleavage of the reduced and pyridylethylated $F(ab')_2$

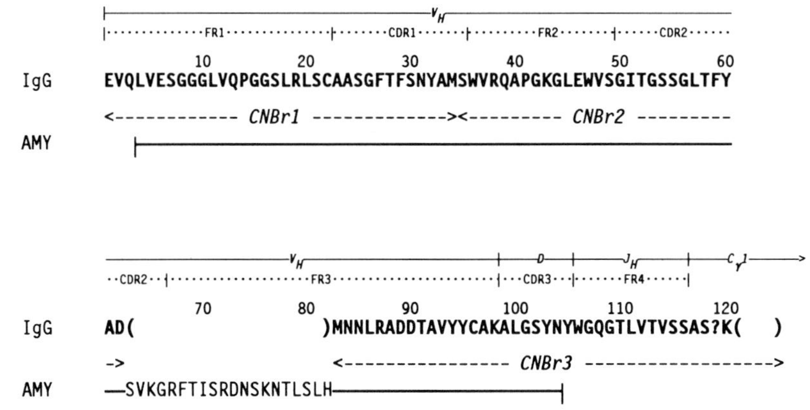

Fig. 4. Comparison of the primary structure of the IgG heavy chain (IgG) and amyloid protein (AMY) from patient MAD. The locations of the cyanogen-bromide (CNBr) peptides derived from cleavage of the IgG protein are indicated. The portion of the IgG heavy chain not sequenced is indicated by parentheses (? denotes residue not identified). Sequence identity between the amyloid protein and IgG heavy chain is denoted by a heavy solid line. The location of the segments encoded by the *V_H*, *D*, *J_H*, and first constant domain ($C_\gamma 1$) heavy-chain genes and of the framework and complementarity-determining regions (FR and CDR, respectively) are indicated.

fragment obtained by pepsin digestion of the IgG protein. The heavy-chain peptides–CNBr1, CNBr2, and CNBr3–encompassed the entire V_H region, including the V_H-, *D*-, and J_H-encoded segments. The amino acid sequence of the V_H and D portions of the IgG heavy-chain MAD was identical to that of the amyloid protein except for the presence of three N-terminal and one additional C-terminal residues (Fig. 4). The heavy chain contained a J_H segment characteristic of that encoded by the J_H4 gene [10]. Sequence analyses of cyanogen-bromide and trypsin peptides derived from the intact IgG protein established the complete nature of the γ heavy chain; i.e., these peptides contained residues typically present in the $C_\gamma1$, hinge, $C_\gamma2$, and $C_\gamma3$ portions of a prototype G1m(a) γ heavy chain of the IgG1 subclass [10].

The V_H3 heavy-chain nature of the amyloid protein derived from the kidney or spleen was also demonstrated in immunoblotting analyses. As is illustrated in Figure 5, this component was recognized by the anti-V_H3-specific antiserum but not by the anti-κ-chain or anti-Fc antisera. That the amyloid protein lacked γ heavy-chain constant-region (C_H) structure was evidenced by its lack of reactivity with an antiserum specific for the Fc portion of human IgG molecules. A similar analysis of the patient's monoclonal IgG protein showed that the heavy chains were also recognized by the specific anti-V_H3 antiserum but, in contrast to the amyloid protein, reacted with the anti-Fc antiserum. The IgG-derived light chains (as well as the urinary Bence Jones protein) reacted with the anti-κ-chain antiserum.

The κ-type Bence Jones protein MAD was classified serologically [6] as a member of the $V_{\kappa II}$ subgroup. This designation was confirmed through automated sequence analysis, which demonstrated that 45 of the first (N-terminal) 51 amino acid residues were identical to those encoded by the $V_{\kappa II}$ germline gene *A2* [10].

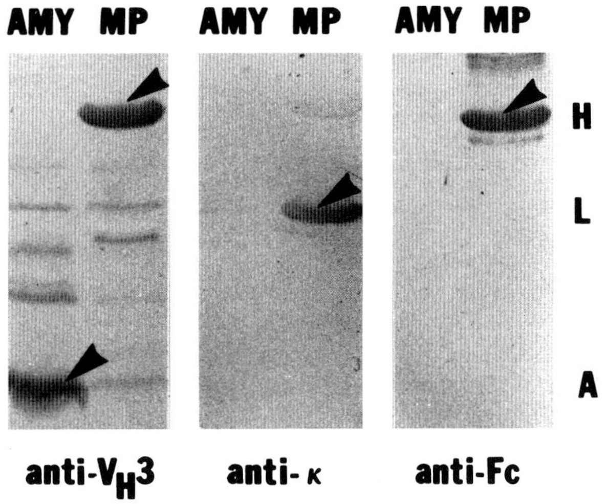

Fig. 5. Immunoblotting analyses of amyloid (AMY) and serum IgGκ (MP) proteins from patient MAD. The reactivity with the anti-V_H3, anti-κ, and anti-Fc antisera of the amyloid (A) and the IgG heavy (H) and light (L) chains are indicated by the arrows.

DISCUSSION

Serological and chemical characterization of the amyloid protein extracted from the kidney or spleen of a patient with systemic amyloidosis who had Bence Jones proteinuria and a serum IgG monoclonal protein established that this material was unexpectedly composed not of light chains but of a heavy chain-related component. This finding was demonstrated through amino acid sequence analyses that revealed the amyloid protein to consist of 101 residues, which included the V_H and D portions of the heavy chain; totally lacking were the J_H segment and the entire C_H region. The fragmentary nature of the amyloid protein was also evidenced by SDS/PAGE. This component had an unusually low M_r of ~11 kd vs. ~55 kd for a complete IgG heavy chain. Furthermore, the V_H3 nature of the amyloid protein evidenced from amino acid sequence was confirmed by immunoblotting experiments. As expected from its chemical composition, this component did not react with anti-Fc or anti-κ-chain antisera. The primary structure of amyloid protein MAD was identical to that of the V_H-D portion of the patient's monoclonal IgG protein, except that the latter had three N-terminal V_H residues and one extra C-terminal D residue (it is not known if this C-terminal tyrosyl residue represented a *D*-gene product or an N-region insertion [11]). Additionally, the IgG MAD heavy chain contained a J_H segment as well as the C_H region characteristic of a protein of the IgG1 subclass [10]. The molecular mass and reactivity with anti-Fc as well as anti-V_H3 antisera also indicated the intact nature of the IgG MAD heavy chain.

More than 80% of all patients with "primary" amyloidosis have a monoclonal gammopathy, most commonly manifested as Bence Jones proteinuria [12]. In such patients, the amyloid protein has been found to contain light chains or, more commonly, fragments corresponding to the entire V_L plus a portion of the light-chain constant region (C_L) [1]. Despite the presence of an apparently typical Bence Jones protein in patient MAD, the amyloid protein contained no light chains; rather, it was composed of a heavy-chain component structurally related to the patient's serum monoclonal IgG protein.

Amyloid protein MAD represented a novel heavy-chain disease-associated molecule. The presence of a virtually intact V_H-encoded region plus a D segment and the lack of J_H or C_H structure distinguished this protein not only from that of the first reported patient with AH amyloidosis [3] but from other cases of γ, α, or μ heavy-chain disease as well [13]. In the latter disorders, the heavy chains are truncated due to extensive V_H as well as C_H structural deletions resulting from either aberrant biosynthesis or postranslational proteolysis [14]. Whether amyloid protein MAD represented a synthetic product or was derived from proteolytic cleavage of the monoclonal IgG molecule remains to be determined. Since the formation of an Ig V_H domain results first from D-J_H-gene recombination followed by linkage of the fused product with a V_H gene [11], it is unlikely that this protein, which consists only of a V_H-D portion of the heavy chain, was formed de novo. The ragged nature of the N-terminus, which lacked up to three N-terminal residues, indicated some degree of proteolysis, as has been noted occasionally in light chain-related amyloid proteins [15]. The homogeneous nature of the heavy chain-related amyloid protein MAD was evidenced by a single C-terminal asparagine that represented the end of a six-residue segment encoded by an as yet unidentified *D* gene [10]. This unusually short D segment and the presence of an adjacent tyrosine in the IgG MAD heavy chain may have resulted in a tertiary structural conformation that rendered the IgG heavy chain unusually sensitive to an endopeptidase capable of cleaving the peptide bond between the asparaginyl and tyrosyl residues [16].

The specific chemical features responsible for the amyloidogenicity of protein MAD are presently unknown. Although the V_H-encoded segments of the two heavy-chain amyloid proteins, MAD and ART [3], were products of a V_H3-related gene, these components differed in the FR1, CDR1, FR2, and CDR2 regions by one, three, zero, and eight residues, respectively (the partial FR3 sequence data on protein ART precluded comparison with protein MAD), and had totally dissimilar D segments. The widely disparate structures of heavy-chain as well as light-chain and non-Ig forms of amyloid indicate the importance of other constituents, e.g., P component, proteoglycans, or amyloid enhancing factor [17], that initiate or facilitate the deposition of these proteins as amyloid. The ability to identify specific amyloidogenic peptides or residues [18,19] and to elucidate particular host factors involved in amyloid formation will further our understanding of the pathogenesis of this disease process.

In addition, the fact that heavy chain-related proteins can form amyloid fibrils raises the possibility that these components can also precipitate in basement membranes, resulting in "heavy-chain deposition disease." Thus heavy chains as well as light chains may be implicated in the pathogenesis of the monoclonal Ig deposition diseases [12].

ACKNOWLEDGMENTS

We thank Dr. Wahid T. Hanna for referral of patient MAD and Dr. Gregg J. Silverman for furnishing the anti-V_H3 antiserum. The helpful discussions with Dr. Blas Frangione, technical assistance of Teresa K. Williams, and manuscript preparation by Julie Ottinger are gratefully acknowledged. This work was supported in part by U.S. Public Health Research Grant CA 10056 from the National Cancer Institute. A.S. is an American Cancer Society Clinical Research Professor.

REFERENCES

1. Glenner GG: Amyloid deposits and amyloidosis: The β-fibrilloses. N Engl J Med 302:1283–1333, 1980.
2. Stone MJ: Amyloidosis: A final common pathway for protein deposition in tissues. Blood 75:531, 1990.
3. Eulitz M, Weiss DT, Solomon A: Immunoglobulin heavy-chain-associated amyloidosis. Proc Natl Acad Sci USA 87:6542, 1990.

4. Natvig JB, Førre Ø, Husby G, Husebekk A, Skogen B, Sletten K, Westermark P (eds): "Amyloid and Amyloidosis 1990. VIth International Symposium on Amyloidosis, August 5–8, 1990, Oslo, Norway." Dordrecht: Kluwer Academic Publishers, 1990.
5. Abe M, Goto T, Kennel SJ, Wolfenbarger D, Macy SD, Weiss DT, Solomon A: Production and immunodiagnostic applications of antihuman light chain monoclonal antibodies. Am J Clin Pathol 100:67, 1993.
6. Solomon A: Light chains of human immunoglobulins. Methods Enzymol 116:101, 1985.
7. Gorevic PD, Prelli FC, Frangione, B: Immunoglobulin Gn (IgG). Methods Enzymol 116:3, 1985.
8. Pras M, Shubert M, Zucker-Franklin D, Rimon A, Franklin EC: The characterization of soluble amyloid prepared in water. J Clin Invest 47:924, 1968.
9. Silverman GJ, Lucas AH: Variable region diversity in human circulating antibodies specific for the capsular polysaccharide of *Haemophilus influenzae*. Preferential usage of two types of VH3 heavy chains. J Clin Invest 88:911, 1991.
10. Kabat EH, Wu Tt, Perry HM, Gottesman KS, Foeller C: "Sequences of Proteins of Immunological Interest, Vol 1, 5th ed." Bethesda, MD: U.S. Department of Health and Human Services (PHS, NIH).
11. Pascual V, Capra JD: Human immunoglobulin heavy-chain variable region genes: Organization, polymorphism, and expression. Adv Immunol 49:1, 1991.
12. Buxbaum JN, Chuba JV, Hellmann GC, Gallo GR, Solomon A: Monoclonal immunoglobulin deposition disease: Light chain and light and heavy chain deposition diseases and their relation to light chain amyloidosis. Clinical features, immunopathology, and molecular analysis. Ann Intern Med 112:455, 1990.
13. Cogne M, Silvain C, Khamlichi AA, Preud'homme J-L: Structurally abnormal immunoglobulins in human immunoproliferative disorders. Blood 79:2181, 1992.
14. Alexander A, Ancito I, Buxbaum J: Gamma heavy chain disease in man. Genomic sequence reveals two noncontiguous deletions in a single gene. J Clin Invest 82:1244, 1988.
15. Eulitz M, Linke R: Amyloid fibrils derived from V-region together with C-region fragments from a λII-immunoglobulin light chain (HAR). Biol Chem Hoppe-Seyler 366:907, 1985.
16. Starkey PM: Elastase and cathespin G; the serine proteinases of human neutrophil leucocytes and spleen. In Barrett AJ (ed): "Proteinases in Mammalian Cells and Tissues." New York: Elsevier/North-Holland Biomedical Press, 1977.
17. Pepys MB: Amyloidosis. In Samter M, Talmage DW, Frank MM, Austen KF, Claman HN (eds): "Immunological Diseases, 4th ed." Boston: Little Brown & Co., 1988.
18. Castaño EM, Frangione B: Biology of disease. Human amyloidosis, Alzheimer disease and related disorders. Lab Invest 48:122, 1988.
19. Westermark P, Engström U, Johnson KH, Westermark GT, Betsholtz C: Islet amyloid polypeptide: Pinpointing amino acid residues linked to amyloid fibril formation. Proc Natl Acad Sci USA 87:5036, 1990.

American Journal of Hematology 45:177–180 (1994)

Treatment of Refractory Undifferentiated Acute Myelogenous Leukemia With All-*Trans*-Retinoic Acid

Jennifer J. Griggs, Susan E. Henley, and Jacob M. Rowe

Department of Medicine (J.J.G., S.E.H.) and Hematology Unit (J.M.R.), Strong Memorial Hospital, University of Rochester, Rochester, New York

A patient is described with undifferentiated acute myeloblastic leukemia refractory to two courses of daunorubicin and cytosine arabinoside. Because some the myeloblasts developed morphologic features of promyelocytes, the patient was treated with all-*trans*-retinoic acid (ATRA) in an attempt to promote maturation. Cytogenetic studies and sensitive molecular analysis did not reveal any abnormality classically associated with acute promyelocytic leukemia. Serial bone marrow biopsies demonstrated myeloid maturation, and the patient uneventfully went into a sustained complete remission. A review of the literature confirms this to be an apparently hitherto undescribed response to ATRA that may have therapeutic implications in similar patients.

Key words: all-trans-retinoic acid, undifferentiated acute myelogenous leukemia

INTRODUCTION

A variety of maturational agents, including all-*trans*-retinoic acid and 13-*cis*-retinoic acid, have been used in an attempt to induce the maturation of myeloblastic cells. Retinoids have been shown to effect maturation of the human promyelocytic cell line HL-60 into mature granulocytes, and clinical responses have been seen in patients with acute promyelocytic leukemia. Patients with acute myelogenous leukemia other than promyelocytic leukemia have not responded to such therapy. We report a patient with primary refractory undifferentiated myeloblastic leukemia who went into complete remission during treatment with all-*trans*-retinoic acid after failing therapy with two courses of daunorubicin and cytosine arabinoside.

CASE REPORT

A 68-year-old woman presented for therapy of acute myelogenous leukemia diagnosed after 8% blasts were seen on her peripheral blood smear. There was no history of fever, chills, easy bruisability, or weight loss. A bone marrow biopsy performed 6 months earlier had revealed morphologic abnormalities consistent with myelodysplasia. Her medical history was otherwise remarkable for unexplained syncope, severe osteoporosis with vertebral compression fractures, esophageal stenosis requiring dilatation, and hypertension. Physical examination revealed a thin but well-appearing woman with an Eastern Cooperative Oncology Group (ECOG) performance status of zero. The skin was without petechiae or ecchymoses. The remainder of the examination was also normal. Pretreatment bone marrow demonstrated 80% blasts and a complete absence of normal progenitors (French-American-British type M0) (Fig. 1). The double esterase stain was negative. Cell marker studies identified two cell populations of differing sizes, both $CD34^+$ and $HLA\text{-}DR^+$, consistent with undifferentiated leukemia. She was placed on a protocol of the Eastern Cooperative Oncology Group (ECOG EST 1490) and was treated with daunorubicin 60 mg/m^2 for 3 days and cytosine arabinoside 100 mg/m^2 for 7 days. Although with mildly decreased cellularity, the day 10 posttreatment bone marrow had 60–70% blasts; she was therefore given, as per protocol, a second course of daunorubicin and cytosine arabinoside (identical dosing schedule). The posttreatment bone marrow, analyzed on day 11 after the second course, again demonstrated no response, with 80% blasts and no significant change in cellularity.

Received for publication April 19, 1993; accepted August 18, 1993.

Address reprint requests to Jacob M. Rowe, MD, Hematology Unit, Box 610, University of Rochester Medical Center, 601 Elmwood Avenue, Rochester, NY 14642.

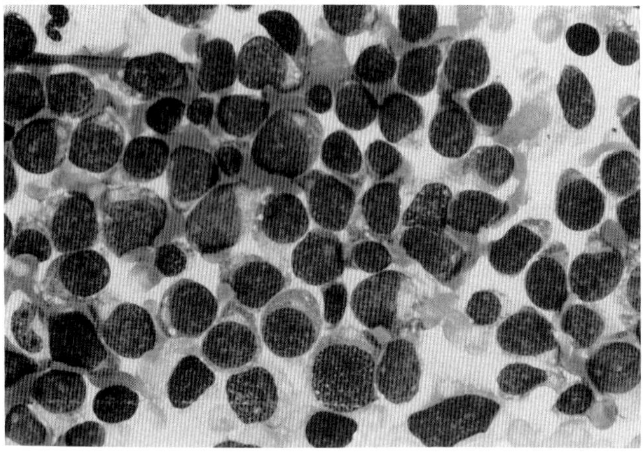

Fig. 1. Pretreatment bone marrow aspirate demonstrating undifferentiated myeloblasts.

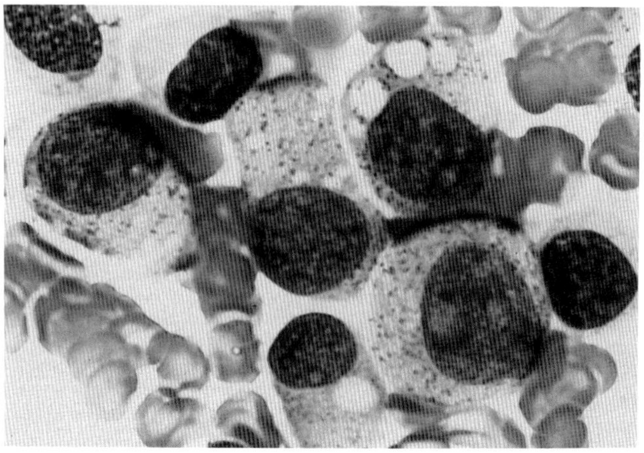

Fig. 2. Bone marrow aspirate after two full-dose courses of daunorubicin and cytosine arabinoside demonstrating blasts with promyelocytic granules. The marrow remained highly cellular.

Repeat bone marrow biopsy done 18 days after the second course of induction therapy had 60% blasts, but on this occasion a number of blasts appeared to have promyelocytic features (Fig. 2). These cells persisted on the marrow biopsy done 1 week later. Cytogenetic studies were normal with, specifically, the absence of the 15;17 translocation. In an attempt further to exclude a PML-RAR rearrangement, a reverse transcriptase polymerase chain reaction (RT-PCR) was performed using oligonucleotide primers known to border the 15;17 translocation breakpoint. The "sense" primer corresponded to nucleotides 975–1001 of the published PML-RAR fusion cDNA [1] (5′-GCGGTACCAGCGCGACTACGAGGAGAT-3′), and the "antisense" primer corresponded to nucleotides 1413–1382 of the same cDNA (5′-GCGGCGGAAGAAGCCCTTGCAGCCCTCACAGG3′).

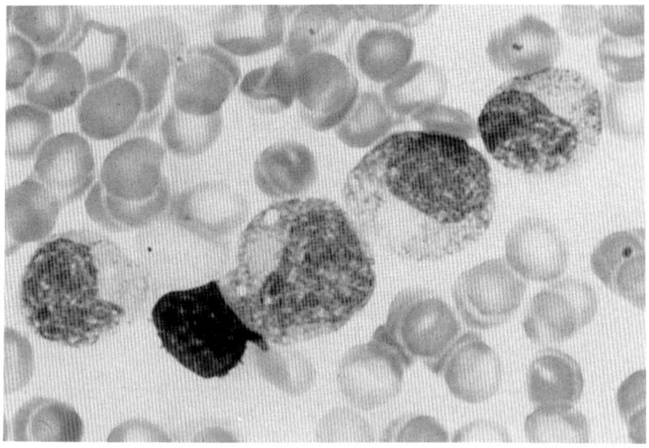

Fig. 3. Metamyelocytes seen on bone marrow aspirate after 34 days of all-*trans*-retinoic acid. Normal erythroid progenitors and megakaryocytes were also seen at this time.

Forty cycles of RT-PCR using an annealing temperature of 55°C failed to amplify any fusion cDNAs.

The patient was started on all-*trans*-retinoic acid (ATRA) 45 mg/m^2 (60 mg) per day on hospital day 38. Six days later, bone marrow demonstrated an increase in the number of blasts with promyelocytic features and a complete absence of mature myeloid forms; cytogenetic studies were again negative for t(15;17). Twice weekly blood work and daily physical examinations were negative for evidence of disseminated intravascular coagulation. Bone marrow biopsy done on day 15 of ATRA demonstrated an increase in the number of myelocytes and occasional segmented neutrophils. Promegakaryocytes and erythroid progenitors were also seen. The marrow on day 22 of ATRA revealed a marked decrease in the number of blasts and a corresponding increase in the number of mature myeloid forms. She was discharged with an absolute neutrophil count of over 1,000/μl. The marrow obtained on day 34 of ATRA demonstrated less than 5% blasts, progressive myeloid maturation, and all stages of erythroid and megakaryocyte development (Fig. 3). She required no blood product support at this time. Two subsequent bone marrow aspirates and biopsies demonstrated complete remission (Fig. 4).

After 90 days of therapy with ATRA, the marrow again revealed less than 5% blasts, and the patient was readmitted for consolidation therapy with mitoxantrone 8 mg/m^2 for 5 days and VP-16 100 mg/m^2 for 5 days, which she tolerated well. ATRA was discontinued upon admission. After recovery of the marrow, bone marrow biopsy again demonstrated remission (Fig. 5). She received granulocyte colony-stimulating factor (G-CSF) for 3 weeks after discharge to maintain an absolute neutrophil count greater than 1,500/μl; this was discontinued after 3 weeks, when the peripheral counts normalized.

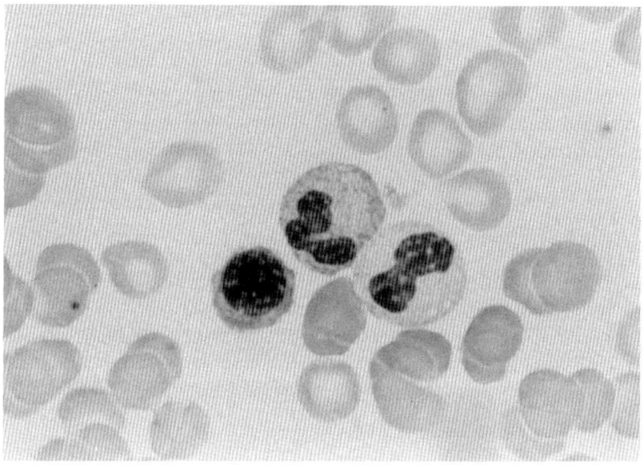

Fig. 4. Bone marrow aspirate after 62 days of all-*trans*-retinoic acid treatment demonstrating continued myeloid maturation. Less than 5% blasts were identified.

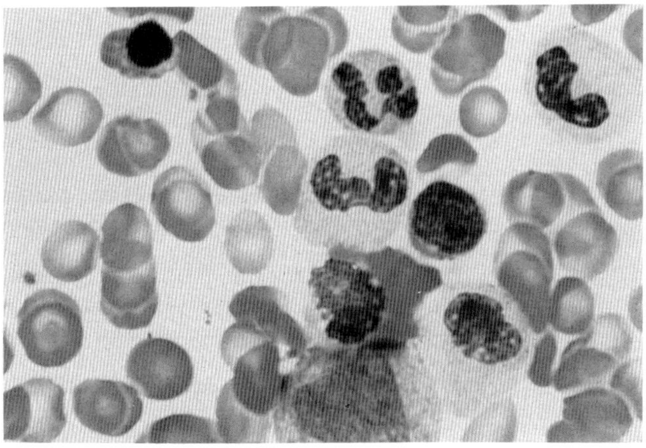

Fig. 5. Normal bone marrow aspirate after marrow recovery following consolidation therapy with mitoxantrone and VP-16.

DISCUSSION

A variety of agents have been used in an attempt to induce maturation of myeloid leukemic cells. Low-dose cytosine arabinoside [2–4], 1,25-dihydroxyvitamin D_3 [5], and two isomers of vitamin A, all-*trans*-retinoic acid (ATRA) and 13-*cis*-retinoic acid (13-cRA) [6,7], have all been used in cell culture and in clinical trials in an attempt to promote the maturation of leukemic clones. With the exception of low-dose cytosine arabinoside, these agents do not induce marrow aplasia, making them attractive agents for study in elderly patients and in those with significant comorbidity.

All-*trans*-retinoic acid induces maturation in patients with acute promyelocytic leukemia (APL) with complete or partial remission rates as high as 100% [8–11]. Because nearly all patients treated solely with ATRA will relapse [8–11], however, treatment with ATRA is generally followed by conventional chemotherapy. A major prospective phase III intergroup study is underway to compare therapy with ATRA and conventional myeloablative chemotherapy with conventional chemotherapy alone. In addition to the improved response rates, early treatment with ATRA attenuates the coagulopathy seen in patients with APL and decreases both the length of hospital stay and the patients' transfusion requirements [8,9]. A recent report describes a patient with APL who demonstrated de novo resistance to two cycles of chemotherapy with daunorubicin and cytosine arabinoside and subsequently entered a complete remission with all-*trans*-retinoic acid [12].

The precise mechanism of action of ATRA on the promyelocytic leukemia cell is unknown, and several possibilities have been raised [13–15]. Both ATRA and 13-cRA inhibit the in vitro growth of the myeloblastic cell line KG-1 and induce maturation of the promyelocytic HL-60 cell line [13–15]. The *trans* isomer appears to be effective at a dose lower than that required for the *cis* isomer, leading investigators to surmise that the interaction between retinoic acid (RA) and its receptor plays an important role in the mechanisms of drug action [16]. Additionally, the gene for one of the RA receptors is located near the 15;17 breakpoint, although no correlation between response to RA and the level of expression of the aberrant RA receptor has been demonstrated [13,16].

In in vitro studies of cells from patients with chronic myelogenous leukemia (CML), both in the chronic phase and in the accelerated or blastic phase, 13-cRA inhibits the clonal growth of the leukemic cells [17]. This inhibition is seen to a greater degree in cell lines from those in the accelerated or blastic phases of the disease, the response in cells from patients in the chronic phase being more heterogenous and thus less predictable. Increased sensitivity of cells to 13-cRA may therefore be a marker of blastic transformation. Additionally, one report describes partial remission in a patient with promyelocytic blast crisis of chronic myelogenous leukemia. While the cells possessed morphologic features of promyelocytes, cytogenetic studies were negative for t(15;17), an abnormality seen in rare cases of CML as a secondary process [18].

Retinoids have been given to patients with myelodysplastic syndromes (MDS) with minimal success. In one report, four patients with MDS were treated with 13-cRA (dosages beginning at 40 mg/day and escalating to 120 mg/day as tolerated). None of the patients demonstrated a response to this therapy [7]. Similarly, a phase I clinical trial of 13-cRA in varying doses demonstrated responses in five of 17 patients, and, while two patients had transient normalization of bone marrow blast counts and an additional three had increases in the white blood cell count, no patient had a documented clinical remission [6].

The reported responses to ATRA and 13-cRA in acute leukemia have been associated almost exclusively with t(15;17). Retinoids have not previously been shown to be effective in patients with undifferentiated myeloid leukemia. In a phase II pilot study, 12 patients over age 65 years were treated with 13-cRA at 100 mg/m^2 with no demonstrated responses [19].

To the best of our knowledge, this is the first reported case of a patient with primary refractory undifferentiated myeloblastic leukemia entering complete remission after therapy with all-*trans*-retinoic acid. It is not known whether the response in this patient is related to the promyelocytic features or whether this is a nonspecific maturational response in an AML patient. Additional studies of ATRA in the treatment of refractory AML may be warranted, particularly if there are concurrent promyelocytic morphologic features.

ACKNOWLEDGMENTS

The authors thank John F. DiPersio, MD, PhD, for performing polymerase chain reaction amplification and Jean A. Shafer for photographing the bone marrow samples.

REFERENCES

1. Kakizuka A, Miller WH, Umesono K, Warrell RP, Frankel SR, Murty VVVS, Dmitrovsky E, Evans RM: Chromosomal translocation t(15;17) in human acute promyelocytic leukemia fuses RARα with a novel putative transcription factor, PML. Cell 6:663, 1991.
2. Castaigne S, Daniel MT, Tilly H, Herait P, Degos L: Does treatment with ara-C in low dosage cause differentiation of leukemic cells? Blood 62:85, 1983.
3. Chomienne C, Abita JP, Balitrand N, Degos L: Drug association including ara-C in myeloid leukemia cell differentiation: In vitro studies. Semin Oncol 12(Suppl 3):60, 1985.
4. Degos L, Castaigne S, Tilly H, Sigaux F, Daniel MT: Treatment of leukemia with low-dose ara-C: A study of 160 cases. Semin Oncol 12(Suppl 3):196, 1985.
5. Koeffler HP, Hirji K, Itri L, and the Southern California Leukemia Group: 1,25-Dihydroxyvitamin D_3: In vivo and in vitro effects on human preleukemic and leukemic cells. Cancer Treat Rep 69:1399, 1985.
6. Gold EJ, Mertelsmann RH, Itri LM, Gee T, Arlin Z, Kempin S, Clarkson B, Moore MAS: Phase I clinical trial of 13-*cis*-retinoic acid in myelodysplastic syndromes. Cancer Treat Rep 67:981, 1983.
7. Hoffman SJ, Robinson WA: Use of differentiation-inducing agents in the myelodysplastic syndrome and acute non-lymphocytic leukemia. Am J Hematol 28:124, 1988.
8. Huang ME, Ye YC, Chen SR, Chai JR, Lu JX, Zhoa L, Gu LJ, Wang ZY: Use of all-*trans* retinoic acid in treatment of acute promyelocytic leukemia. Blood 72:567, 1988.
9. Castaigne S, Chomienne C, Daniel MT, Ballerini P, Berger R, Fenaux P, Degos L: All-*trans* retinoic acid as a differentiation therapy for acute promyelocytic leukemia. I. Clinical results. Blood 76:1704, 1990.
10. Warrell RP, Frankel SR, Wilson HM, Scheinberg DA, Itri LM, Hittelman WN, Vyas R, Andreef M, Tafuri A, Jakubowski A, Gabrilove J, Gordon M, Dmitrovsky E: Differentiation therapy of acute promyelocytic leukemia with tretinoin (all-*trans*-retinoic acid). N Engl J Med 324:1385, 1991.
11. Chen ZX, Xue YQ, Zhang R, Tao RF, Xia XM, Li C, Wang W, Zu WY, Yao XZ, Ling BJ: A clinical and experimental study on all-*trans* retinoic acid-treated acute promyelocytic leukemia patients. Blood 78:1413, 1991.
12. Mulvey K, Dahut W, Frame J, Phares J: All-*trans* retinoic acid (ATRA) is effective induction therapy in de novo chemo-resistant acute promyelocytic leukemia. Blood 80(10):423A, 1992.
13. Douer D, Koeffler HP: Retinoic acid: Inhibition of the clonal growth of human myeloid leukemia cells. J Clin Invest 69:277, 1982.
14. Gallagher RE, Bilello PA, Ferrari AC, Chang CS, Yen RWC, Nickols WA, Muly EC III: Characterization of differentiation-inducer-resistant HL-60 cells. Leukemia Res 9:967, 1985.
15. Gallagher RE, deCuevillas F, Chang C-S, Schwartz EL: Variable regulation of sensitivity to retinoic acid-induced differentiation in wild-type and retinoic acid-resistant HL-60 cells. Cancer Commun 1:45, 1989.
16. Chomienne C, Ballerini P, Balitrand N, Daniel MT, Fenaux P, Castaigne S, Degos L: All-*trans* retinoic acid in acute promyelocytic leukemias. II. In vitro studies: Structure-function relationship. Blood 76:1710, 1990.
17. Januszewicz E, Rabizadah E, Maimon Z, Zaizov R, Shaklai M: Inhibition by retinoic acid of myeloid progenitors in chronic myeloid leukemia and myeloproliferative disease: Increased sensitivity in blastic phase of chronic myeloid leukemia. Pathology 20:1, 1988.
18. Wiernik PH, Dutcher JP, Paietta E, Hittelman WN, Vyas R, Strack M, Castaigne S, Degos L, Gallagher RE: Treatment of promyelocytic blast crisis of chronic myelogenous leukemia with all-*trans*-retinoic acid. Leukemia 5:504, 1991.
19. Kramer ZB, Boros L, Wiernik PH, Anderson J, Bennett JM, Cassileth P, Oken M: 13-*cis*-retinoic acid in the treatment of elderly patients with acute myeloid leukemia. Cancer 67:1484, 1991.

American Journal of Hematology 45:181–184 (1994)

Expression of the Thrombospondin Receptor (CD36) on the Cell Surface in Megakaryoblastic and Promegakaryocytic Leukemias: Increment of the Receptor by Megakaryocyte Differentiation In Vitro

Nobutaka Imamura, Hiromi Ota, Kazuhiro Abe, and Atsushi Kuramoto

Department of Internal Medicine, Research Institute for Nuclear Medicine and Biology, Hiroshima University, Hiroshima, Japan

In this report we describe four cases of acute megakaryocytic leukemia demonstrated by the presence of megakaryocyte-platelet-related cell-surface antigens. These were detected utilizing flow cytometry and monoclonal antibodies in addition to both platelet peroxidase activity, which was shown by ultrastructural cytochemistry, and emergence of differentiation antigens, while culturing these leukemic cells. The blasts of one patient possessed both platelet GpIb and GpIIb/IIIa cell-surface antigens detected by AN51(CD42b), J15, P2, and HPL2(CD41), respectively, whereas the remaining three patients almost completely lacked GpIb cell-surface antigen. Hence the former were diagnosed as immature(pro)megakaryocytic leukemia and the latter as acute megakaryoblastic leukemia from the viewpoint of immunophenotypic analysis. While we cultured these leukemic cells in conditioned medium prepared from phytohemagglutinin-stimulated leukocytes and interleukin 3, expression of CD36(OKM5) antigen (thrombospondin receptor) increased gradually according to the differentiation and maturation of these cells. Finally, all leukemic cells differentiated to mature megakaryocytes. The function of CD36 on these cells remains to be elucidated.

Key words: CD36(OKM5), cell culture, flow cytometric analysis, acute megakaryoblastic and promegakaryocytic leukemia

INTRODUCTION

Thrombospondin (TSP) is an adhesive 450 kD multifunctional glycoprotein composed of three identical disulphide-linked chains [1]. TSP has a broad tissue distribution and is synthesized by endothelial cells, fibroblasts, smooth muscle cells, alveolar pneumocytes, monocytes, and neuroglial cells. It is known to bind heparin, fibrinogen, fibronectin, histidine-rich glycoprotein, collagen, and plasminogen.

OKM5 monoclonal antibody (CD36; obtained courtesy of Ortho Diagnostic Systems K.K., Tokyo, Japan) is reactive with platelets, endothelial cells, and monocytes [2]. It identifies an 88 kD glycoprotein and has recently been found to inhibit the specific binding of TSP to C32 melanoma cells and HT1080 fibrosarcoma cells. It also reacts with the cellular receptor for TSP [3]. The expression of CD36 antigen (TSP receptor) on the cell surface of megakaryoblastic leukemia is described during differentiation in an in vitro cell culture.

MATERIALS AND METHODS

Diagnosis and Samples

Diagnosis was established by examining peripheral blood and bone marrow smears, treated with May-Grünwald-Giemsa and myeloperoxidase (MPO) stainings. Morphological criteria were based on the French-American-British (FAB) classification of acute lymphocytic leukemia (ALL) cells. Among the 67 ALL cases, four patients whose blasts did not express T-cell and B-cell antigens but did express the megakaryocyte- and platelet-associated cell-surface antigens OKM6 and CD41 were selected for further analysis.

Received for publication April 1, 1993; accepted June 30, 1993.

Address reprint requests to Dr. Nobutaka Imamura, Hematology/Oncology Group, Department of Internal Medicine, Research Institute for Nuclear Medicine and Biology, Hiroshima University, 1-2-3 Kasumi, Minami-Ku, Hiroshima 734, Japan.

Cell Separation

Mononuclear cells were isolated from heparinized peripheral blood and/or bone marrow of patients with acute leukemia by a density-gradient technique (Ficoll/sodium metrizoate d = 1.077 g/cm^3).

Monoclonal Antibodies

Monoclonal antibodies (MAbs) AN51 and J15 were obtained from Prof. A.J. McMichael (Nuffield Department of Clinical Medicine), HPL2 and HPL5 were obtained from Prof. H. Shiku (Department of Oncology, Nagasaki University), and OKM6 was obtained from Dr. G. Goldstein (Ortho Pharmaceutical Co., Raritan, NJ). All the other monoclonal antibodies were obtained either commercially or courtesy of Ortho Diagnostic Systems (Tokyo, Japan), Japan Scientific Instrument Co. (Tokyo, Japan), and Fujisawa Pharmaceutical Co. (Osaka, Japan).

Indirect Immunofluorescence Testing

Indirect immunofluorescence test was carried out as previously described [4–6].

Flow Cytometric Analysis

Fluorescent-positive cells were analyzed in a fluorescence-activated cell sorter (FACS IV; Becton Dickinson, Mountain View, CA) as described previously [4–6].

Cell Culture

The cells were seeded in Falcon 3013 plastic tissue culture flasks (Falcon, Division of Becton Dickinson, Oxnard, CA) at 10^6/ml in 8 ml RPMI culture medium (Grand Island Biochemical Co., Grand Island, NY) supplemented with 20% heat inactivated fetal calf serum (FCS; Irvine Scientific, Santa Ana, CA), aqueous penicillin G (200 U/ml), streptomycin (50 μg/ml), and 2 mM L-glutamine and sodium bicarbonate and then were incubated at 37°C with a humidified atmosphere of 5% CO_2 in an incubator. The stimulation factors were conditioned medium from leukocytes stimulated by phytohemagglutinin (PHA) and recombinant interleukin 3 (Genzyme Corporation, Boston, MA). Cultures were fed twice weekly by partial replacement of spent medium with the fresh material.

RESULTS

Cell-Surface Phenotype

The blastoid cells from the four cases selected did not react with any lymphocyte-associated antigens detected by B1 (CD20), B2 (CD21), B3 (CD22), B4 (CD19), T3 (CD3), T4 (CD4), T8 (CD8), T6 (CD1), T11 (CD2), T1 (CD5), and Ti(TCRα/β). The blasts from cases 1, 2, and 4 did not possess the platelet-associated antigen GPIb, which is detectable by AN51 (CD42b), but the blasts from case 3 did express this antigen on the cell surface. Nonetheless, blasts from all the cases expressed the megakaryocyte and platelet-associated cell-surface antigens detected by OKM6, HPL5 and Plt-1, and GPIIb/IIIa complex detected by J15, P2, and HPL2 (CD41). Ia (HLA-DR) antigen were also expressed strongly in cases 1, 2, and 4 and weakly in case 3.

Cell-Surface Phenotype in Cultured Cells

Approximately 10 days after the beginning of the culture of cells from cases 1, 2, and 4, blastoid cells gradually differentiated to mature magakaryocytic cells. On day 15, many multinucleated cells were found with abundant neutrophilic cytoplasm, including many azurophilic granules (Fig. 1A). The antigen reacting with AN51 (CD42b) MAb, which can detect GPIb of platelets, emerged suddenly; however, Ia-like antigen (HLA-DR) decreased gradually on cell surfaces. Positivity for J15, P2, and HPL2 (CD41) did not change in expression on the cell surface. The antigen for TSP-receptor reacting with OKM5(CD36) increased gradually on their cell-surface during the megakaryocytic differentiation, as shown in Figure 1B.

DISCUSSION

TSP, a 450 kD multifunctional glycoprotein with a broad tissue distribution, is secreted following platelet stimulation. It binds to the activated platelet surface and supports platelet aggregation, which is mediated by TSP receptor. CD36, an 88 kD glycoprotein, is an integral plasma membrane protein present on platelets, endothelial cells, and monocytes. CD36 is one of the cell surface receptors for TSP, and the CD36-TSP interaction plays a role in mediating platelet-platelet and platelet-monocyte cell adhesion [3,7] as well as cell attachment to matrix [8]. The expression of TSP receptor in the megakaryocyte lineage leukemias is described, and it is shown that the expression of TSP receptor increased with differentiation and maturation of megakaryocyte lineage cells in in vitro cell culture.

Recently, Leung et al. [9] identified the CD36 sequence 139–155 as part of the OKM5 epitope using synthetic peptides and proposed a two-step process of CD36-TSP interaction. We previously demonstrated the different expression of CD36 antigen molecule on the surface of megakaryocyte lineage leukemias and megakaryocyte leukemia cell lines. We suggested that TSP-mediated adhesion represents an alternative pathway for cytoadherence and that CD36 expression on various kinds of cells may lack some essential modifications or components necessary for the TSP receptor activity [10]. Our experimental results clearly support this proposal. In this report, we demonstrated that the expression of TSP

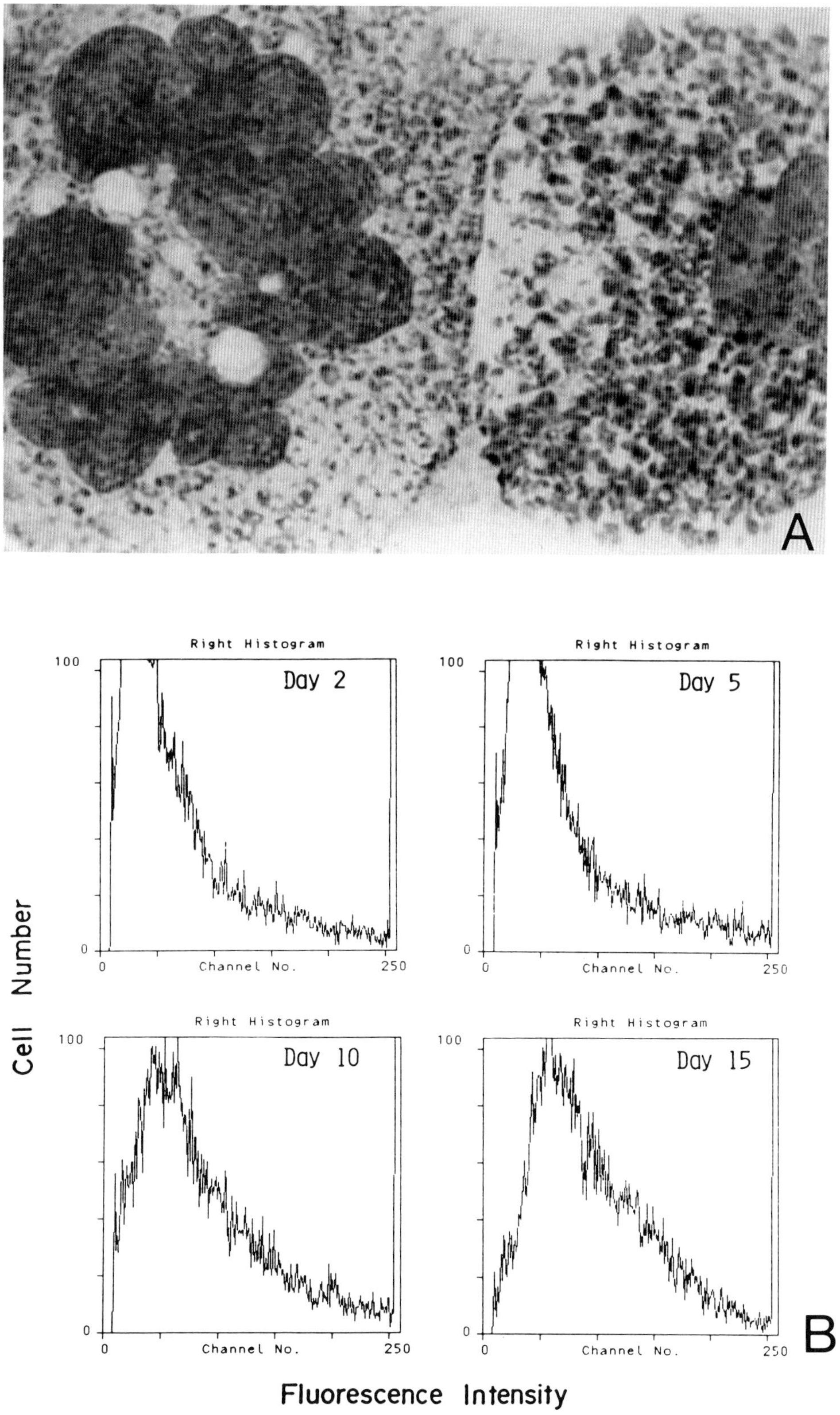

Fig. 1. Morphologic and immunophenotypic analysis of cultured cells from the patient with megakaryoblastic leukemia. A: May-Grünwald-Giemsa staining of cultured cells (day15). Mature megakaryocytes having large, multiple, and convoluted nuclei with many granules in a neutrophilic cytoplasm were seen. B: Flow cytometric analysis of cultured cells with CD36(OKM5) MAb. Increment of CD36 antigen was obvious.

receptor, OKM5 epitope, increased with differentiation and maturation of megakaryocyte lineage cells. The function of the CD36 molecule on these cells remains to be elucidated.

REFERENCES

1. Lawler J, Derick LH, Connolly JE, Chen JH, Chao FC: The structure of human platelet thrombospondin. J Biol Chem 260:3762, 1985.
2. Talle MA, Rao PE, Westberg E, Allegan N, Makowski M, Mittler RS, Goldstein G: Patterns of antigenic expression on human monocytes as defined by monoclonal antibodies. Cell Immunol 78:83, 1983.
3. Asch AS, Barnwell J, Silverstein RL, Nachman RL: Isolation of the thrombospondin membrane receptor. J Clin Invest 79:1054, 1987.
4. Imamura N, Kajihara H, Kuramoto A: Flow cytometric analysis of peroxidase negative acute leukemias by monoclonal antibodies. II. Acute megakaryoblastic and acute pro-megakaryocytic leukemias. Leukemia Res 12:279, 1988.
5. Imamra N, Kuramoto A: Analysis of peroxidase negative acute leukemias by monoclonal antibodies. III. Acute lymphoblastic leukemia. J Clin Lab Anal 3:88, 1989.
6. Imamura N, Kusunoki Y, Kawa-Ha K, Yumura K, Hara J, Oda K, Abe K, Dohy H, Inada T, Kajihara H, Kuramoto A: Aggressive natural killer cell leukaemia/lymphoma; Report of four cases and review of the literature. Possible existence of a new clinical entity originating from the third lineage of lymphoid cells. Br J Haematol 75:49, 1990.
7. McGregor JL, Catimel B, Parmentier S, Clezardin P, Dechavanne M, Leung LLK: Rapid purification and partial characterization of human platelet glycoprotein IIIb. Interaction with thrombospondin and its role in platelet aggregation. J Biol Chem 264:501, 1989.
8. Asch AS, Tepler J, Silbiger S, Nachman RL: Cellular attachment to thrombospondin. Cooperative interactions between receptor system. J Biol Chem 266:1740, 1991.
9. Leung LLK, Li WX, McGregor JL, Albrecht G, Howard RJ: CD36 peptides enhance or inhibit CD36-thrombospondin binding. A two-step process of ligand-receptor interaction. J Biol Chem 267:18244, 1992.
10. Imamura N, Mtasiwa DM, Inada T, Kuramoto A: Different expression of CD36 antigen molecule on the surface of megakaryocyte lineage leukemias and megakaryocyte leukemia cell lines MEG-01 and HEL. Leukemia 4:525, 1990.

American Journal of Hematology 45:185–186 (1994)

Molecular Abnormality of a Unique Japanese Glucose-6-Phosphate Dehydrogenase Variant (G6PD Kobe) With a Greatly Increased Affinity for Galactose-6-Phosphate

Akira Hirono, Shiro Nakayama, Hisaichi Fujii, and Shiro Miwa

Okinaka Memorial Institute for Medical Research, Tokyo (A.H., S.M.), Department of Medicine, Kobe Municipal Center Hospital, Kobe (S.N.), and Department of Blood Transfusion Medicine, Tokyo Women's Medical College, Tokyo (H.F.), Japan

Systematic molecular analysis of a Japanese class 1 glucose-6-phosphate dehydrogenase (G6PD) variant (G6PD Kobe) cDNA revealed a unique nucleotide substitution (1318 C to T) in exon 11, which predicts a substitution of leucine for phenylalanine at residue 440. This substitution is located in a region surrounding the putative structural NADP-binding domain. The markedly abnormal kinetics of glucose-6-phosphate (G6P) of G6PD Kobe suggest the interaction between both NADP and G6P binding sites.

Key words: G6PD deficiency, mutation, variant, hemolytic anemia

INTRODUCTION

Glucose-6-phosphate dehydrogenase (G6PD) deficiency is one of the most common genetic disorders, and ~400 variant enzymes have so far been identified enzymologically [1]. Some of these variants are of great interest for their unique properties. Recent progress in molecular biology has elucidated some important structure-function relationships in these variants [2]. G6PD Kobe is particularly unique because of its extremely high utility of a substrate analogue galactose-6-phosphate (Gal-6P) and reduced affinity for the normal substrate glucose-6-phosphate (G6P) [3]. We speculated that this variant has a structural abnormality in the binding domain for substrate G6P. In the present paper, we report the molecular analysis of this unique Japanese G6PD variant.

MATERIALS AND METHODS

The case history of the patient and the enzymatic characterization of G6PD Kobe have been reported elsewhere [3]. There were no other relatives with hemolytic anemia.

A fresh blood sample was obtained from the subject with G6PD Kobe by venipuncture following informed consent. Leukocyte RNA was extracted using guanidine isothiocyanate. The first strand cDNA containing an entire coding sequence was synthesized using an oligonucleotide primer, 5′-AGGAATGTGCAGCTGAGGTCAAT using the method described by Kanno et al. [4]. Two overlapped DNA segments containing the exon (2–9) region and the exon (7–13) region, respectively, were then amplified by polymerase chain reaction (PCR) [5] using two pairs of primers, 5′-CGCGGAGGGCGACGACGACGAAGCG and 5′-ACATCATGGAACTGCAGCCTCA, and 5′-ATTTGCCAACAGGATCTTCGGC and 5′-AGGAATGTGCAGCTGAGGTCAAT. Artificial Eco RI sites were introduced to the each end of the amplified DNA segments by reamplification with modified primers and subcloned into pBluescript (Stratagene, La Jolla, CA). Nucleotide sequencing was performed by the dideoxy chain-termination method [6] using primers described previously [7].

The 169 bp fragment including nucleotide 1318 was amplified from the patient's and from 22 unrelated Japanese subject's genomic DNAs using primers 5′-ACTCCACATGGTGCAGGCAG and 5′-CATAGCCCACAGGTATGC. The amplified DNAs were digested with Aor 51HI (Takara Shuzo, Japan) according to the manufacturer's instructions. The digested DNA fragments were sep-

Received for publication May 28, 1993; accepted June 30, 1993.

Address reprint requests to Akira Hirono, MD, Okinaka Memorial Institute for Medical Research, 2-2-2 Toranomon, Minato-ku, Tokyo 105, Japan.

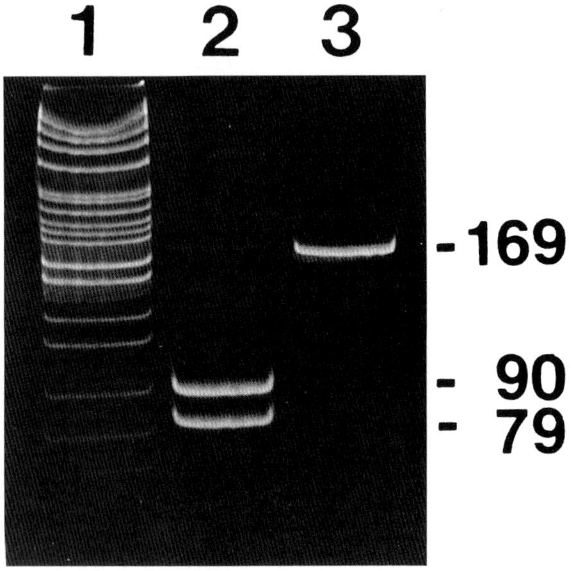

Fig. 1. Aor 51HI cleavage of the PCR segment containing the G6PD Kobe mutation site. The 169 bp amplified fragment of G6PD Kobe was cleaved to 90 bp and 79 bp fragments at an Aor 51HI site created by the nucleotide substitution at 1318. Lane 1: Size marker (Msp I digest of pBR322 DNA). Lane 2: G6PD Kobe. Lane 3: Normal control.

arated by 12% polyacrylamide gel electrophoresis and visualized by ethidium bromide staining.

RESULTS AND DISCUSSION

Direct sequencing of the entire coding region of G6PD Kobe revealed a C to T substitution at nucleotide 1318 in exon 11. Because the nucleotide change creates an Aor 51HI recognition site, we were able to confirm the mutation directly in genomic DNA (Fig. 1). We also examined 22 unrelated Japanese subjects for this mutation using Aor 51HI cleavage and found that none of them had the substitution (data not shown). Since no other base substitution or other sequence abnormality existed at the cDNA level, we concluded that this C to T substitution was responsible for the enzymatic abnormality of G6PD Kobe. This nucleotide substitution predicts a leucine to phenylalanine substitution at amino acid 440.

Among 21 different mutations known to result in hereditary chronic hemolytic anemia, 16 are clustered in the region surrounding a putative NADP-binding domain [8]. The mutation found in our G6PD Kobe is also located in this region. Although several variants that have mutations in this region are characterized by reactivation due to high concentrations of $NADP^+$ [9], we found no restoration of the enzyme activity even with $NADP^+$ concentrations as high as 2 mM.

G6PD Kobe is characterized by the reduced affinity for its normal substrate G6P and the extremely high rate of utilization of a substrate analogue, Gal-6P. It might be reasonable to expect that structural change occurs at the portions inducing conformational changes of the G6P-binding site of the enzyme. Beutler et al. [9] and Filosa et al. [10] reported that some variants, which have mutations in the region surrounding a putative NADP-binding domain, revealed very high Km for substrate G6P. They suggested the interaction between $NADP^+$ and G6P binding site in the native, folded state of the enzyme. The abnormal kinetics for substrate G6P in our present case might support their hypothesis.

ACKNOWLEDGMENTS

We thank Y. Okamura, A. Kawaguchi, M. Hoshino, and K. Hirono for their technical assistance. This work was supported in party by a Scientific Research Grant from the Ministry of Education, Science and Culture, Japan, and by a Research Grant for Specific Diseases from the Ministry of Health and Welfare, Japan.

REFERENCES

1. Beutler E, Yoshida A: Genetic variation of glucose-6-phosphate dehydrogenase: A catalog and future prospects. Medicine 67:311–334, 1988.
2. Hirono A, Miwa S: Human glucose-6-phosphate dehydrogenase: Structure and function of normal and variant enzymes. Haematologia 25:85–97, 1993.
3. Fujii H, Miwa S, Tani K, Takegawa S, Fujinami N, Takahashi K, Nakayama S, Konno M, Sato T: Glucose 6-phosphate dehydrogenase variants: A unique variant (G6PD Kobe) showed an extremely increased affinity for galactose 6-phosphate and a new variant (G6PD Sapporo) resembling G6PD Pea Ridge. Hum Genet 58:405–407, 1981.
4. Kanno H, Fujii H, Hirono A, Miwa S: cDNA cloning of human R-type pyruvate kinase (PK) and identification of a single amino acid substitution (Thr^{384} → Met) affecting enzymatic stability in pyruvate kinase variant (PK Tokyo) associated with hereditary hemolytic anemia. Proc Natl Acad Sci USA 88:8218–8221, 1991.
5. Saiki RK, Gelfand DH, Stoffel S, Scharf SJ, Higuchi R, Horn GT, Mullis KB, Erlich HA: Primer-directed enzymatic amplification of DNA with a thermostable DNA polymerase. Science 239:487–491, 1988.
6. Sanger F, Nicklen S, Coulson AR: DNA sequencing with chain terminating inhibitors. Proc Natl Acad Sci USA 74:5463–5467, 1977.
7. Hirono A, Fujii H, Miwa S: Molecular abnormality of G6PD Konan and G6PD Ube, the most common glucose-6-phosphate dehydrogenase variants in Japan. Hum Genet 91:507–508, 1993.
8. Beutler E: Glucose-6-phosphate dehydrogenase deficiency. N Engl J Med 324:169–174, 1991.
9. Beutler E, Kuhl W, Gelbart T, Forman L: DNA sequence abnormalities of human glucose-6-phosphate dehydrogenase variants. J Biol Chem 266:4145–4150, 1991.
10. Filosa S, Calabro V, Vallone D, Poggi V, Mason P, Pagnini D, Alfinito F, Rotoli B, Martini G, Luzzatto L, Battistuzzi G: Molecular basis of chronic non-spherocytic haemolytic anaemia: A new G6PD variant (393 Arg→His) with abnormal Km^{G6P} and marked in vivo instability. Br J Haematol 80:111–116, 1992.

American Journal of Hematology 45:187–188 (1994)

Reversible Encephalopathy After Cryopreserved Peripheral Blood Stem Cell Infusion

Madhav Dhodapkar, Stuart L. Goldberg, Ayalew Tefferi, and Morie A. Gertz
Division of Hematology and Internal Medicine, Mayo Clinic, Rochester, Minnesota

We report two patients who experienced severe reversible encephalopathy following infusion of peripheral blood stem cells cryopreserved in 10% dimethylsulfoxide (DMSO). In one patient, reduction of DMSO level with plasmapheresis resulted in marked improvement in encephalopathy. Infusion of large volumes of cryopreserved stem cells may result in a significant toxic reaction. Plasmapheresis may be a treatment option for patients with significant toxicity related to DMSO.

Key words: dimethylsulfoxide toxicity, encephalopathy, perpheral blood stem cell transplant

INTRODUCTION

Infusion of cryopreserved autologous peripheral blood stem cells (PBSC) has been associated with a number of infusion related toxicities [1]. Frequency of these side effects correlates with the volume of infused cells, dose of cryopreservative dimethylsulfoxide (DMSO), and volume of infused red cells. However, there have been no reports of significant neurologic toxicity as a complication of PBSC infusion. We report two patients who experienced encephalopathy after infusions of DMSO-cryopreserved stem cells.

CASE REPORTS

Case 1

A 54-year-old man underwent a PBSC transplant for refractory IgA multiple myeloma. The conditioning regimen consisted of high-dose melphalan, corticosteroids, cyclophosphamide, and total body irradiation, which was well tolerated, with the exception of mild renal insufficiency (serum creatinine 2.0 mg/dl). He received 2,254 cc of PBSC cryopreserved in 10% DMSO (mononuclear cells, 11.3×10^8/kg) infused over 10 hr. On the day following the infusion, he became oliguric and developed pulmonary edema related to fluid overload and rapid atrial fibrillation. He became extremely somnolent and was poorly responsive to verbal commands. Neurologic examination and a CT scan of the head revealed no focal abnormalities. Echocardiogram revealed normal left ventricular function. His hemodynamic status stabilized over the next 24 hr with supportive care, including dialysis. However, 5 days following the PBSC infusion, he remained poorly responsive. He was not receiving any sedatives, and his electrolytes, liver enzymes, and arterial blood gases were unremarkable. The only significant metabolic abnormality was renal insufficiency with a serum creatinine of 3.5 mg/dl. On day 6, a DMSO level was determined by HPLC in view of persistent garlic odor and was 388 μg/ml. Plasmapheresis was performed to remove the DMSO. Immediately following the plasmapheresis, the DMSO level was reduced to 78 μg/ml, and, by 24 hr following the procedure, no DMSO could be detected. The patient's mental status improved dramatically immediately following the plasmapheresis; he was able to follow simple commands. Unfortunately, over the next several days, he developed additional problems with progressive pulmonary infiltrates and sepsis and ultimately died on day 24.

Case 2

A 46-year-old man-underwent a PBSC transplant for refractory IgG multiple myeloma. The patient had mild renal insufficiency (creatinine 1.7 mg/dl) but was otherwise doing fairly well at the time of the stem cell infusion. The conditioning regimen was identical to that used for case 1. The patient received 1,198 cc of PBSC cryo-

Received for publication June 23, 1993: accepted June 30, 1993.

Address reprint requests to M.A. Gertz, MD, W-10, Mayo Clinic, 200, 1st St. S.W., Rochester, MN 55905.

preserved with 10% DMSO (mononuclear cells, 21.4×10^8/kg). Six hours following infusion, the patient became extremely lethargic and somnolent. He was arousable and was responsive to direct stimulation. On detailed neurologic examination, there were no focal findings. There was no evidence of any metabolic abnormality to explain his encephalopathy. However, gradual improvement in neurologic status back to baseline occurred over the next 5–6 days without specific therapy.

DISCUSSION

Infusion of DMSO-cryopreserved autologous PBSC is generally well tolerated, although it may occasionally be associated with a variety of side effects, including abdominal bloating, hypertension, and tachycardia [1,2]. In addition to its use as a cryopreservative, DMSO has been utilized in a variety of medical treatments, including cerebral edema, head injury, and spinal cord trauma primarily due to its hyperosmolar properties [3–5]. The use of DMSO in other settings has been associated with toxic effects, including abnormalities of liver enzymes, hemolysis, renal insufficiency, and, most notably encephalopathy [6–8].

Our cases represent the first reports of encephalopathy following DMSO-cryopreserved stem cell infusion. The development of encephalopathy shortly following the stem cell infusion, the lack of additional significant metabolic or focal neurologic abnormalities, and the dramatic resolution following reduction of DMSO levels by plasmapheresis support DMSO as the causative agent. Although other medical complications in case 1 could have contributed to encephalopathy, this would not be expected to resolve dramatically following plasmapheresis with any other etiology. The presence of renal insufficiency may have predisposed our patients to the development of neurologic toxicity by delaying the excretion of DMSO and its metabolites. It should be noted that the volume of infused cells in these cases was rather high. The main reason for this was the high incidence of graft failure noted in earlier patients with heavily pretreated refractory myeloma (M.A. Gertz et al., unpublished data). Since these patients were treated, we have limited the amount of DMSO used for cryopreservation in this protocol, and subsequent patients have experienced minimal toxicity related to stem cell infusion.

In summary, infusion of large volumes of cryopreserved stem cells may be associated with significant toxicities related to DMSO, including encephalopathy. Attempts to limit the amount of DMSO infused should be considered in patients receiving such volumes of stem cells, particularly those with renal insufficiency. Plasmapheresis may be a treatment option for these patients.

REFERENCES

1. Kessinger A, Schmit-Pokorny K, Smith D, Armitage J: Cryopreservation and infusion of autologous peripheral blood stem cells. Bone Marrow Transplant 5(Suppl 1):25–27, 1990.
2. Davis JM, Rowley SD, Hayden BG, Piantadosi S, Santos GW: Clinical toxicity of cryopreserved bone marrow graft infusion. Blood 75:781–786, 1990.
3. Ashwood-Smith MJ: Radioprotective and cryoprotective properties of DMSO. In Jacob SW, Rosenbaum EE, Wood DC (eds): "Basic Concepts of DMSO." New York: Marcel Dekker, 1971, pp 147–188.
4. John H, Laudahn G: Clinical experiences with the topical application of DMSO in orthopedic diseases: Evaluation of 4180 cases. Ann NY Acad Sci 141:506–516, 1967.
5. De La Torre JC, Kawanaga HM, Johnson CM, et al.: DMSO in central nervous system trauma. Ann NY Acad Sci 243:362–389, 1975.
6. Yellowlees P, Greenfield C, Mcintyre N: Dimethylsulphoxide induced toxicity. Lancet ii:1004–1006, 1980.
7. Bond GR, Curry SC, Dahl DW: Dimethylsulphoxide induced encephalopathy (letter). Lancet i:1134–1135, 1989.
8. Brobyn RB: The human toxicology of dimethylsulphoxide. Ann NY Acad Sci 243:497–506, 1975.

American Journal of Hematology 45:189–190 (1994)

A Possible Survival Advantage in Adults With Acute Leukemia Receiving ABO-Identical Platelet Transfusions

Joanna Mary Heal, Naomi Kenmotsu, Jacob M. Rowe, and Neil Blumberg

Transfusion Medicine, Departments of Pathology and Laboratory Medicine (N.K., N.B.), Hematology Units, Department of Medicine (J.M.H., J.M.R.), University of Rochester Medical Center, and American Red Cross Blood Services, Rochester Region (J.M.H.), Rochester, New York

In a small cohort of leukemic patients participating in a randomized trial of ABO-identical vs. ABO-unmatched platelet transfusions, a statistically significant decrease in remission duration and increase in mortality were observed in patients receiving ABO-unmatched platelet transfusions. This difference was unexplained by previously described prognostic factors for remission duration and survival. Further study of this association is warranted.

Key words: blood transfusion, adverse effects; blood platelets, immunology; neoplasms, treatment

Due to controversy regarding the role of ABO in platelet transfusion [1], a randomized, controlled study of ABO-identical vs. ABO-unmatched platelet transfusions was performed in accordance with a human subjects review board-approved protocol during 1987–1989 [2]. The investigation was designed to determine whether administration of ABO-identical platelets reduced the number of platelet transfusions required. However, an apparent survival advantage to those in the ABO-identical arm was noted. Adults with acute leukemia had been randomized to receive ABO-identical (n = 21) or ABO-unmatched (n = 19) platelets. Of these patients, 30 had acute myeloid leukemia (AML) and ten acute lymphoid (ALL). Fifteen patients in each arm had AML. Minimal follow-up was 34 months from diagnosis.

The actual survival curves for the 24 patients alive at 3 months who achieved a complete remission (CR) are shown in Figure 1 (one patient in the identical group died in remission during the initial 3 months). Significance at each time point was determined by a one-tailed, randomized Fisher's exact test using a computer program written by Dr. William Engels of the Genetics Department of the University of Wisconsin, Madison ("Fish 6—v. 1.001"). Similar results were obtained when patients not achieving CR were included in the analysis or when ALL and AML patients were analyzed separately. Mean survival for those achieving CR was 25 months for ABO-identical recipients and 13 months for unmatched recipients ($P = 0.02$ by one-tailed t test).

To evaluate whether these survival differences could be explained by known prognostic factors, a blinded observer retrospectively collected data on the following: age, cytogenetics, type of leukemia, white cell and platelet counts on admission, underlying medical problems, and infection or bleeding on admission. Of these factors, only unfavorable cytogenetics were correlated with failure to achieve a complete remission. Unfavorable cytogenetics were present in six of 21 (29%) patients receiving ABO-identical platelets vs. three of 19 (16%) patients receiving unmatched platelets. Mean age was greater in the ABO-identical group (55 years) than in the unmatched group (52 years). One patient in the ABO-identical group had a history of myelodysplasia. Diabetes was present in three of 21 ABO-identical recipients vs. one of 19 unmatched recipients. The mean white cell count on initial admission was 18,800/μl in the ABO-identical group vs. 14,100 in the unmatched group. None of these differences was statistically significant. In all instances, the unfavorable prognostic findings were more frequent or pronounced in those transfused with ABO-identical platelets. The CR rates were 62% in the identical group and 63% in the unmatched group. CR rates overall were

Received for publication August 4, 1993; accepted August 18, 1993.

Address reprint requests to Neil Blumberg, MD, University of Rochester Medical Center, 601 Elmwood Avenue—Box 608, Rochester, NY 14642.

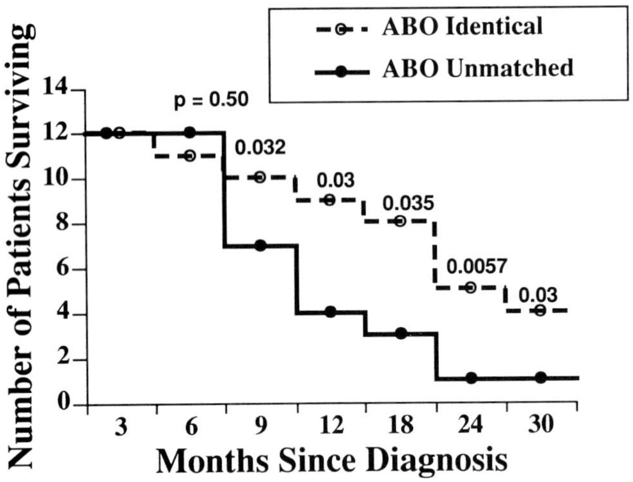

Fig. 1. Patient survival data.

57% in AML (17 of 30) and 80% in ALL (eight of ten; $P = 0.35$). Mean duration of remission overall was 384 days in AML and 587 in ALL ($P = 0.14$).

Finally, a logistic regression (performed using JMP software for the Macintosh; SAS Institute, Cary, NC) found that receipt of ABO-identical platelets was the best predictor of prolonged survival. Included in this regression were cytogenetics ($P = 0.29$), age ($P = 0.20$), white cell ($P = 0.38$) and platelet ($P = 0.69$) counts on admission, infection ($P = 0.58$) or bleeding ($P = 0.56$) on admission, and receipt of ABO-identical platelets ($P = 0.038$).

In this small cohort of leukemic patients, repetitive transfusion of ABO-unmatched platelets was associated with shorter remission and survival, unexplained by known prognostic factors. The patients receiving ABO-identical platelets had better outcomes despite the fact that they were older, had higher white cell counts, and were more likely to have diabetes and unfavorable cytogenetics. Thus receipt of ABO-unmatched platelets not only may lead to earlier platelet refractoriness [2,3] but may be associated with earlier death. Caution is warranted in interpreting this finding due to the small number of patients studied and because this is an unexpected observation from a randomized trial intended to study another endpoint. Nonetheless, it would be worthwhile to confirm or refute this relationship by studying larger cohorts of patients.

Transfusion of ABO-unmatched platelets leads to increased levels of circulating immune complexes [4]. There is evidence that immune complexes can interfere with immunologic function [5]. If transfusion of ABO-mismatched platelets contributes to leukemia recurrence, one might speculate that the mechanism involves impaired immune defenses against leukemia due to immune complexes. Levels of immune complexes have been linked to duration of remission in acute leukemia [6].

ACKNOWLEDGMENTS

The authors acknowledge the assistance of Dr. Charles Geilfuss, MD, in the collection of some of the data reported here. This study was supported in part by funds from the American Red Cross.

REFERENCES

1. Anonymous: ABO incompatibility and platelet transfusion. Lancet 335:142, 1990 (editorial).
2. Heal JM, Rowe JM, McMican A, Finke C, Blumberg N: The role of ABO matching in platelet transfusion. Eur J Haematol 50:110, 1993.
3. Carr R, Hutton JL, Jenkins JA, Lucas GF, Amphlett NW: Transfusion of ABO-mismatched platelets leads to early platelet refractoriness. Br J Haematol 75:408, 1990.
4. Heal JM, Masel D, Blumberg N: Circulating immune complexes involving the ABO system in patients refractory to platelet transfusions. Transfusion 31(Suppl 1):30S, 1991 (abstract) [full paper in press, Br J Haematol].
5. Virgin HW, Unanue ER: Immune complexes suppress cellular immunity. Ann NY Acad Sci 437:16, 1984.
6. Larson RA, Lukin CL, Daly KM, Mick R, Gore S, Le Beau M: Circulating immune complexes correlate with remission duration in acute myeloid leukemia. Leukemia 5:131, 1991.

American Journal of Hematology 45:191–197 (1994)

LETTERS AND CORRESPONDENCE

Letters and correspondence submitted for possible publication must be identified as such. Text length must not exceed 500 words and five bibliographic references. A single concise figure or table may be included if it is essential to support the communication. Letters not typed double-spaced will not be considered for publication. Letters not meeting these specifications will not be returned to authors. Letters to the Editor *are utilized to communicate a single novel observation or finding.* Correspondence *is to be used to supplement or constructively comment on the contents of a publication in the journal and cannot exceed the restrictions for Letters to the Editor. The Editor reserves the right to shorten text, delete objectional comments and make other changes to comply with the style of the journal. Permission for publication must be appended as a postscript. Submissions must be sent to Marcel E. Conrad, M.D., Associate Editor, American Journal of Hematology, USA Cancer Center, Mobile, Alabama 36688 to permit rapid consideration for publication.*

Acquired Ichthyosis as a Manifestation of Abdominal Recurrence of Non-Hodgkin's Lymphoma

To the Editor: Acquired ichthyosis (AI) is known as a rare complication of Hodgkin's disease (HD), and only nine such cases have been reported in the literature [1,2]. The complication has never, however, been described in patients with non-Hodgkin's lymphoma (NHL). We identified a unique patient with T-cell type NHL who developed AI as a manifestation of abdominal recurrence after a transient spontaneous regression.

A 42-year-old female was referred to the Gunma University Hospital in October, 1990, because of fever, weight loss, nausea, vomiting, and left cervical and supraclavucular lymph node swelling. No abnormal data were obtained from routine laboratory examinations. A CT scan revealed no thoracic or abdominal masses. A diagnosis of NHL (diffuse large cell, T-cell) was made following cervical lymph node biopsy. Since she had a high fever, clavulanic acid ticarcillin (3.2 g/day) was administered, and the fever abated within 1 week. Interestingly, the enlarged lymph nodes also decreased in size. She was judged to have had a spontaneous regression and was discharged without chemotherapy in November, 1990. In December, 1990, eczema craquele appeared on both sides of her shins, thighs, legs, and abdomen (Fig. 1). In January, 1991, she was hospitalized again for severe diarrhea and overall abdominal pain. A CT scan demonstrated mesenteric and paraaortic lymph nodes swelling and bulky intestinal involvement. A skin biopsy revealed hyperorthokeratosis and absence of the granular layer, suggesting acquired ichthyosis. Combination chemotherapy consisting of CPM, VCR, PCZ, BLM, ADM, PSL, MIT, VP-16, VDS, and MTX dramatically improved her clinical symptoms and the ichthyosis. At the same time, the complete disappearance of the abdominal lymph node swelling was confirmed by serial CT scans. These findings strongly suggest that the ichthyosis was a complication associated with NHL. However, the patient developed pleural effusion, including lymphoma cells, which became refractory to chemotherapy in May, 1991, and died of pneumonia in June, 1991.

There are two possibilities to explain the relationship between an ichthyosis and Hodgkin's disease. Cooper et al., [2] described increased serum cholesterol levels in seven patients with ichthyosis complicating Hodgkin's disease. They postulated that impaired dermal lipogenesis is one of the causes of the ichthyosis complicating Hodgkin's disease. In the course of our case, however, the serum cholesterol level was 135 mg/dl (normal 140–230). Alternatively, Dykes and Marks [3] reported a Hodgkin's disease case complicated with ichthyosis. They considered that one of the causes of desquamation was malnutrition. The clinical course of our patient, in whom diarrhea, abdominal pain, and AI were improved in parallel with the complete disappearance of abdominal tumor, suggested that the intestinal involvement of NHL caused malnutrition, resulting in the development of AI. Chance association cannot be excluded, however.

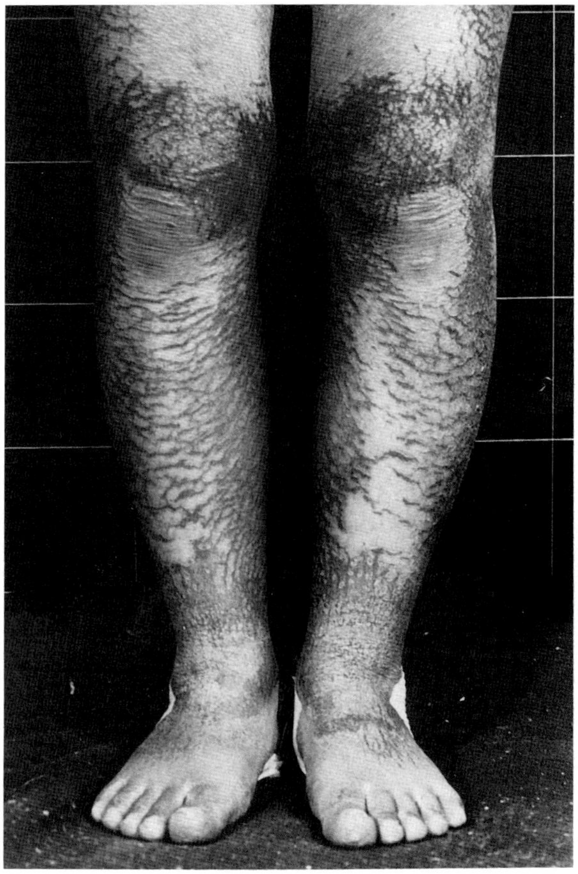

Fig. 1. Acquired ichthyosis of legs was seen with the abdominal recurrence of NHL.

Jun'ichi Tamura
Masahiko Shinohara
Takafumi Matsushima
Morio Sawamura
Hirokazu Murakami
Kazuo Kubota
Third Department of Internal Medicine, Gunma University School of Medicine, Maebashi, Gunma, Japan

References

1. Barker DJ, Cotterill JA: Generalized eczema craquele as a presenting feature of lymphoma. Br J Dermatol 97:323–326, 1977.
2. Cooper MF, Wilson PD, Hartop PJ, Shuster S: Acquired ichthyosis and impaired dermal lipogenesis in Hodgkin's disease. Br J Dermatol 102:689–693, 1980.
3. Dykes PJ, Marks R: Acquired ichthyosis: Multiple causes for an acquired generalized disturbance in desquamation. Br J Dermatol 97:327–334, 1977.

Cyclosporin Therapy for Pure Red Cell Aplasia in Patients With Chronic Lymphocytic Leukemia

To the Editor: We read with interest the recent article published by Chikkappa et al. [1] entitled "Cyclosporin and prednisone therapy for pure red cell aplasia in patients with chronic lymphocytic leukaemia." We would like to make a few comments. We agree that pure red cell aplasia (PRCA) in B cell CLL patients is an underdiagnosed entity and a correct diagnosis of the condition would avoid unnecessary and inappropriate therapy.

Our experience suggests that cyclosporin A (CyA) with or without prednisone is effective in inducing and maintaining remission of PRCA for patients with B CLL [2]. However, the mechanism of action of CyA in this context remains unclear. As was mentioned in the article, CyA inhibits production of cytokines such as interleukin-2 (IL-2) and γ-interferon that are known to cause inhibition of erythropoiesis [3]. Chikkappa et al. speculate that the lack of or decreased production of IL-2, interleukin-4, and IL-2 receptors from $CD4^+$ cells under the influence of CyA results in decreased proliferation of T cells including the abnormal T cells. They also state that the speculated reduction in abnormal T cell numbers in response to CyA treatment has not been demonstrated in PRCA associated with B-CLL. The clinical and laboratory features documented before and after treatment with CyA in one of our patients previously described [2] provide support for their speculation that CyA does cause reduction of the abnormal T cell population.

The patient was a 74-year-old white woman diagnosed as having stage A B-CLL in 1987, who remained well without treatment. The lymphocyte count was 50×10^9/liter. She had no lymphadenopathy or hepatosplenomegaly. In late 1990, she developed a rapid-onset anaemia (hemoglobin 5.6 g/dl) and reticulocytopenia, with no new clinical features. A marrow examination revealed total absence of red cell precursors despite adequate myelopoiesis. She had no evidence of parvovirus infection, and autoantibody screen was negative. Gene rearrangement studies showed, as expected, a rearranged immunoglobulin heavy chain gene and, in addition, evidence of presence of a clonal T-cell population with rearranged T-cell receptor δ chain genes. She was treated with CyA (5 mg/kg). This resulted in a reticulocyte response within 4 weeks. The dose was reduced to 3 mg/kg and was later discontinued after 3 months of therapy. The patient's PRCA relapsed after 6 months, and cyclosporin (3 mg/kg) was given again, with good effect. The cyclosporin was not discontinued again (apart from for 1 month), and the patient died of chronic obstructive airways disease and congestive failure 2 years later, in remission from PRCA. The repeat gene rearrangement studies carried out during remission showed persistence of the immunoglobin heavy chain gene rearrangement, but the clonal T-cell population had disappeared. These studies were not repeated when she relapsed.

It is possible that the clonal T-cell population demonstrated in this patient prior to treatment was responsible for the development of PRCA. Mangan et al. [4] demonstrated that accumulation of T γ cells (T cell with the receptors for IgG) in B-CLL patients leads to suppression of erythropoiesis. It is tempting to speculate that CyA suppressed the clonal T cell population, resulting in removal of inhibition of erythropoiesis and remission of PRCA in our case. This view is supported by reports of CyA efficacy in the treatment of some cases of T-cell malignancies, e.g., cutaneous T-cell lymphoma [5].

Whatever the mechanisms of action of CyA, it promises to be a useful therapeutic agent in the treatment of PRCA in B-CLL cases. However, the use of CyA should be carefully monitored because of its side effects, in particular renal toxicity, increased incidence of opportunistic infections, and the potential risk of developing other neoplasia. In view of the latter two risks, it would be reasonable to use CyA in a standard dose (5 mg/kg) with or without prednisone to induce remission and then to use a combination of prednisone and the smallest possible dose of CyA to maintain the remission.

M. Sivakumaran
Department of Haematology, Leicester Royal Infirmary, Leicester, United Kingdom
M. Bhavnani
Department of Haematology, Royal Albert Edward Infirmary, Wigan, United Kingdom

References

1. Chikkappa G, Pasquale D, Zarrabi MH, Weiler RJ, Divakara M, Tsan MF: Cyclosporin and prednisone therapy for pure red cell aplasia in patients with chronic lymphocytic leukaemia. Am J Haematol 41:5–12, 1992.
2. Bhavnani M: Cyclosporin A treatment of pure red cell aplasia associated with B-CLL. Br J Haematol 79:137–139, 1991.
3. Kahan BD: Drug therapy—Cyclosporin. N Engl J Med 321:1725–1738, 1989.
4. Mangan KF, Chikkappa GR, Farley DC: T gamma (Tγ) cells suppressing growth of erythroid colony forming units in vitro in the pure red cell aplasia of B-CLL chronic lymphocytic leukaemia. J Clin Invest 70:1148–1156, 1982.
5. Knusli C, Buchnev S, Gudat R, Obrecht J-P: Treatment of cutaneous T cell lymphoma with cyclosporin A—Case report and literature review. Leukaemia Lymphoma 4:4, 1991.Serum and Red Cell Ferritin: Diagnostic Tools and Pathophysiologic Clues

Serum and Red Cell Ferritin: Diagnostic Tools and Pathophysiologic Clues

To the Editor: Many malignant, infectious or inflammatory disorders are complicated by anemia. Anemia of chronic disorders (ACD) is most commonly involved, but this diagnosis can be made only by exclusion. The detection of iron-deficiency anemia (IDA) has been subject of many studies [1,2], including that by Balaban et al. [3]. Of the disorders listed in the latter study, it must be realized that IDA is only one diagnostic problem. Gastrointestinal blood loss [carcinoma, lymphoma, rheumatoid arthritis (RA)] does not necessarily lead to IDA, and, in addition, it can be masked by increased ferritin levels. Hemolysis may be present in lymphoma, carcinoma, certain infections, and inflammatory disorders. Bone marrow invasion occurs in lymphoma, carcinoma, and myeloma. Drug-induced anemia (chemotherapy, long-acting antirheumatic drugs, NSAIDs) may be present in any kind of chronic disorder. Therefore, before we have to differentiate between ACD and IDA, a number of laboratory tests and, in selected cases, bone marrow morphology or gastrointestinal examinations should be carried out to rule out any other cause of anemia.

Regarding the detection of IDA, Balaban et al. [3] have accurately compared the diagnostic value of serum (SERFER) and red blood cell ferritin (RBCFER). RBCFER sensitivity and specificity were not fully conclusive. Thus the poor validity, the inappropriately high levels in certain disorders, and the more cumbersome procedure limit the clinical usefullness of RBCFER as compared to SERFER. It is likely that the underlying disorders in their study have different effects on iron metabolism. Especially, malignant disorders may carry very high ferritin levels due to cellular leakage, whereas the isoferritin pattern also varies between disorders affecting the iron contents of the molecule. It is thought that RBCFER is determined by plasma transferrin iron delivery and the rate of heme synthesis [4]. Therefore, probably not only the level at which erythropoiesis and heme synthesis are impaired but also the isoferritin pattern determine RBCFER and iron storage in erythroid precursors. In a study among RA patients, RBCFER did not differ between those with IDA and ACD, whereas SERFER did [5]. Apart from the wide range of RBCFER values, the lack of difference may indeed be explained by an impaired iron delivery to erythroblasts, which is the case not only in IDA but also in ACD, as the number of transferrin receptors and affinity for iron is decreased in RA [6]. Among the RA population, it was found that the combination of MCV, SERFER, and transferrin levels at their cutoff levels resulted in 100% validity. It must be realized, however, that a considerable number of patients have different combinations with levels below and above the cutoff point of these three parameters. This may also be the case in the evaluation by Balaban et al. when combining SERFER and RBCFER levels, but data were not shown. Ferguson et al. [2] demonstrated that serum transferrin receptor (sTfR) level is a reliable parameter of iron stores, clearly differentiating between IDA and ACD. sTfR levels are less dependent on factors such as acute-phase response and inappropriately high ferritin levels in malignancy due to leakage. The exact role of sTfR determinations for diagnostic purposes can be established only in large, unselected studies.

In certain disorders, RBCFER may be a valuable diagnostic tool, but in others its value is limited. RBCFER in combination with SERFER may shed some light on the level at which iron metabolism and transport are impaired in a specific disease. SERFER reflects ferritin synthesis in response to iron stores or acute-phase reaction or is increased by cellular leakage. RBCFER points to the amount taken up by erythroblasts, available for heme synthesis. The respective levels may, to some extent, determine at what level iron metabolism and heme synthesis are affected. In both parameters, the pattern of isoferritin and iron content is also influenced by the underlying disease. Thus assessing cutoff levels for both parameters for categories of disorders (malignant, infectious and inflammatory), instead of for all kinds of diseases with concomitant anemia, may be helpful in increasing the validity of these parameters.

Gerard Vreugdenhil
Division of Hematology, Department of Internal Medicine, University Hospital, Nijmegen, The Netherlands

References

1. Cash JM, Sears DA: The anemia of chronic disease: spectrum of associated diseases in a series of unselected hospitalized patients. Am J Med 87:683–644, 1989.
2. Ferguson BJ, Skikne BS, Simpson KM, Baynes RD, Cook JD: Serum transferrin receptor distuinguishes the anemia of chronic disease from iron deficiency anemia. J Lab Clin Med 19:385–390, 1992.
3. Balaban EP, Sheehan RG, Demian SE, Cox JV, Frenkel EP: Evaluation of bone marrow iron stores in anemia associated with chronic disease: A comparative study of serum and red cell ferritin. Am J Hematol 42:177–181, 1993.
4. Cazzola M, Ascari E: Red cell ferritin as a diagnostic tool. Br J Haematol 62:209–213, 1986.
5. Vreugdenhil G, Baltus CAM, Van Eijk HG, Swaak AJG: Anaemia of chronic disease: diagnostic significance of erythrocyte and serological parameters in iron deficient rheumatoid arthritis patients. Br J Rheumatol 29:105–110, 1990.
6. Feelders RA, Vreugdenhil G, Van Dijk JP, Swaak AJG, Van Eijk HG. Decreased affinity and number of transferrin receptors on erythroblasts in the anemia of rheumatoid arthritis. Am J Hematol 43:200–204, 1993.

Author's Reply

To the Editor: We certainly concur that the potential causes of anemia in patients with malignant, infectious, or inflammatory disorders are numerous. However, the thrust of our study [1] was not related to the differential diagnosis of anemia in these settings. We addressed the more limited question of whether one could reliably determine the status of (bone marrow) iron stores in this diverse group of patients without requiring a bone marrow examination. More specifically, would measurement of red cell ferritin help overcome the lack of reliability of the serum ferritin that is due to the diverse effects of these diseases on iron metabolism, as carefully detailed by Dr. Vreugdenhil. Dr. Vreugdenhil is also quite correct in suggesting that our patients had different combinations of values above and below the cutoff levels. The point of our conclusion was that certain specific combinations were highly predictive of the presence or absence of iron deficiency. The remaining patients, not fulfilling those parameters, would require a different approach to define the status of their iron stores.

The isoferritin issue has been investigated in a variety of normal and abnormal iron metabolic states [2–5]. The emerging consensus is that the basic (liver) isoferritin (which we measured solely) is the more stable isoferrtiin, more closely related to heme synthesis [compared to the acidic (heart) subtype], and may represent an "intracellular depot of iron which is in excess of that required for heme synthesis" [3].

Ed Balaban
Richard Sheehan
Eugene P. Frenkel
Hematology-Oncology Division, Simmons Cancer Center, University of Texas Southwestern Medical Center at Dallas, Dallas, Texas

References

1. Balaban EP, Sheehan RG, Demian SE, Cox JV, Frenkel EP: Evaluation of bone marrow iron stores in anemia associated with chronic disease: A comparative study of serum and red cell ferritin. Am J Hematol 42:177, 1993.
2. Hodgetts J, Peters SW, Hoy TG, Jacobs A: The ferritin content of normoblasts and megaloblasts from human bone marrow. Clin Sci 70:47, 1986.
3. Cazzola M, Arosio P, Barosi G, Bergamaschi G, Dezza L, Ascari E: Ferritin in the red cells of normal subjects and patients with iron deficiency and iron overload. Br J Haematol 53:659, 1983.
4. Cazzola M, Dezza L, Bergamaschi G, Barosi G, Bellotti V, Caldera D, Ciriello MM, Quaglini S, Arosio P, Ascari E: Biologic and clinical significance of red cell ferritin. Blood 62:1078, 1983.
5. Peters SW, Jacobs A, Fitzsimons E: Erythrocyte ferritin in normal subjects and patients with abnormal iron metabolism. Br J Haematol 53:211, 1983.

Antiphospholipid Antibodies in Sickle Cell Disease

To the Editor: We read with interest the article by Kucuk et al. [*Am J Hematol* 42:380–383, 1993] entitled "Antiphospholipid antibodies in sickle cell disease." Their statement that their work was the first to describe an association between antiphospholipid (aPL) antibody formation and sickle cell disease is inaccurate; we have reported this previously [1].

Clearly, aPL antibodies are not limited to patients with lupus and have now been described in malignant, drug-induced, and infectious disorders. However, the majority of these patients have low-titer positive tests, which are often transient and of little clinical importance.

Although both Kucuk et al.'s study and our study have shown an increased prevalence of anticardiolipin (aCL) antibodies in homozygous sickle cell disease, there was no relationship between the increase of the level of aPL antibodies and clinical manifestations. It has recently been suggested that aPL antibodies in autoimmune diseases require a protein cofactor for maximal binding to cardiolipid in the ELISA system [2]. This cofactor has been identified as β_2-glycoprotein I, which is present in normal plasma and was shown to have anticoagulant properties [3]. The use of 10% adult bovine serum (our study) or calf serum (Kucuk et al. study) in the ELISA would provide enough cofactor for aCL antibodies to have maximal binding. Infection-induced aCL antibodies can bind to anionic phsopholipids in the absence of β_2-glycoprotein I. In contrast, binding of aCL antibodies from patients with autoimmune diseases is significantly enhanced by β_2-glycoprotein I [4]. Thus a distinction should be made between aPL antibodies that appear in patients with autoimmune diseases (pathogenic) and aPL antibodies in patients with infectious and other diseases (nonpathogenic). It is possible that aPL antibodies that appear in sickle cell disease are of the nonpathogenic type and do not require the presence of the cofactor. This hypothesis has not been ruled out in Kucuk et al.'s study or our study.

Munther A. Khamashta
Graham R. V. Hughes

Lupus Research Unit, The Rayne Institute, St Thomas' Hospital, London, United Kingdom

References

1. DeCeular K, Khamashta MA, Harris EN, Serjeant GR, Hughes GRV: Antiphospholipid Antibodies in homozygous sickle cell disease. Ann Rheum Dis 51:671–672, 1992.
2. Galli M, Comfurius P, Maassen C, et al.: Anticardiolipin antibodies directed not to cardiolipin but to plasma protein cofactor. Lancet 335:1544–1547, 1990.
3. McNeil HP, Simpson RJ, Chesterman CN, Krilis SA: Antiphospholipid antibodies are directed against a complex antigen that includes a lipid-binding inhibitor of coagulation: β 2-glycoprotein I (apolipoprotein H) Proc Natl Acad Sci USA 87: 4120–4124, 1990.
4. Hunt JE, McNeil HP, Morgan GJ, Crameri RM, Krilis SA: A phospholipid-β_2-glycoprotein I complex is an antigen for anticardiolipin antibodies occurring in autoimmune disease but not with infection. Lupus 1:75–81, 1992.

Author's Reply

To the Editor: In regard to the correspondence from Drs. Khamashta and Hughes, I would mention that we had made at least two searches of the medical literature during the preparation of our paper and did not find reference to their work [1]. I would also mention that we had previously reported our work at the 16th annual meeting of the National Sickle Cell Disease Program on March 24, 1991. In response to the comment on the levels of antiphospholipid antibody titers in sickle patients, we observed that titers varied from high to low, with some titers being distinctly elevated as shown in Table 1 in our paper [2]. We agree that it could be of interest to determine the pathogenicity or nonpathogenicity of the increased aPL titers using the protein cofactor β_2-glycoprotein I.

M.P. Westerman

Division of Hematology/Oncology, Department of Medicine, University of Health Sciences/The Chicago Medical School, Mount Sinai Hospital Medical Center, Chicago, Illinois

References

1. De Ceular K, Khamashta MA, Harris EN, Serjeant GR, Hughes GRV: Antiphospholipid antibodies in homozygous sickle cell disease. Ann Rheum Dis 51:671, 1992.
2. Kucuk O, Gilman-Sachs A, Beaman K, Lis LJ, Westerman MP: Antiphospholipid antibodies in sickle cell disease. Am J Hematol 42:380, 1993.

Circulating Late-Stage Erythroid Progenitors in a Patient With Agnogenic Myeloid Metaplasia

To the Editor: Agnogenic myeloid metaplasia (AMM) is a chronic myeloproliferative disorder of clonal origin, characterized by myelofibrosis and extramedullary hematopoiesis. Increased CFU-GM but not CFU-E has been found in the peripheral blood of patients with this disorder [1,2]. Here we present a patient with AMM who had large numbers of CFU-Es in the peripheral blood; CFU-Es accounted for as many as 2% of all the peripheral blood mononuclear cells of this patient.

The patient was a 50-year-old man with a 1 year history of exertional dyspnea and easy fatiguability. Physical examination revealed hepatomegaly and splenomegaly of 15 cm below the left costal margin in the midclavicular line. Bone tenderness was present in the upper arms and legs. Medical history was unremarkable. The clinical laboratory date are shown in Table I.

The patient was diagnosed as having Philadelphia chromosome-negative CML in accelerated phase and was treated briefly with vincristine, predonisone, and α-interferon, which resulted in relict of symptoms and hepatosplenomgaly. However, by December, 1991, the spleen had enlarged into the pelvis, and nonhemolytic aneamic was prominent (see Table I). The patient was treated with periodic red cell transfusion.

The peripheral blood cells were cultured in methylcellulose as described by Shibuya et al. [3]. The cells were separated by Ficoll-Metrizoate centrifugation, and 2×10^5nucleated cells were cultured in α medium, 30% fetal calf serum, 2 U/ml rhEpo, 10 ng/ml rhGM-CSF and rhG-CSF, and 0.8% methylcellulose. On average, 11 CFU-G and 18.5 CFU-GM per 5×10^4 mononuclear cells plated developed in the presence of G-CSF and GM-CSF, respectively. This is not different from the number of myeloid progenitors found in normal individuals and in previous reports [1,4] (this patient). In contrast, the numbers of 7 and 14 day hemoglobinized colonies was greatly increased, with mean values of 123 and 29.5 CFU-E and BFU-E per 5×10^4 mononuclear cells, respectively (Fig. 1). The peripheral blood from normal volunteers contained 10.5 BFU-E colonies per 2×10^5 mononuclear cells. No CFU-E were grown from normal peripheral blood.

The clinical features and pathological findings in this patient indicated that he had AMM. Of particular interest in this case was the finding of large numbers of both early and late erythroid precursors in the peripheral blood, which is quite different from what is found in normal individuals. Previous studies by others have revealed the presence of BFU-E but not CFU-E in the peripheral blood of normal individuals and patients with other proliferative disorders [1,2,4]. The presence of circulating erythroid progenitors in AMM has previously been measured; in those studies, increased numbers of BFU-E but not CFU-E were noted [1,2,4,5]. The finding of increased numbers of CFU-E that could fully mature in culture in our patient is therefore unusual. However, the patient suffered from severe anemia. The mechanism responsible for the anemia is unknown, but in addition to the splenomegaly it is possible that the premature release of erythroid precursors and subsequent failure to mature played a role in the anemia. This require further study.

Hua-Kang Wu
Shigeru Chiba
Ken Inamori
Hiroyuki Mano
Tsuyoshi Tange
Yoshio Yazaki
Hisamaru Hirai

Third Department of Internal Medicine, Department of Pathology, Faculty of Medicine, University of Tokyo, Tokyo, Japan

TABLE I. Laboratory Data

	November, 1990 (diagnosis)	December, 1991
Peripheral blood count		
Red blood cell		
Hemoglobin	96 g/liter	47 g/liter
Orthochromatic erythroblasts	(−)	100 erythroblasts per 100 leukocytes
White blood cell	116.4×10^9/liter	5.9×10^9/liter
Myeloblasts	2%	8%
Myelocytes	27%	
Metamyelocytes	5%	
Mature neutrophils	52%	
Eosinophils	6%	
Basophils	6%	
Lymphocytes	2%	
Platelet count	112×10^9/liter	23×10^9/liter
Lactate dehydrogenase	543 U/liter (80–166)	
Neutrophil alkaline phosphatase	30 scores	
Bone marrow histology	a. cellular hyperplasia with increased myelopoiesis and megakaryopoiesis b. An increase in reticulin fiber content	a. Megakaryocytic hyperplasia b. Cellular marrow with intense fibrosis
Cytogenetic analysis	$46XY,3q^+,-5,10p^+,13q^-,15q^+$, + mar	
Philadelphia chromosome	(−)	(−)
RT-PCR for *cr-abl* rearrangement	(−)	(−)

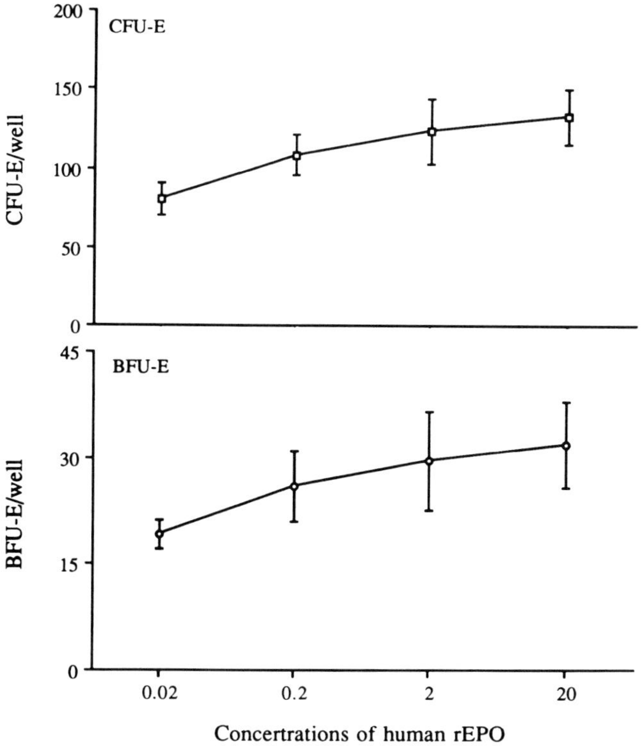

Fig. 1. Influence of increasing concentrations of rhEpo (U/ml) on erythroid colonies growth from the blood (5×10^4 cells/well) of a patient with agnogenic myeloid metaplasia. Results are expressed as mean number of colonies ±SD.

MARK D. MINDEN
Department of Medical Biophysics, Ontario Cancer Institute/Princess Margaret Hospital, University of Toronto, Toronto, Ontario, Canada

REFERENCES

1. Douer D, Fabian I, Cline MJ: Circulation puripotent haemopoietic cells in patients with myeloproliferative disorders. Br J Haematol 54:373–381, 1983.
2. Kornberg A, Fibach E, Treves A, Goldfarb A, Rachmilewitz EA: Circulating erythroid progenitors in patients with "spent" polycythaemia vera and myelofibrosis with myeloid metaplasia. Br J Haematol 52:573–578, 1982.
3. Shibuya K, Chiba S, Hino M, Kitamura T, Miyagawa K, Takaku F, Miyazano K: Enhancing effect of ubenimex (Bestatin) on proliferation and differentiation of hematopoietic progenitor cells, and the suppressive effect on proliferative of leukemia cell lines via peptidasa regulation. Biomed Pharmacother 45:71–80, 1991.
4. Selleri C, Catalano L, De Rosa G, Fontana R, Notaro R, Rotoli B: Danazol: in vitro effects on human haemopoiesis and in vivo activity in hypoplastic and myelodysplastic disorders. Eur J Haematol 47:197–203, 1991.
5. Ogawa M, Grush OC, O'Dell RF, Hara H, MacEachern D: Circulating erythropoietic precursors assessed in culture: Characterization in normal men and patients with hemoglobinopathies. Blood 50:1081–1092, 1977.

Translocation (3;3)(q21;q26)

To the Editor: In a recently published paper (April issue) entitled "New translocation involving homologous chromosome 3 in acute myelogenous

TABLE I. Published Reports of t(3;3)

Karyotype	Diagnosis	References
45,XX,−7,t(3;3) (q21;q26)	AML	Bitter et al. [*Blood* 66:1362, 1986]
46,XX,t(3;3) (q21;q26)	AML	Bitter et al. [*Blood* 66:1362, 1985]
45,XX,t(3;3)(q21;q26)	AML-M1	Mahoney et al. [*Am J Pediatr Hematol Onc* 11:153, 1989]
45,XX,−7,ins(3;3) (q21;q21q26)	AML-M2	Rowley et al. [*Blood* 58:759, 1981]
45,XX,−7,ins(3;3) (q21;q21q26)	AML-M2	Larson et al. [*Cancer Genet Cytogenet* 39:167, 1989]
45,XY,t(3;3) (q21;q21q26)/2 patients	AML-M4	Gascoyne et al. [*Cancer Genet Cytogenet* 10:219, 1983]
46,XY,t(3;3) (q21q26)	AML-M4	Jenkins et al. [*Cancer Genet Cytogenet* 39:167, 1989]
46,XX,t(3;3) (q21;q26),del(7) (q22q36)	RAEB-T	Bellomo et al. [*Cancer Genet Cytogenet* 59:138,1992]
46,XX,t(3;3) (q21;q26),del(5) (q31)	AML-M2	Golomb et al. [*Blood* 60:404, 1982]
45,XX,−7,t(3;3) (q21;q26)	Biphenotypic leukemia	Oval et al. [*Blood* 76:1369, 1990]
46,XY,t(3;3) (q21;q26)/2 patients	AML-M4	Grigg et al. [*Br J Haematol* 83:158, 1993]
46,XX,t(3;3) (q21;q26)	AML-M5a	Grigg et al. [*Br J Haematol* 83:158, 1993]
46,XY,t(3;3) (q21;q26)del(7) (q22)	AML-M5a	Grigg et al. [*Br J Haematol* 83:158, 1993]
45,XX,−7,t(3;3) (q21;q29)	AML	Whang-Pang et al. [*Blood* 71:403, 1988]
46,XY,t(3;3) (q26;q29)	AML	Bernstein et al. [*Cancer Genet Cytogenet* 6:187, 1982]
47,XX,+14,del(3) (q21→q26), dup(3) (q21→q26)t(3;3) (q21;q26)	AML-M1	Najfeld et al. [*Br J Haematol* 80:560, 1992]

leukemia (M2)," the authors, R.S. Verma, M. Da Costa, S.K. Gogineni, and G. Palermo [1], stated that "balanced translocation involving both chromosomes 3 has not been reported earlier." As is shown in Table I, 15 patients with the identical translocation (3;3) (q21;q26) described by the authors have been reported thus far in the literature. Two additional patients with t(3;3) had different breakpoints, and one additional patient had t(3;3) with a duplication q21→q26. In total, 18 documented patients have been described in the literature with translocation involving both homologous chromosome 3. An additional four patients with t(3;3) have been described, but the breakpoints were not reported [2].

Two recent papers included review of over 100 patients with abnormalities of the long arms of chromosome 3, citing clinical hematological and cytogenetic evidence for the existence of 3q21q26 syndrome [3,4]. Most of the published reports cited in Table I are complied in the *Catalog of Chromosome Aberrations in Cancer* by Mitelman [2]. All karyotypically abnormal patients published in the world literature are compiled in this catalog by disease and by abnormal or rearranged chromosome. The purpose of the catalog is to provide a quick reference for cancer cytogeneticists when they are faced with a single patient showing an unusual abnormal karyotype. Dr. Verma did cite Mitelman's catalog as reference 1.

For hematologists with diverse interests, a single leukemic patient with a rearranged karyotype may be of profound importance not for their particular subspecialty but for their academic and scholarly interests. Their interests, however, may have been misled given that at least 18 such patients have been described.

Vesna Najfeld
Tumor Cytogenetic Laboratory, Medicine/Hematology, Mount Sinai School of Medicine, New York, New York

References

1. Verma RS, da Costa M, Giogineni SK, Palermao G: New translocation involving homologous chromosome 3 in acute myelogenous leukemia (M2). Am J Hematol 42:398–399, 1993.
2. Mitelman F: "Catalog of Chromosome Aberrations in Cancer, Ed. 4. New York: Wiley-Liss, 1991.
3. Bellomo MJ, Parlier V, Muhlematter D, Grob JP, Beris P: Three new cases of chromosome 3 rearrangement in band q21 and q26 with abnormal thrombopoiesis bring further evidence to the existence of a 3q21q26 syndrome. Cancer Genet Cytogenet 59:138–160, 1992.
4. Grigg AP, Gascoyne RD, Phillips GL, Horsman DE: Clinical hematological and cytogenetic features in 24 patients with structural rearrangements of the q arm of chromosome 3. Br J Haematol 83:158–165, 1993.

Author's Reply

To the Editor: Neither of the two additional publications [1,2] cited by Najfeld was available through Medline or Index Medicus at the time the article was submitted. Obviously, she has missed the point that the balanced translocation in AML-M2 is a significant finding, and, when chromosome 3 is involved, band 3q26 is most often the breakpoint. Her letter could confuse hematologists; she has pooled together other abnormalities along with chromosome 3 in relation to different subsets of FAB in Table I.

Ram S. Verma
Division of Genetics, Long Island College Hospital, SUNY Health Science Center, Brooklyn, New York

References

1. Bellomo MJ, Parlier V, Muhlematter D, Grob JP, Beris PH: Three new cases of chromosome 3 rearrangement in band q21 and q26 with abnormal thrombopoiesis bring further evidence to the existence of a 3q21q26 syndrome. Cancer Genet Cytogenet 59:138–160, 1992.
2. Grigg AP, Gascoyne RD, Phillips GL, Horsman DE: Clinical Hematological and cytogenetic features in 24 patients with structural rearrangements of the q arm of chromosome 3. Br J Haematol 83:158–165, 1993.

Factor VIIa Levels Are Decreased in Patients With Hemophilia B

To the Editor: Factor VII (FVII) has an important role in the extrinsic blood coagulation pathway [1]. Very recently, Wildgoose et al. [2] reported that

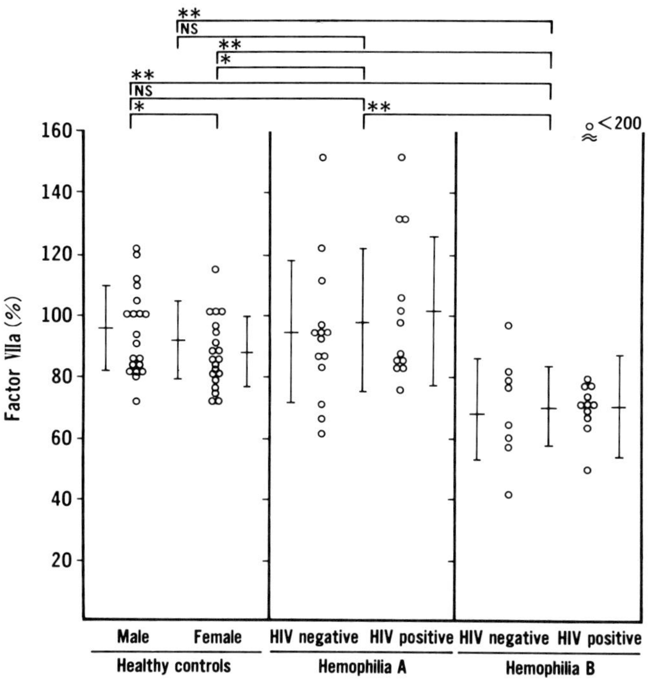

Fig. 1. Plasma factor VIIa (FVIIa) levels in the patients with hemophilia A and B. **$P < 0.01$, *$P < 0.05$, NS; not significant.

the plasma FVIIa level was lower in patients with hemophilia B than in those with hemophilia A and speculated that factor IX (FIX) was the important activator of FVII under normal conditions. We conducted this study to confirm their findings in hemophiliacs, including those with human immunodeficiency type 1 (HIV-1) infection.

The subjects were 46 hemophiliacs aged 18–42 years. They included 26 patients with hemophilia A, of whom 12 had asymptomatic HIV-1 infection (AC) and 20 had a factor VIII (FVII):C level <1% (1–4% in remaining four). The other 20 patients had hemophilia B and included 11 AC patients. FIX: C levels were <1% in 16 patients and 1–4% in the remaining four. They had not received antihemophilic factor concentrate treatment within the 7 days before this study. The plasma FVII antigen (FVII:Ag) level was measured using an FVII:Ag ELISA kit (Diagnostica Stago France). The plasma FVIIa level was assayed according to the method of Seligsohn et al. [3].

The mean FVII:Ag level was higher in the total control group (97.5% ± 9.6%; $P < 0.01$; Student's t test) than in the patients with hemophilia A ($P < 0.01$) and hemophilia B ($P < 0.01$). Male controls (100.5% ± 6.7%) had higher FVII:Ag levels than both the hemophilia A and B patients and the female controls ($P < 0.01$). The mean FVIIa concentration was higher in the patients with hemophilia A (96.4 ± 23.4%; $P < 0.01$) than in those with hemophillia B (68.2% ± 12.6%; $P < 0.01$; Fig. 1). The total control group (91.1 ± 13.0%) had a higher FVIIa level than the patients with hemophilia B ($P < 0.01$). Male controls had a higher FVIIA level than the female controls (87.3 ± 11.1%). Female controls had a lower FVIIa level than both the hemophilia A patients ($P < 0.05$) and the hemophilia B patients ($P < 0.01$). There was no difference between the patient groups with or without HIV-1 infection.

We found that the plasma FVIIa level was lower in hemophilia B patients than in hemophilia A patients. This finding was in agreement with the report of Wildgoose et al. [2]. However, the plasma FVIIa level in seven of the 26 patients with hemophilia A was lower than the mean FVIIa (±SD) level in the patients with hemophilia B. In addition, one hemophilia B patient had a very high FVIIa level (>200%) despite this severe FIX deficiency (<1%). These findings suggest that there may be regulatory influences other than FIX that modulate the plasma FVIIa level. It is possible that this change in FVIIa is caused by a concomitant decrease in other serine proteases capable of activating FVII, such as thrombin and factor Xa [2,4].

Thus we conclude that FIX is not the sole regulator of the in vivo activation of FVII under normal conditions, although it is important. However, further investigation is needed to clarify this point and to determine whether the FVIIa levels differ between males and females [5].

Juzo Matsuda
Noriko Saitoh
Kengo Gohchi
Miyo Tsukamoto
Moritaka Gotoh
Department of Medicine, Teikyo University School of Medicine, Tokyo, Japan

Hideji Hanabusa
Minoru Inagaki
Department of Pediatrics, Ogikubo Hospital, Tokyo, Japan

References

1. Nagasaki T, Foster DC, Derkner KL, Kisiel W: Initiation of the extrinsic pathway of blood coagulation: Evidence for the tissue factor dependent autoactivation of human blood coagulation factor VII. Biochemistry 30:10819, 1991.
2. Wildgoose P, Nemerson Y, Lyng L, Nielsen FE, Glazer S, Hendner U: Measurement of basal levels of factor VIIa in hemophilia A and B patients. Blood 80:25, 1992.
3. Seligsohn U, Osterud B, Rapaport SI: Coupled amidolytic assay for factor VII: Its use with a clotting assay to determine the activity state of factor VII. Blood 52:978, 1978.
4. Miller BC, Hultin MB, Jesty J: Altered factor VII activity in hemophilia. Blood 65:845, 1985.
5. Kario K, Matsuo T, Kario T, Kobayashi H: Sex-related differences in the relationship between plasma factor VII levels and serum lipids, lipoproteins, and apolipoproteins. Thromb Res 64:769, 1991.

American Journal of Hematology 45:201–204 (1994)

A New Deletional α-Thalassemia Detected in Yemenites With Hemoglobin H Disease

Lea Shalmon, Chava Kirschmann, and Rina Zaizov
Basil and Gerald Felsenstein Medical Research Center (FMRC), Sackler School of Medicine, Rogoff Medical Research Institute and Sambur Center for Pediatric Hematology-Oncology, Beilinson Medical Center, Petah Tikva, Israel

A new large deletion from the human α-globin gene cluster is characterized. It involves at least 39 kb and includes the two α-globin genes, the ϑ 1-gene, all the pseudogenes, and the two hypervariable regions (HVRs), interzeta-HVR and α-globin 3′HVR. The conserved ζ-globin gene has been identified in various restriction fragments of abnormal size. The new deletion was found in four unrelated Israeli patients with Hb H disease, all originating in Yemen, and has been designated $--^{YEM}$. It is the only two-gene deletion identified in this ethnic group.

Key words: gene deletion, α-globin genes, two-gene deletion, Hb H disease

INTRODUCTION

α-Thalassemia (α-thal) is an α-globin deficiency that results from a partial or complete inactivation of the duplicated α-globin genes. Generally, partial inactivation arises from short deletions that involve one of the α-globin genes or from nondeletional mutations and is designated α-thal-2, whereas complete inactivation arises from deletions of both α-genes and is designated α-thal-1. The interaction of α-thal-2 and α-thal-1 produces hemoglobin (Hb) H disease, the most severe clinical form of α-thal compatible with survival into adult life. In the course of a study of the genetic background for α-thal in Yemenite Jews, we have found ζ-specific restriction fragments of abnormal size in DNA from four unrelated patients with Hb H disease. The studies reported here revealed that these patients have a new form of deletional α-thal.

MATERIALS AND METHODS

Hematological data and globin chain synthesis ratios were determined by standard methods. Restriction analysis of DNA from leukocyte nuclei [1] was performed with Southern blot technology [2,3] using the following probes: a 1.5 kb Pst I fragment of pα1Pst for α-globin genes [4], a 1.9 kb Hinf I fragment of pBRζ for the ζ- and ψζ-genes [5], a 1.16 kb Bgl II/Pvu II fragment of pBRζ for exon 1 and IVS-I of the ζ- and ψζ- genes [6], an 0.3 kb Eco RI/Sac I fragment of pBRζ for the interzeta-hypervariable region (IZHVR) [7], and a 4 kb Hinc II fragment of pα3′HVR.64 for the α-globin 3′ hypervariable region (3′HVR) [8]. Autoradiograms were scanned in a soft laser scanning densitometer (Biomed Instruments, Inc.).

RESULTS

Family, Clinical, and Hematological Data

The patients, three females and one male, belong to the Yemenite community now living in Israel; two of the families came from the city of Aden. The clinical pictures of the patients were similar and conformed with thalassemia intermedia; hematological studies revealed that the patients have Hb H disease. The data given in Table I show that the patients had moderate anemia, marked microcytosis and hypochromia, and low α-/β-globin synthesis ratios. The mother of patient 1 had moderate anemia, with less pronounced alterations in red cell parameters and reduced α-globin synthesis, and the father showed normal hematological data and slightly diminished α-globin synthesis. These findings and the results of DNA analyses described below show that the father of patient 1 carries the common one-gene deletion $-\alpha^{3.7}$, the mother has α-thal trait and carries the new

Received for publication February 15, 1993; accepted June 30, 1993.

Address reprint requests to Chava Kirschmann, PhD, Rogoff Medical Research Institute, Beilinson Medical Center, 49100 Petah-Tikva, Israel.

TABLE I. Hematological Data and α-Globin Gene Genotypes*

Patient	Hb (g/dl)	RBC (10^{12}/liter)	MCV (fl)	MCH (pg)	HbH (%)	α/β Synthesis	α-Globin genotype
1	9.6	6.47	68	17.5	8	0.29	$-\alpha^{3.7}/--^{YEM}$
Mother of 1	10.2	4.90	71	20.8	—	0.66	$\alpha\alpha/--^{YEM}$
Father of 1	14.3	5.23	72	27.3	—	0.81	$\alpha\alpha/-\alpha^{3.7}$
2	10.9	6.29	62	17.3	6.6	0.24	$-\alpha^{3.7}/--^{YEM}$
3	9.6	5.71	66.9	16.8	17.8	0.16	$\alpha\alpha^{T}/--^{YEM}$
4	10.0	5.01	68.1	20.0	+++	0.36	$\alpha\alpha^{T}/--^{YEM}$

*Abbreviations: Hb, hemoglobin; RBC, red blood cells; MCV, mean corpuscular volume; MCH, mean corpuscular hemoglobin; α^T, α-thalassemia.

TABLE II. Sizes of ζ-Specific Restriction Fragments (kb)

Enzyme	Haplotype αα	Haplotype $--^{YEM}$
Eco RI	4.6 (23)[a]	11.0
Hind III	13.5 (16–19)	13.0
Hpa I	12.3 (10.8–11.7)	17.5
Acc I	7.3 (7.1–8.0)	7.3
Xba I	20.3 or 16 (16)	14.3
Bgl II	10.5–12.0 (12.6)	10.8
Sph I	16.4	14.0

[a]ψζ-Specific fragments are given in parentheses.

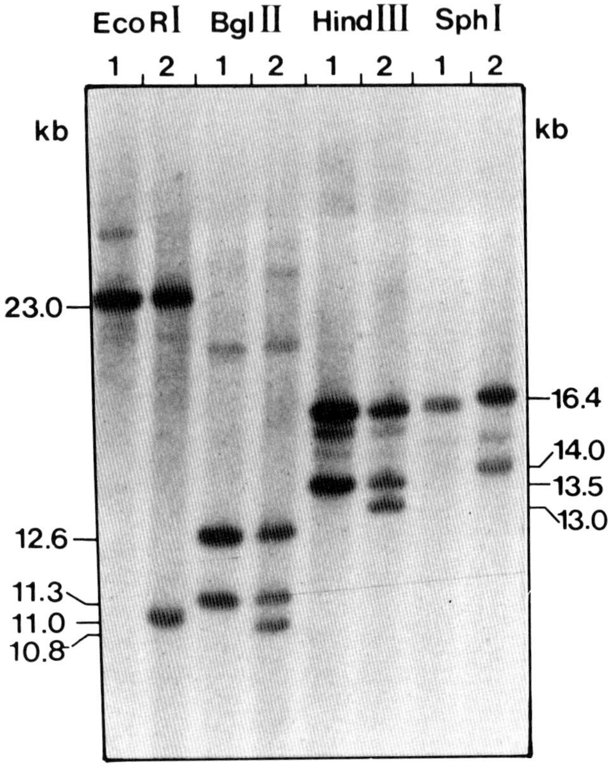

Fig. 1. Autoradiogram of ζ-specific fragments obtained by four restriction enzymes. Lanes 1: Nonthalassemic DNA (αα/αα). Lanes 2: DNA from patient 4 ($\alpha\alpha^{T}/--^{YEM}$).

deletion designated $--^{YEM}$, and their daughter has inherited the two defects.

DNA Restriction Analysis

With the α-specific probe, DNA blots of patients 1 and 2 showed one Eco RI fragment of 19 kb and one Bgl II fragment of 16 kb, consistent with a 3.7 kb deletion on their α-thal-2 chromosomes, and no α-globin genes on the α-thal-1 chromosomes. Blots from patients 3 and 4 showed normal Eco RI and Bgl II fragment patterns, suggesting a nondeletional mutation on one chromosome and no α-genes on the other. The new deletion was positively identified in DNA from the four patients and from the mother and maternal aunt of patient 1 with the ζ-specific probe. Following digestion with seven different restriction enzymes fragments of abnormal size appeared on their hybridization blots, these are listed in Table II. Figure 1 shows an 11 kb Eco RI fragment, a 10.8 kb Bgl II fragment, a 13 kb Hind III fragment, and a 14 kb Sph I fragment that represent the new deletion. The abnormal fragments did not appear when a probe for the IZHVR was used, indicating inclusion of this region in the deletion. The presence of a ψζ-globin gene on chromosomes affected by the new deletion was studied by densitometry of a hybridization blot of Sac I fragments (Fig. 2A). ζ-had ψζ-genes show in 5.8 and 1.86 kb bands, respectively. The father of patient 1 (genotype $\alpha\alpha/-\alpha^{3.7}$; lane 1) and a ψζ/ζ density ratio of 1.38, while the mother (genotype $\alpha\alpha/--^{YEM}$; lane 2) had a ratio of 0.74. Since the father has two ψζ-genes, the mother has one on her normal chromosome and none on the α-thal-1 chromosome. The presence of an α-globin 3′HVR on chromosomes that carry the new deletion was studied in Pvu II digested DNA. Figure 2B shows that the father of patient 1 (lane 1) carries two distinct 3′HVRs of 5.4 and 4.1 kb, while the mother and the patient (lanes 2 and 3) have only one each, of 2.1 and 4.1 kb, respectively. Thus the patient has inherited a chromosome with a 4.1 kb 3′HVR from her father and an α-thal-1 chromosome that has no α3′HVR from her mother.

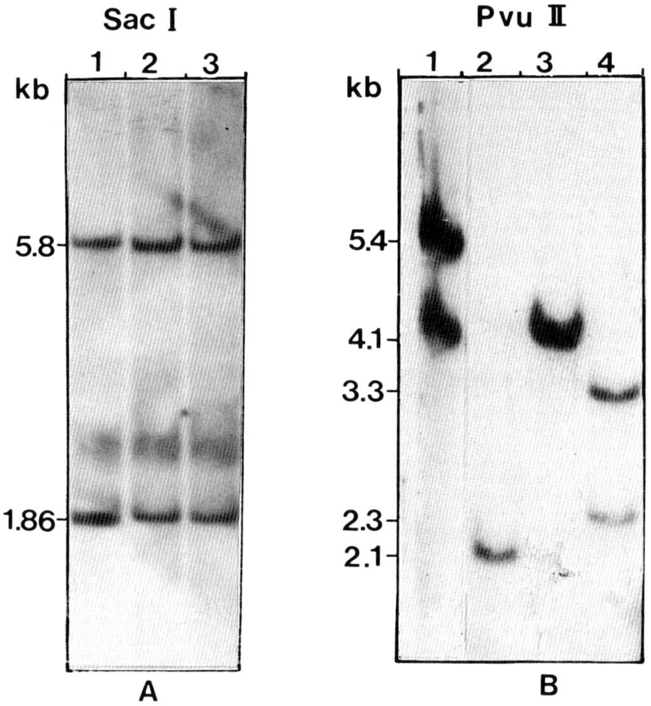

Fig. 2. Quantitative analysis of ψζ-globin genes and 3′HVRs in DNA from carriers of the Yemenite deletion. A: Sac I fragments obtained by a 1.16 kb probe for the 5′-parts of the ζ- and ψζ-globin genes. Lane 1: Father of patient 1 ($-\alpha^{3.7}/\alpha\alpha$). Lane 2: Mother of patient 1 ($--^{YEM}/\alpha\alpha$). Lane 3: Maternal aunt of patient 1 ($-\alpha^{3.7}/--^{YEM}$). B: Pvu II fragments obtained by a 4 kb probe for α3′HVRs. Lane 1: Father of patient 1 ($-\alpha^{3.7}/\alpha\alpha$). Lane 2: Mother of patient 1 ($--^{YEM}/\alpha\alpha$). Lane 3: Patient 1 ($-\alpha^{3.7}/--^{YEM}$). Lane 4: A patient with Hb H disease ($-\alpha^{3.7}/--^{MED}$).

Definition of Breakpoint Regions

Figure 3 shows a map of the normal α-globin gene cluster, restriction sites of ten different enzymes [9] and the sizes of seven abnormal ζ-specific restriction fragments that characterize the new deletion. The bottom line in Figure 3 shows that the deletion includes the two HVRs (IZHVR and α3′HVR) and all the genes and pseudogenes that lie between them, leaving only the ζ-globin gene. The 5′-breakpoint of this deletion should be located between the ζ-globin gene and the IZHVR. Since both the Bam HI and Sac I fragment patterns were normal, while Eco RI, Hind III, and Hpa I produced abnormal ζ-fragments, this breakpoint has been mapped between the restriction sites of Sac I and Eco RI, which are 1.3 kb apart. The 3′-breakpoint must be located downstream of the deleted 3′HVR. The restriction sites of Xba I and Bgl II at coordinates 37 and 37.2 are too close to the 3′HVR to accommodate the respective ζ-fragments of 14.3 and 10.8 kb, so they are included in the deletion. Consequently, the restriction sites of Sph I and Acc I that lie 4–5 kb further downstream should also be included in the deletion. The restriction site of Hind III at coordinate 43.3 may well be the 3′-end of a 13 kb Hind III fragment, of which 12 kb is located upstream of the deletion. However, since the region beyond this site has not been mapped, the possibility cannot be excluded that the 3′-end of the deletion lies close to some other Hind III site, further downstream. Thus the map in Figure 3 shows that the Yemenite deletion involves 39 kb, but its total length has not been determined.

DISCUSSION

A new form of deletional α-thal has been found in four Yemenite patients with Hb H disease. The Yemenite community in Israel is known to carry α-thalassemia at a moderately high rate; elevated levels of Hb Bart's have been found in 17% of Yemenite newborns [10,11]. Although this community numbers 152,000, only a few cases of Hb H disease have been diagnosed, and the hydrops fetalis syndrome has not been reported. Thus the frequency of the new mutation in this ethnic group is rather low. It is noteworthy that this is the only α-thal-1 determinant detected in 13 unrelated Yemenite patients with α-thal.

The phenotypic expression of the Yemenite deletion is similar to that of α-thal-1 found in other populations. The heterozygote has α-thal trait, with significant microcytosis and hypochromia and an α/β-globin chain synthesis ratio of 0.66, while interaction with the 3.7 kb deletion or with a nondeletional mutation results in Hb H disease. The most severe hematologic alterations were found in patient 3, one of the two patients with a nondeletional mutation. This difference in expression may correlate with two distinct mutations in the two patients. We have not identified these mutations.

The Yemenite deletion includes the IZHVR and the α3′HVR; its length is either 39 kb or longer, and it is the largest ψζα-thal deletion from the α-globin gene cluster. The 5′-breakpoint of the deletion is located between the restriction sites of Sac I and Eco RI, 1.2–2.5 kb downstream of the conserved ζ-globin gene. Thus it lies within a known breakpoint cluster region [9], in close proximity to the 5′-ends of the 20.5 kb deletion [12] and the 27 kb British deletion [13]. The 3′-breakpoint maps outside of the gene cluster, probably close to the restriction site of Hind III at coordinate 43.3. So far, only three large deletions from the α-globin gene cluster that encompass the 3′HVR have been described. They are the 47 kb deletion found in a German family [14], the 27 kb deletion found in a Spanish family [15], and the 37 kb deletion found in British patients [16]. Sequence analysis around the ends of these deletions and of the Yemenite deletion has not been performed, and the mechanism for their generation remains unclear.

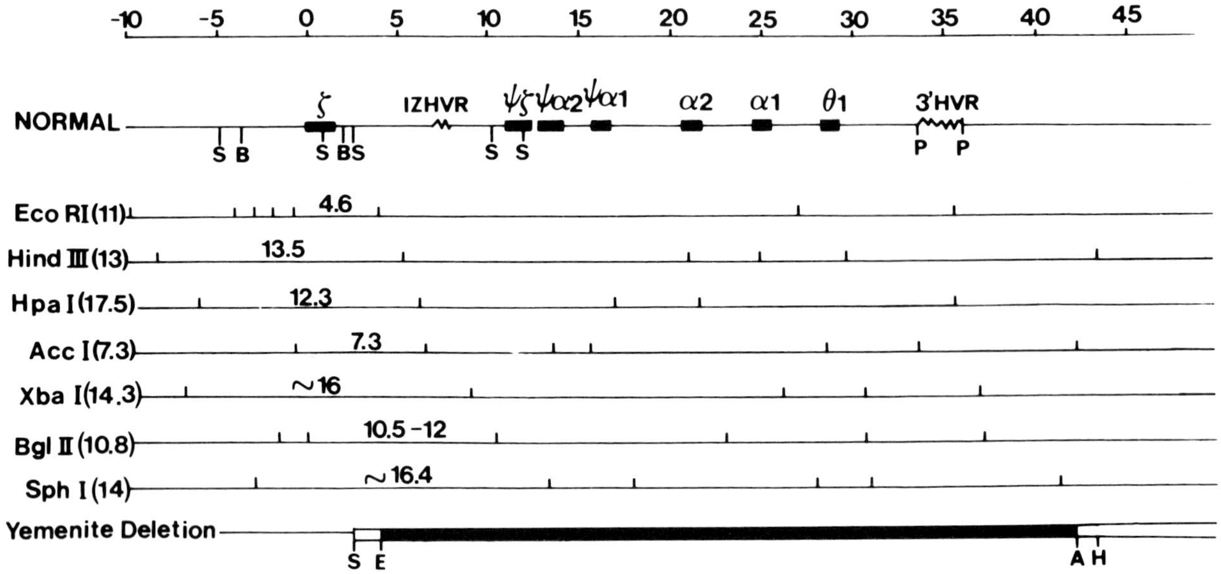

Fig. 3. Restriction maps of the normal α-globin gene cluster and location of the Yemenite deletion. The restriction sites of Sac I (S), Bam HI (B), and Pvu II (P) are shown on the map. The restriction sites of seven other enzymes are given separately under the map, and the sizes of the normal ζ-specific fragments are indicated. The sizes of the abnormal ζ-specific fragments are given in parenthesis at left. The solid bar at the bottom shows the location of the deletion, and the open bars indicate the limits of the breakpoints.

ACKNOWLEDGMENTS

We thank Drs. T. Maniatis and D.R. Higgs for gifts of recombinant plasmids and Dr. A. Ravid for densitometric analysis of autoradiograms.

REFERENCES

1. Bell GI, Karam JH, Rutter WJ: Polymorphic DNA region adjacent to the 5′ end of the human insulin gene. Proc Natl Acad Sci USA 78:5759, 1981.
2. Southern E: Detection of specific sequences among DNA fragments separated by gel electrophoresis. J Mol Biol 98: 503, 1975.
3. Wahl GM, Stern M, Stark GR: Efficient transfer of large DNA fragments from agarose gels to diazobenzyloxymethyl-paper and rapid hybridization by using dextran sulfate. Proc Natl Acad Sci USA 76: 3683, 1979.
4. Michelson AM, Orkin SH: Boundaries of the gene conversion within the duplicated human α-globin genes. J Biol Chem 258:15245, 1983.
5. Felice AE, Cleek MP, McKie K, McKie V, Huisman THJ: The rare α-thalassemia-1 of Blacks is a ζα-thalassemia-1 associated with deletion of all α- and ζ-globin genes. Blood 63:1253, 1984.
6. Lauer J, Shen C-K J, Maniatis T: The chromosomal arrangement of human α-like globin genes: Sequence homology and α-globin gene deletions. Cell 20:119, 1980.
7. Winichagoon P, Higgs DR, Goodbourn SEY, Lamb J, Clegg JB, Weatherall DJ: Multiple arrangements of the human embryonic zeta globin genes. Nucleic Acids Res 10:5853, 1982.
8. Jarman AP, Nicholls RD, Weatherall DJ, Clegg JB, Higgs DR: Molecular characterization of a hypervariable region downstream of the human α-globin gene cluster. EMBO J 5:1857, 1986.
9. Nicholls RD, Fischel-Ghodsian N, Higgs DR: Recombination at the human α-globin gene cluster: Sequence features and topological constraints. Cell 49:369, 1987.
10. Halbrecht I, Ben Porat S: The incidence of Bart's hemoglobin in the cord blood of 3218 newborns of different ethnic groups in Israel. Harefuah 73:254, 1967.
11. Zaizov R, Matoth Y: α-Thalassemia in Yemenite and Iraqi Jews. Israel J Med Sci 8:11, 1972.
12. Nicholls RD, Higgs DR, Clegg JB, Weatherall DJ: α°-thalassemia due to recombination between the α1-globin gene and an Alu I repeat. Blood 65:1434, 1985.
13. Higgs DR, Ayyub H, Clegg JB, Hill AVS, Nicholls RD, Teal H, Wainscoat JS, Weatherall DJ: α-Thalassaemia in British people. Br Med J 290:1303, 1985.
14. Fortina P, Delgrosso K, Rappaport E, Poncz M, Ballas SK, Schwartz E, Surrey S: A large deletion encompassing the entire α-like globin gene cluster in a family of Northern European extraction. Nucleic Acids Res 16:11223, 1988.
15. Gonzalez-Redondo JM, Diaz-Chico JC, Malcorra-Azpiazu JJ, Balda-Aguirre MI, Huisman THJ: Characterization of a newly discovered α-thalassaemia-1 in two Spanish patients with Hb H disease. Br J Haematol 70:459, 1988.
16. Higgs DR, Vickers MA, Wilkie AOM, Pretorius I-M, Jarman AP, Weatherall DJ: A review of the molecular genetics of the human α-globin gene cluster. Blood 73:1081, 1989.

American Journal of Hematology 45:205–211 (1994)

von Willebrand's Disease: Use of Collagen Binding Assay Provides Potential Improvement to Laboratory Monitoring of Desmopressin (DDAVP) Therapy

Emmanuel J. Favaloro, Mark Dean, Linda Grispo, Tom Exner, and Jerry Koutts

Haemostasis and Thrombosis Research Unit, Department of Haematology, Institute of Clinical Pathology and Medical Research (ICPMR), Westmead Hospital, Westmead, New South Wales, Australia

This report describes studies investigating the use of a collagen binding assay to improve the laboratory monitoring of desmopressin (DDAVP) therapy in patients with von Willebrand's disease (vWD). We evaluated the response of seven patients with vWD (four type I, three type IIA) to DDAVP, administered using a standard protocol, by assessing levels of von Willebrand factor (vWF) and factor VIII, as well as performing skin bleeding times (SBT) prior to, and at sequential time points following, DDAVP administration. The study employed the following assays: von Willebrand factor antigen assay (vWF:Ag; determined by ELISA); a novel functionally based collagen binding assay (CBA; determined by ELISA); ristocetin cofactor assay (RCof; determined by platelet aggregometry); von Willebrand factor multimer analysis (using SDS-agarose gels); factor VIII coagulant (FVIIIC; determined by clotting assay); and factor VIII antigen (FVIIICAG; determined by ELISA). All patients showed an initial incremental increase in vWF/FVIII levels using all assays above, and some showed some correction in SBT. Although the absolute levels of vWF/FVIII antigen or activity varied between patients, the CBA was found to provide consistently the greatest proportional incremental increases (i.e., -fold) compared to baseline (pre-DDAVP) levels. Accordingly, we consistently observed an increase in the CBA to vWF:Ag ratio for all patients evaluated. This supplements previous findings that have suggested a unique ability of our CBA procedure to bind preferentially to higher molecular weight (i.e., more functionally active) forms of vWF. We therefore propose that the use of the above test combination (e.g., vWF:Ag plus CBA) may provide the basis for more accurate estimation of a patient's functional responsiveness to DDAVP therapy in future studies.

Key words: von Willebrand's disease, von Willebrand factor, desmopressin, DDAVP, collagen binding assay

INTRODUCTION

Von Willebrand factor (vWF) has two primary roles in haemostasis. First, it permits adhesion of platelets to sites of vascular damage, and, second, it acts to stabilise factor VIII within blood [1–4]. Patients suffering defects in, or reduced level of, vWF are diagnosed as having von Willebrand's disease (vWD) and are typed according to classification protocols involving both clinical observations and laboratory analysis of patient plasma [1,2]. Indeed, vWD is now reported to be the most common inherited bleeding disorder [see, e.g., 4–6]. Laboratory investigation usually involves a battery of tests, including determination of (skin) bleeding times, vWF antigen (vWF:Ag) levels, functional activities such as factor VIII coagulant (FVIIIC) and ristocetin cofactor (RCof), and vWF multimetric analysis [1,2].

Generally, type I vWD patients suffer from a quantitative reduction in all vWF multimers present, with concurrently decreased levels of vWF:Ag and RCof activity (typically in similar proportions). Alternatively, type II vWD is characterised by qualitative abnormalities of

Received for publication February 2, 1993; accepted July 20, 1993.

Address reprint requests to Dr. E.J. Favaloro, Department of Haematology, Westmead Hospital, NSW, 2145 Australia.

vWF multimers. Although at least four subtypes have been characterised, these patients generally exhibit a prolongation in their bleeding time, normal to slightly reduced levels of both factor VIII and vWF:Ag, reduced RCof activity, and an absence of intermediate to large vWF multimers. Classification of the patient's vWD is important not only because the biological activity of vWF is related to its multimer profile, but also since subsequent clinical management may differ substantially on this basis [5–8]. In order to improve and simplify our laboratory's diagnostic procedure for vWD, we developed a novel functional collagen-based ELISA assay for vWF. Based on previous observations that vWF binds to collagen, with preference for high-molecular-weight forms, this assay is capable of sensitive discrimination between plasma derived from type II vWD patients, and that derived from either type I vWD patients, or from normal individuals [9,10]. The current study extends the findings of these reports, by analysing, in parallel, changes that occur in both von Willebrand factor and factor VIII in patients administered desmopressin (DDAVP) and utilising our improved laboratory procedure. This study is thus the first to report on the use of this CBA in such treatment procedures and suggests that this laboratory test, in association with other standard procedures (such as the vWF:Ag assay), may more properly reflect true functional changes to vWF following DDAVP than do currently existing laboratory protocols.

MATERIALS AND METHODS

Patient Samples

These were derived from patients previously assessed as having von Willebrand's disease type I or type IIA, but whose DDAVP responsiveness had not been established. All assays were performed using plasma isolated from venous blood collected into 0.012 M sodium citrate (9 parts blood, 1 part citrate), and centrifuged (1,500 *g*; 15 min) to remove cellular components, according to standard procedures. In addition to patient samples, a large number of individual normal plasma samples were also obtained from healthy volunteers and were utilised for control purposes and to provide a large pool (PNP; >60 individuals) for assay calibration. All plasma samples collected were snap frozen (at −70°C) to permit multiple analysis by various assays.

DDAVP (Desmopressin) Infusion and Blood Collection/Testing Protocol

This was a standard protocol for administration of desmopressin (0.3 μg desmopressin/kg i.v.; administered over a 30 min period). After we obtained informed consent, blood samples were drawn prior to DDAVP administration and at selected time intervals following completed administration, and specifically at plus 30 min, and then +1 hr, +2 hr, +4 hr, and +6 hr. Tests performed were as stated below, plus monitoring of routine coagulation parameters (prothrombin time, PT; activated partial thromboplastin time, APTT). A blood sample was also collected into EDTA at these times to permit monitoring of routine haematology parameters (platelet counts, white cell counts, red cell counts, haemoglobin, haematocrit, etc). Skin bleeding time (SBT) estimations were performed prior to DDAVP administration, and repeated at time plus 2 hr following administration.

Laboratory Protocol for Assessment of DDAVP Therapy

Assays for von Willebrand factor (vWF) antigen levels (vWF:Ag), ristocetin cofactor (RCof) functional activity, a functional collagen binding assay (CBA), and assays for factor VIII coagulant (FVIIIC), and factor VIII antigen (FVIIICAG) were as described below and elsewhere [9,10]. To permit comparative evaluation, and to allow derivation of assay to assay ratios (e.g., CBA to vWF:Ag ratio), the lower limit of sensitivity for each assay was arbitrarily set at 0.1%. Skin bleeding times were performed using Simplate II devices according to manufacturer's instructions (AKZO/Organon Teknika, Australia), and multimer analysis was performed as indicated below.

ELISA assay for vWF:Ag. This assay, a sandwich, indirect 96-well plate procedure, has been described in detail elsewhere [9]. Test plasma values for vWF:Ag were calculated with reference to PNP.

Ristocetin cofactor assay. This assay has also been described in detail elsewhere [9] and utilises platelet aggregometry.

Collagen binding assay for vWF. This assay, together with a detailed analysis of assay variables, has been outlined previously [9] and is based on modifications to the assay originally described by Brown and Bosak [11].

Factor VIII coagulant levels. These were assessed using a standard clotting based semiautomated procedure, utilising mixing tests with factor VIII deficient plasma (AKZO/Organon Teknika, Australia), and the ACL-300R automated coagulation analyser (Coulter, Australia). Factor VIII coagulant activity was calculated with respect to a commercial standard plasma (Verify plasma; AKZO/Organon Teknika, Australia); PNP was used as a secondary reference plasma source.

Factor VIII antigen assay. This was performed as an ELISA procedure, which utilised reagents similar to those previously described for vWF:Ag and CBA [9,10]. Specific modifications were as follows: Fresh 96-well plates were coated (overnight, 4°C) with antisera to factor VIII (immunoglobulin fraction derived and purified from a patient with factor VIII inhibitor; diluted according to previously established titre experiments). Plates were then washed three times using BSA ELISA buffer [9], blocked using 5% BSA (1 hr, 22°C), and rewashed twice. Patient plasma was then introduced (at final 1:10 dilution in BSA ELISA buffer containing 0.1% sodium azide), and plates were left overnight (22°C) and rewashed five times. Biotinilated antisera (obtained from previously biotinilated immunoglobulin fraction derived and purified from patient above) were then introduced (using previously established dilution) in BSA ELISA buffer containing 0.1% sodium azide, and plates were again left overnight (22°C). Plates were rewashed six times, and wells were then incubated with a suitable dilution (typically 1:1,000) of commercially prepared streptavidin-HRP (Dakopatts, Denmark; 2 hr, 22°C). Plates were rewashed six times and colour visualised as per the vWF:Ag ELISA [9]. A calibration curve utilising PNP was set up with each plate to extend from 0% to 400%, with respect to PNP at final dilution 1:10 being equivalent to 100% of the normal level of FVIII CAG [see 9].

Multimer analysis. This was performed as previously described [12,13].

RESULTS

General Observations

A total of seven vWD patients were evaluated in this study (four type I, three type IIA). All patients tolerated DDAVP well, and all showed an initial incremental increase in vWF and FVIII levels using all relevant assays, although the sensitivity in the respective assays to detect such changes varied, both between patients and between assays. Some patients also showed some correction in their skin bleeding times following DDAVP infusion (see below). No patient showed any consistent change in any routine haematology (noncoagulation) parameter (e.g., white cell count, red cell count, platelet count, haemoglobin, haematocrit, etc.; data not shown). Monitoring of routine coagulation tests showed a small, but consistent, fall in the APTT for all patients following DDAVP infusion, whereas the PT did not change appreciably for any patient (data not shown).

Changes in vWF Parameters Following DDAVP

All patients evaluated in the current study showed an initial incremental increase in the levels of vWF in patient plasma following DDAVP, as detected by each of the four vWF assays employed (see below and Figs. 1, 2). However, patients differed markedly in respect to the magnitude of response on both a patient to patient and on an assay to assay basis. In this regard, then, type I vWD patients tended to show greatest absolute release responses (see Fig. 1) compared to type IIA vWD patients (Fig. 2). Most striking in the DDAVP response in type I vWD patients was the incremental increases observed in CBA values, which markedly overshadowed the vWF response detected using any other assay type (Fig. 1). This is further strikingly depicted in Figure 3, where changes have been shown as -fold increases over baseline (i.e., pre-DDAVP) levels. Even in type IIA patients, where the absolute quantitative increase in CBA was not as marked (Fig. 2), changes, when expressed as -fold increase over baseline levels, tended to be most striking (Fig. 4). As a result of this differential pattern, the ratio of CBA-derived values to vWF:Ag-derived values for each patient is observed to increase following DDAVP infusion (and particularly for type I vWD patients).

Changes in FVIII Parameters Following DDAVP

All patients evaluated in the current study showed increases in the levels of FVIII in patient plasma following DDAVP, as detected by the two FVIII assays employed (see Figs. 1, 2). Differences detected between patients in their response to DDAVP in terms of factor VIII levels were not as marked as those observed for vWF above. Thus, all patients gave a good response in terms of both FVIII coagulant activity and antigen, with similar upward changes between patients (even between type I and type IIA patients). Responses were generally more striking with respect to functional (FVIII coagulant) activity (see Figs. 1, 2). Changes expressed as -fold increase over baseline levels also tended to be fairly consistent between patients (see Figs. 3, 4).

Time Course of Changes to vWF and FVIII

Peak responsiveness to DDAVP was observed for most patients, and using most assays, at between 30 min and 2 hr post-DDAVP (see Figs. 1–4). Levels remained elevated even at 6 hr post-DDAVP infusion (Figs. 3, 4). While there were minor differences between patients and between assays, there did not appear to be any consistent major differences in the pattern of changing levels with time as assessed by using the different assays. Thus, peak levels of vWF, or of FVIII, as assessed by all assays, and for each patient, occurred at a similar time point (usually between 30 and 60 min post-DDAVP), and fell subsequently at rates that we could not determine to be different. One patient's responsiveness was assessed for a longer time frame (type I vWD). In this patient, values for vWF and FVIII fell to baseline levels by 24 hr; at this time the patient was rechallenged with DDAVP and showed a smaller, but significant, response as detected by all assays (data not shown).

SBT Changes Following DDAVP

All three type IIa patients evaluated had initial prolonged SBTs (each >15.0 min), and two of these (patients shown in Fig. 2A,B, respectively) showed some correction (to 8.5 min and 12.0 min) following DDAVP. Of the four type I patients evaluated in this study, only one (patient shown in Fig. 1C) was determined to have an

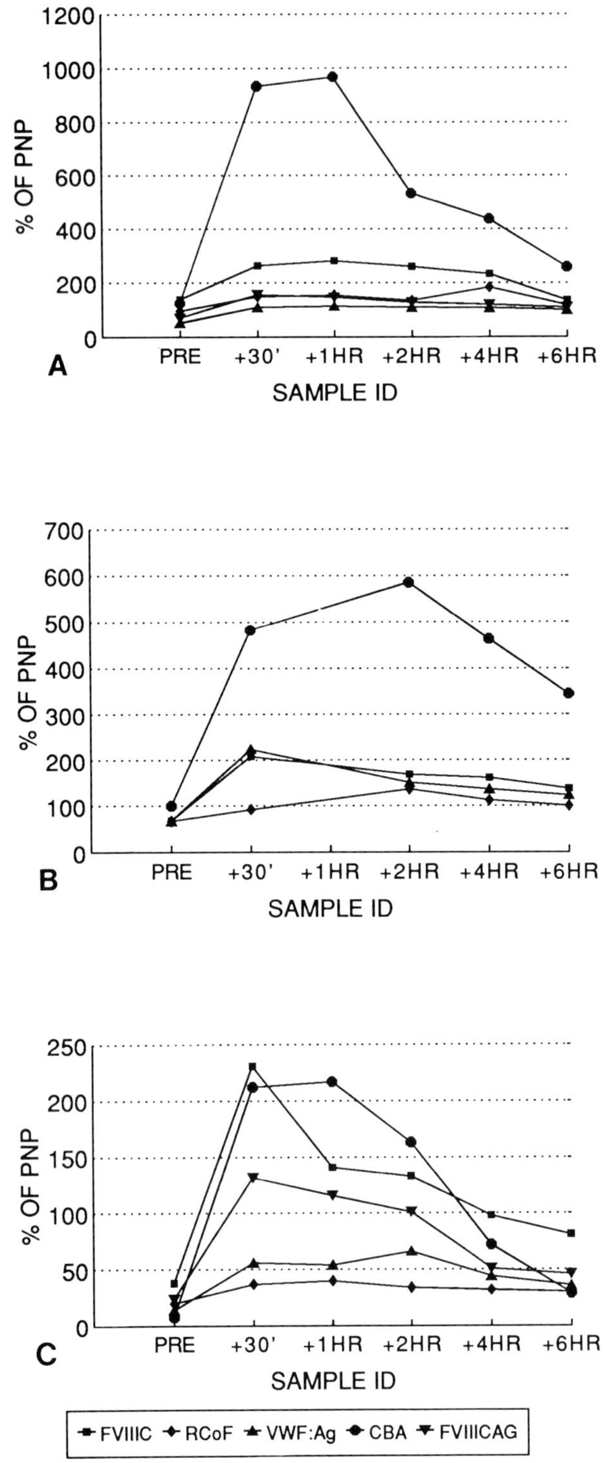

Fig. 1. Changes in vWF and FVIII levels following DDAVP infusion, as detected using five separate assay procedures, for three separate patients (A–C) with type I vWD. Results are expressed as a percentage of PNP value (assigned to equal 100%). Samples were collected preinfusion (PRE) and at indicated times following infusion (+30 min [= +30]; + 1 hr; + 2 hr; + 4 hr; + 6 hr). All patients showed initial upward increases using all tests but consistently showed the greatest upward change in CBA assay values. A fourth type I vWD patient evaluated yielded data essentially similar to those for the patient shown in C.

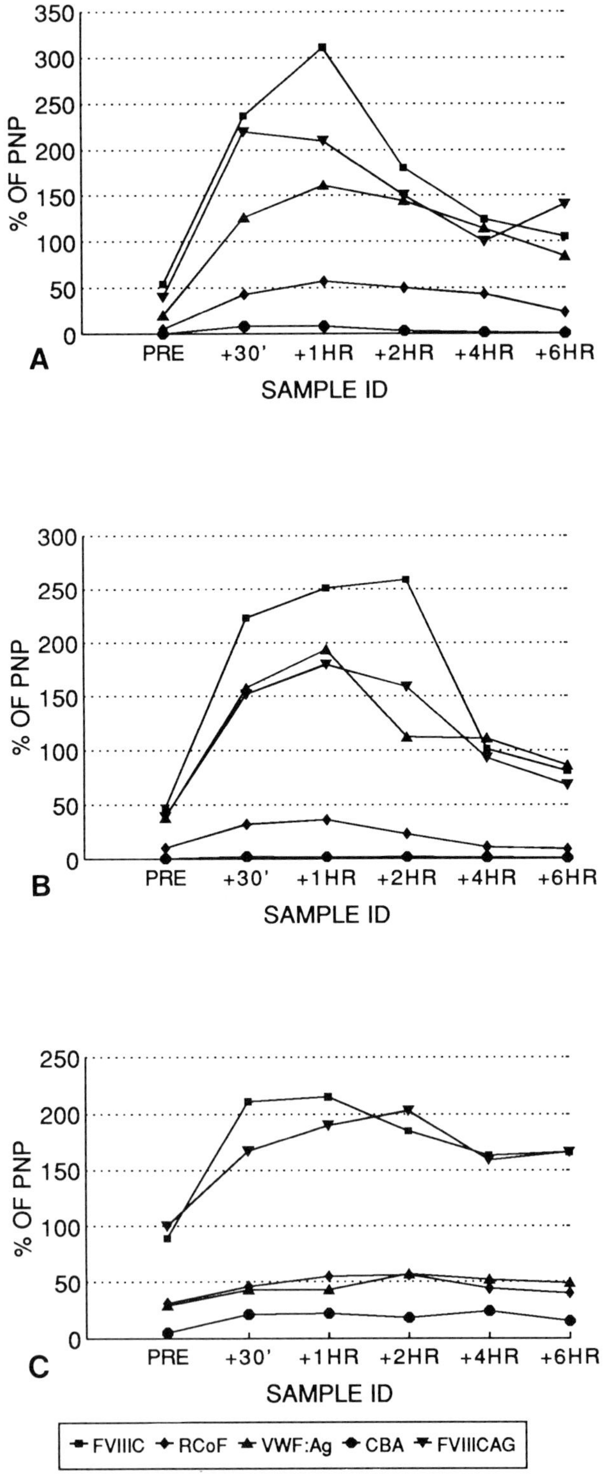

Fig. 2. Changes in vWF and FVIII levels following DDAVP infusion, as detected using five separate assay procedures, for three separate patients (A–C) with type IIA vWD. Results are expressed as a percentage of PNP value (assigned to equal 100%). Sampling times are as in Figure 1. All patients showed initial upward increases using all tests.

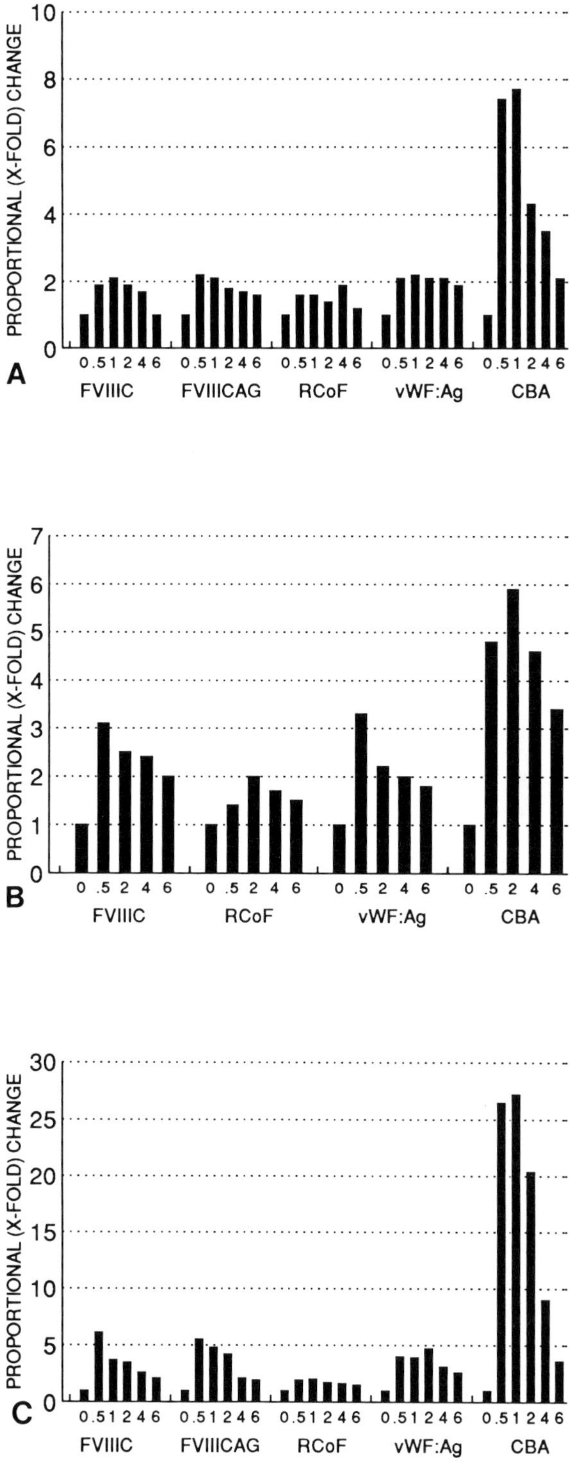

Fig. 3. Changes in vWF and FVIII levels following DDAVP infusion for vWD type I patients (A–C) shown in Figure 1, with results expressed as proportional changes compared to baseline values (i.e., -fold change over baseline = 1.0). All patients showed initial upward increases using all tests, but note the consistently greater upward change using the CBA. X axis abbreviations: 0 = pre DDAVP; 0.5 = + 30 min post-DDAVP; 1 = + 1 hr post-DDAVP; 2 = + 2 hr post-DDAVP; etc. Fourth type I vWD patient evaluated yielded data essentially similar to those for the patient shown in C.

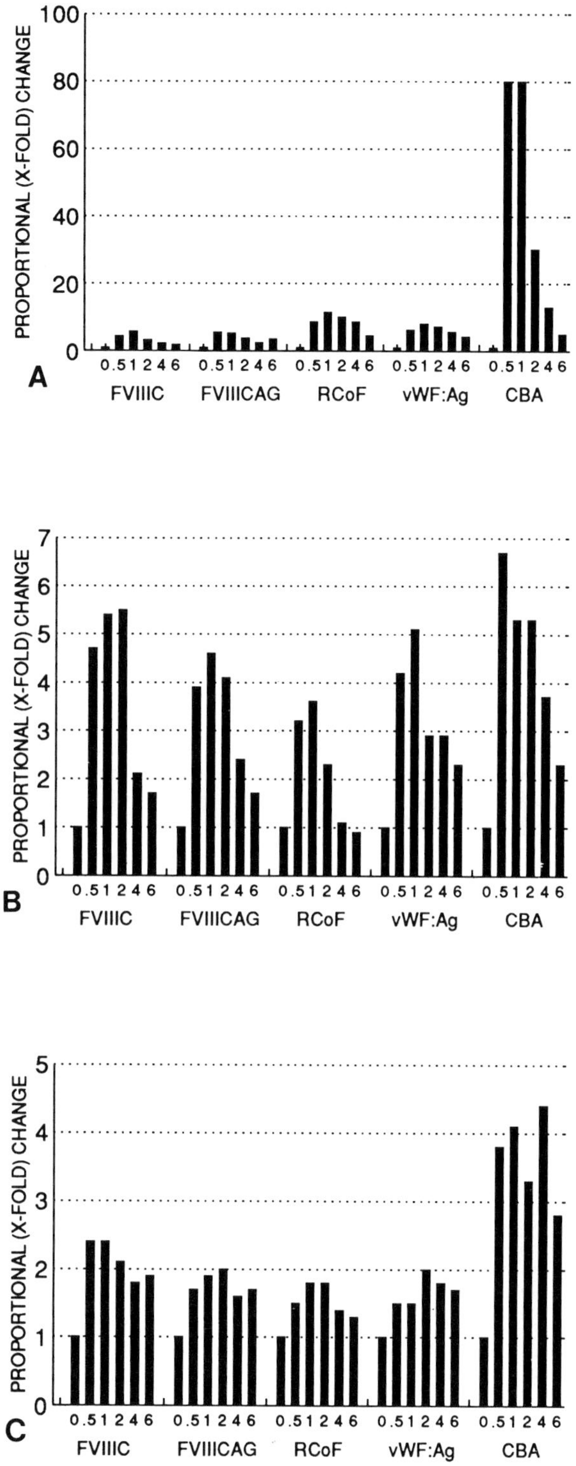

Fig. 4. Changes in vWF and FVIII levels following DDAVP infusion for vWD type IIA patients (A–C) shown in Figure 2, with results expressed as proportional changes compared to baseline values (i.e., -fold change over baseline = 1.0). All patients showed initial upward increases using all tests and, despite the low absolute CBA levels depicted in Figure 2, showed consistently high upward change (as -fold increase) using the CBA compared to baseline values. Abbreviations are as in Figure 3.

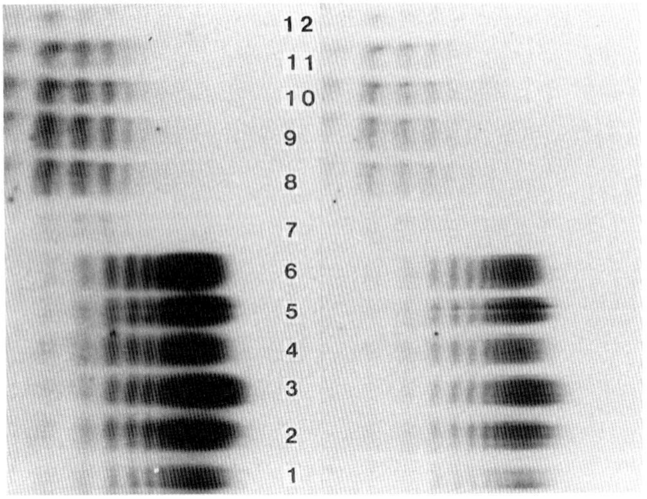

Fig. 5. Sample multimer patterns, obtained using plasma from two vWD patients (type I vWD patient) [depicted in Figs. 1A, 3A] and lanes 1–6 this figure; type IIA vWD patient [depicted in Figs. 2A, 4A] and lanes 7–12 this figure). Left and right segments show the same gel results with high and low autoradiography exposure to improve resolution of both qualitative and quantitive changes observed following DDAVP infusion. Lanes 1–6: Type I vWD patient: lanes 1 = pre-DDAVP sample; 2 = +30 min post-DDAVP; 3 = +1 hr; 4 = +2 hr; 5 = +4 hr; 6 = +6 hr. Lanes 7–12: = Type IIA vWD patient: lanes 7 = pre-DDAVP sample; 8 = +30 min post-DDAVP; 9 = 1 hr; 10 = +2 hr; 11 = +4 hr; 12 = +6 hr.

abnormal SBT prior to DDAVP (>15.0 min), and this showed correction (to 7.0 min) following DDAVP.

Multimer Analysis

Sample results are depicted in Figure 5. DDAVP infusion resulted in the expression within plasma of both increased levels of vWF (quantitative change; represented in Fig. 5 by the darker intensity of resultant multimer bands in post-DDAVP sample lanes) and in the expression or appearance of higher molecular weight multimer forms of vWF (qualitative change; represented in Fig. 5 by the appearance of multimer bands in post-DDAVP sample lanes, which are not visible in pre-DDAVP sample lanes).

DISCUSSION

This report is the first to describe the use of the newly developed [9] collagen binding assay, a novel functional assay for von Willebrand factor, in the assessment of the responsiveness of patients with von Willebrand's disease to DDAVP infusion. This assay has previously proved its worth [9,10] by its unique ability to allow effectively separation of type I and type II vWD patients (the two most common subtypes of vWD).

In type I vWD patients (four evaluated in the current study), responsiveness to DDAVP in terms of vWF release, as detected using the CBA, consistently overshadowed levels of vWF assessed by other standard laboratory procedures (Figs. 1, 3). Interestingly, in this group of patients, responsiveness as assessed using the standard functional vWF assay, the ristocetin cofactor assay, showed least effect among the group of tests employed. Responsiveness to DDAVP, as assessed using factor VIII coagulant assays, were generally concordant with that assessed using the vWF:Ag assay. That the CBA showed the most striking initial proportional changes in these patients following DDAVP infusion is significant for a number of reasons. First, and simply, the CBA appears to be more sensitive to such changes (i.e., detection of vWF levels following DDAVP) than existing standard and utilised assay systems (vWF:Ag, RCof). Second, the CBA is a functional assay, which measures an "adhesive" ability of vWF and selectively enables the measurement of (collagen) binding to higher molecular weight (i.e., more functional) forms of vWF. It follows, then, that levels of vWF detected using the CBA more likely reflect a true functional responsiveness of the patient to DDAVP infusion. In simple terms, the CBA is detecting vWF more functionally relevant than that detected using other vWF assays.

In type IIA vWD patients (three evaluated), absolute quantitative changes in CBA values following DDAVP (Fig. 2) were less marked than those observed in type I vWD patients (Fig. 1). Despite this, however, initial proportional (i.e., -fold) increases in CBA tended to be more striking than those observed using other assays (Fig. 4). In this group of patients, proportional changes in vWF or factor VIII assessed by other assays tended to be similar to each other.

While our CBA has not been previously used to evaluate vWD patients' responsiveness to DDAVP, there are many reports of studies utilising the other assay systems described here [see, e.g., 5–8]. In two recent reviews [6,7], the use of DDAVP is advocated for all suitable (and trialed) vWD patients (e.g., most type I, and some type IIA patients benefit haemostatically following DDAVP infusion, but DDAVP is not effective in type III vWD and is contra indicated in type IIB or pseudo-vWD). It is also generally concluded that, if DDAVP is able to correct factor VIII coagulant levels, this might be sufficient to ensure satisfactory haemostasis in most cases of haemorrhagic complications. The obvious exceptions are cases of mucosal bleeding, which are more difficult to predict, and it is in these cases when the use of the CBA to evaluate DDAVP responsiveness may be of further relevance, particularly as a proposed marker of vWF/platelet/subendothelial activity. It is a functional vWF assay, and it is capable of far more sensitive discrimination of DDAVP-induced changes than the standard vWF functional assay (the RCof assay). Since it has never been previously evaluated, one cannot be certain what correction in the CBA would be required to enable prediction of satisfactory haemostasis in such cases.

With respect to the current study, some measure of clinical responsiveness (i.e., correction of potential mucosal bleeding) following DDAVP was evaluable in three patients. While it may be premature to attempt to draw any firm conclusion regarding the clinical relevance of these findings, we can confirm that (at least for these patients) effective haemostasis was evident post-DDAVP. In a similar manner, correction of SBT was also evident in some patients. Only further work in this area will allow clarification of the relationship between CBA levels and effective haemostasis for both minor and major surgery/trauma.

In conclusion, the CBA is a novel functional assay for vWF, whose use should now be extended from that of a test to distinguish type I and type II vWD patients [9,10] to that of monitoring the responsiveness of such patients to DDAVP therapy. We propose that it may reflect more accurately the true functional vWF responsiveness of such patients, and we have determined it to be a sensitive procedure for detection of such changes.

ACKNOWLEDGMENTS

The authors thank clinicians who referred to us patients or patient samples for evaluation in this study. In particular we relay our gratitude to Dr. Keith Jones and Margaret Aboud (at Royal North Shore Hospital), Prof. Peter Castaldi (Westmead Hospital), Dr. Warwick Benson (Westmead Hospital), and Dr. David Gottlieb (Blacktown Hospital). In addition, we convey our gratitude to Judith Maybin for expert assistance in the preparation of the manuscript.

REFERENCES

1. Ruggeri ZM, Zimmerman TS: von Willebrand factor and von Willebrand disease. Blood 70:895–904, 1987.
2. Giddings JC, Peake IR: The investigation of factor VIII deficiency. In Thompson JM (ed): "Blood Coagulation and Haemostasis." New York: Churchill Livingstone, 1985, pp 135–207.
3. Girma J-P, Meyer D, Verweij CL, et al.: Structure-function relationship of human von Willebrand factor. Blood 70:605–611, 1987.
4. Sadler JE: Review: Von Willebrand factor. J Biol Chem 266:22777–22780, 1991.
5. Mannucci PM, Altieri D, Faioni E. Vasopressin analogues: Their role in disorders of haemostasis. Ann NY Acad Sci 509:71–81, 1987.
6. Rodeghiero F, Castamann G, Mannucci PM: Clinical indications for desmopressin (DDAVP) in congenital and acquired von Willebrand disease. Blood Rev 5:155–161, 1991.
7. Mannuci PM: Desmopressin: A nontransfusional form of treatment for congenital and acquired bleeding disorders. Blood 72:1449–1455, 1988.
8. Mannucci PM: Desmopressin (DDAVP) for treatment of disorders of haemostasis. Progr Hemostas Thromb 8:19–43, 1986.
9. Favaloro EJ, Grispo L, Exner T, Koutts J: Development of a simple collagen based ELISA assay aids in the diagnosis of, and permits sensitive discrimination between, type I and type II, von Willebrand's disease. Blood Coag Fibrinolysis 2:285–291, 1991.
10. Favaloro EJ, Grispo L, Dinale A, Berndt M, Koutts J: von Willebrand's disease: Laboratory investigation using an improved functional assay for von Willebrand factor. Pathology 25:152–158, 1993.
11. Brown JE, Bosak JO: An ELISA test for the binding of von Willebrand antigen to collagen. Thromb Res 43:303–311, 1986.
12. Exner T, Hill P, Cleland J, et al.: Studies on an unusual von Willebrand's variant-type IID. Aust NZ J Med 20:553–557, 1990.
13. Ruggeri ZM, Zimmerman TS: Variant von Willebrand's disease: Characterization of two subtypes by analysis of multimer composition of factor VIII/von Willebrand factor in plasma and platelets. J Clin Invest 65:1318–1235, 1980.

American Journal of Hematology 45:212–216 (1994)

Detection of PML-Retinoic Acid Receptor-α Fusion Transcripts in Acute Promyelocytic Leukemia With Trisomy 8 but Without t(15;17)

Kazuma Ikeda, Kazunori Sasaki, Taizo Tasaka, Masami Nagai, Koichi Kawanishi, Jiro Takahara, and Shozo Irino

Department of Transfusion Medicine (K.I., K.K.) and the First Department of Internal Medicine (K.S., T.T., M.N., J.T.), Kagawa Medical School (S.I.), Kagawa, Japan

Chromosome translocation t(15;17), the breakpoints of which are in the PML gene on chromosome 15 and retinoic acid receptor-α (RARα) gene on chromosome 17, is specifically found in acute promyelocytic leukemia (APL). Clinically typical APL without t(15;17) and with the PML-RARα fusion transcripts or rearrangements in PML and/or RARα gene has been reported, suggesting submicroscopic changes at the molecular level without apparent t(15;17) or observation of normal metaphases. Trisomy 8 is common in APL as a secondary chromosomal abnormality in addition to t(15;17), as well as in acute myelogenous leukemia in general, but it is rare as a sole chromosomal anomaly in APL. PML-RARα fusion transcript was detected in an APL case with trisomy 8 but without t(15;17), indicating that the leukemic cells lacked t(15;17) and still expressed the PML-RARα fusion transcripts. This indicates that the same submicroscopic molecular changes as in APL with t(15;17) do occur in APL without t(15;17) and supports the use of molecular analysis for PML-RARα fusion in APL.

Key words: PML, APL, trisomy 8, t(15;17)

INTRODUCTION

Chromosome translocation t(15;17), the breakpoints of which are in the PML gene on chromosome 15 and retinoic acid receptor-α (RARα) gene on chromosome 17 [1–3], is specifically found in acute promyelocytic leukemia (APL) [4,5]. APL without t(15;17) has been reported, and PML-RARα fusion transcripts [6] and rearrangement of PML and/or RARα gene [7] have been detected in some of APL patients without t(15;17). Correlation between the presence of the fusion transcripts and the responsiveness to all-*trans*-retinoic acid has also been claimed in APL with or without t(15;17) [6]. Trisomy 8 is common in APL as a secondary chromosomal abnormality in addition to t(15;17), as well as in acute myelogenous leukemia in general, but it is rare as a sole chromosomal anomaly in APL [8]. We detected the PML-RARα fusion transcripts in an APL case with trisomy 8 but without t(15;17), in which trisomy 8 excludes the possibility that the karyotype of normal nonneoplastic cells was detected, and in which the PML-RARα fusion transcript suggests that the same submicroscopic molecular events as in APL with t(15;17) do occur in APL without t(15;17).

CASE REPORT

Pancytopenia with 30% promyelocytes in peripheral blood leukocytes was found in a 26-year-old Japanese woman in April, 1988. On physical examination, pallor, swollen left tonsil, and systolic ejection murmur were noticed. Her laboratory data revealed a leukocyte count of 1.4×10^6/ml with 40% promyelocytes, anemia, moderate thrombocytopenia, slightly increased lactate dehydrogenase (LDH), and prolonged prothrombin time. Her bone marrow was normocellular with 73% promyelocytes, some of which had numerous Auer rods (Fig. 1). The abnormal cells were positive for myeloperoxidase and AS-D chloroacetate esterase and positive for CD13 and CD33 on cytofluorometric analysis. A diagnosis of APL was made, and she was treated with combination chemotherapy including daunorubicin hydrochloride,

Received for publication March 3, 1993; accepted July 20, 1993.

Address reprint requests to Kazuma Ikeda, Assistant Professor, Department of Transfusion Medicine, Kagawa Medical School, Ikenobe, Miki, Kagawa 761-07, Japan.

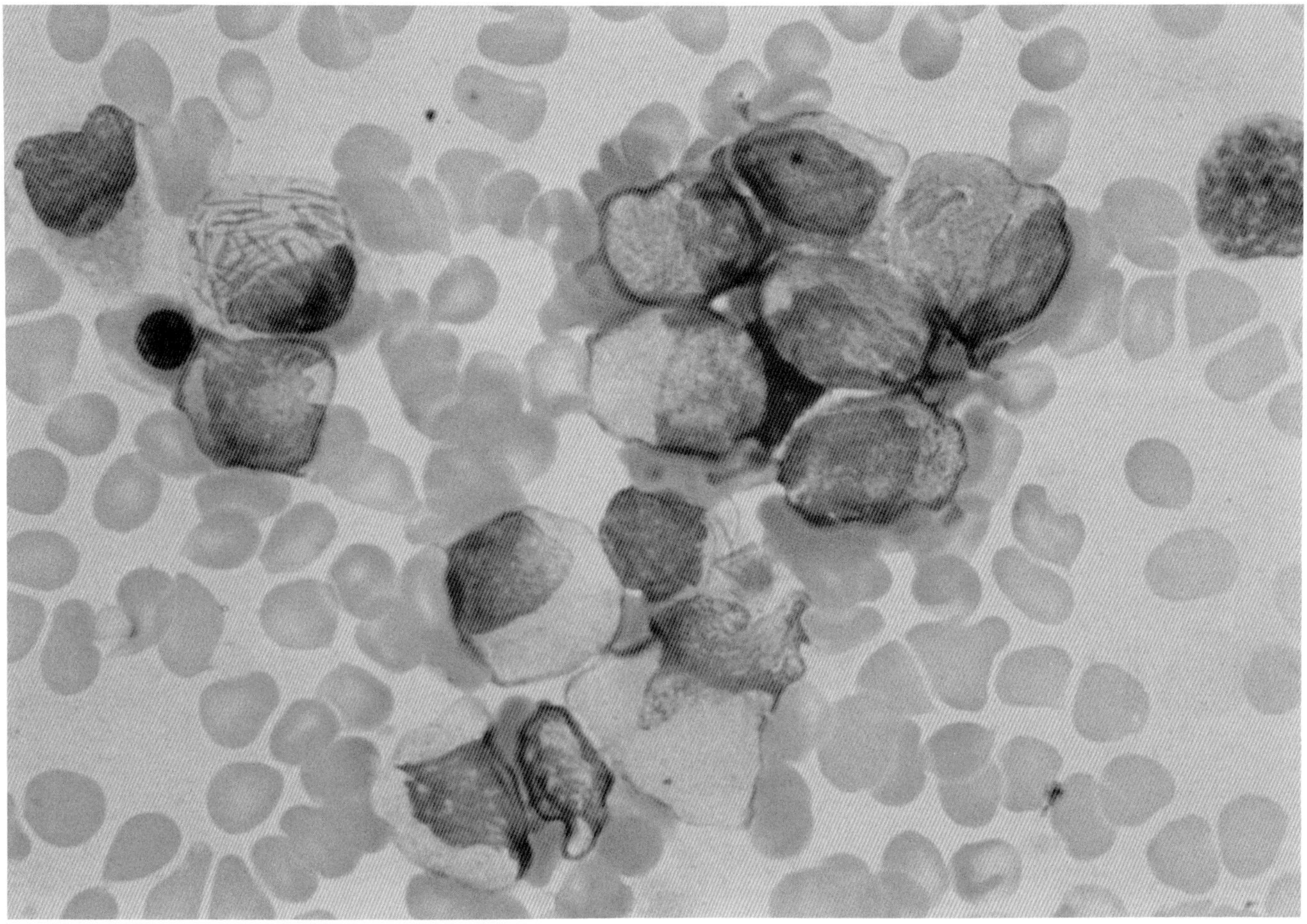

Fig. 1. May-Giemsa staining of the bone marrow film obtained on the patient's initial presentation. Some promyelocytes include numerous Auer rods.

enocitabine, and mercaptopurine. Complete remission was achieved, but her clinical course was complicated by heart failure due to anthracyclin-induced cardio-myopathy. Because low-voltage and negative T waves on electro-cardiography and hypokinesis and decreased wall thickness on echocardiography persisted, she was followed without maintenance chemotherapy until April, 1992, when relapse developed. Again her leukemic cells showed findings typical for APL. Chemotherapy consisting of etoposide, cytarabine, and mitoxantrone hydrochloride was given, but the patient died of respiratory failure caused by pneumonia in July, 1992.

MATERIALS AND METHODS

Bone marrow mononuclear cells were collected via Ficoll/Hypaque density centrifugation. Cytogenetic studies were performed on unstimulated bone marrow cultures by Giemsa banding [9] (Fig. 2). Total RNA was isolated from bone marrow mononuclear cells and from hemopoietic cell line K562 [10]. Random hexanucleotide-primed cDNA of 1 μg RNA was synthesized in 10 μl reaction mixture with reagents supplied by Amersham Japan, (Tokyo, Japan). One microliter of cDNA synthesis reaction mixture was subjected to polymerase chain reaction (PCR) in a 10 μl reaction mixture consisting of 500 μM each of primers M5 and R2, 0.25 unit of Taq polymerase, 500 μM of dNTP mix, 10 mM Tris-HCl (pH 8.3), 50 mM KCl, 1.5 mM $MgCl_2$, 0.01% (v/w) gelatin on a DNA Thermal Cycler PJ2000 (Perkin-Elmer/Cetus) [11]. The PCR cycle consisted of denaturation at 90°C for 1 min, annealing at 60°C for 45 sec, and extension at 72°C for 2 min, and the cycle was repeated 50 times. Oligonucleotide primers for PCR were synthesized on a Cyclone Plus DNA synthesizer (MilliGen/Biosearch). PCR product was run through a 2% Nusieve/1% SeaKem agarose (FMC BioProducts, Rockland, ME) gel and transferred to a nylon membrane. The membrane was probed with a biotin-labeled oligonucleotide and FLASH detection system (Staratagene). Briefly, the oligonucle-

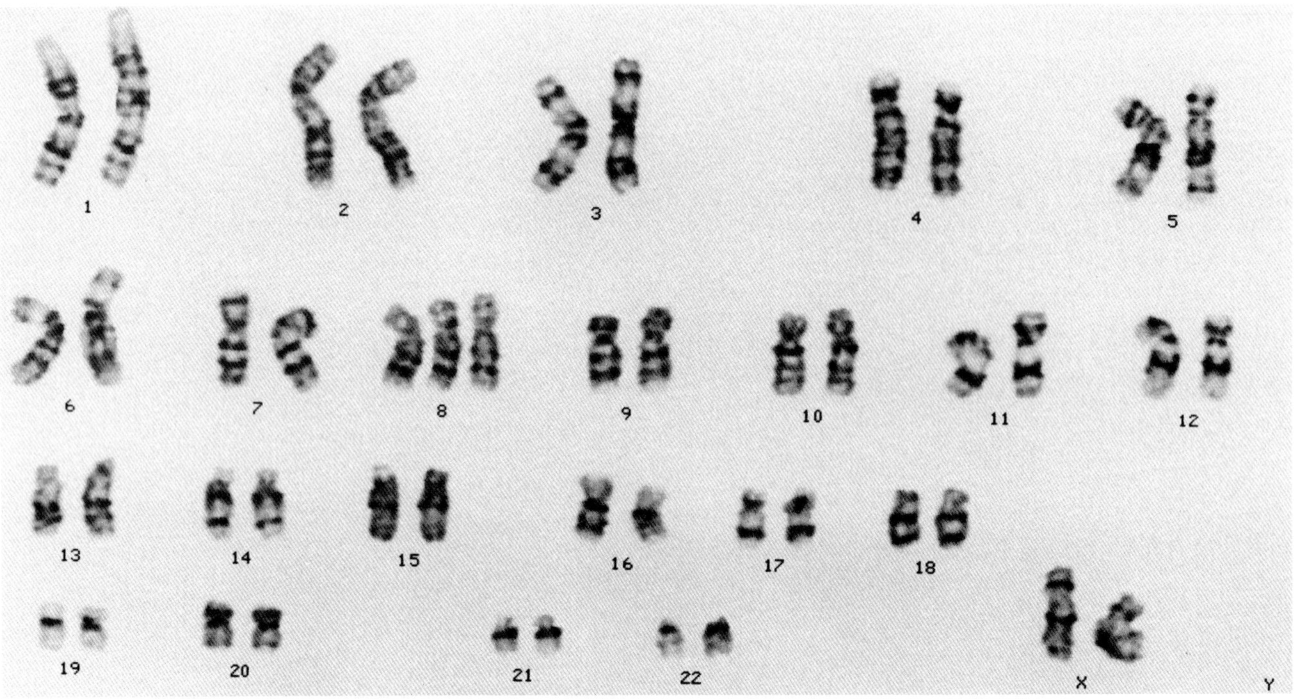

Fig. 2. Chromosome analysis on relapse, which showed trisomy 8 but no t(15;17) in all of 60 metaphases analyzed. Karyotype on initial presentation was also trisomy 8 without t(15;17) in 20 of 21 metaphases analyzed and 46,XX in the remaining one metaphase.

otide probe was synthesized as described above for the PCR primers, except that biotin was added to 5′ end by Biotin-On Phosphoramidite (Clontech) and was hybridized to the membrane. After avidin-alkaline phosphatase conjugate was bound to biotin, chemiluminescent substrate was added, and the light signal was recorded on X-omat AR film (Eastman Kodak). The sequences of the primers and the probe were as follows: M5;GACCCTATTGACGTTGACCT, R2;CCTCCAAGGCAGTCTCACCA, probe:biotin-GCTCAAAGTCAGATGCTACT (Fig. 3A).

For sequencing the amplified DNA fragment, the PCR product was cloned into pCR vector (TA Cloning System, Invitrogen, CA), and the dideoxynucleotide sequencing reaction was carried out with biotinylated M13 oligonucleotides (New England Biolab, Boston, MA) or the biotinylated oligonucleotide probe described above as primers. Sequencing products were run on a 6% polyacrylamide-7.67 M urea denaturing gel, and DNA sequence was determined using Uniplex sequence kit (MilliGen/Biosearch).

RESULTS

Chromosome analysis on the patient's initial presentation showed 47, XX, +8 in 20 of 21 metaphases analyzed and one metaphase with 46, XX. All 60 metaphases analyzed at relapse revealed 47, XX, +8 (Fig. 2).

The breakpoint in the PML gene is reported to be either upstream (within intron 3) or downstream (within exon 6 or intron 6) [1–3,12]. RT-PCR for PML-RARα fusion transcript amplified fragments of three sizes compatible with the fusion transcripts with the downstream PML breakpoint and alternative splicing of exon 5 or exons 5 and 6 (Fig. 3). DNA sequencing of the largest amplified fragment confirmed the fusion between the 3′ end of exon 6 of the PML gene and the 5′ end of the third exon (region B) of the RARα gene [1,2] (Fig. 4), indicating that the PML breakpoint in this patient was in intron 6 [1,2,12].

DISCUSSION

Trisomy 8 is a fairly common secondary chromosomal abnormality in APL in addition to t(15;17) [8], as well as in acute myelogenous leukemia in general. However, APL with trisomy 8 but without t(15;17) is rare. Berger et al. [8] reported cytogenetic studies of 105 APL patients, in which t(15;17) with or without additional abnormalities was observed in 101 cases; three had only normal karyotype, and trisomy 8 (41 metaphases) and trisomies of 8 and 21 (19 metaphases) were observed in one pa-

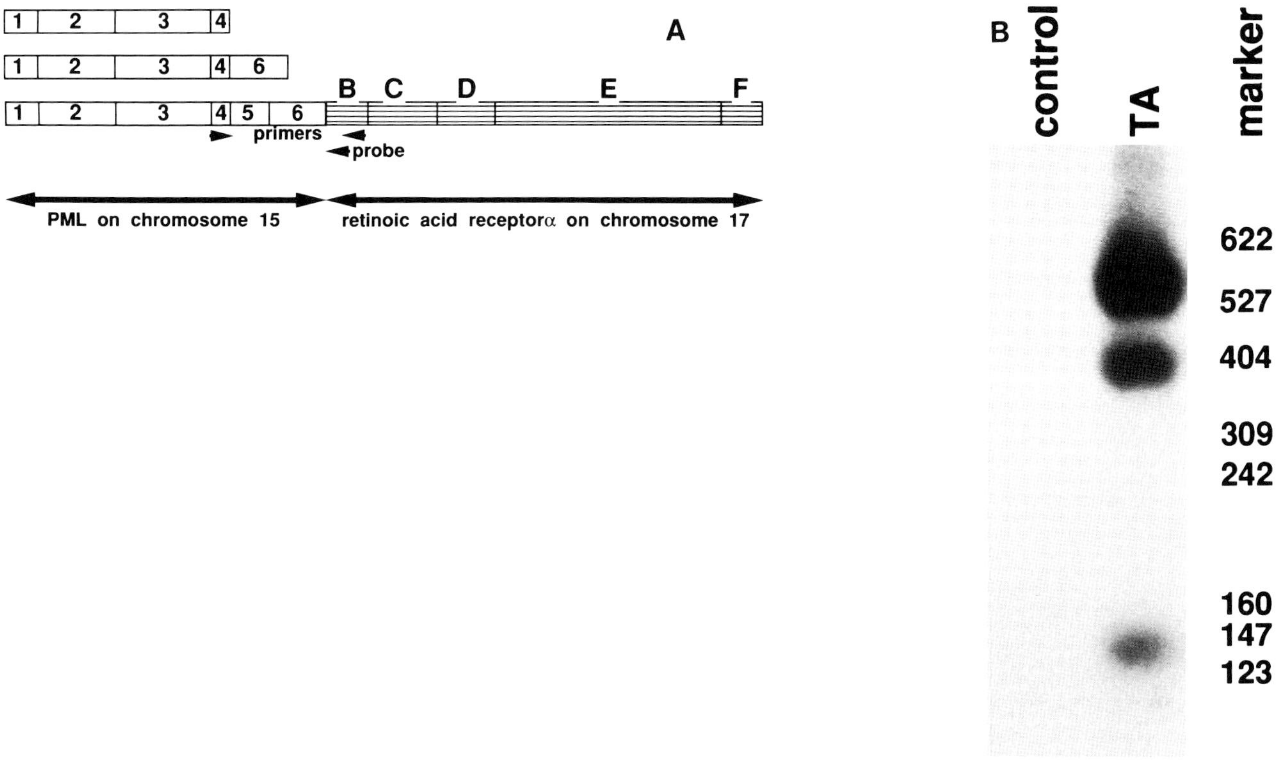

Fig. 3. A: Schema showing the fusion between PML and RARα gene. Open boxes with numbers indicate exons of the PML gene, and hatched boxes with letters indicate regions of the RARα gene. The primers for gene amplification were in exon 4 of PML and in exon 3 (region B) of RARα, and the probe was in the 5′ end of exon 3 of the RARα gene. B: RT-PCR amplified fragments of three sizes compatible with the fusion with the downstream PML breakpoint with alternative splicing of exon 5 or exons 5 and 6. TA, the patient. Control, K562 as negative control. Marker, in base pairs.

tient. Clinically typical APL without t(15;17) has been reported, and the PML-RARα fusion transcripts [6] or rearrangements in PML and/or RARα genes [7] in such patients have been proved. These might result from submicroscopic changes at the molecular level without apparent t(15;17) or observation of normal metaphases. Miller et al. [6] studied 36 clinically diagnosed APL and reported that eight of 36 cases had normal karyotype, four of whom had PML-RARα fusion transcripts and another four did not. They also observed that APL cases with the fusion transcripts responded to all-*trans*-retinoic acid but those without did not, suggesting that clinically diagnosed APL without the PML-RARα fusion transcripts is of a different etiology [6]. In trisomy 8 on karyotype analysis, metaphase of leukemic cells, not of normal cells, was observed. Detection of PML-RARα fusion transcript in APL with trisomy 8 but without t(15;17) showed that the leukemic cells lacked t(15;17) and still expressed the PML-RARα fusion transcripts. Morris et al. [13] showed that a part of chromosome 9 that contained the 3′ portion of the ABL gene was inserted into the major breakpoint cluster region of the BCR gene, resulting in apparently normal karyotype and typical BCR-ABL fusion gene in a Ph-negative chronic myelogenous leukemia patients. Similar mechanisms might explain the presence of PML-RARα fusion transcripts without t(15;17) in our patient. Our observation not only indicates that the same molecular changes as in APL with t(15;17) occur in APL without typical t(15;17) but also further indicate the necessity of molecular analysis in clinically diagnosed APL, considering the reported correlation between the presence of the PML-RARα fusion and the responsiveness to all-*trans*-retinoic acid [6].

ACKNOWLEDGMENTS

This work was supported in part by Grants-in-Aid from the Ministry of Education, Science and Culture of Japan. Excellent technical assistance from Kiyo Ueeda is appreciated.

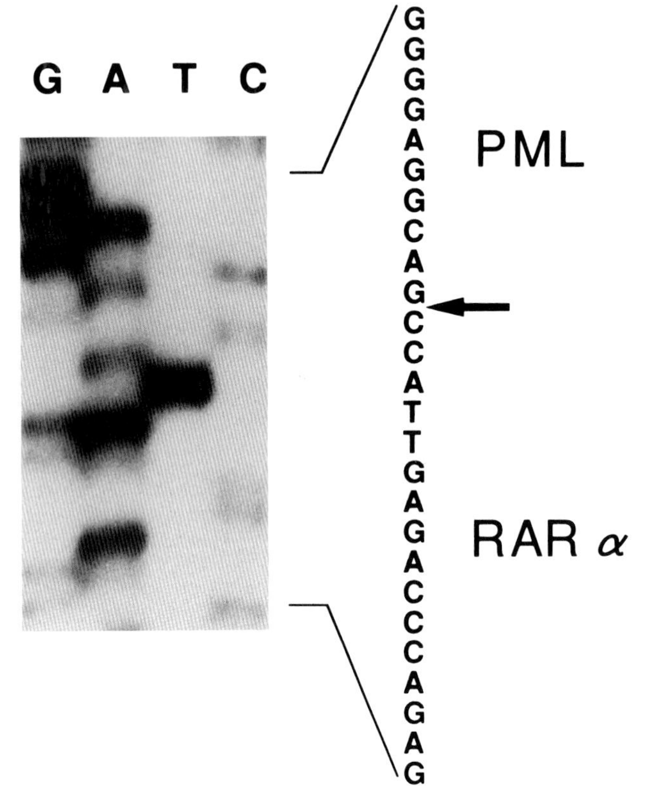

Fig. 4. Nucleotide sequence of the amplified fragment of the largest size showed that the 3′ end of PML exon 6 was fused to 5′ end of RARα exon 3, indicating that the breakpoint in PML gene was in intron 6.

REFERENCES

1. de The H, Lavau C, Marchio A, Chomienne C, Degos L, Dejean A: The PML-RARα fusion mRNA generated by the t(15;17) translocation in acute promyelocytic leukemia encodes a functionally altered RAR. Cell 66:675, 1991.
2. Pandolfi PP, Grignani F, Alcalay M, Mencarelli A, Biondi A, LoCoco F, Grignani F, Pelicci PG: Structure and origin of the acute promyelocytic leukemia myl/RARα cDNA and characterization of its retinoid-binding and transactivation properties. Oncogene 6:1285, 1991.
3. Kakizuka A, Miller WHJ, Umesono K, Warrell RPJ, Frankel SR, Murty VVVS, Dmitrovsky E, Evans RM: Chromosomal translocation t(15;17) in human acute promyelocytic leukemia fuses RARα with a novel putative transcription factor, PML. Cell 66:663, 1991.
4. Rowley JD, Golomb HM, Dougherty C: 15/17 Translocation, a consistent chromosomal change in acute promyelocytic leukemia. Lancet 1:549, 1977.
5. Bennet JM, Catovksy D, Daniel MT, Flandrin G, Galton DAG, Gralnick HR, Sultan C: Proposed revised criteria for the classification of acute myeloid leukemia. Br J Haematol 33:451, 1976.
6. Miller WH, Jr, Kakizuka A, Frankel SR, Warrell RP, Jr, DeBlasio A, Levine K, Evans RM, Dmitrovsky E: Reverse transcription polymerase chain reaction for the rearranged retinoic acid receptor α clarifies diagnosis and detects minimal residual disease in acute promyelocytic leukemia. Proc Natl Acad Sci USA 89:2694, 1992.
7. Lo Coco F, Diverio D, D'Adamo F, Avvisati G, Alimena G, Nanni M, Alcalay M, Pandolfi PP, Pelicci PG: PML/RAR-α rearrangement in acute promyelocytic leukaemias apparently lacking the t(15;17) translocation. Eur J Haematol 48:173, 1992.
8. Berger R, Le Coniat M, Derre J, Vecchione D, Jnveaux P: Cytogenetic studies in acute promyelocytic leukemia: A survey of secondary chromosomal abnormalities. Genes Chromosomes Cancer 3:332, 1991.
9. International System for Human Cytogenetic Nomenclature (ISCN). Report of the Standing Committee on Human Cytogenetic Nomenclature. Birth Defects 21:1, 1985.
10. Chomczynski P, Sacchi N: Single-step method of RNA isolation by acid guanidinium thiocyanate-phenol-chloroform extraction. Anal Biochem 162:156, 1987.
11. Saiki RK, Gelfand DH, Stoffel S, Scharf SJ, Higuchi R, Horn GT, Mullis KB, Erlich HA: Primer-directed enzymatic amplification of DNA with a thermostable DNA polymerase. Science 239:487, 1988.
12. Pandolfi PP, Alcalay M, Fagioli M, Zangrilli D, Mencarelli A, Diverio D, Biondi A, Lo Coco F, Rambaldi A, Grignani F, Rochette-Egly C, Gaube MP, Chambon P, Pelicci PG: Genomic variability and alternative splicing generate multiple PML/RARα transcript that encode aberrant PML proteins and PML/RARα isoforms in acute promyelocytic leukemia. EMBO J 11:1397, 1992.
13. Morris CM, Heisterkamp N, Kennedy MA, Fitzgerald PH, Groffen J: Ph-negative chronic myeloid leukemia: Molecular analysis of ABL insertion into M-BCR on chromosome 22. Blood 76:1812, 1990.

American Journal of Hematology 45:217–223 (1994)

Stability of Factor VIII Concentrates After Reconstitution

Sam Schulman, Sanford Gitel, and Uri Martinowitz
The National Hemophilia Center, Chaim Sheba Medical Center, Tel Hashomer, Israel

Adjusted-dose continuous infusion of factor VIII (F VIII) has recently been shown to reduce the doses of the factor in patients undergoing surgery by 50–75%. The main limitation of this method has been the instability of factor concentrates. All manufacturers are recommending infusion of the concentrate within hours after reconstitution. We studied the stability of 15 different lyophilized F VIII products. Reconstituted samples were stored for periods of 4, 24, and 72 hr and 1, 2, 3, and 4 weeks at temperatures of 4–8°C, 20–23°C, and 37°C in their original glass containers and in plastic tubes and then frozen. Assays were performed in duplicate, using a one-stage clotting method and a chromogenic assay for F VIII, with all samples from a single concentrate in the same run. Activation of the coagulation factor occurred in some concentrates, more often at 4–8°C than at 20–23°C or 37°C. The stability of all products was substantially better than that declared by the manufacturers. Several concentrates maintained factor activities above 80% of baseline for the entire period of 4 weeks at 4–8°C or at 20–23°C. The results demonstrate that many of the F VIII concentrates may be used for continuous infusion.

Key words: factor VIII, concentrates, stability, hemophilia A

INTRODUCTION

The prophylaxis against or treatment of hemorrhage in patients with hemophilia is based on substitution of the missing coagulation factor. Concentrates of these factors have generally been administered as bolus injections. An alternative mode of administration is by continuous infusion, which was described by McMillan et al. [1] with cryoprecipitate or glycine precipitated plasma fractions and later with lyophilized factor concentrates [2–5]. It is obvious that, whereas bolus injections require high peak levels in order to keep the troughs above a minimum level, below which there is an imminent risk of bleeding, continuous infusion can allow maintenance of a constant level slightly above this minimum. The latter method requires 50–75% less factor concentrate in, for example, postoperative settings [6]. In previous reports on continuous infusion, the factor concentrate was resuspended in a large volume (e.g., 500 ml saline). In most concentrates, when a stabilizing substance has been added, such a dilution could affect the stability of the concentrate. By using an infusion minipump, which can administer volumes as low as 0.1 ml/hr, no dilution other than the reconstitution, as recommended by the manufacturer, is necessary. Using this system, we have been able to limit refilling to once daily and sometimes even less frequently [6]. In this context it is of paramount importance to assess the stability of the concentrate after reconstitution. Only limited data on this topic have been published previously [7]. The manufacturers have usually performed stability tests before and after reconstitution and at different temperatures, but the recommendations are to use the concentrate immediately or within 1 or 3 hr after reconstitution, depending on the concentrate. Our preliminary observations indicated that some concentrates are stable for a considerably longer period. Furthermore, it is not always possible or necessary to inject the full contents of a bottle immediately after reconstitution, for example, when there are difficulties with venepuncture or in infants. In such cases, if the remaining reconstituted concentrate could be stored until the next injection, significant savings would result. In this report we present data on long-term stability after reconstitution of 15 different investigational or currently used factor VIII (F VIII) concentrates stored at different temperatures.

Received for publication March 18, 1993; accepted July 20, 1993.

Address reprint requests to Dr. Uri Martinowitz, Head, The National Hemophilia Center, The Chaim Sheba Medical Center, Tel Hashomer 52621, Israel.

TABLE I. Factor Concentrates Studied and the Method of Viral Inactivation/Elimination Used, Potency, Specific Activity, and Stability After Reconstitution, as Claimed by the Manufacturer

No.	Name	Viral inactiv/ elim[a]	Manufacturer	Potency (IU/ml)	Specific activity (IU/mg protein)	Stability (hr)
1	Beriate HS (F VIII:C)	P	Behringwerke	25	≈5 (alb)[b]	3
2	Haemate P (HS)	P	Behringwerke	25	4–6 (alb)[b]	3
3	Hemofil M	SD&IC	Baxter	24	2–15 (alb)[b]	1
4	Kryobulin TIM 3	S	Immuno	25	1–5	3
5	Monoclate	DH&IC	Armour	110	5–10 (alb)[b]	3
6	Monoclate P	P&IC	Armour	110	5–10 (alb)[b]	3
7	Factonord	P	Novo Nordisk	50	2 (alb)[b]	1
8	Octa-V.I.	SD	Octapharma	25	>2.5	—
9	Octavi	SD	Octapharma	25	≥50	—
10	Octaliquid[c]	SD	Octapharma	50	≈150	—
11	Octonativ-M	SD&IC	Kabi Pharmacia	101	25 (alb)[b]	1
12	Profilate HS	P	Alpha	48	4	0
13	Profilate OSD	SD	Alpha	24	12	3
14	Recombinate[c]	IC	Baxter	110	10 (alb)[b]	—
15	8Y	DH	BPL	27.5	1.1	1

[a]P, pasteurization; S, steam heat; DH, dry heat; SD, solvent-detergent; IC, immunoaffinity chromatography.
[b]Specific activity after addition of albumin as stabilizer.
[c]Investigational products at the time of the study.

MATERIALS AND METHODS

Factor Concentrates

In total, 15 different F VIII concentrates, some obtained as gifts from the manufacturers, were examined. The names, manufacturers, declared potencies, specific activities, and stabilities after reconstitution are shown in Table I. Octaliquid and Recombinate were investigational products at the time of the study.

The concentrates were reconstituted according to the recommendations of the manufacturers, using the utensils provided whenever available. Half of the volume was stored in the original bottles and the remainder aliquoted into polypropylene Eppendorf tubes for storage at the different temperatures and time periods. At times 0, 4, 24, and 72 hr and 1, 2, 3, and 4 weeks, samples were taken from the bottles and added to a second set of Eppendorf tubes, which, together with tubes from the previous group, were frozen and kept at −70°C until assayed. We have tested the effect of freezing and thawing on four concentrates. There was no consistent difference between fresh and frozen-thawed samples taken at time 0, all deviations being within the variations of the assay. We could not exclude, however, that after 7 days the F VIII activity is sensitive to freezing and thawing, since there was a trend to lower values compared to unfrozen samples.

The reconstituted factor concentrates were kept in the dark 1) in a refrigerator (4–8°C), 2) at room temperature (20–23°C), and 3) in an incubator at body temperature (37°C). Care was taken to handle the reconstitution and storage under sterile conditions to avoid bacterial contamination.

Factor Assays

All samples were diluted in saline containing 30% F VIII-deficient plasma to obtain a calculated concentration of 0.7–0.8 U/ml. All assays were performed in duplicate. F VIII-deficient plasma was obtained from a patient with severe hemophilia A (<1% F VIII, with no measurable inhibitor to F VIII). Two lots of plasma from the same patient were used to perform all the F VIII activity assays. Normal control plasma was a pool of plasma from 30 healthy donors, stored at −70°C in small aliquots. Normal control plasma at several dilutions (undiluted 100% and diluted to 50% and 25%) were assayed at the beginning, during, and at the end of each run. The results of the normal control plasma were used to normalize the results of the test materials.

For a normal test run of a single F VIII concentrate, the coefficient of variation was determined to be ±5%, using six separate dilutions of a F VIII concentrate. In the preparation of the sample, there is also an error of 5%. For the one-stage F VIII method the standard aPTT based assay was used employing Actin FS (Dade, Miami, FL) as the aPTT reagent, Tris-buffered saline, pH 7.3, as the sample diluent, in an MLA Electra 1000 coagulation analyzer (Medical Laboratory Automation, Inc, Pleasantville, NY). The chromogenic assay for F VIII was performed with the Dade chromogenic reagent for F VIII (Dade, Düdigen, Switzerland), according to the instructions for use with the MLA Electra 1000. All 44 samples from the same concentrate were tested together in a single run.

Statistical Analyses

The activity measured at time 0 was normalized to 100%, and subsequent results were compared to this. It was decided to set the lower limit for the criterion of a stable concentrate at 80% of the activity at time 0, since a variation of ±20% is allowed according to the U.S. Pharmacopaeia.

RESULTS

The decays of F VIII activities according to the one-stage clotting assay for the different factor concentrates are depicted in Figure 1. Activities, as measured with the chromogenic F VIII assay, decreased more rapidly than in the one-stage assay, the only exceptions being concentrates 11 and initially also 4. A comparison of the results of the one-stage clot assay and the chromogenic assay of the F VIII concentrates is shown in Figure 2. No results of the chromogenic assay of Monoclate (concentrate 5) are available due to malfunction of the assay, but this product is no longer manufactured. The duration of good stability, defined as at least 80% of initial activity, of F VIII in the concentrates is shown in Figure 2. If the activity decreased below 80% at any single point in time and then increased, the low value was disregarded both for Figure 2 and in the following discussion. Bacterial growth or other abnormalities were not visually observed in any bottles or tubes.

Influence of Time

There was generally a loss of activity with time, although several concentrates remained above 80% for all 4 weeks at 4–8°C (Fig. 2). Some concentrates remained above 80% activity also at 20–23°C (Fig. 2). On the other hand temporary increments of one-stage clot activity were also observed. Some of these occurred in samples at an isolated time point and could have been due to technical errors. Other elevations were observed in successive samples of concentrates 4–6, 9–11, 14, and 15 (see also Fig. 1). The elevation seen in concentrates 4 and 11 differed from the other F VIII products in that high one-stage clotting levels were paralleled by corresponding or often even higher chromogenic results.

Influence of Temperature

As expected, storage at 37°C caused the most rapid drop in activity. Concentrations below 80% were reached in less than 4 hr in products 11 and 14 in plastic and glass, respectively. However, some concentrates retained their activities for up to 2 weeks at 37°C in plastic containers (Fig. 2). Stability at 20–23°C was as good as that at 4–8°C in several concentrates (Fig. 2). Interestingly, activities of concentrates stored at 4–8°C dropped more rapidly than at 20–23°C in a few concentrates (Fig. 2).

Influence of the Material of the Container

In the one-stage assay, storage in plastic containers (Eppendorf tubes) was not superior to storage in glass (the original bottles) at 4–8°C (plastic better than glass n = 2; glass better than plastic n = 2). At 20–23°C (plastic better than glass n = 6; glass better than plastic n = 3) and at 37°C (plastic better than glass n = 5; glass better than plastic n = 0), plastic containers seemed to be superior to glass.

DISCUSSION

Only very limited observations on the stability of immunoaffinity-purified F VIII (Monoclate) for 12 hr after reconstitution [7] and on fibrinogen in thawed cryoprecipitate at 1–6°C for 1 month [8] have previously been published. In a recent report, the stability of Octaliquid at 4°C for 5 months and at 37°C for 2 weeks was also mentioned [9]. In our study we included many of the F VIII concentrates currently used as well as some investigational ones. With the relatively large number of concentrates studied, the cost of the material prohibited us to study more than one batch of each. However, we have substantial clinical experience with two concentrates (Monoclate P and Octavi), which showed minimal batch to batch variation in the analyses of F VIII levels of the contents in the infusion bags after 1–3 days. It is obvious from our results that the stability after reconstitution of all factor concentrates exceeds that declared by the manufacturers.

The most pertinent data with respect to continuous infusion with a minipump are the results at 20–23°C. The vessel to be filled with factor concentrate in these pumps is a sterile plastic bag. Our study demonstrates that all F VIII concentrates tested will retain an activity (by the one-stage clotting assay) above 80% of baseline in a plastic container at 20–23°C for at least 24 hr. If Profilate HS and Profilate OSD are excluded, the stability is sufficient for at least 1 week. The plastic container in our study was made of polypropylene, and it is possible that the stability could differ in bags and connection lines made of polyvinyl chloride or other plastic materials. Before application, the stability of the concentrate intended for usage should be tested in the plastic bag and connection lines available to confirm our results. If the concentrate is stable under these conditions, it will be possible to fill the pump with enough factor concentrate to last for an extended period, for example, over a weekend. Although this study presents only in vitro data, which is no evidence for the preservation of normal in

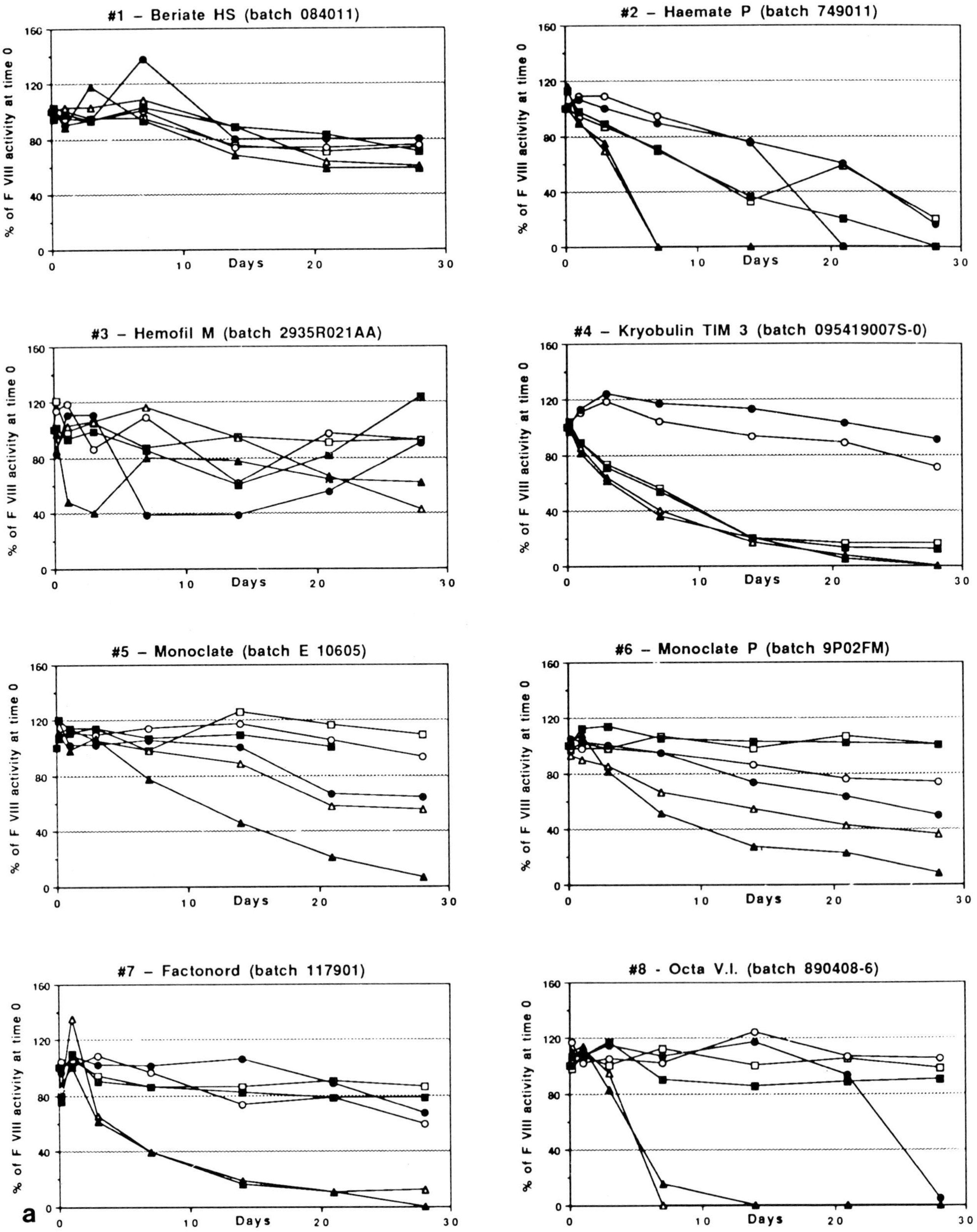

Fig. 1. a,b: Decays of F VIII activities according to the one-stage clotting assay. Open symbols, storage in plastic; solid symbols, storage in glass; squares, at 4–8°C; circles, at 20–23°C; triangles, at 37°C.

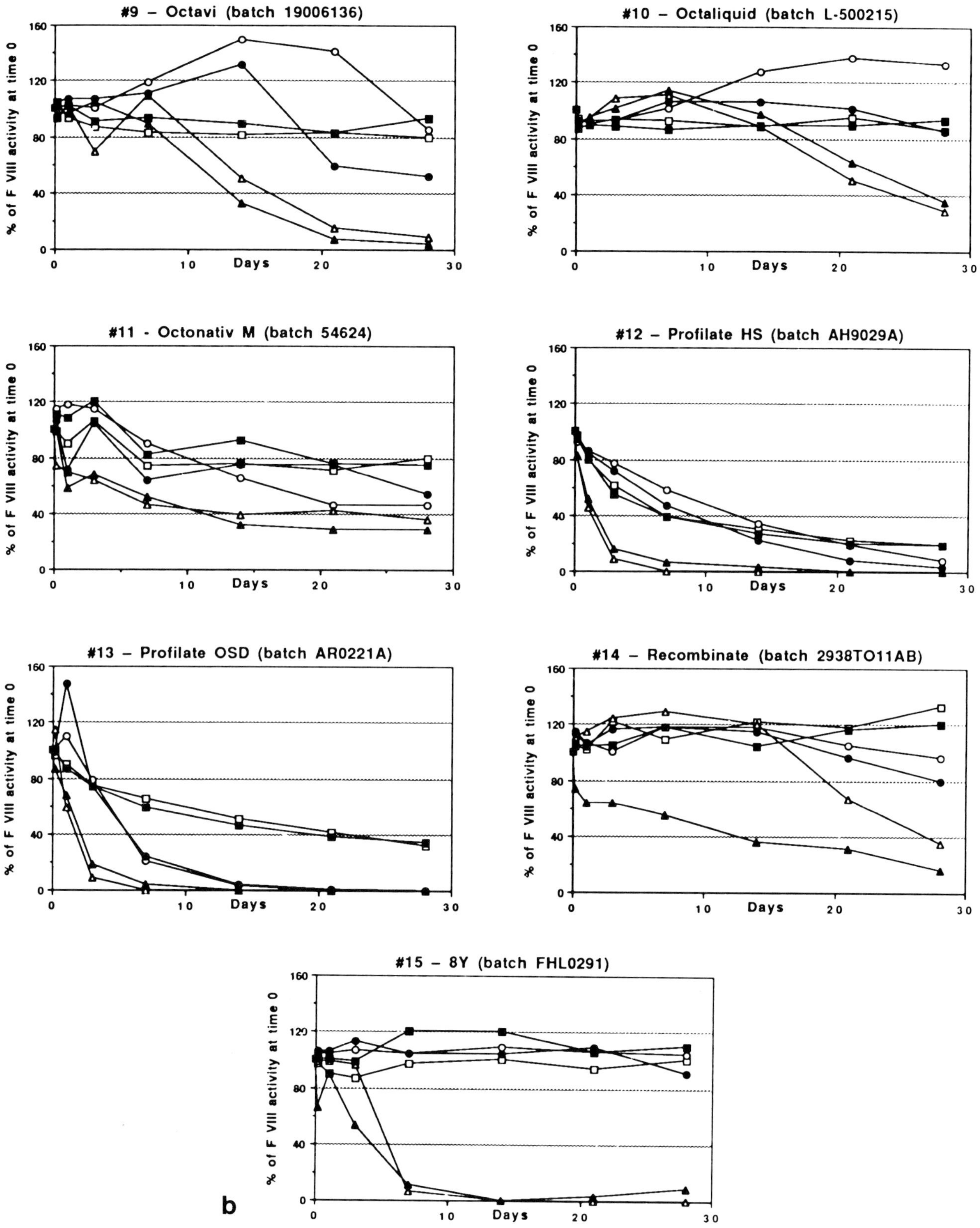
#9 – Octavi (batch 19006136)
#10 – Octaliquid (batch L-500215)
#11 - Octonativ M (batch 54624)
#12 – Profilate HS (batch AH9029A)
#13 – Profilate OSD (batch AR0221A)
#14 – Recombinate (batch 2938TO11AB)
#15 – 8Y (batch FHL0291)
% of F VIII activity at time 0
Days
0
10
20
30
40
80
120
160
b

Fig. 1. b.

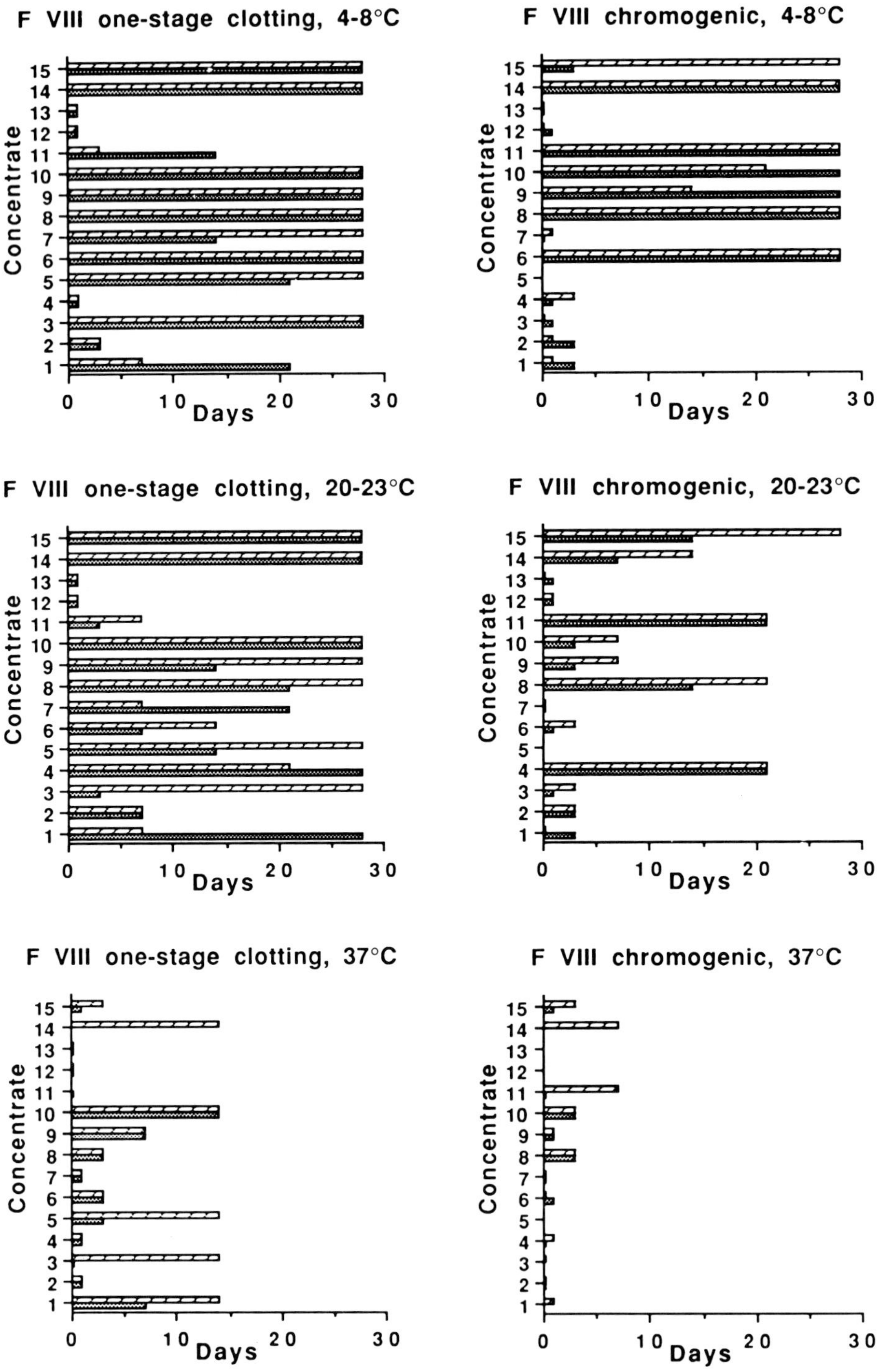

Fig. 2. Duration of retained F VIII activity of at least 80%, according to the one-stage clotting and chromogenic assay. Hatched bars, storage in plastic; shaded bars, storage in glass.

vivo recovery, we have recently published clinical results obtained with one of the concentrates (Octavi), which clearly demonstrated that the F VIII levels obtained in the patients during continuous infusion were as expected [6]. Indeed, there was a progressive decrease in the clearance of F VIII during continuous infusion over 5 days, and we have now confirmed this observation with two more concentrates (Monoclate P and Octonativ M, unpublished results).

We examined the stability at body temperature with the

anticipation that a totally implantable venous access system, similar to a port-A-cath, in combination with a micropump, might be available in the future for regular prophylaxis with factor concentrates. Our data show that five F VIII concentrates (Beriate HS, Hemofil M, Monoclate, Octaliquid, and Recombinate) are stable enough in polypropylene containers to allow refilling once in 2 weeks. To avoid large volumes, concentrates for such use would, however, have to be of higher potency after reconstitution than the present products. This should be technically feasible with the ultrapure products presently available. Admittedly, our data would not be valid for new and more concentrated products, which would have to undergo similar stability tests. Still, the results indicate that such a development is possible.

The increments in activity in the one-stage clotting assay, especially when unparalleled by increments in the chromogenic assay results, may indicate an activation of F VIII. This was not observed more often in glass than in plastic containers. It seemed to be more common at 4–8°C (n = 6) than at 20–23°C (n = 3) or 37°C (n = 1). Although the clinical significance of this increase in activity is unclear, it did not occur at 20–23°C in plastic containers before 1 week and should thus not affect the therapy with continuous infusion from an extracorporeal pump. The concomitant rise in activities with one-stage clotting as well as with chromogenic assay observed for Kryobulin TIM 3 and Octonativ M after storage for 24 and 4 hr, respectively, is puzzling. Since we do not know the cause of the more rapid drop in activity of most F VIII concentrates with the chromogenic than with the one-stage clotting assay, we are unable to provide an interpretation of this observation. It may seem surprising that Octonativ M did not behave in the same way as Hemofil M, since they share the same methods of purification and viral inactivation, but there are some differences in the manufacturing process between the two.

It was somewhat unexpected that activation occurred more often at 4–8°C and that the stability of some concentrates was better at 20–23°C than at 4–8°C. It is highly unlikely that the cause would be cold activation of F VII, known to occur in plasma, since all these F VIII concentrates were purified by immunoaffinity chromatography. Our results demonstrate that if a bottle of factor concentrate has been reconstituted, but for some reason cannot be administered at once, it is not necessarily advantageous to store it in the refrigerator. We have looked for some common features among the concentrates with the best stability data, but we were not able to detect any consistency with regard either to the degree of purification or to the mode of viral inactivation.

In conclusion, we found that the factor concentrates studied maintain their original activity after reconstitution for longer periods than officially declared. We therefore suggest that the manufacturers update their monographs and package inserts, even when the data exceed official requirements. Provided that sterility is guaranteed, many of these products may be kept for days and some even for a week at room or body temperature, allowing convenient continuous infusion. In our clinical experience from over 1 year with continuous infusion in the hospital as well as home treatment, no infectious complications have been observed. The microbiological safety of continuous infusion should be further investigated in future studies.

ACKNOWLEDGMENTS

The study was supported by ALEH, the Israeli Hemophilia Association.

REFERENCES

1. McMillan CW, Webster WP, Roberts HR, Blythe WB: Continuous intravenous infusion of factor VIII in classic haemophilia. Br J Haematol 18:659–667, 1970.
2. Blatt PM, White GC II, McMillan CW, Roberts HR: Treatment of anti-factor VIII antibodies. Thromb Hemostas 38:514, 1977.
3. Levin J, Ness PM, Bell WR: Continuous infusion of factor VIII concentrate for therapy of hemophilia A. Blood 58:220a, 1981.
4. Hathaway WE, Christian MJ, Clarke SL, Hasiba U: Comparison of continuous and intermittent factor VIII concentrate therapy in hemophilia A. Am J Hematol 17:85–88, 1984.
5. Bona RD, Weinstein A, Weisman SJ, Bartolomeo A, Rickles FR: The use of continuous infusion of factor concentrates in the treatment of hemophilia. Am J Hematol 32:8–13, 1989.
6. Martinowitz U, Schulman S, Gitel S, Horoszowski H, Heim M, Varon D: Adjusted dose continuous infusion of factor VIII in patients with haemophilia A. Br J Haematol 82:729–734, 1992.
7. Weinstein RE, Bona RD, Rickles FR: Continuous infusion of monoclonal antibody-purified factor VIII. Am J Hematol 36:211–212, 1991.
8. Howard PL, Bovill EG, Golden E: Postthaw stability of fibrinogen in cryoprecipitate stored between 1 and 6 degrees C. Transfusion 31:30–31, 1991.
9. Peerlinck K, Arnout J, Vermylen J: Factor VIII solutions in pre-filled syringes. Lancet 2:303–304, 1992.

American Journal of Hematology 45:224–231 (1994)

Effects of Interleukin-2 Administration on Platelet Function in Cancer Patients

Leslie Oleksowicz, Dina Zuckerman, Zbigniew Mrowiec, Elena Puszkin, and Janice P. Dutcher

Departments of Medical Oncology (L.O., Z.M., J.P.D.) and Pathology (E.P.), Montefiore Medical Center Hospital, Albert Einstein College of Medicine, Bronx, New York; Department of Pediatric Hematology-Oncology, Cornell Medical Center, New York, New York (D.Z.)

Platelet function in 16 patients with metastatic renal cell carcinoma and melanoma was studied sequentially over the first 96 hr of treatment with moderate and high-dose interleukin-2 (IL-2). During the first 96 hr of therapy, an increased *ex vivo* platelet maximal aggregation (MA) response to ADP, epinephrine, and arachidonic acid was paralleled by a decrease in the peripheral platelet count. Plasma specimens from patients receiving the moderate dose schedule showed a significant IL-2 induced secretory response of the platelet α-granule components β-thromboglobulin (BTG) and platelet factor 4 (PF4) and the eicosanoid thromboxane B_2 (TBX_2) as measured by RIA. The increase in TXB_2 was highly correlated with MA when analyzed by bivariate regression analysis, whereas the addition of PF4 to TXB_2 in a multiple regression analysis further increased their correlation to MA. The observed decrease in peripheral platelet count correlated significantly with MA and PF4 secretion. High-dose IL-2-treated patients showed a statistically significant increase in the percentage of large platelets exceeding 12 fl in diameter and platelet responsiveness to hypotonic shock. These observations suggest that IL-2 therapy results in a reduced peripheral platelet pool, with an increased proportion of the remaining pool of platelets larger, more viable, and activated.

Key words: platelet, interleukin-2, platelet aggregation, platelet factor 4, β-thromboglobulin, thromboxane B2

INTRODUCTION

Hemostatic abnormalities are frequently observed in patients receiving interleukin-2 (IL-2) as immunotherapy for metastatic cancer. Serious episodes of deep vein thrombosis [1], mesenteric thrombosis [2,3], thrombocytopenia [4,5], and, less commonly, hemorrhagic complications [5] have been reported. Although these clinically observed IL-2-induced hemostatic abnormalities have been attributed generally to IL-2 induced disturbances in coagulation [2,6,7], fibrinolysis [2], or reduced hepatic synthesis of clotting factors [8], recent work in rodent models has shown increases in intracapillary platelets associated with thrombus formation following IL-2 treatment [9]. In view of this and the finding that IL-2 induces alterations of whole blood platelet aggregation and secretion in vitro [10], we considered platelets to be potentially important in the pathogenesis of such complications.

Optical platelet aggregometry is an established in vitro measure of platelet-platelet cohesive abilities in response to an agonist challenge. In this study, platelet-rich plasma (PRP) specimens from IL-2-treated patients were subjected to optical aggregometry studies to assess the platelet aggregation response ex vivo to the agonists ADP, epinephrine, and arachidonic acid. The kinetics of secretion of platelet specific α-granule components, platelet factor 4 (PF4) and β-thromboglobulin (BTG), as well as thromboxane B2 (TXB_2) secretion, were quantified from patient's plasma specimens corresponding to collection times of aggregation specimens. Increased plasma levels of BTG and PF4, secreted exclusively from α-granules, occur as a consequence of platelet activation [11]. In order to asses further the functional and morphologic characteristics of the pool of peripheral platelets in these patients, platelet size parameters were analyzed as well as

Received for publication February 3, 1993; accepted August 18, 1993.

Address reprint requests to Leslie Oleksowicz, MD, Department of Medical Oncology, Montefiore Medical Center, 111 East 210th Street, Bronx, NY 10467.

hypotonic shock response (HSR). HSR, an indicator of membrane integrity measured as the ability to maintain cationic gradients, predicts platelet viability [12]. Furthermore, HSR is of value in assessing the age of the platelet population, as larger (younger) platelets are considerably more resistant to osmotic stress [13,14]. The studies reported here demonstrate alterations in platelet functional and morphologic characteristics that may contribute to hemostatic abnormalities in patients undergoing immunotherapy with IL-2.

MATERIALS AND METHODS

Patients

Sixteen patients, two females and 14 males, with histologically proven metastatic renal cell carcinoma (13) or melanoma (three) were entered in the study after informed consent was obtained. Ages ranged from 36 to 70 years, with a mean age of 55 years. IL-2 was administered as a continuous IV infusion of 30×10^6 IU/m^2 daily for 5 days in four patients, as a daily subcutaneous injection in four patients at 30×10^6 IU/m^2 daily for 5 days, or as high-dose bolus therapy, 21.7×10^6 IU/m^2 every 8 hr for a 5 day course of 14 doses in eight patients. The experimental protocol was approved by the institution's Investigational Review Board. In patients treated with moderate IL-2 therapy, administration of nonsteroidal antiinflammatory agents, aspirin, rinitidine, or other platelet inhibitors was avoided. Due to severe fever, chills, and gastric symptoms occuring with high-dose IL-2 therapy, these patients were treated with indomethacin, 25 mg PO every 8 hr and rinitidine 150 mg PO every 12 hr throughout the course of therapy. Specimens for aggregation, secretion, and peripheral platelet counts were collected at time 0, prior to the initiation of any medication, and then at 24 hr intervals over 96 hr of treatment. Given that the plasma half-lives of indomethacin and rinitidine are short (4.5 and 3.5 hr, respectively), 24 hr interval specimens were collected immediately prior to the scheduled dose of indomethacin and rinitidine in order to minimize any platelet-inhibitory effects of these agents. A similar schedule of specimen collection was utilized for moderate-dose IL-2 patients.

Preparation of Platelet-Rich Plasma (PRP) and Optical Aggregation

Blood for in vitro platelet aggregation studies was drawn by atraumatic technique with a 19-gauge needle into a plastic syringe containing 3.8% trisodium citrate as an anticoagulant and then centrifuged at 160*g* for 10 min at room temperature, and the buffy coat of platelets was collected with a serologic pipette. Platelet counts were determined via cell counter (Technicon 1; Laboratory Information System, Tarrytown, NY) and were confirmed, when platelet counts were less than 100,000/μl, by manual platelet counts. The specimen was diluted to a final platelet count of 250,000–350,000/μl using platelet-poor plasma that was obtained by centrifuging the remaining aliquot of identical PRP at 800*g* for 20 min. If the platelet count of the PRP was below 250,000, no further dilution was carried out.

Aggregometry studies were performed with a PAP-4 platelet aggregometer (BioData Corporation, Hatboro, PA). Adenosine diphosphate (ADP), 0.050 ml, (Sigma Chemical Co., St. Louis, MO) was added as an aggregating agonist to a final concentration of 4 μM in all patients. PRP specimens from patients receiving high-dose bolus IL-2 therapy were also subjected to aggregation assays using epinephrine (Sigma) and arachidonic acid (BioData Corp.) at final concentrations of 1 μM and 500 μg/ml, respectively. These reagents were added in 0.050 ml aliquots to 0.450 ml PRP. Each patient served as his or her own control (time 0, pretreatment), and each patient sample was analyzed in duplicate on one channel of the aggregometer. Aggregation activity is expressed as maximal aggregation as measured in millimeters divided by the platelet count of the PRP specimen to control for the variance in the platelet concentration between samples.

Eicosanoids and α-Granule Components

Blood specimens drawn by venipuncture simultaneously with aggregation samples were placed in siliconized tubes prepared with EDTA 2.5% and platelet inhibitors—2 chloroadenosine 0.025%, procaine HCl 7.0%—and put immediately on ice. These specimens were centrifuged at 1,500*g* for 20 min at 4°C, and supernatants were collected for radioimmunosassay (RIA) determinations. RIA using ^{125}I-labeled tracers was carried out according to the TXB_2 (New England Nuclear, Boston, MA; limits of sensitivity, 0.5 pg/ml), BTG (Amersham, Arlington Heights, IL; 10 ng/ml), or PF4 (Abbott, North Chicago, IL; 10 ng/ml) assays, respectively.

Mean Platelet Volume (MPV), Platelet-Large Cell Ratio (P-LCR), and Platelet Hypotonic Shock Response (HSR) and Platelet ATP Levels

For patients receiving high-dose IL-2 therapy, specimens were analyzed with a Sysmex K-100 cell analyzer (Baxter Diagnostics Inc., of McGraw Park, IL). Platelet size parameters were determined by sizing all platelets between 2 and 30 fl, sorting particles into bins of 1 fl increments, and plotting data on a platelet size distribution curve, with the mean determined by the machine's computer. The parameter P-LCR is the ratio of the quantity of platelets larger than 12 fl divided by the total platelet population. Platelet response to hypotonic shock was evaluated with a 4053 Kinetics Spectrophotometer (Pharmacia LKB Biotechnology Inc., Piscatawa, NJ) by the method of Handlin et al. [15]. Platelet ATP levels were determined with an enzymatic assay (Sigma).

Statistics

A kinetic analysis of the variables was performed with the paired Student's t test. MA, TXB_2, BTG, PF4, and peripheral platelet counts were analyzed through a comparison against pretreatment values. In cases when variance precluded Student's t test, a Wilcoxon sign rank test was used.

Separate investigations examining MA, PF4, and peripheral platelet count utilized regression analysis. For analyses examining TXB_2 correlation to MA, two measures of TXB_2 and MA, expressed as ratios to baseline values, were utilized. These measures corresponded to the minimal TXB_2 and maximal TXB_2, the independent variable. In order to ascertain the interactive effect of other variables, a step-up multiple regression analysis was implemented. Similarly, an examination of MA and PF4 correlation to peripheral platelet count involved bivariate regression analysis in which two measures of MA and PF4 (minimal and maximal values) were correlated with peripheral platelet count.

RESULTS

PRP specimens from patients undergoing IL-2 immunotherapy were subjected to optical aggregometry studies as described in Methods and Materials. Figure 1 shows the aggregation curve of a patient receiving high-dose IL-2 as immunotherapy using epinephrine (A) and ADP (B) as agonists. The curves illustrate a substantial increase in ADP and epinephrine platelet responsiveness (curves b compared with a baseline curves a), with the epinephrine aggregation curve developing biphasic characteristics at 96 hr after the initiation of IL-2 treatment. Kinetics of platelet aggregation response to ADP, epinephrine, and arachidonic acid are summarized in Figure 2. A significant increase in platelet aggregation response, compared to baseline values, can be observed, with a 50% increase in ADP-induced MA at 24 hr of study ($P = 0.008$), a 72% increase in epinephrine-induced MA at 24 hr of study ($P = 0.060$), and a 138% increase in arachidonic-induced MA at 48 hr of study ($P = 0.020$). A 2.4-, 4.2-, and 8.4-fold increase in agonist-induced MA could be observed by 96 hr of study (ADP, $P = 0.004$; epinephrine, $P = 0.067$; arachidonic acid, $P = 0.066$, respectively). The graph of the kinetics of peripheral platelet count (Fig. 2, inset) shows a significant linear reduction over the 96 hr of study ($P < 0.001$ for all time points compared to baseline). Furthermore, a consistent, significant decrease in peripheral platelet count was observed over each 24 hr period ($P < 0.02$). Regression analysis using peripheral platelet count as the independent variable and ADP-induced MA as the dependent variable showed a significant negative linear correlation in these patients treated with high-dose IL-2 ($r^2 = 0.66$, $P < 0.0009$; plot not shown).

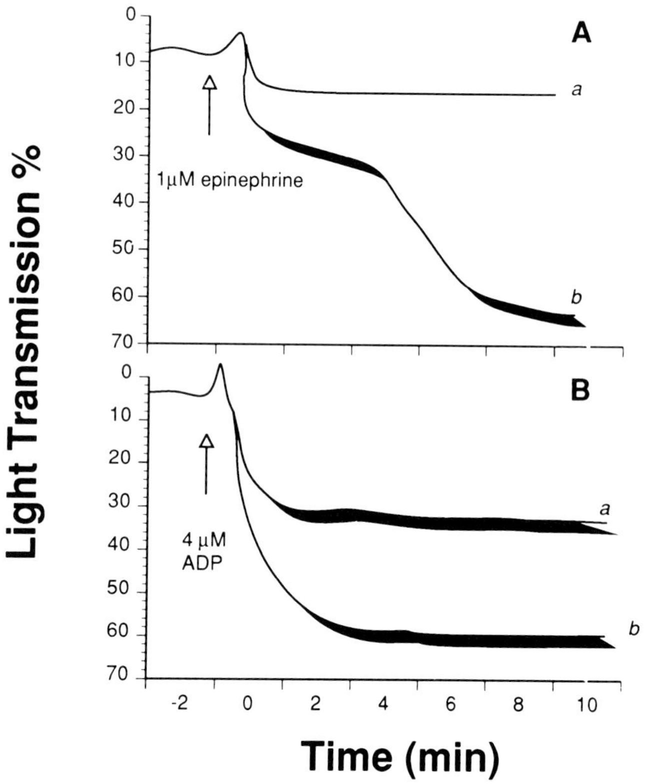

Fig. 1. Representative tracings of the aggregation response of platelets ex vivo to epinephrine (A) and ADP (B). Curves labeled *a* represent PRP obtained from the patient prior to high-dose IL-2 treatment, while curves labeled *b* represent PRP obtained at 96 hr after the initiation of treatment. Note the substantial increase in maximal aggregation in both ADP and epinephrine *b* curves as well as the biphasic characteristics of the epinephrine *b* curve.

Analysis of hematologic parameters was studied in 12 patients receiving high-dose bolus IL-2 therapy. Total leukocyte count did not change significantly from a mean baseline of 7,800 ± 450/μl to 7,460 ± 970/μl at 96 hr of therapy. Both hemoglobin levels and hematocrit showed a significant drop over the course of treatment, 13.4 ± 0.43 g/dl and 39% ± 1.0% prior to therapy, which decreased to 12.12 ± 0.6 g/dl ($P < 0.016$) and 34% ± 1.6% ($P < 0.005$) at 96 hr, respectively. The platelet count showed a similar significant decrease from a mean of 244,000 ± 17,000/μl prior to therapy to 82,800 ± 8,800/μl at 96 hr ($P < 0.0009$).

Figure 3A shows the kinetics of ADP-induced MA in patients receiving moderate dose IL-2 as immunotherapy over a 96 hr period. A 66% increase in platelet ADP-responsiveness was observed on day 2, which reached a plateau at approximately 1.7 times control values throughout 96 hr of study (Fig. 3A). Parallel plasma

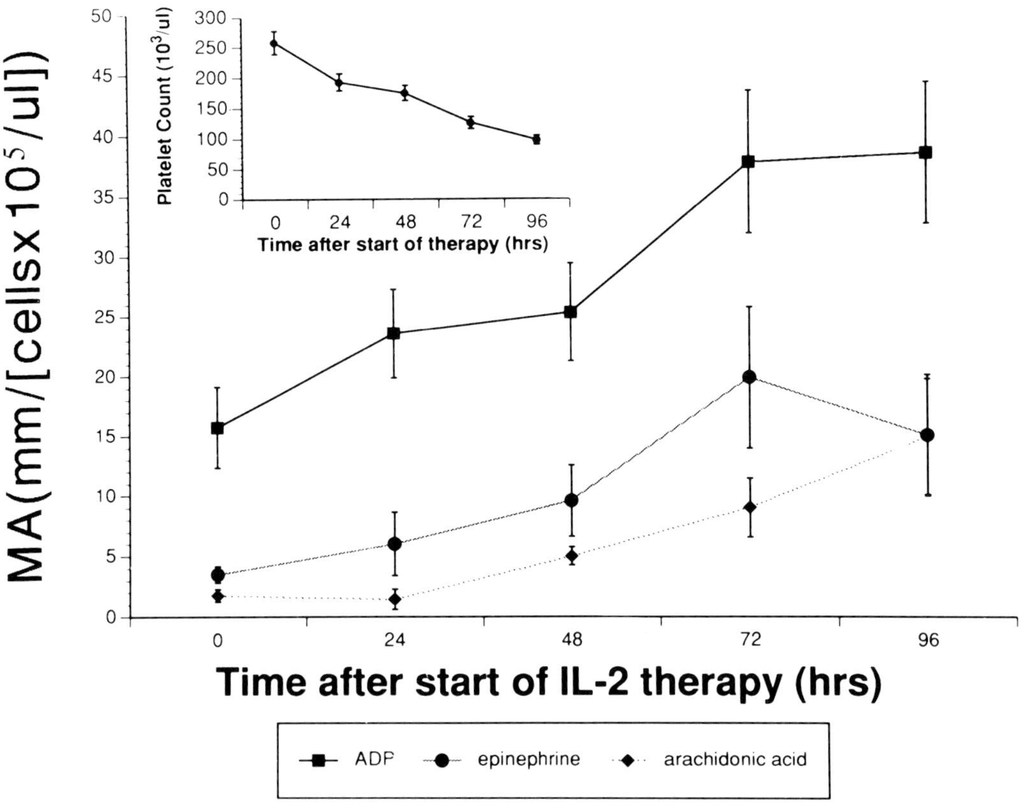

Fig. 2. Kinetics of optical aggregation in patients treated with high-dose IL-2 measured as MA in response to ADP, epinephrine, and arachidonic acid; 0.050 ml of each agonist was added to 0.45 ml PRP to final concentrations of 4 μM ADP, 1 μM epinephrine, and 500 μg/ml arachidonic acid as described in Materials and Methods. MA was calculated as the maximal change in optical density as expressed in millimeters at the time of the curve's plateau. Aggregation activity is expressed as MA (mm) divided by the platelet count of the PRP sample to control for the variance in the platelet concentration between samples. Each curve represents the mean from eight patients. Solid bars represent SEM. Inset: Kinetics of peripheral platelet count over 96 hr of study. The curve represents the mean from eight patients receiving high-dose IL-2 therapy.

specimens were drawn from patients at the same time intervals and assayed for platelet α-granule proteins, BTG, PF4, and the eicosanoid TXB_2. As Figure 3B–D demontrates, all patients showed significant increases in TXB_2, PF4, and BTG over the 96 hr of study, respectively. As with high-dose IL-2 therapy, a significant time-dependent decrease in peripheral platelet count was observed over the 96 hr course of the study (Fig. 3E).

Examination of the extent and time course of platelet morphologic and functional changes in patients receiving high-dose IL-2 therapy is described in Table I, top. A 24% ($P = 0.033$) and a 28% ($P = 0.010$) increase in P-LCR and HSR were observed in high-dose IL-2-treated patients, with corresponding peaks at 70 and 76 hr, respectively. These findings were also confirmed by a 7% increase ($P = 0.035$) in mean platelet volume, this parameter peaking at 75 hr (data not shown). A 5.9-, 8.4-, and 2.7-fold increase in epinephrine ($P = 0.018$), arachidonic acid ($P = 0.066$), and ADP ($P = 0.009$)-induced maximum aggregation was observed, with mean times to peak of 72, 84, and 75 hr, respectively.

In patients treated with moderate-dose IL-2, the mean peaks for ADP-induced MA, PF4, TXB_2, and BTG were statistically significant at 2.29, 2.4, 8.3, and 6.1 times control values, respectively (Table I, bottom). The mean times to peak for ADP-induced MA, TXB_2, and BTG were similar at 57, 50, and 58 hr, respectively. The mean time to peak for PF4 occurred earlier, at 33 hr. Furthermore, when values for high-dose and moderate-dose ADP-induced MA are compared, a 20% dose-dependent increase in peak MA values was observed when variables were expressed as the ratio of peak to control to account for variation in baseline values. Similarly, an increase of approximately 18 hr for ADP-induced MA in high-dose IL-2-treated patients (75 hr) compared to the moderate dose ADP-induced MA peak (57 hr) was evident.

Platelet ATP levels were also examined prior to and upon conclusion of IL-2 therapy. Table I shows a signifi-

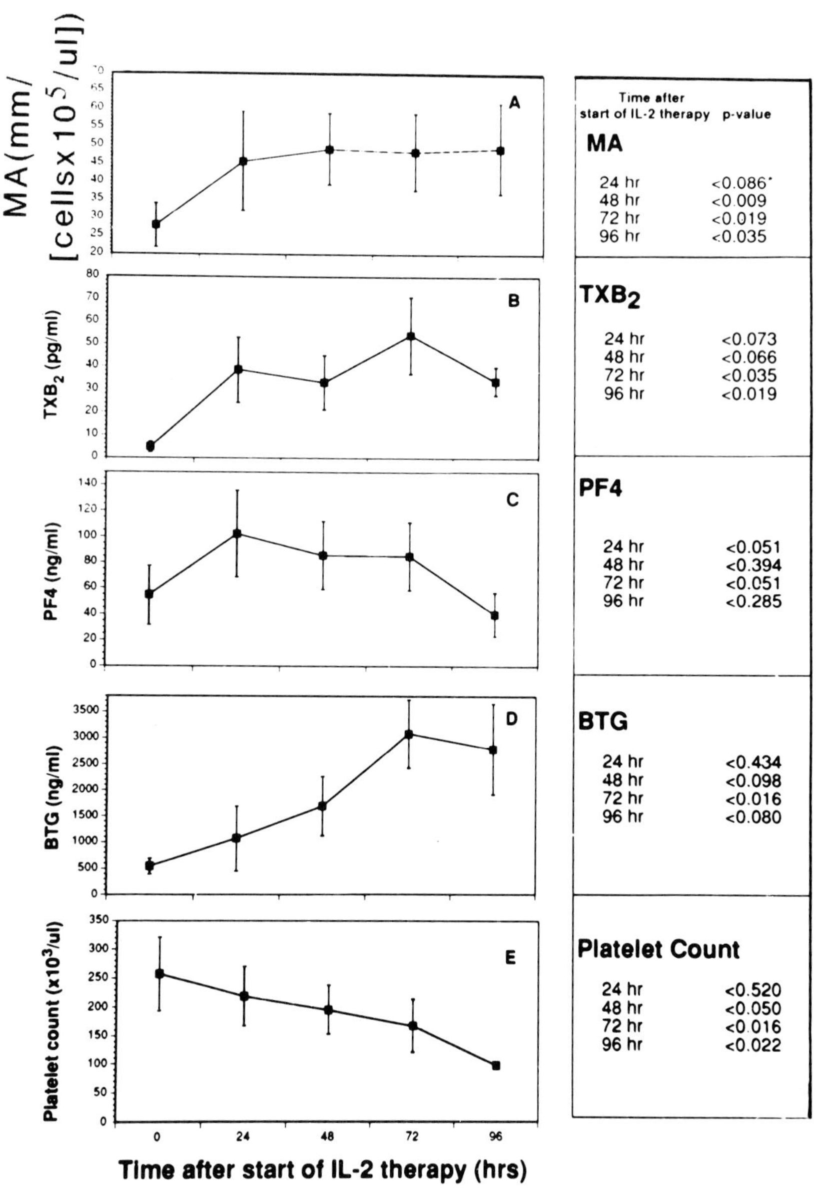

Fig. 3. Kinetics of ADP-dependent optical aggregation measured as MA (A); secretion of TXB_2 (B), PF4 (C), or BTG (D); and peripheral platelet count (E) in patients undergoing immunotherapy with moderate-dose IL-2. Each curve represents the mean from eight patients. Solid bars represent SEM. The *P* values were obtained by paired Student's t test, comparing time 0 to time 24, 48, 72, and 94 hr. In cases when variable distribution precluded the use of Student's t test, the *P* value (*) was calculated by the nonparametric Wilcoxon signed rank test.

cant increase in mean platelet ATP from 10.4 ± 0.85 μmol/10^{11} platelets prior to therapy to 22.5 ± 0.69 μmol/10^{11} platelets at 96 hr of therapy ($N = 5$; $P < 0.0009$).

These observations were corroborated by the findings illustrated in Figure 4. A significant positive linear correlation was observed between TXB_2 secretion and ADP-induced MA in patients receiving moderate-dose IL-2, by regression analysis ($P = 0.002$, $r^2 = 0.66$). When simple regression analyses were carried out using PF4, BTG, and TXB_2 as independent variables, only TXB_2 provided a statistically significant correlation to MA in this analysis. However, when a multiple regression analysis was performed using TXB_2 and PF4 as independent variables, the inclusion of PF4 increased the coefficient of correlation to 0.77 ($P = 0.001$) for this multivariate model. This analysis is strongly supportive of an interactive effect between TXB_2 and PF4 in determing MA.

We further investigated the relationship between the peripheral platelet count in patients receiving moderate-dose IL-2 and MA and PF4 of parallel specimens. Figure 5A demonstrates a significant negative correlation be-

TABLE I. Morphologic and Functional Characteristics of Platelets During IL-2 Therapy*

	N	Control	Peak	*P* value	Mean time to peak (hr)
P-LCR (%)	7	13.7 ± 2.0	17.02 ± 2.6	0.033	70
HSR (%)	5	75.0 ± 14.9	95.9 ± 8.7	0.010	76
MA_{epi} (mm/[cells × 10^5/μl])	6	3.50 ± 0.66	20.92 ± 5.37	0.018	72
MA_{AA} (mm/[cells × 10^5/μl])	5	1.76 ± 1.76	14.80 ± 4.78	0.066	84
MA_{ADP} (mm/[cells × 10^5/μl])	8	15.73 ± 3.4	43.15 ± 4.12	0.0009	75
MA_{ADP} (mm/[cells × 10^5/μl])	8	35.49 ± 6.60	81.46 ± 16.1	0.005	57
PF4 (ng/ml)	7	47.29 ± 21.6	115.50 ± 32.1	0.060	33
TXB_2 (pg/ml)	7	7.04 ± 3.22	58.71 ± 15.6	0.018	50
BTG (pg/ml)	6	0.620 ± 0.14	3.71 ± 0.73	0.010	58
ATP (μmol/10^{11} platelets)	5	10.40 ± 0.85	22.46 ± 0.69	0.0009	—

*Assays for P-LCR (platelet-large cell ratio), hypotonic shock response (HSR), agonist-induced maximal aggregation (MA), and secretion of PF4, TXB_2, and BTG, and platelet ATP levels were performed as described in Materials and Methods. MA_{epi}, epinephrine-induced maximal aggregation; MA_{AA}, arachidonic acid-induced maximal aggregation; MA_{ADP}, ADP-induced maximal aggregation. Platelet ATP levels were assayed at time 0 and at 96 hr of therapy. *P* values are from paired Student's t tests comparing control (time 0) to peak value for each patient. Top half shows assays performed with specimens from patients receiving high-dose IL-2 therapy, while bottom half shows those from patients receiving moderate-dose IL-2 therapy.

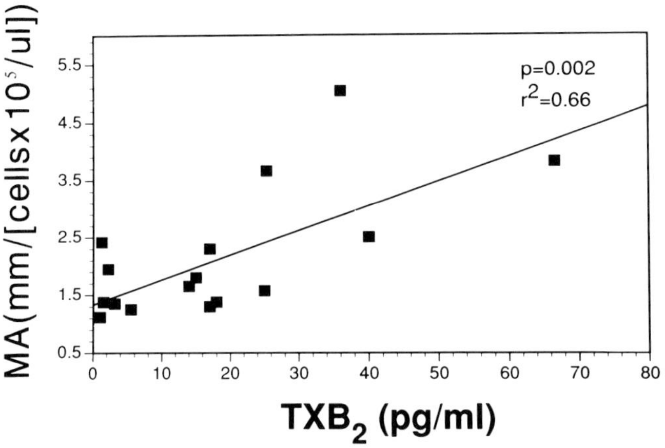

Fig. 4. Regression analysis correlating TXB_2 secretion with MA. Both variables are expressed as ratio of experimental values to control (time 0) for each patient.

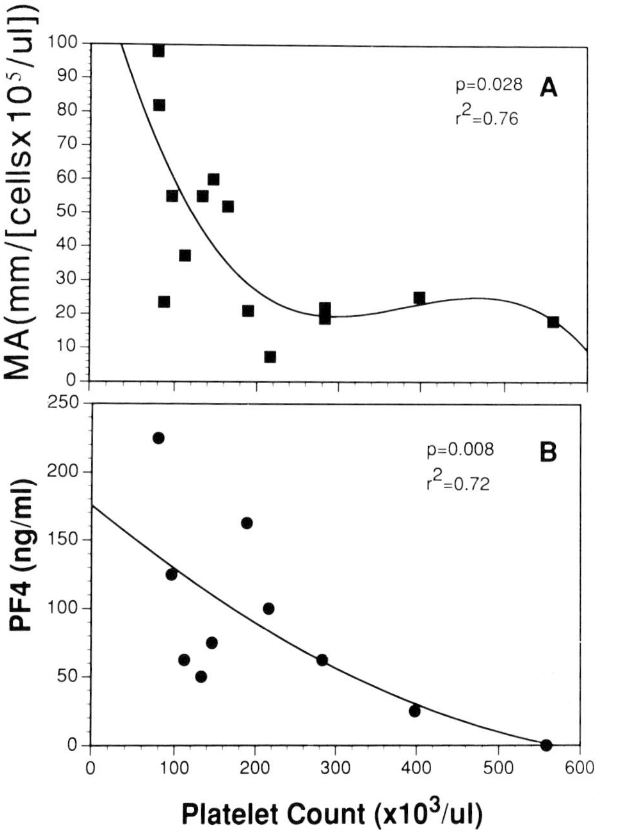

Fig. 5. Regression analysis correlating peripheral platelet count with MA (A) and PF4 (B) for each patient.

tween peripheral platelet count and MA, with MA increasing exponentially as the peripheral platelet count decreased ($P = 0.028$, $r^2 = 0.76$). Furthermore, MA values increased at the greatest rate at a peripheral platelet count threshold of approximately 200,000/μl. Figure 5B shows the relationship between peripheral platelet count and PF4. The relationship between these two variables showed a negative second-degree polynomial correlation ($P = 0.008$, $r^2 = 0.72$). Neither BTG nor TXB_2 was significant in a similar analysis.

DISCUSSION

IL-2, a lymphokine involved in immune regulation and T-cell activation, has been used clinically as immunotherapy in renal cell carcinoma, melanoma, lymphoma, and other neoplasms [16]. Although IL-2-induced secondary cytokine secretion of TNF, IL-1, and γ-interferon has been postulated as a mechanism contributing to vascular toxicities associated with IL-2 therapy [17,18], the pathophysiologic basis for hematologic toxicities associated with IL-2 administration has not been clarified. In this study we identified aberrations in platelet function consequent to the initiation of IL-2 as immunotherapy, observed as alterations from baseline agonist-induced platelet aggregation responsiveness and platelet α-granule secretion. Changes in these parameters occurred concomitantly with peripheral thrombocytopenia. The peripheral platelet pool in these IL-2-treated patients showed an increase in the percentage of large platelets, which were more viable as demonstrated by increased membrane stability to HSR and an increase in platelet ATP levels. Given that HSR has been shown to decrease as platelets senesce [12,14] and that increased ATP levels are observed in younger platelets [12], our findings are consistent with a mechanism of increased platelet turnover resulting in a population of younger, activated platelets.

Platelet-specific proteins, such as BTG and PF4, are found exclusively in platelets and are secreted in response to a variety of agonists. Hence their presence in the plasma of circulating blood is regarded as a measure of platelet activation in vivo. In the present work, secretion of these α-granule components in patients undergoing immunotherapy with moderate-dose IL-2 was observed to peak at 30 hr for PF4 and at 51 hr for BTG. Such observations suggest that IL-2 therapy influences the differential secretion of α-granule components. Also, the peak of aggregation activity corresponded closely with the peak of thromboxane secretion, yet the mean peak for PF4 secretion occurred before changes in optical aggregation could be observed. The phenomenon of IL-2-induced aggregation perturbations being observed after secretion occurred was confirmed in our earlier in vitro work [10]. It may be concluded that, under conditions of both in vivo and in vitro IL-2 stimulation, platelet aggregation and secretion are two distinct processes, with changes in secretion observable before changes in platelet activity an be detected by optical aggregometry.

Secretion of TXB_2, the stable conversion product of the potent aggregating agent TXA_2, was temporally associated and highly correlated with increased platelet activity as expressed by maximum aggregation in moderate-dose IL-2 regimes. Interestingly, this correlation was strengthened with PF4 secretion, suggesting an interactive effect. Recent work has demonstrated the presence of high-affinity PF4 binding sites on platelets, which result in increasing sensitivity to aggregating agents such as ADP and arachidonic acid when bound by PF4 [19]. The observation that the PF4 secretion peak occurred early in the course of IL-2 therapy, whereas the TXB_2 peak was a later event (33 and 50 hr, respectively), further implicates a PF4 platelet-modulating effect in IL-2-treated patients.

The source of thromboxane from plasma specimens drawn from patients undergoing immunotherapy with IL-2 remains unclear. Metabolically active platelets aggregate, liberate arachidonate from membrane phospholipids, and metabolize it to thromboxane A2, which is short-lived and subsequently is converted to TXB_2. However, we and others have shown that mononuclear cells stimulated with IL-2 in vitro secrete thromboxane [10,20]. Further complicating this issue is the finding of increased thromboxane levels in sera of patients with head and neck carcinoma [21], in cultures derived from human lung adenocarcinomas [22], and in tissue cultures of human ovarian carcinoma [23]. Whether the increased thromboxane levels are due to increased platelet activity, to IL-2 induced mononuclear cell activation, or to the release from lysing tumor cells in patients treated with IL-2 is a question awaiting clarification.

We have further shown a statistically significant negative correlation between PF4 secretion and peripheral platelet count in patients undergoing IL-2 immunotherapy. Given the recent evidence implicating PF4 in the inhibition of megakaryopoiesis in vitro [24], the finding of elevated platelet secretory PF4 levels in these patients could imply a central PF4-induced mechanism of megakayopoietic suppression involved in the observed thrombocytopenia. Attempts to explain the IL-2-induced thrombocytopenia have invoked a peripheral destructive mechanism [5] as well as an inhibitory effect of IL-2 [25] and LAK cells [26] on hematopoietic progenitors. Because hematologic parameters were found to be within normal limits in these patients prior to cytokine therapy, bone marrow examinations were not performed due to the low index of suspicion of marrow infiltration by metastatic tumor. Other groups have noted an absence of bone marrow precursor cells in bone marrow examinations of IL-2-treated patients [4]. Observations from early clinical studies demonstrated clumping of platelets on peripheral smears in IL-2-treated patients [27], potentially implicating an increase in these inactive platelet aggregates in the etiology of IL-2-induced thrombocytopenia. Although the results described herein provide correlative data supporting a central mechanism for thrombocytopenia in IL-2-treated patients, further work is necessary to determine the spectrum of its pathogenesis.

Evidence indicates that platelet function is impaired in cancer patients. Ex vivo platelet studies in these patients have shown depletion of dense granule ADP and serotonin (5-HT) [28], while in vivo studies have shown increased basal secretion of BTG [29,30] and PF4 [29]. In some subsets of cancer patients, ex vivo platelet aggregation studies have shown a decreased response to epinephrine and ADP [30], with more recent in vitro work implicating a tumor-derived nitric oxide factor in such inhibition [31]. These findings were also evident in our population of patients, in whom baseline epinephrine- and arachidonic acid-induced aggregation were modest and baseline serum levels of PF4 were substantially increased. That the epinephrine curve developed biphasic features after 96 hr of study suggests a secondary secretion-dependent platelet aggregation response. Given that the mean time to peak for epinephrine also corresponded closely with mean times to peak of P-LCR and HSR further implicates a metabolically intact population of larger, younger platelets induced by IL-2 treatment.

The results of the current study suggest that IL-2 therapy is associated with significant stimulation of platelet function, as measured as increases in both sensitivity to agonist-induced aggregation and secretion activity. Although our study has not examined the role of tumor-released procoagulants in contributing to these observations, our earlier in vitro work has shown that IL-2 perturbs platelet function in the absence of tumor [10]. This supports a mechanism of IL-2-induced platelet stimulation independent of coagulation system activation by tumor cell products. Despite these findings in our patients, clinically significant episodes of severe bleeding and thrombosis were rare, suggesting in vivo compensatory factors. Additional studies will be necessary to elucidate the specific contributions of these factors, but increased understanding of these phenomena could be of value in both the prediction and the prevention of hemostatic complications of IL-2 treatment.

ACKNOWLEDGMENTS

L.O. is a recipient of an American Cancer Society Clinical Oncology Career Development Award (CDA 93-52). This study was further supported by Cancer Center Core Grant P30CA1330-21 provided by the National Cancer Institute.

REFERENCES

1. Sculier JP, Bron D, Verboven N, Klastersky J: Multiple organ failure during IL-2 administration and LAK cell infusion. Intes Care Med 14:666, 1988.
2. Fleischman JD, Shingeleton WB, Gallegher C, Ratnoff OP, Chahine A: Fibrinolysis, thrombocytopenia, and coagulation abnormalities complicating high-dose interleukin-2 immunotherapy. J Lab Clin Med 117:76, 1991.
3. Sporano JA, Dutcher JP, Kaleya R, Caliendo G, Fiorito J, Mitsudo S: Colonic ischemia complicating immunotherapy with Interleukin-2 and alpha-interferon. Cancer 68:1538, 1991.
4. Ettinghausen SE, Moore JC, Whilte DE, Platanias L, Young NS, Rosenberg SA: Hematologic effects of immunotherapy with lymphokine activated killer cells and recombinant IL-2 in cancer patients. Blood 69:1654, 1987.
5. Paciucci PA, Mandeli J, Oleksowicz L, Holland JH: Thrombocytopenia during immunotherapy with IL-2 by constant infusion. Am J Med 89:308, 1990.
6. Hack HC, Wagstagg J, Strack von Schnijndel RJ, Pinedo HM, Thijs LG, Niojens JH: Studies on contact system of coagulation during therapy with high doses of recombinant IL-2: Implications for septic shock. Thromb Hemostas 65:497, 1991.
7. Richard V, Bernier M, Themelin L, Brion D, Sculier JP: Blood coagulation abnormalities during adoptive immunotherapy with interleukin-2 (r-MET hu IL-2 [ala 125]). Ann Oncol 2:67, 1991.
8. Strack M, Sussman I, Grima K, et al.: Unique pattern of change of coagulation factors during interleukin-2. Blood 78:485a, 1991 (abstract).
9. Edwards MJ, Miller FN, Sims DE, Abney DL, Schuschke DA, Corey TS: Interleukin 2 acutely induces platelet and neutrophil-endothelial adherence and macromolecular leakage. Cancer Res 52:3425, 1992.
10. Oleksowicz L, Paciucci PA, Zuckerman D, Colorito A, Rand JH, Holland JF: Alterations in platelet function induced by IL-2. J Immunother 10:363, 1991.
11. Holmsen H: Platelet secretion. In Coleman RW, Hirsh J, Marder VJ, Salzman EW (eds): "Hemostasis and Thrombosis." Philadelphia: J.B. Lippincott, 1987.
12. Karpatkin S: Human platelet senescence. Annu Rev Med 23:101, 1972.
13. Karpatkin S: Heterogeneity of human platelets. II. Functional evidence suggestive of young and old platelets. J Clin Invest 48:1073, 1969.
14. Holme S, Heaton A, Momoda G: Evaluation of a new, more oxygen-permeable polyvinylchloride container. Transfusion 29:159, 1989.
15. Handlin RI, Fortier NL, Valeri CR: Platelet response to hypotonic stress after storage at 4°C or 22°C. Transfusion 10:305, 1970.
16. Rosenberg SA, Lotz MT, Mool LM, Leitman S, Chang AE, Ettinghausen SE: Observations on the systemic administration of autologous lymphokine-activated killer cell and recombinant IL-2 to patients with metastatic cancer. N Engl J Med 313:1485, 1985.
17. Martin S, Maruta K, Burkart V, Gillis S, Kolb H: IL-1 and IFN-gamma increase vascular permeability. Immunology 64:301, 1988.
18. Amador JF, Vazquez AM, Cabrera L, Barral AM, Gendelman R, Jondal M: Toxic effects of interleukin-2-activated lymphocytes on vascular endothelial cells. Nat Immun Cell Growth Regul 10:207, 1991.
19. Capitanio AM, Niewiarowski S, Rucinski B, et al.: Interaction of platelet factor 4 with human platelets. Biochim Biophys Acta 839:161, 1985.
20. Remich DG, Larrick JW, Ngugen DT, Kunkel SL: Stimulation of prostaglandin E2 and thromboxane B2 production by human monocytes in response to IL-2. Biochem Biophys Res Commun 147:86, 1987.
21. Slotman GJ: Plasma thromboxane A2 and prostacyclin concentrations in squamous cell carcinoma of the head and neck. J Surg Oncol 38:33, 1988.
22. Hubbard WC, Alley MC, McClemore TL, Boyd MR: Evidence for thromboxane biosynthesis in established lines derived from human lung adenocarcinoma. Cancer Res 48:2674, 1988.
23. Aitokallio-Tallberg AM, Viinikka LU, Ylinkarkala RO: Increased synthesis of prostaglandin and thromboxane in human ovarian malignancy. Cancer Res 48:2396, 1988.
24. Hans ZC, Sensébe L, Abgrall JF Briére J: Platelet factor 4 inhibits human magakaryocytopoiesis in vitro. Blood 75:1234, 1990.
25. Liue Shu-Jun, Ascensao JL, Podack E, et al.: Cellular interactions in hematopoiesis. Blood Cells 13:101, 1987.
26. Guarini A, Sanavio F, Novarino A, Gillio Tos A, Aglietta M, Foa R: Thrombocytopenia in acute leukemia patients treated with IL-2: cytolytic effect of LAK cells on megakaryocytic progenitors. Br J Haematol 79:451, 1991.
27. Oleksowicz L, Paciucci PA, Rand J, Holand JF: Effects of IL-2 in vitro and in vivo on platelet function. Proc Am Assoc Cancer Res 30:330, 1989 (abstract).
28. Mannucci PM, Cattaneo M, Canciani MT, Maniezzo M, Vaglini M, Cascinelli N: Early presence of activated ("exhausted") platelets in malignant tumors (breast adenocarcinoma and malignant melanoma). Eur J Cancer Clin Oncol 25:1413, 1989.
29. Al-Mondhiry H, Manni A, Owen J, Gordon R: Hemostatic effects of hormonal stimulation in patients with metastatic prostate cancer. Am J Hematol 28:141, 1988.
30. Yahara Y, Okawa S, Onozawa Y, Motomiya T, Tanoue K, Yamazaki H: Activation of platelets in cancer, especially with reference to genesis of disseminated intravascular coagulation. Thromb Res 29:27, 1983.
31. Mollace V, Salvemini D, Anggard E, Vane J: Cultured astrocytoma cells inhibit platelet aggregation by releasing a nitric oxide-like factor. Biochem Biophys Res Commun 172:564, 1990.

American Journal of Hematology 45:232–236 (1994)

Elevated Plasma Tissue Factor Antigen Level in Patients With Disseminated Intravascular Coagulation

Hideo Wada, Tsutomu Nakase, Ryusuke Nakaya, Kouzou Minamikawa, Yoshihiro Wakita, Toshihiro Kaneko, Michiaki Ohiwa, Katsumi Deguchi, and Shigeru Shirakawa

The Second Department of Internal Medicine (H.W., K.M., Y.W., T.K., M.O., S.S.) and College of Medical Science (T.N., R.N.), Mie University School of Medicine Mie, Japan; Department of Internal Medicine, Nagai Hospital, Nagai, Japan (K.D.)

The plasma tissue factor (TF) antigen level was measured in patients with disseminated intravascular coagulation (DIC). The plasma TF antigen was detected in normal volunteers, and it was significantly higher in DIC patients than in non-DIC patients. However, in some patients with DIC, the plasma TF antigen level was within the normal range. The plasma TF antigen level in patients with DIC significantly decreased after therapy, but it was not correlated with organ failure or outcome. The plasma TF antigen level in patients with DIC was not correlated with other hemostatic markers. The plasma TF antigen level tended to be higher in DIC patients with nonlymphoid leukemia than in those with lymphoid tumor. TF might be implicated in the occurrence and progression of DIC.

Key words: TF, DIC

INTRODUCTION

The tissue factor (TF) is the primary cellular initiator of the coagulation protease cascade, which serves as the receptor and essential cofactor for factor VII and VIIa [1]. As a potent initiator of coagulation. TF is believed to have a critical function in hemostasis and thrombogenesis [2–4]. Physiologic and pathologic mediators can induce TF expression in monocytes or endothelial cells, suggesting an integral involvement of TF in the pathologic processes of inflammation and thrombogenesis [4–7].

Disseminated intravascular coagulation (DIC) [8,9] is often associated with severe bleeding tendency due to secondary fibrinolysis and organ failure due to thrombosis. Since DIC in acute leukemia is considered to be caused by the TF production in leukemic cells [10,11]. TF may play an important role in the onset of DIC in other diseases [12,13]. We examined the plasma TF antigen in patients with DIC by a recently developed enzyme-linked immunosorbant assay (ELISA).

MATERIALS AND METHODS

Our subjects were 55 DIC patients [13 with acute lymphoblastic leukemia (ALL), 11 with acute promyelocytic leukemia (APL), 12 with acute nonlymphoblastic leukemia (ANLL) other than APL, 13 with solid cancer, two with sepsis, and four with other diseases], 15 pre-DIC patients (five with ALL, two with ANLL other than APL, four with solid cancer, and four with other diseases), ten non-DIC patients (one with ALL, three with ANLL other than APL, one with solid cancer, one with sepsis, and four with other diseases), and 12 normal volunteers. The diagnosis of DIC was based on the criteria established by the Japanese Ministry of Health and Welfare (Table I) [14]. Pre-DIC was defined as five or six points in the DIC score in nonleukemia or three points in leukemia, and the non-DIC patient group consisting of patients with associated underlying DIC diseases had lower DIC scores than the pre-DIC patients. The lungs were considered to be in a state of organ failure when the PaO_2 was 50 mm Hg or less and for the kidney when creatinine was 3 mg/dl or higher, when symptoms of shock from heart failure were present, and when the patient was in a coma or responded only to pain. These patients were treated with gabesate mesilate (FOY) [15,16] or with a combination of FOY and heparin. Of the DIC patients, 31 showed a good outcome after treatment, with the DIC score descreasing

Received for publication March 29, 1993; accepted August 18, 1993.

Address reprint requests to Hideo Wada, MD, The Second Department of Internal Medicine, Mie University School of Medicine, 2-174 Edobashi, Tsu-city, Mie-ken 514, Japan.

TABLE I. Diagnostic Criteria for DIC*

Criteria	Values		Points
PT (sec)	15<	<20	1
	20<		2
Fibrinogen (mg/dl)	100<	>150	1
		<100	2
FDP (μg/ml)	10<	<20	1
	20<	<40	2
	40<		3
Platelet count ($\times 10^4/\mu l$)	8<	<12	1
	5<	<8	2
		<5	3
Bleeding symptoms			1
Organ failure due to thrombosis			1

*In the leukemic patients, the sum of the scores 1, 2, 3, and 6 was 3 or higher. In nonleukemic patients, the sum of the scores for 1, 2, 3, 4, 5, and 6 was 6 or higher.

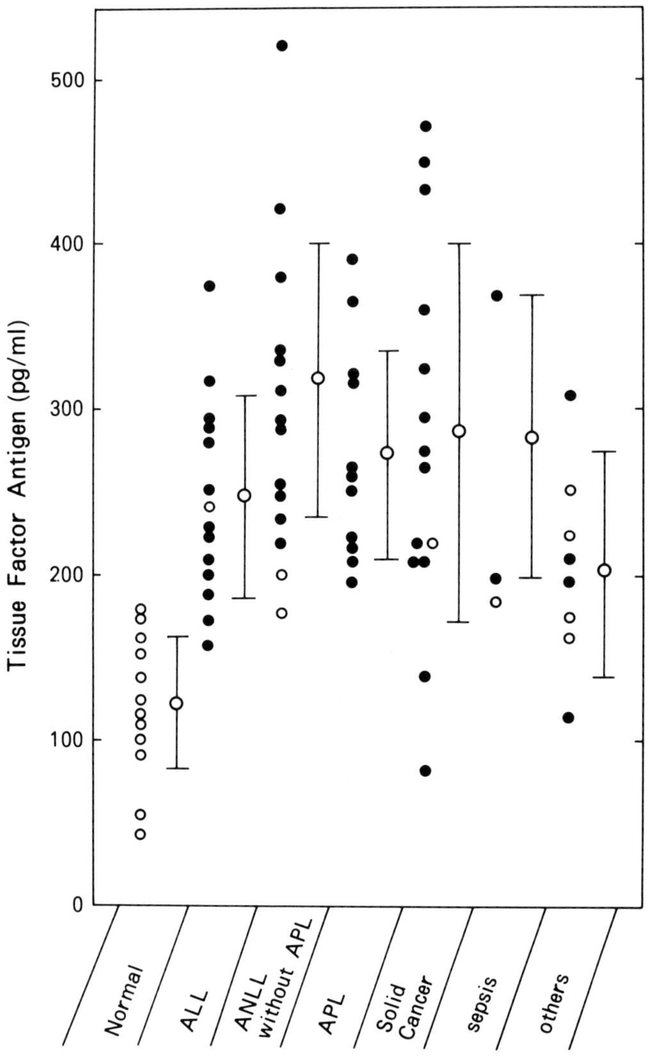

Fig. 1. Plasma level of tissue factor antigen in patients with DIC. ●, DIC patients; ○, non-DIC patients.

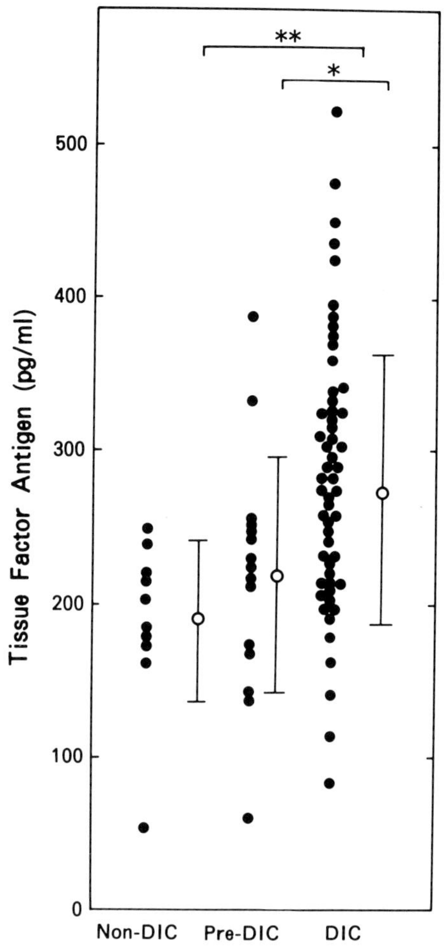

Fig. 2. Plasma level of tissue factor antigen in patients with non-DIC, pre-DIC, and DIC.$P < 0.02$, *$0.02 < P < 0.05$.**

by more than three points, and the other 24 patients were considered to have a poor outcome.

Blood specimens were collected at the diagnosis of DIC and 2 weeks after treatment (or after 1 week in patients who died within 2 weeks). Whole blood was anticoagulated by addition of 9 volumes to 1 volume of 3.8% trisodium citrate solution and centrifuged for 15 min at 1,500 rpm. The plasma was used for TF assay, and the TF antigen was detected in neither platelets nor the leukocytes fraction from 10 ml normal blood. Hematological tests were conducted in our laboratory as described below. The thrombin-antithrombin III complex (TAT), plasmin-α2 plasmin inhibitor complex (PIC), and FDP-D-dimer levels were determined using Enzygnostic-TAT (Behringwerke AG) [17], PIC-test (Teijin) [18], and Frelisa D-dimer (Agen), respectively. The plasma tissue-type plasminogen activator (t-PA) and plasminogen activator inhibitor I (PAI-I) levels were measured using a one-step sandwich ELISA (Fujirebio, Ltd.) and Imulyse PAI-I (Biopool AB), respectively. The plasma TF antigen was measured using the IMUBIND Tissue

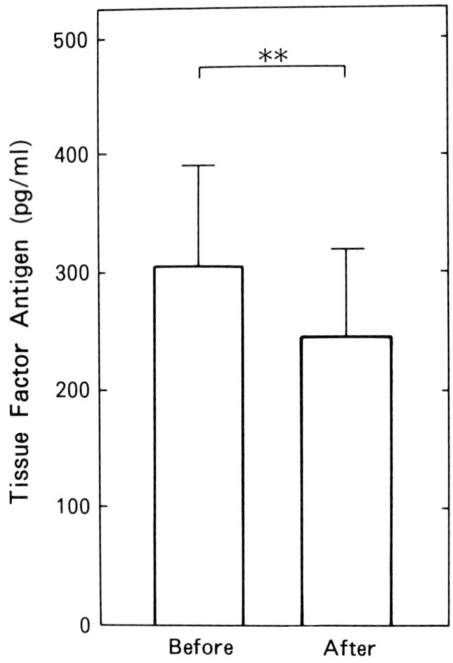

Fig. 3. Plasma level of tissue factor antigen in DIC patients at before and after treatment for DIC. **$P < 0.02$.

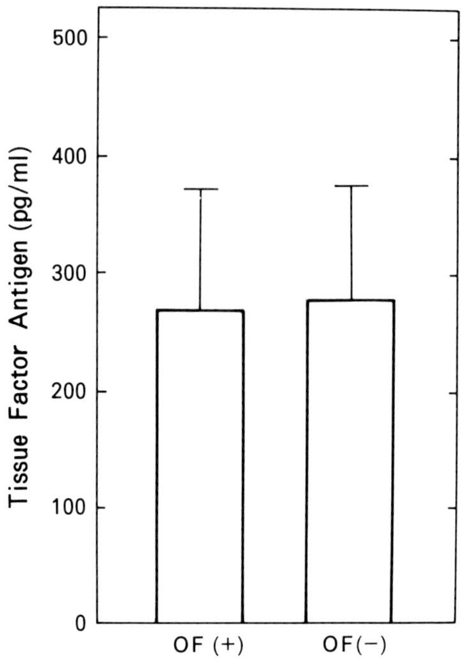

Fig. 4. Plasma level of tissue factor antigen in DIC patients with or without organ failure (OF).

Factor ELISA Kit (ADI). The test specimen was diluted 1/80 in 0.05 M Tris, pH 7.5, with 2% bovine serum albumin and 0.05% Tween 20 buffer, to eliminate the matrix effect of undiluted plasma. The monoclonal antibody in this kit was the murine immunoglobulin G_1 for tissue factor from the human brain, detecting the TF-apoprotein complex, TF, and TF-FVII complex [19,20]. Values are expressed as mean ± standard deviation, and the significance of the difference between two groups was assessed by Student's nonpaired t test.

RESULTS

Plasma TF antigen was detected in normal volunteers (126 ± 41 pg/ml), and it was increased in DIC patients with ALL (252 ± 60 pg/ml), APL (279 ± 64 pg/ml), ANLL other than APL (326 ± 85 pg/ml), solid cancer (292 ± 116 pg/ml), sepsis (288 ± 87 pg/ml), and other diseases (208 ± 69 pg/ml; Fig. 1). The TF antigen level was higher in DIC patients (281 ± 90 pg/ml) than in pre-DIC patients (223 ± 77 pg/ml; $P < 0.05$) and non-DIC patients (192 ± 53 pg/ml; $P < 0.02$; Fig. 2). However, it was within the normal range in four patients with DIC. There was no significant difference in plasma TF antigen levels between DIC patients with (268 ± 103 pg/ml) and without (276 ± 74 pg/ml) organ failure (Fig. 3). After treatment of DIC, the TF antigen was significantly reduced (246 ± 75 pg/ml; $P < 0.02$; Fig. 4). There was no marked difference in plasma TF antigen level between good outcome (286 ± 94 pg/ml) and poor outcome (282 ± 94 pg/ml; Fig. 5) patients. Plasma TAT, PIC, FDP-D-dimer, t-PA and PAI-I antigen levels were increased in patients with DIC compared to pre-DIC and non-DIC patients (Table II). The plasma TF antigen level was not correlated with these hemostatic markers.

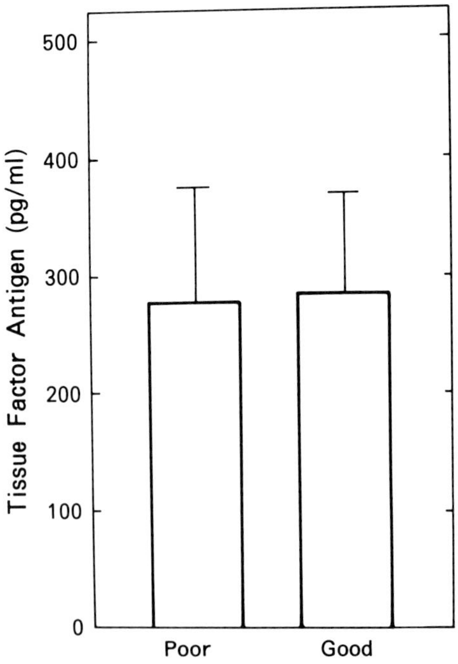

Fig. 5. Plasma level of tissue factor antigen in DIC patients with poor outcome or good outcome.

TABLE II. Hemostatic Markers in DIC, Pre-DIC, and Non-DIC Patients

Marker	DIC	Pre-DIC	Non-DIC
TAT (ng/ml)	51.6 ± 9.7	28.9 ± 9.2	11.5 ± 10.1
PIC (μg/ml)	3.67 ± 0.44	2.65 ± 0.51	1.35 ± 0.33
t-PA (ng/ml)	29.6 ± 4.6	24.6 ± 4.6	17.3 ± 4.6
PAI-I (ng/ml)	91.5 ± 7.3	28.4 ± 6.2	24.5 ± 7.9
FDP-D-dimer (ng/ml)	3,205 ± 514	1,428 ± 284	657 ± 47

DISCUSSION

Since TF is the main initiator for onset of DIC in acute leukemia [10,11], the presence of TF in the plasma has been considered to be the pathologic state. However, the plasma TF antigen was detected not only in DIC patients but also in normal volunteers. Since the TF antigen was not detected in the platelets or leukocytes without stimulation, the plasma TF was suggested to be physiologically released from locally stimulated monocytes or endothelial cells. In vitro, the TF activity in mononuclear cells and vascular endothelial cells is enhanced by addition of endotoxin or several cytokines [21,22]. The TF antigen level was significantly higher in DIC patients than in pre-DIC or non-DIC patients. The plasma TF antigen in DIC patients with ANLL was higher than that in those with ALL. The TF activity in leukemic cell lysates was reported to be higher in ANLL than in ALL cell lysates [11]. In DIC with leukemia, plasma TF has been considered to be produced by the leukemic cells. The increase of TF might play an important role in the onset of DIC. TF was increased in DIC patients with ALL, ANLL, solid cancer, sepsis, and other diseases. In sepsis and solid cancer, elevated plasma cytokine levels have been reported [12,13], and the elevated cytokines might increase the TF synthesis by the monocytes or vascular endothelial cells. However, the plasma TF level was within the normal range in four patients with DIC. Other factors such as infections may be required for the onset of DIC in such patients.

There was no significant difference in plasma TF antigen level between DIC patients with organ failure and those without organ failure, suggesting that organ failure may not increase the plasma TF level. Since the TF antigen was significantly reduced after treatment for DIC, the malignant cycle in the DIC state might increase the plasma TF level further. These findings suggested that the treatment of DIC should be begun at an early stage. There was no marked difference in the plasma TF antigen level between good outcome and poor outcome, suggesting that TF might initiate DIC, but it might not be responsible for the outcome after treatment of DIC. The plasma TF antigen level was slightly associated ($r = 0.323$) with the plasma TAT level, probably because TF initiates the activation of the extrinsic pathway of blood coagulation and finally activation of prothrombin to thrombin.

ACKNOWLEDGMENTS

This work was supported in part by a Grant-In-Aid for cancer Research from the Ministry of Education, Science and Culture, Japan.

REFERENCES

1. Nemerson Y, Bach R: Tissue factor revisited. Progr Hemostas, 6:237–261, 1982.
2. Nemerson Y: Tissue factor and hemostasis. Blood 71:1–8, 1988.
3. Weiss HJ, Lages B: Evidence for tissue factor-dependent activation of the classic extrinsic coagulation mechanism in blood obtained from bleeding time wounds. Blood 71:629–635, 1988.
4. Rodgers GM: Hemostatic properties of normal and perturbed vascular cells. FASEB J 1:116–123, 1988.
5. Conkling PR, Greenberg CS, Weinberg JB: Tumor necrosis factor induces tissue factor-like activity in human leukemia cell line U939 and peripheral blood monocytes. Blood 72:128–133, 1988.
6. Colucci M, Balconi G, Lorenzet R, Pietra A, Locati D, Donati MB, Semerara N: Cultured human endothelial cell generate tissue factor in response to endotoxin. J Clin Invest 71:1893–1986, 1983.
7. Tannenbaum SH, Finko R, Cines DB: Antibody and immune complexes induce tissue factor production in human endothelial cells. J Immunol 137:1532–1537, 1986.
8. Colman RT, Robboy SJ, Minna ID: Disseminated intravascular coagulation (DIC): An approach. Am J Med 52:679–689, 1974.
9. Gralnick HR, Bargrey J, Abrell E: Heparin treatment for the hemorrhagic diathesis of acute promyelocytic leukemia. Am J Med 52:167–174, 1972.
10. Gralnick HR, Abrell E: Studies on the procoagulant and fibrinolytic activity of promyelocytic leukemia. Br J Haematol 24:89–98, 1973.
11. Wada H, Nagano T, Tomeoku M, Kuto M, Karitani Y, Deguchi K, Shirakawa S: Coagulant and fibrinolytic activities in the leukemic cell lysates. Thromb Res 30:315–322, 1982.
12. Cybulsky MI, Chan MKW, Movat HZ: Acute inflammation and microthrombus induced by endotoxin, interleukin-1, and tumor necrosis factor and their implications in gram-negative infection. Lab Invest 58:365–378, 1988.
13. Wada H, Tamaki S, Tanigawa M, Takagi M, Mori Y, Deguchi A, Katayama N, Yamamoto T, Deguchi K, Shirakawa S: Plasma level of IL-1β in disseminated intravascular coagulation. Thromb Haemostas 65:364–368, 1991.
14. Kobayashi N, Maegawa T, Takada M, Tanaka H, Gonmori H: Criteria for diagnosis of DIC based on the analysis of clinical and laboratory findings in 345 DIC patients collected by the Research Committee on DIC in Japan. Bibliogr Haematol 49:265–275, 1987.

15. Ohno H, Kosaki G, Kambayashi J, Imaoka S, Hirata F: FOY; [ethyl p-(6-guanidinohexanoxyloxy) benzoate] methaneslfonate as a serine protease inhibitor. I. Inhibition of thrombin and factor Xa in vitro. Thromb Res 19:579–588, 1980.
16. Ohno H, Kambayashi J, Chang SW, Kosaki G: FOY; [ethyl p-(6-guandinohexanonxyloxy) benzoate] methaneslfonate as a serine protease inhibitor. II. In vivo effect on coagulofibrinolytic system in comparison with haparin or aprotinin. Thromb Res 24:445–452, 1981.
17. Asakura H, Saito M, Ito K, Jokaji Y, Uotani C, Kumabashiri I, Matsuda T: Levels of thrombin-antithrombin III complex in plasma in cases of acute promyelocytic leukemia. Thromb Res 50:895–899, 1988.
18. Mimuro J, Koike Y, Sumi Y, Aoki N: Monoclonal antibodies to discrete regions in α2-plasmin inhibitor. Blood 69:446–453, 1987.
19. Morrissey JH, Fair DS, Edgington TS: Monoclonal antibody analysis of purified and cell-associated tissue factor. Thromb Res 52:247–261, 1988.
20. Drake TA, Morrissey JH, Edgington TS: Selective cellular expression of tissue factor in human tissue. Am J Pathol. 134:1087–1096, 1989.
21. Charsen E, Flatmark A, Prydz H: Cytokine-induced procoagulant activity in monocytes and endothelial cells. Transplantation 46:575–580, 1988.
22. Wada H, Tanigawa M, Wakita Y, Nakase T, Minamikawa K, Kaneko T, Ohiwa M, Kageyama S, Kobayashi T, Noguchi T, Deguchi K, Shirakawa S: Increased plasma level of interleukin-6 in disseminated intravascular coagulation. Blood Coagulation Fibrinolysis (in press).

American Journal of Hematology 45:237–239 (1994)

Erythropoietin in the Treatment of Delayed Immune Hemolysis of a Major ABO-Incompatible Bone Marrow Transplant

J. López, J.L. Steegmann, G. Pérez, M.J. Otero, M. Berberana, R. Cámara, M. Lamana, M.J. Fernández Villalta, and J.M. Fernández-Rañada

Hematology Department, Hospital de La Princesa, Madrid, Spain

Delayed immune hemolysis can be observed after major ABO-incompatible bone marrow transplants (BMT). The management of these hemolytic episodes includes transfusion of group O red blood cells and increases of immunosuppression. Here we report the case of a 25-year-old patient who developed overt immune hemolysis on day +50 after a HLA-identical ABO-incompatible BMT. To avoid added immunosuppression, erythropoietin was started: an increase in reticulocytes sufficient to maintain hemoglobin despite persistent hemolysis was observed. We conclude that erythropoietin may have a role in the management of delayed-onset hemolysis of major ABO-incompatible BMT, especially when added immunosuppression is undesirable.

Key words: immune hemolysis, hemolysis, HLA types, BMT, erythropoietin

INTRODUCTION

Major ABO incompatibility between donor and recipient exists in ~10–20% of allogeneic bone marrow transplants (BMT). Although ABO incompatibility is not a barrier to successful BMT, prolonged reticulocytopenia, delayed onset of erythropoiesis with increased dependence of red blood cells transfusions, and pure red cell aplasia occasionally occur in these transplants [1,2]. Delayed immune hemolysis due to persistence of receptor ABO isohemagglutinins has also been reported, mainly in patients who received cyclosporine for graft-versus-host-disease (GVHD) prophylaxis [3].

Erythropoietin (EPO) has been successfully used in the management of other immunohematologic complications of ABO-incompatible transplants [4,5] and in the therapy of hemolytic episodes of different etiologies [6]. Yet, as far as we know, the drug has not been used in the treatment of delayed hemolysis associated with major ABO-incompatible grafts. We report here our successful experience with EPO in a patient with ABO-incompatible hemolysis who, while receiving methotrexate-cyclosporine as GVHD prophylaxis, developed overt delayed hemolysis in the second month post-BMT.

CASE REPORT

A 25-year-old man with first chronic phase chronic myeloid leukemia underwent a BMT from his HLA-identical sister. There was major ABO incompatibility between the patient and his donor (donor: A; receptor: O). The conditioning regime included cyclophosphamide (120 mg/kg) and fractionated total body irradiation (12 Gy divided in six fractions over 3 days). GVHD-prophylaxis consisted on cyclosporine and a short course of methotrexate (Seattle).

On day 0, a red blood cell-depleted graft (obtained by processing the graft with an IBM Code-2991 cell separator) containing 2.9×10^8 nucleated cells/kg and 8 ml ABO-incompatible red blood cells was infused without significant clinical problems.

The patient received EPO therapy between days 0 and +36 because he was included in a prospective, randomized protocol to test usefulness of EPO in BMT (EPO

Received for publication March 4, 1993; accepted May 13, 1993.

Address reprint requests to Dr. Javier López Jiménez, Hospital de La Princesa, C/Diego de León 62, Madrid, Spain.

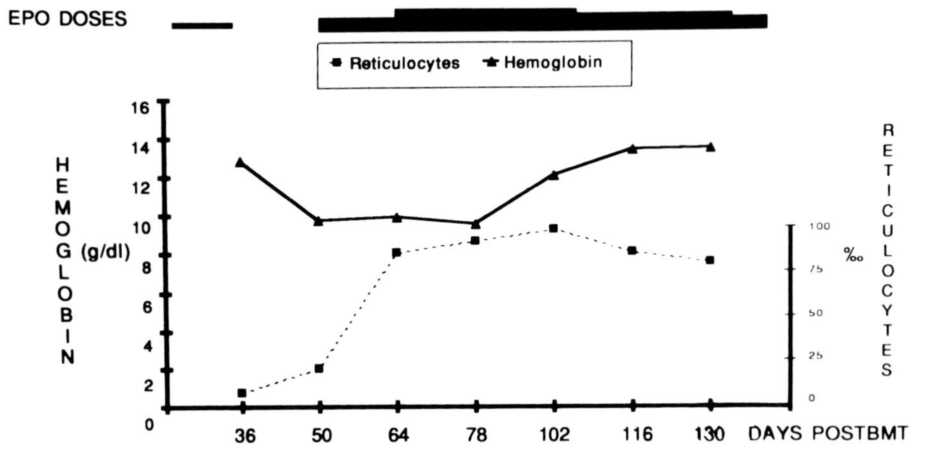

	36	50	64	78	102	116	130	NORMAL RANGE
LDH (U/L)	381	860	751	574	451	419	347	<360
Bilirubin (mg/dl)	1.2	N.T.	0.9	N.T.	0.7	0.7	0.6	0.3-1.3
Haptoglobin (U/L)	N.T.	0	0	0	N.T.	106	145	50-150
Serum EPO levels (mU/ml)	128	28	186	N.T.	N.T.	156	310	4-28

Fig. 1. Top: Response of hemoglobin and reticulocytes to EPO administration. Bottom: Serum EPO levels and parameters of hemolysis before and after EPO therapy. N.T., not tested.

doses: days 0–7: 100 units/kg/day; days 7–36: 150 units/kg/day. EPO was always administered as a single daily bolus injection). Neutrophil and platelet engraftment were observed, respectively, on days +16 and +23. The patient reached reticulocytes >5‰ on day +21. After transplant, anti-A was detectable in the patient's serum until day +175. No clinical GVHD was observed.

On day +50 mild jaundice was observed, but bilirubin levels were not determined. Hemoglobin levels had fallen to 9.7 g/dl and haptoglobin was 0, while reticulocyte count and LDH had increased to 20‰ and 860 IU/liter (Fig. 1). Direct antiglobulin test, previously negative, was positive for C_3. Anti-A was eluated from red blood cells and was also found in the patient's serum. Schistocytes were not observed in a blood smear.

The patient was followed on cyclosporine therapy, and no change in the dose was attempted. EPO (100 units/kg/day i.v. daily as a bolus injection) was reassumed. Two weeks later, reticulocyte count increased to 90‰ and hemoglobin did not fall further, in spite of persistent hemolysis (LDH 751 IU/liter; haptoglobin 0 IU/liter. The EPO dose was increased to 125 U/kg/day. One month later hemoglobin rose to 12.4 g/dl, and a normalization of the hemolytic parameters was observed. EPO was tapered to 125 units/kg/day twice per week and discontinued on day +150. No new hemolytic episodes were observed during follow-up.

DISCUSSION

We report a major ABO-incompatible BMT patient with a hemolytic crisis due to persistence of recipient isohemagglutinins on day +50 post-BMT who responded to EPO therapy. Isohemagglutinin production from residual recipient cells seems to be the cause of hemolysis, although cytogenetic analysis showed complete chimerism. However, the sensitivity of these methods is not high enough for the detection of residual receptor immunocompetent cell [2]. Passive administration of ABO antibody in red blood cell/platelet transfusions does not seem to be a plausible explanation, since the last transfusion was received 1 month before the hemolytic episode.

Data in the literature about these hemolytic episodes are very similar to the data described here: a median onset on day +65, with a drop in hemoglobin levels between 1.5 and 4 g/dl and a median duration of hemolysis of 36 days. Hemolysis has been found more often among patients treated with cyclosporine, and it is usually managed with transfusion of group O red blood cells and/or increases in the dose of prednisone [3].

However, the question raised by some groups of an increased relapse rate in BMT patients when cyclosporine-methotrexate is employed as GVHD prophylaxis [7] and the experience of our group and others with EPO after BMT [8,9] prompted us to use EPO as therapy for the hemolytic crisis instead of adding potent immunosuppressive drugs such as prednisone. Moreover, Locatelly et al. [5] have demonstrated that recombinant EPO may be useful in correcting anemia after allogeneic bone marrow transplantation when endogenous EPO levels are inappropriately low for the degree of anemia, as was observed in our patient.

After the start of EPO therapy (Fig. 1) 1) a prompt increase (near 500%) in the reticulocyte count could be observed; 2) hemoglobin levels, that had fallen down from 12.8 to 9.7 g/dl, did not fall further in spite of persisting hemolysis (LDH and haptoglobin levels remained high and low, respectively; and 3) when hemolysis ceased, the reticulocyte count was as high as 80‰ in spite of hemoglobin levels between 13.5 and 13.8 g/dl. Thus, hemoglobin levels rose, although anti-A persisted in serum (anti-A titers on day +141: IgM, 1/8; IgG, 1/16).

Treatment with EPO seems to have contributed to the successful management of the hemolytic episode in our patient. EPO has been shown to be effective against hemolytic anemia in NZB mice and in the recovery period from anemia in PHZ mice [10]. The increase in red blood cell mass induced by EPO may reduce hemolysis through isohemagglutinin adsorption mechanisms. Finally, EPO may modestly reduce cellular as well as humoral systemic immunity [11,12]. In summary, we believe that EPO may have a beneficial role in the delayed onset hemolysis of major ABO-incompatible BMT, especially in those high-relapse-risk patients in whom added immunosuppression may be undesirable.

REFERENCES

1. Bensinger WI, Buckner CD, Thomas ED, Clift RA: ABO-incompatible marrow transplants. Transplantation 33:427, 1982.
2. Gmür JP, Burger J, Schaffuer A, et al: Pure red cell aplasia of long duration complicating major ABO-incompatible bone marrow transplantation. Blood 75:290, 1990.
3. Sniecinski IJ, Oien L, Petz LD, Blume KG: Immunohematologic consequences of major ABO-mismatched bone marrow transplants. Transplantation 45:530, 1988.
4. Heyll A, Aul C, Runde V, Arning M, Schneider W, Wernet P: Treatment of pure red cell aplasia after major ABO-incompatible bone marrow transplantation with recombinant erythropoietin. Blood 77: 906, 1991.
5. Locatelly F, Pedrazzoli P, Barosi G, et al: Recombinant human erythropoietin is effective in correcting erythropoietin-deficient anaemia after allogeneic bone marrow transplantation. Br J Haematol 80:545, 1992.
6. Kornowski R, Schwartz D, Jaffe A, Pines A, Aderka D, Levo Y: Erythropoietin therapy obviates the need for recurrent transfusions in a patient with severe hemolysis due to prosthetic valves. Chest 102:315, 1992.
7. Aschan J, Ringdén O, Sundberg B, Gahrton G, Ljungman P, Winiarski J: Methotrexate combined with cyclosporin A decreases graft-versus-host disease, but increases leukemic relapse compared to monotherapy. Bone Marrow Transplant 7:113, 1991.
8. Link H, Diedrich H, Ebell W et al. Recombinant human erythropoietin after allogeneic bone marrow transplantation. Bone Marrow Transplant 5(Suppl 2):113, 1990.
9. Steegmann JL, López J, Otero MJ, De la Cámara R, Berberana M, Lamana ML, Díaz A, Fernández-Rañada JM. Erythropoietin treatment in allogeneic bone marrow transplantation: A prospective, controlled and randomized study. Bone Marrow Transplant 10:541, 1992.
10. Cynshi O, Shimonaka Y, Higuchi M, et al: Effects of recombinant human erythropoietin on haemolytic anaemia in mice. Br J Haematol 76:414, 1990.
11. Kiball PM, Kerman RH. Erythropoietin: A potential immunomodulator? Transplant Proc 23:336, 1991.
12. Grimm PC, Sekiya NM, Robertson LS, Robinson BJ, Ettenger RB: Recombinant human erythropoietin decreases anti-HLA sensitization and may improve renal allograft outcome: involvement of anti-idiotypic antibody. Transplant Proc 23:407, 1991.

American Journal of Hematology 45:240–243 (1994)

Spontaneous Factor VIII Inhibitor Occurring in Association with Chronic Graft-Versus-Host Disease

Christopher W. Seidler, Letha E. Mills, Mary E.D. Flowers, Keith M. Sullivan

Norris Cotton Cancer Center and the Dartmouth-Hitchcock Medical Center, Lebanon, New Hampshire (C.W.S., L.E.M.); Fred Hutchinson Cancer Research Center and the University of Washington, Seattle (M.E.D.F., K.M.S.)

The development of spontaneously acquired Factor VIII inhibitors is rare and may lead to serious hemorrhagic sequelae. We report here the case of a patient who acquired a Factor VIII inhibitor two years after an allogeneic bone marrow transplant for CML. This occurred in association with a flare of chronic graft versus host disease (GVDH). He responded to corticosteroid therapy. A review of autoimmune phenomena associated with chronic GVDH and the treatment of Factor VIII inhibitors is discussed.

Key words: Factor VIII inhibitors, chronic graft versus host disease

INTRODUCTION

The development of factor VIII inhibitors in nonhemophiliacs is rare and may lead to serious or even fatal hemorrhage by inhibition of endogenous factor VIII activity. Spontaneously acquired factor inhibitors have been reported to occur in several clinical situations: autoimmune diseases, lymphoproliferative disorders, allergic drug reactions, uncomplicated childbirths, and occasionally spontaneously in otherwise healthy elderly individuals [1,2]. We describe a patient who developed an acquired factor VIII inhibitor occurring in association with chronic graft-versus-host disease (GVHD) 2 years after allogeneic bone marrow transplantation for chronic myelogenous leukemia.

CASE REPORT

A 27-year-old white man presented to Dartmouth-Hitchcock Medical Center with complaints of abdominal pain and fatigue. On physical examination he had marked splenomegaly and a white blood cell count of 235,200/μl, with predominantly mature myeloid forms. A bone marrow biopsy demonstrated a hypercellular marrow with typical features of chronic myelogenous leukemia in chronic phase. Cytogenetic analysis of 30 marrow metaphases revealed 100% Philadelphia chromosome-positive cells. There was no history of a bleeding disorder, and routine coagulation tests were normal.

He was briefly treated with γ-interferon but discontinued treatment within 1 week due to toxicity. Oral hydroxyurea (1 g/day) was started with a gradual decrease in the white count to 13,500/μl over several months and resolution of splenomegaly.

Five months after diagnosis, while still in chronic phase, the patient underwent allogeneic marrow transplantation at the Fred Hutchinson Cancer Research Center, Seattle, Washington. Both the patient and the donor (his brother) were HLA type A28,29; B44; DR1,7. The preparative chemotherapy regimen consisted of oral Busulfan (16 mg/kg) and intravenous cyclophosphamide (120 mg/kg). GVHD prophylaxis consisted of intravenous cyclosporine and methotrexate [3]. Trilineage engraftment was noted by day 36.

The early posttransplant course was complicated by venocclusive disease of the liver, with a peak bilirubin of 5.8 mg/dl on day 13. Neutropenic fevers without documented infection responded to intravenous antibiotics and amphotericin B. He had no evidence of acute GVHD. A Hickman catheter infection and *Clostridium difficile* enterocolitis responded to appropriate antibiotic therapy.

The clinical course after hospital discharge was uncomplicated. He remained on a tapering dose of oral cyclosporine and had no evidence of GVHD on screening studies at 100 days posttransplant [4]. Cyclosporine was

Received for publication November 10, 1992; accepted July 20, 1993.

Address reprint requests to Letha E. Mills, MD, Norris Cotton Cancer Center, Dartmouth-Hitchcock Medical Center, One Medical Center Drive, Lebanon, NH 03756.

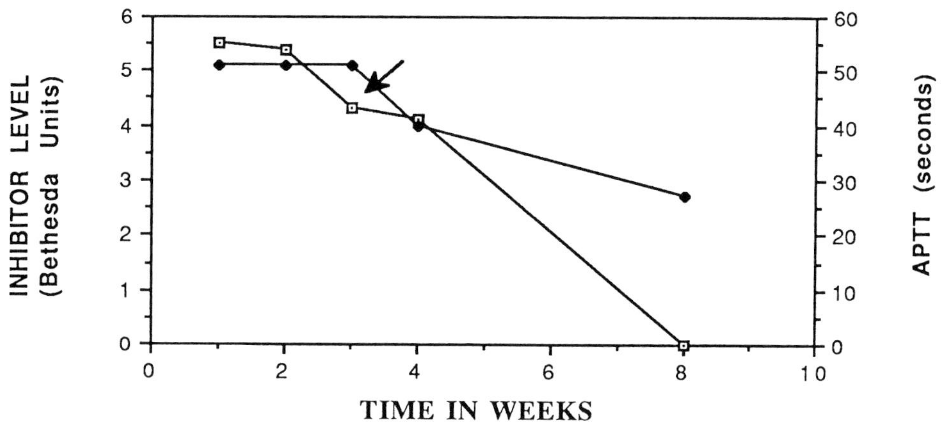

Fig. 1. Factor VIII inhibitor level vs. time since inhibitor detection. Arrow marks start of prednisone therapy (1 mg/kg/day).

tapered off gradually over 6 months and did well for the next 3 months with no immunosuppressive medications.

Nine months after transplant, the patient developed oral leukoplakia, a mild skin rash, dry eyes, and jaundice. Laboratory tests revealed marked elevation of serum transaminases (AST 638 U/liter, alkaline phosphatase 454 U/liter) and bilirubin (3.3 mg/dl). Hepatitis A, B, C, and cytomegalovirus (CMV) antibody titers were all negative. Modest declines in the platelet count (138,000/μl) and white count (2,600/μl) were noted. A skin biopsy showed chronic inflammation and lichenoid changes consistent with grade II chronic GVHD.

The patient was started on prednisone (1 mg/kg) for chronic GVHD and twice daily infection prophylaxis with trimethoprim/sulfamethoxazole, which led to rapid resolution of symptoms and improvement in laboratory parameters. A bone marrow biopsy obtained 1 year after the transplant revealed normal marrow morphology and cytogenetics. A repeat skin biopsy performed 4 months after initiation of prednisone revealed no evidence of GVHD. The prednisone was gradually tapered and discontinued over 9 months. He did well in the interim 4-month period off corticosteroids and antibiotics with only mild elevation of transaminases and no evidence of skin disease.

Two years after the transplant, the patient began again to develop symptoms of chronic GVHD manifested by dry skin rash and dry eyes. He also noted increased bruising with minimal trauma. A repeat bone marrow biopsy was performed and revealed a remission marrow with normal cytogenetics. However, he continued to bleed from the bone marrow biopsy site for 2 weeks and required suturing and compression dressings to maintain local hemostasis. An activated partial thromboplastin time (APTT; normal range 19–34 sec) was markedly prolonged (53.0 sec), with a normal prothrombin time (PT) of 12.1 sec (normal range (11–13 sec) and a normal thrombin time (TT) of 13 sec (normal range 10–15 sec). There was no evidence for disseminated intravascular coagulation (negative D-dimer test, fibrinogen 332 mg/dl). Further investigation detected a factor VIII inhibitor of 5.4 Bethesda units and decreased factor VIII activity of 6.0% (Fig. 1). A PTT mixing study with dilutions of 10%, 50%, and 90% normal plasma demonstrated immediate and progressive inhibition at 60 min. A platelet neutralization procedure was negative. The modified dilute Russell viper venom test was also normal, indicating that this was not a lupus-like anticoagulant. The factor IX activity was 70%. Testing of the marrow donor revealed a normal PT and PTT and no factor VIII inhibitor. The donor has no history of a bleeding diathesis. The patient's inhibitor showed little inhibition of porcine factor VIII activity in vitro. Mixing studies revealed that the patient's plasma was able to inhibit the donor's coagulation system, with prolongation of his PTT.

The patient developed worsening of the oral leukoplakia and skin rash. Liver function test results became elevated, similar to the first episode of chronic GVHD. Mild hypogammaglobulinemia (0.6 g/dl) and thrombocytopenia (133,000/μl) were also noted. This constellation of findings was consistent with a flare of chronic GVHD activity.

The patient's factor VIII inhibitor persisted, and the symptoms of chronic GVHD worsened, although no clinically significant bleeding occurred. Four weeks after the inhibitor was first detected, the patient was started on prednisone therapy (1 mg/kg/day). Treatment was complicated by an episode of steroid psychosis, which required reduction of the prednisone dose to 0.5 mg/kg/day. With this therapy the patient had a decrease in the factor VIII inhibitor level to less than 1.0 BU within 3 weeks (Fig. 1). The PTT normalized, and he has had no clinical evidence of bleeding. Two months after restarting of steroids, his oral leukoplakia and skin rash have resolved and liver function tests have returned to baseline. He is currently being maintained on prednisone (0.5 mg/kg QOD) and trimethoprim/sulfamethoxazole prophylaxis (3 times per week). He remains without evidence of factor VIII inhibitor 6 months after restarting of therapy with prednisone.

DISCUSSION

To our knowledge this is the first report describing the development of an acquired factor VIII inhibitor occurring in association with chronic GVHD. Chronic GVHD occurs in 33% of patients after HLA-identical marrow transplantation [5]. Clinical manifestations include chronic cholestatic liver disease, skin disease, keratoconjunctivitis, ocular sicca, oral mucositis, small and large intestinal involvement, and pulmonary insufficiency [6–8]. Poikiloderma and scleroderma occur and may lead to joint contracture [9,10]. A number of "autoimmune" conditions occur in the setting of chronic GVHD [7,9,11–14]. These include clinical manifestation resembling systemic lupus erythematosus, lichen planus, progressive systemic sclerosis, Sjögren syndrome, primary biliary cirrhosis, and eosinophilic fasciitis [15].

Patients with chronic GVHD have been treated with prednisone, cyclosporine, azathioprine cyclophosphamide, and thalidomide as single drugs or in combination [16–18]. Early treatment (before functional impairment) is more effective than late treatment in preventing disability.

The mechanisms leading to the formation of spontaneous factor VIII inhibitors in the nonhemophilic population are not known. Inhibitors have been detected in a variety of "autoimmune" conditions, including systemic lupus erythematosus, rheumatoid arthritis, dermatitis herpetiformis, erythema multiforme, reginal enteritis, ulcerative colitis, bronchial asthma, and penicillin allergy [1,2,19–21]. In many respects, chronic GVHD resembles autoimmune disorders [11,12,15]. This may reflect impaired autoregulatory cell function or cytokine generation [22]. Factor VIII inhibitors are not reported to occur with any increased frequency in patients on chronic immunosuppressive therapy or in primary immunosuppressed states.

Treatment of factor VIII inhibits is initially directed toward controlling local hemorrhage and achieving hemostasis and then eliminating the inhibitor. The available modes of therapy are immunosuppressive drugs, factor VIII concentrates (human or porcine), factor IX complex concentrates, activated factor IX complex concentrates, intravenous high-dose gammaglobulin, and plasma exchange [2,19–21].

Cyclophosphamide, prednisone, and azathioprine have been reported to be effective singly or in combination in decreasing inhibitor levels [2,19,20]. The optimal immunosuppressive treatment of factor VIII inhibitors is not known. Certain subsets of patients are reported to respond better to corticosteroids, particularly postpartum and in elderly patients without underlying disease [2]. Inhibitors developing in patients with underlying autoimmune conditions such as rheumatoid arthritis are often resistant to steroid therapy and require the use of cytotoxic agents, particularly cyclophosphamide, either alone or in combination with corticosteroids [2,23].

Immunosuppressive drugs are not useful in the management of acute bleeding in patients with inhibitors. When the inhibitor titer is <5 BU, large, saturating doses of factor VIII can be infused to overcome the inhibitor effects and achieve hemostasis [2,19–21,24]. In patients with a high titer of inhibitor, porcine factor VIII (Hyate: C), factor IX complex concentrates (Konyne-HT and Proplex-T), or activated factor X complexes (FEIBA VH and Autoplex HT) can be used [2,19–21,24]. However, since factor IX complex concentrates have more risks associated with their use (possible transmission of hepatitis B and hepatitis C, disseminated intravascular coagulation, thromboembolism, and acute myocardial infarction), these agents are used infrequently [25]. Intravenous gammaglobulin has also been reported to be effective [26].

Since our patient did not have clinically significant bleeding, we initially chose to observe him. However, with the passage of time, additional manifestations of GVHD became apparent, and the inhibitor persisted. Immunosuppressive therapy with prednisone alone was effective in rapidly lowering the inhibitor level.

The development of factor VIII inhibitor in this patient has practical implications. In any patient who has received an allogeneic marrow transplant, factor VIII inhibitor should be considered if a bleeding diathesis occurs in the setting of chronic GVHD. Physicians who routinely care for patients with chronic GVHD should be aware of this late complication. Furthermore, this patient's inhibitor was rapidly responsive to prednisone therapy and did not require additional cytotoxic agents. The inhibitor showed little activity against porcine factor VIII, which could be a therapeutic option should the hemostatic need arise.

ACKNOWLEDGMENTS

This study was supported in part by grants (CA 18221, CA 18029, CA 15704, and CA 23108) from the National Institutes of Health, DHHS. We appreciate comments on and review of the manuscript by Dr. Arthur Thompson of the Puget Sound Blood Center.

REFERENCES

1. Green D, Lechner K: A Survey of 215 Non-hemophilic patients with inhibitors to factor VIII. Thromb Hemostas 45:1981.

2. Coleman RW, et al. (eds): Acquired inhibitors against factor VIII and other clotting proteins. In: Hemostasis and Thrombosis 2nd ed. New York: Springer Verlag, 1990.
3. Storb R, Deeg HJ, et al.: Methotrexate and cyclosporine compared with cyclosporine alone for prophylaxis of acute graft versus host disease after marrow transplantation for leukemia. N Engl J Med 314:12, 1986.
4. Loughran TP, Sullivan KM, Morton T, et al.: Value of day 100 screening studies for predicting the development of chronic graft-versus-host disease after allogeneic bone marrow transplantation. Blood 76:a, 1990.
5. Sullivan KM, Agura E, Anasetti C, et al.: Chronic graft-versus-host disease and other late complications of bone marrow transplantation. Semin Hematol 28:3, 1991.
6. Shulman HM, Sullivan KM, Wieden PL, et al.: Chronic graft-versus-host syndrome in man. a long-term clinicopathologic study of 20 Seattle patients. Am J Med 69: 1980.
7. Epstein O, Sherlock S, Thomas HC: Primary biliary cirrhosis is a dry gland syndrome with features of graft-versus-host disease. Lancet 1:8179, 1980.
8. Clark JG, Crawford SW, Madtes DK, Sullivan KM: Obstructive long disease after allogeneic marrow transplantation. Ann Intern Med 111, 1989.
9. Lawley TJ, Peck GL, Moutsopoulos HM, Gratwohl AA, Deisseroth AB: Scleroderma, Sjögren-like syndrome, and chronic graft-versus-host disesae. Ann Intern Med 87: 1977.
10. Sullivan KM, Shulman HM, Storb R, et al.: Chronic graft-versus-host disease in 52 patients: Adverse natural course and successful treatment with combination immunosuppression. Blood 57:267–277, 1981.
11. Fialkow PJ, Gilchrist C, Allison AC: Autoimmunity in chronic graft-versus-host disease. Clin Exp Immunol 13, 1973.
12. Graze PR, Gale RP: Chronic graft versus host disease: A syndrome of disordered immunity. Am J Med 66, 1979.
13. Dighiero G, Intrator L, Cordonnier C, Tortevoye P, Vernant J: High levels of Anti-cytoskeleton Autoantibodies are Frequently Associated with Chronic GVHD. Br J Haematol 67, 1987.
14. Rouquett-Gally AM, Goyeldieu D, Prost AC, Glockman E: Autoimmunity after allogeneic bone marrow transplantation. Transplantation 46:2, 1988.
15. Shulman HM, Sullivan KM: Graft-versus-host disease: Allo- and autoimmunity after bone marrow transplantation. Concepts Immunopathol 6, 1988.
16. Sullivan KM, Witherspoon RP,Storb R, et al.: Prednisone and azathioprine compared with prednisone and placebo for treatment of chronic graft-versus-host disease: Prognostic influence of prolonged thrombocytopenia afer allogeneic marrow transplantation. Blood 72:2, 1988.
17. Sullivan KM, Witherspoon RP, Storb R, Deeg HJ: Alternating-day cyclosporine and prednisone for treatment of high-risk chronic graft-v-host disease. Blood 72:2, 1988.
18. Vogelsang GB, Farmer ER, Hess AD, et al.: Thalidomide for the treatment of chronic graft-versus-host disease. N Engl J Med 326:16, 1992.
19. Lusher JM: Factor VIII inhibitors: Etiology, characterization, natural history and management. Ann NY Acad Sci 509:89, 1987.
20. White GC, McMillan CW, Blatt PM, et al.: Factor VIII inhibitors: A clinical review. Am J Hematol 13:335, 1982.
21. Kasper CK: Management of inhibitors to factor VIII. Progr Hematol 12, 1981.
22. Ferrara JLM, Deeg HJ: Graft-versus-host disease. N Engl J Med 324: 10, 1991.
23. Spero JA, Lewis JH, Hasiba U: Corticosteroid therapy for acquired factor VIII inhibitors. Br J Haematol 48: 1981.
24. Kentrowitz JL, Lee ML, McClure DA, et al.: Early experience with the use of anti-inhibitor coagulant complex to treat bleeding in hemophiliacs with inhibitors to factor VIII. Clin Ther 9:405, 1987.
25. Green D, Kasper CK, and Lusher JM: Acquired hemophilia—A continuing education monograph. Los Angeles: Orthopaedic Hospital, 1991, pp. 62–63.
26. Zimmermann R, Kommerell B, Harenber J, et al.: Intravenous IgG for patients with spontaneous inhibitor to factor VIII. Lancet 1: 1985.

American Journal of Hematology 45:244–247 (1994)

Malignant Histiocytosis Associated With Autoimmune Thrombocytopenia

Tatsuharu Ohno, Tateo Sugiyama, Hiroo Furukawa, Takafumi Ishibashi, and Minoru Okuma
Hematology Unit, Department of Internal Medicine, Ohtsu Red Cross Hospital, Shiga (T.O., T.S., H.F.), and The First Division, Department of Internal Medicine, Faculty of Medicine, Kyoto University, Kyoto (T.I., M.O.), Japan

We describe a patient with malignant histiocytosis whose serum contained an autoantibody against platelet protein. The patient was admitted because of nasal bleeding and high-grade fever. The clinical course was fulminantly progressive and terminated with cerebral hemorrhage. Bone marrow aspirate showed the proliferation of large atypical cells, some of which exhibited phagocytic activity. At postmortem examination, there was diffuse infiltration of these atypical cells in the liver, spleen, kidney, and bone marrow. Morphological, cytochemical, immunohistochemical, and genotypic characteristics suggested that the proliferating cells were derived from the monocyte-macrophage system. Western blot analysis revealed the presence of autoantibody against an ~88 kd molecule of platelet proteins. Although the relationship of cause and effect remains to be clarified, this autoantibody appeared to have stimulated thrombophagocytosis of the neoplastic cells.

Key words: malignant histiocytosis, autoimmune thrombocytopenia, autoantibody

INTRODUCTION

Malignant histiocytosis (MH) is a systemic, progressive, and invasive proliferation of neoplastic cells resembling histiocytes and frequently displaying phagocytic activity [1]. The disease was renamed from the former term, *histiocytic medullary reticulosis* [2]. Major clinical manifestations include fever, wasting, pancytopenia, hepatosplenomegaly, and lymphadenopathy. Thrombocytopenia has been reported in >90% of cases [3]. Although cases of MH associated with Coombs-positive autoimmune hemolytic anemia have been reported [4,5], to our knowledge, no study has reported the cause of thrombocytopenia in MH. In the present paper, we describe a case of MH with severe thrombocytopenia conceivably influenced by the autoantibody against platelet protein.

CASE REPORT

A 55-year-old man was admitted to the Ohtsu Red Cross Hospital because of nasal bleeding, upper abdominal pain, and high-grade fever, which had worsened during the previous 3 weeks. His clinical history was noncontributory, and no special medication was taken before admission. Physical examination revealed a temperature of 39.5°C and icteric conjunctiva. The liver was palpable 5 cm below the right costal margin, while the spleen was not palpable and superficial lymph nodes were not swollen. Laboratory results disclosed an erythrocyte sedimentation rate (ESR) of 40 mm/hr. The levels of total and direct bilirubin were 6.3 and 4.6 mg/dl, respectively. SGOT was 370 IU/liter, SGPT 126 IU/liter, A1P 81.2 IU/liter, LAP 640 IU/liter, γGTP 130 IU/liter, and LDH 4,035 IU/liter (I 3.7%, II 22.1%, III 41.8%, IV 24.0%, V 8.2%). Ferritin concentration was 430.2 ng/ml, and that of lysozyme was 8.0 μg/ml in the serum. RBC was $438 \times 10^4/\mu l$, Hb 12.3 g/dl, Ht 36.4%, and leukocyte count 5,100/μl, with 28% bands, 56% segmented forms, 3% monocytes, and 13% lymphocytes. The platelet count was $2.2 \times 10^4/\mu l$. The bleeding time was 7.5 min by Duke's method, PT 11.9 sec (66%), fibrinogen 169 mg/dl, and FDP 10 μg/ml, while fibrin monomer was not detectable.

The bone marrow puncture disclosed the proliferation of large neoplastic cells (32.6%) resembling histiocytes

Received for publication February 18, 1993; accepted July 20, 1993.

Address reprint requests to Tatsuharu Ohno, MD, Hematology Unit, Department of Internal Medicine, Ohtsu Red Cross Hospital, 1-35, 1 Chome, Nagara, Ohtsu 520, Japan.

in the markedly hypoplastic myelogram. Nasal bleeding, high-grade fever, and thrombocytopenia persisted despite the administration of high-dose corticosteroid. Furthermore, anemia, leukocytopenia, and jaundice progressed. He died of cerebral hemorrhage on the thirteenth hospital day.

At postmortem examination, the liver weighed 1,950 g, with infiltration of neoplastic cells in the periportal area and hepatic sinusoid. The spleen weighed 535 g and was congested. The white pulp was not recognizable, and pulp cords and splenic sinusoids were infiltrated with neoplastic cells. The kidney was also infiltrated with neoplastic cells in the interstitial space. Lymph nodes in the mediastinum and in the peritoneal cavity were not swollen.

MATERIALS AND METHODS

Cell Morphology, Cytochemistry, and Immunohistochemistry

Cell morphology was examined on May-Grünwald-Giemsa-stained smears of bone marrow aspirates. Cytochemical studies included peroxidase (POX), periodic acid-Schiff (PAS), acid phosphatase (AcP), naphtol ASD chloracetate esterase (CAE), and α-naphthyl butylate esterase (αNBE) activities.

Autopsy specimens fixed gently in paraffin were employed for the immunohistochemical detection of cell surface and cytoplasmic antigens using the following antibodies: rabbit antihuman CD3 antibody (Ab), C3D-1 (CD15), L-26 (CD20), 1F8 (CD21), Ber-H2 (CD30), UCHL-1 (CD45RO), KP-1 (CD68), antileukocyte common antigen (LCA), antilysozyme, and anti-S100 protein (DAKO Japan, Kyoto, Japan).

Southern and Western Blot Analyses

Southern blot hybridization was performed as described previously [7]. Briefly, DNA exracted from the patient's spleen and digested with EcoRI, BamHI, or HindIII was fractionated on agarose gels and transferred to nitrocellulose membranes. The membrane-bound DNA fragments were then hybridized to ^{32}P-labeled probes, washed with appropriate stringency, and visualized on autoradiograms. The probes used were germline HindIII-EcoRI fragments containing the first C and J region of TCRβ (Cβ1)- and γ (Jγ1)-chain genes, and the J region of immunoglobulin heavy-chain (J_H) gene, respectively.

Western blot analysis was performed as described elsewhere [8]. Briefly, isolated pooled platelets (3×10^9) were lysed in 1 ml 1% NP-40 in 50 mM Tris HCl buffer, pH 7.4, containing protease inhibitors. The cell lysate was analyzed via sodium dodecyl sulfate (SDS)-polyacrylamide gel electrophoresis (PAGE) in a 7.5% slab gel. Platelet proteins separated by the SDS-PAGE were transblotted to nitrocellulose paper (Bio-Rad, Richmond, CA). The paper strips were incubated with 5% bovine skim milk, followed by overnight reaction with 2.5 ml of serially diluted patient's or control serum. After extensive washings, the strips were incubated with biotinylated goat antihuman IgG at room temperature for 2 hr and then were washed. Then, the bound antibody was visualized via the ABC peroxidase system using diaminobenzidine as a substrate (Vectastain ABC kit; Funakoshi Chemicals Co., Tokyo, Japan).

RESULTS

Characterization of the Proliferating Cells

May-Grünwald-Giemsa-stained smears of bone marrow aspirate taken on the eighth hospital day showed proliferation of large bizarre cells against a the background of hypoplastic normal marrow components. As is shown in Figure 1, a spectrum of histiocytic cells was present, ranging from relatively differentiated cells to immature and overtly malignant cells (Fig. 1). POX, PAS, AcP, and CAE were negative, while αNBE was weakly to strongly positive depending on the stage of differentiation of these atypical cells. Immunohistological stain was performed using an autopsy specimen as described elsewhere [6]. The proliferating cells in the spleen were negative for CD3, CD20, CD21, CD30, CD45RO, and S100 protein, while lysozyme, LCA, CD15, and CD68 were positive in these cells. To negate further the possibility of lymphocytic derivation of these cells, Southern blot hybridization was performed using the probes for TCRβ, TCRγ, and IgH genes as described previously [7]. BamH1, EcoR1, and HindIII digests of DNA from the spleen displayed an intact germline configuration for these genes.

Western Blot Analysis for Autoantibody to Platelet-Associated Antigen

Because severe thrombocytopenia was a unique hematological abnormality on admission, the patient's serum was analyzed via Western blotting for the presence of autoantibody against platelet-associated protein. As is shown in Figure 2, while several unidentified bands other than platelet-associated IgG were obtained in both control and patient lanes, the patient's serum recognized an ~88 kd protein of pooled platelet lysate under nonreducing conditions.

DISCUSSION

Thrombocytopenia was one of the most prominent clinical features in this patient, and intractable hemorrhagic diathesis due to thrombocytopenia was the initial and final manifestation. This clinical characteristic prompted us to investigate the cause of thrombocytope-

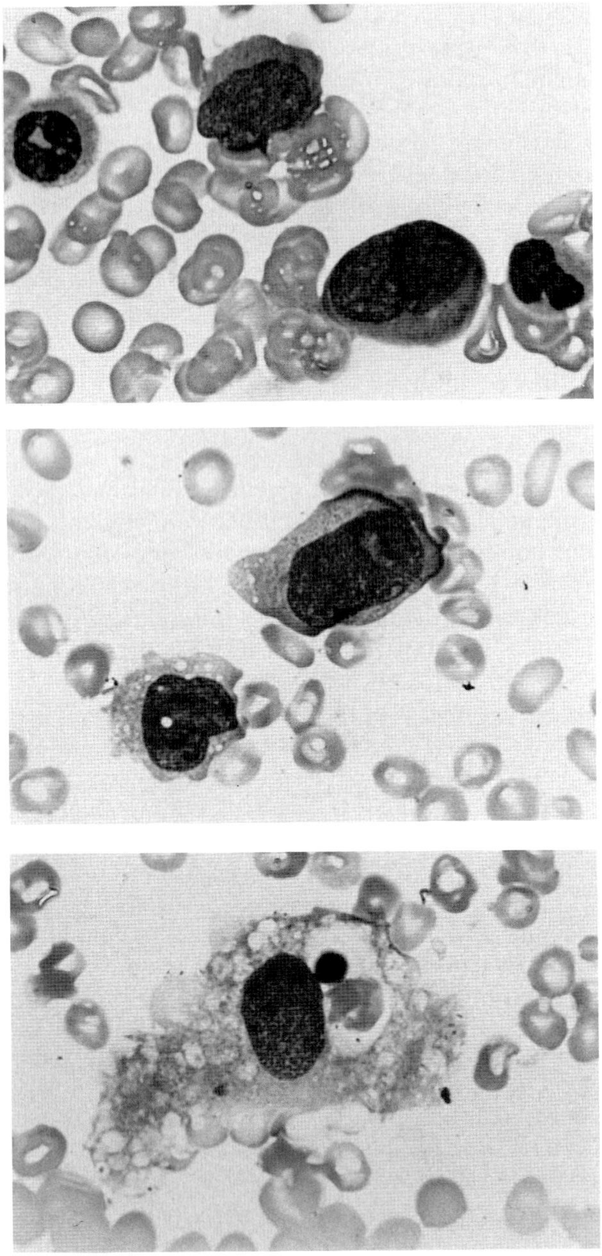

Fig. 1. Morphologic characteristics of the proliferating cells in the bone marrow. May-Grünwald-Giemsa stain. ×1000. Top: Large immature cells with irregular clumping of the nuclear chromatin, prominent multiple nucleoli, and basophilic scarce cytoplasm. Middle: Immature histiocytic cells with vacuolated and less basophilic cytoplasm. Bottom: A huge histiocytic cell with nuclear atypia and abundant cytoplasm, which phagocytose erythroblast, erythrocyte, and platelets.

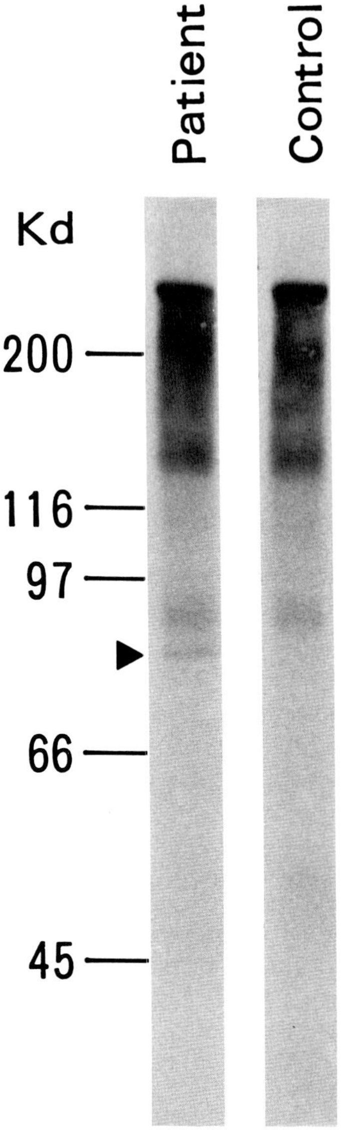

Fig. 2. Western blot analysis showing an autoantibody against platelet protein. An ~88 kd molecule (arrowhead) was recognized in the patient's serum. Among several nonspecific bands, the broad band around 200 kd appears to be platelet-associated IgG. Twenty-five micrograms of the 1% NP40 lysate of pooled platelets was applied and run on the 7.5% SDS-PAGE under nonreduced conditions. Size-fractionated protein was transferred onto the nitrocellulose membrane. The membrane was incubated with 100-fold diluted patient's or control serum and developed with the ABC peroxidase system.

nia, and Western blot analysis revealed that the patient's serum recognized one specific molecule of platelet proteins, the molecular weight of which was comparable to that of GPIV or GPV [9]. A single band of similar molecular weight was also observed under reduced conditions (data not shown). A cursory review of the literature revealed that this is the first MH case in whom it was shown that the serum contained an autoantibody against the platelet protein. Although it should be determined whether this autoantigen was derived from surface or cytoplasmic proteins, the fact that the unique hematological abnormality was thrombocytopenia suggests surface derivation of this autoantigen; thus the proliferating neoplastic histiocyte rapidly cleared the opsonized platelets from the peripheral blood.

It is not likely that the ~88 kd molecule is a platelet-specific alloantigen, because the patient was an adult man with no history of transfusion with blood products. While GPIIb-IIIa complex and GPIb are the most common autoantigens found in patients with chronic idiopathic thrombocytopenic purpura [10–17], autoantibody against GPV has also been reported, especially in patients with acute syndrome [18,19]. GPIV is the receptor for thrombospondin, the binding of which is inhibited by OKM5 monoclonal antibody (MoAb), and GPV is a thrombin substrate [20–22].

Is the presence of autoantibody against platelet-associated protein in this patient coincidence? One possibility is the cross-reactivity of antibody against virus-associated antigen. However, the patient did not have any prodromal episode, and there was no significant elevation of titer of antibodies against viruses examined so far. Another explanation is that the appearance of autoantibody was the result of thrombophagocytosis. With phagocytosis of platelets, incompletely digested and probably denatured protein components were shed from neoplastic cells and sensitized lymphocytes to produce autoantibody. However, the clinical course was fulminant, and thrombocytopenia is presumed to have occurred only shortly before the admission. It is attractive, but might be unjustified, to assume that the whole course of humoral immune response was completed in such a short period. The third possibility is that the defective immunosurveillance system of this patient permitted a forbidden clone to regenerate as well as allowing the proliferation of malignant histiocytes. Regardless of speculations on the etiology, the presence of autoantibody against platelet-associated protein was the likely cause of the patient's severe thrombocytopenia.

ACKNOWLEDGMENTS

We thank Dr. T. Kanoh (First division, Department of Internal Medicine, Faculty of Medicine, Kyoto University) for his critical reading of the manuscript and Dr. Y. Tani (DAKO Japan, Kyoto) for technical assistance.

REFERENCES

1. Scott RB, Robb-Smith AHT: Histiocytic medullary reticulosis. Lancet ii:194, 1939.
2. Byrne GE, Rappaport H: Malignant histiocytosis. In: "Malignant Disease of the Hematopoietic System." Gann Monograph on Cancer Research, Vol 15. Tokyo: University of Tokyo Press, 1973, p 145.
3. Sonneveld P, van Lom K, Kappers-Klunne M, Prins MEF, Abels J: Clinicopathological diagnosis and treatment of malignant histiocytosis. Br J Haematol 75:511, 1990.
4. Willcox DRC: Haemolytic anaemia and reticuloses. Br Med J 1:1322, 1952.
5. Kalderon AE: Histiocytic medullary reticulosis associated with cytomegalic inclusion disease. A case report. Cancer 27:659, 1971.
6. Wilson MS, Weiss LM, Gatter KC, Mason DY, Dorfman RF, Path FRC, Warnke RA: Malignant histiocytosis. A reassessment of cases previously reported in 1975 based on paraffin section immunophenotyping studies. Cancer 66:530, 1990.
7. Ohno T, Kanoh T, Arita Y, Fujii H, Kuribayashi K, Masuda T, Horiguchi Y, Taniwaki M, Nosaka T, Hatanaka M, Uchino H: Fulminant clonal expansion of large granular lymphocytes. Characterization of their morphology, phenotype, genotype, and function. Cancer 62: 1918, 1988.
8. Sugiyama T, Okuma M, Ushikubi F, Sensaki S, Kanaji K, Uchino H: A novel platelet aggregating factor found in a patient with defective collagen-induced platelet aggregation and autoimmune thrombocytopenia. Blood 69:1712, 1987.
9. Fitzgerald LA, Phillips DR: Structure and Function of Platelet Membrane Glycoproteins. In Kunicki TJ, George JN (eds): "Platelet Immunology." Philadelphia: JB Lippincott, 1989, p 9.
10. van Leeuwen EF, van der Ven JThM, Engelfriet CP, von dem Borne AEGKr: Specificity of autoantibodies in autoimmune thrombocytopenia. Blood. 59:23, 1982.
11. Varon D, Karpatkin S: A monoclonal anti-platelet antibody with decreased reactivity for autoimmune thrombocytopenic platelets. Proc Natl Acad Sci USA 80:6992, 1983.
12. Beardsley DJS, Spiegel JE, Jacobs MM, Hamdin RI, Lux SE: Platelet membrane glycoprotein IIIa contains target antigens that bind antiplatelet antibodies in immune thrombocytopenias. J Clin Invest 74: 1701, 1984.
13. Woods VL, Kurata Y, Montgomery RR, Tani P, Mason D, Oh EH, McMillan R: Autoantibodies against platelet glycoprotein Ib in patients with chronic immune thrombocytopenic purpura. Blood 64:156, 1984.
14. Woods VLJr, Oh EH, Mason D, McMillan R: Autoantibodies against the platelet glycoprotein IIb/IIIa complex in patients with chronic idiopathic thrombocytopenic purpura. Blood 63:368, 1984.
15. Szatkowski NS, Kunicki TJ, Aster RH: Identification of glycoprotein Ib as a target for autoantibody in idiopathic (autoimmune) thrombocytopenic purpura. Blood 67:310, 1986.
16. Nugent DJ: Identification of antiplatelet antibody idiotypes associated with glycoprotein Ib specificity, present in ITP plasma and produced by human hybridomas from ITP spleen cell fusions. Thromb Haemostas 58a:531, 1987.
17. Tomiyama Y, Kurata Y, Mizutani H, Kanakura Y, Tsukakio T, Yonezawa T, Tarui S: Platelet glycoprotein IIb as a target antigen in two patients with chronic idiopathic thrombocytopenic purpura. Br J Haematol 66:535, 1987.
18. Beardsley DJS, Ho J, Beyer EC: Varicella associated thrombocytopenia: Antibodies against an 85kD thrombin sensitive protein (?GPV). Blood 66:1030a, 1985.
19. Stricker RB, Koerper MA, Bussel J, Shuman MA: Target platelet antigens in childhood immune thrombocytopenic purpura. Blood 68: 118A, 1986.
20. Fitzgerald LA, Phillips DR: Platelet membrane glycoproteins. In Colman RW, Hirsh J, Marder VJ, Salzman EW (eds): "Hemostasis and Thrombosis: Basic Principles and Clinical Practice," 2nd ed. Philadelphia; JB Lippincott, 1987, p 572.
21. Asch AS, Barnwell J, Silverstein RL, Nachman RL: Isolation of the thrombospondin membrane receptor. J Clin Invest 79:1054, 1987.
22. George JN: The role of membrane glycoproteins in platelet function. Transfusion Med Rev 1:34, 1987.

American Journal of Hematology 45:248–251 (1994)

α-Interferon Treatment for Idiopathic Hypereosinophilic Syndrome

Paula L. Bockenstedt, John T. Santinga, and Steven F. Bolling

Divisions of Hematology/Oncology (P.L.B.) and Geriatrics (J.T.S.), Department of Internal Medicine, and Department of Thoracic Surgery (S.F.B.), University of Michigan Medical Center and Ann Arbor VA Medical Center, Ann Arbor

Idiopathic hypereosinophilic syndrome (HES) is a poorly understood disorder characterized by a markedly elevated peripheral blood eosinophil count in the absence of known associated causes of hypereosinophilia. Idiopathic hypereosinophilic syndrome is associated with eosinophil-induced organ damage, including endomyocardial and pulmonary fibrosis, stroke, and gastrointestinal disease. Treatment of idiopathic HES is centered on the reduction of peripheral circulating eosinophils in an effort to diminish tissue infiltration and destruction. Multiple cytotoxic agents have been tried, with variable results. Prednisone and hydroxyurea have remained the therapies of choice in long term treatment of idiopathic HES. We report here the successful 2 year treatment of aggressive idiopathic HES, refractory to hyroxyurea and prednisone, with α-interferon.

Key words: α-interferon, idiopathic hypereosinophilic syndrome, Loeffler's syndrome

INTRODUCTION

Idiopathic hypereosinophilic syndrome (HES) is a serious, often fatal disorder characterized by a markedly elevated blood eosinophil count and evidence of eosinophil induced peripheral end-organ damage involving the heart, lungs, gastrointestinal tract, and central nervous system [1–3]. The etiology of idiopathic HES is unknown. Eosinophilia occurs in response to certain parasitic infestations such as with *Toxocara canis, Trichinella spirella,* or *Ascaris* [4]. Autoimmune disorders such as eosinophilic fasciitis, vasculitis, and the L-tryptophan syndrome may display variable degrees of peripheral blood eosinophilia [5]. The most striking eosinophilia is encountered in idiopathic hyperesoinophilic syndrome and with malignancy, such as in acute lymphocytic leukemia [6,7], lung cancer [8], eosinophilic leukemia [9], and myeloproliferative disorders [10].

Treatment of idiopathic HES is centered on the reduction of total circulating eosinophils in an effort to diminish tissue infiltration and damage by eosinophil-derived basic and acidic proteins. Several different therapies have been reported for HES, including steroids [2], hydroxyurea [1], vincristine [11], etoposide [12], and 6-mercaptopurine [13] as well as other antitumor agents. With each of these cytotoxic agents, there has generally been a reduction in clinical symptoms in association with reduction of total eosinophil count. In some instances, however, the disease process has become refractory to the cytotoxic agent, or, due to bone marrow suppression, an alternate therapeutic regimen has been required. Three recent reports have described the successful use of α-interferon for the treatment of HES refractory to steroids and hydroxyurea [1]. We report a case of aggressive idiopathic HES treated successfully for 2 years with α-interferon.

CASE REPORT

The patient is a 28-year-old male fruit farmer who presented in August, 1989, with abdominal pain, nausea, and vomiting most pronounced after ingestion of alcohol. He had a 3 month history of easy fatiguability and 10 pound weight loss but no fever, night sweats, pruritus, or musculoskeletal complaints. There was no history of L-tryptophan exposure.

Received for publication March 8, 1993; accepted July 20, 1993.

Address reprint requests to Paula L. Bockenstedt, MD, University of Michigan Medical Center, Simpson Memorial Building, 102 Observatory, Ann Arbor, MI 48109-0724.

On physical examination, vital signs were normal, and the patient was afebrile. The chest was clear to auscultation, and there were no cardiac murmurs. The liver was normal in span, and the spleen was not palpable. There was no pedal edema or skin rash. Neurological examination was normal.

Laboratory studies revealed mild anemia with an hematocrit (Hct) 38.5% and normal red blood cell indices. His white blood count (WBC) was 16,400/mm^3, with 60% eosinophils, 19% polymorphonuclear leukocytes, 5% bands, 13% lymphocytes, 2% metamyelocytes, and 1% myelocytes. PT and PTT were normal. Liver function tests, uric acid, creatinine, and BUN were all normal, with the exception of an LDH of 362. Sedimentation rate, rheumatoid factor, antineutrophil antibodies, and leukocyte alkaline phosphatase were all normal. Stool parasite examination was negative, as were serologic tests for *Toxocara, Strongyloides, Trichinella,* and *Ascaris*. Bone marrow aspirate and biopsy showed a hypercellular marrow with increased numbers of granulocytic precursors consisting of predominantly eosinophilic myelocytes, bands, and mature eosinophils. Bone marrow cytogentic studies were negative, using both conventional techniques and polymerase chain reaction (PCR) studies for the bcr/abl locus. Small bowel biopsy showed infiltration of eosinophils, plasma cells, and occasional lymphocytes in the lamina propria throughout the jejunum and proximal ileum, gradually decreasing toward the terminal ileum. Allergy testing was negative, and serum IgE level was normal. Chest X-ray, EKG, echocardiogram, and abdominal CT scan were all normal.

He was treated with prednisone 60 mg/day, with marked decrease in peripheral eosinophilia and improvement in platelet count. Three months later however, his WBC became increasingly difficult to control and hydroxyurea was added. In January, 1990, he developed bilateral hilar adenopathy, splenomegaly, and intraabdominal lymphadenopathy and underwent splenectomy and nodal biopsy in evaluation of possible lymphoma. Pathological specimens did not reveal any evidence of lymphoma or myeloproliferative disease at that time. Following surgery, there was a transient decrease in peripheral WBC and eosinophilia. Peripheral blood counts, chest X-ray, EKG, and echocardiogram were obtained every 3 months. One year later, despite escalating doses of hydroxyurea and steroids, the total peripheral WBC and eosinophils remained elevated, with a cyclical rise in total eosinophil count and prominent drop in platelet count every 6–8 weeks. Following an episode of transient monocular blindness with evidence of a retinal microembolus on flourescein examination, a grade four holosystolic murmur was noted, and the patient was found to have fulminant mitral regurgitation.

Cardiac catheterization revealed a mean right atrial pressure of 9 mm Hg, right ventricular pressure of 58/12 mm Hg, pulmonary artery pressure of 58/25 mm Hg (mean 39), pulmonary capillary wedge pressure of 29 mm Hg, and cardiac output of 13.5 liters/min by thermal dilution. Transesophageal echocardiography demonstrated 4+ mitral regurgitation, with reversal of flow in the pulmonary veins. There was only moderate enlargement of the left atrium, indicating that this was a fairly acute process. Left ventricular function was well maintained. The patient underwent emergency mitral valve replacement. On inspection of the mitral valve, the posterior leaflet was noted to be completely destroyed, with no identifiable posterior annulus, leaflet, or chordal structures. The anterior leaflet was much less affected. The papillary muscles were intact but appeared to be fused into a large mass of fibrotic granular debris, which on pathology was shown to be a leaflet infiltrated with eosinophils. The left ventricular cavity did not have a marked fibrotic response. A porcine mitral valve was placed using pledgeted 2-0 Ethibond sutures.

Repeat bone marrow biopsy again showed marked eosinophilia, with granulocytic hyperplasia consistent with, but not diagnostic of, a myeloproliferative etiology. Bone marrow and peripheral blood cytogenetics were normal. He was then cross-matched for potential bone marrow transplantation and was begun on α-interferon 6 million units 3 times per week. Within 6 weeks, the widely fluctuating granulocytosis and eosinophilia were controlled and by 2 months, the patient noted clinical improvement (see Fig. 1A, B.) The dose of interferon was reduced to 3 million units three times per week because of increased fatiguability 6 months later. The patient has since been clinically stable and fully functional. His WBC is 8,500/mm^3, with 50% polymorphonuclear leukocytes, 3% bands, 10% eosinophils, 10% monocytes, and 27% lymphocytes. His platelet count and hemoglobin are normal. Serial EKGs, echo, MUGA, and pulmonary function tests have shown no evidence of progression of cardiac or pulmonary disease for 23 months since the institution of interferon treatment. The patient has two HLA-matched siblings available as bone marrow transplant donors but declines transplant at this time.

DISCUSSION

The treatment of idiopathic HES has, until recently, been highly individual and largely directed at controlling end-organ damage. When hypereosinophilia is associated with acute lymphocytic leukemia or Philadelphia chromosome-positive myeloproliferative disease, therapy may be appropriately aggressively directed to the primary bone marrow malignancy. Often, as in this case, although a myeloproliferative disorder is suspected, there is no clear evidence of malignancy and treatment is dictated by peripheral blood eosinophilia and extent of clinical symptoms. In some cases HES leads a more aggres-

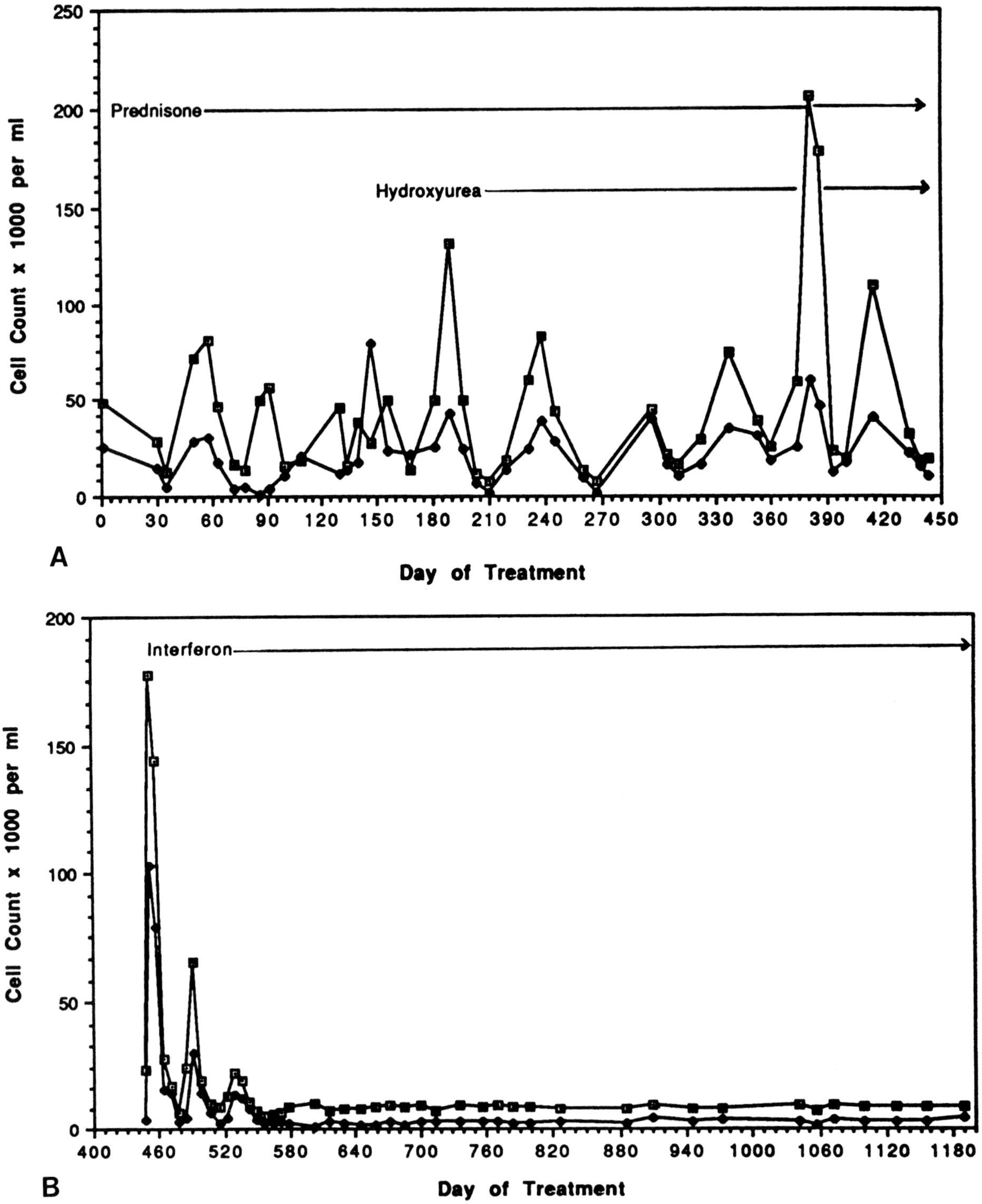

Fig. 1. Response of total peripheral white blood count (open squares) and eosinophil count (solid squares) to hydroxyurea and prednisone (A) **and alpha interferon** (B).

sive course and fails to respond to hydroxyurea or prednisone, subsequently requiring a more cytotoxic therapy. The prognosis in untreated hypereosinophilic syndrome is poor, with a 9 month median survival. With therapy designed to control peripheral eosinophilia, an improved survival can be expected [1].

The majority of deaths in idiopathic HES are due to intractable congestive heart failure. Progressive subendocardial fibrosis with thrombosis formation occurs, leading to a restrictive cardiomyopathy and valvular disease [14]. Cardiac disease may develop fulminantly, as in this patient, when the peripheral eosinophilia is poorly controlled. However, progression of cardiac disease has been documented despite well controlled eosinophil levels [15]. Selection of the valvular prosthesis poses a difficult problem in patients with HES, most of whom present at a young age and with small left ventricular cavities due to endomyocardial fibrosis. Furthermore, valve replacement in HES has been complicated by thrombosis and ongoing fibrosis in and around the prosthesis [14–17], requiring anticoagulation with warfarin [18]. Since this patient had severe thrombocytopenia associated with HES, a contraindication to anticoagulation, a porcine bioprosthesis was selected. The rapid control of peripheral eosinophilia with interferon may have played a role in avoiding valvular thrombosis.

Since both α and γ-interferon are potent activators of eosinophil cytotoxicity in previously stimulated eosinophils in culture [2,18,19], an adverse acceleration of eosinophil-mediated tissue damage may, in theory, be possible when interferon is used in treatment of HES. The 25 month follow-up of interferon treatment for nearly fatal idiopathic HES in this patient does not demonstrate any progression of cardiac or pulmonary disease, suggesting that α-interferon does not promote increased eosinophil cytotoxic activity in this disease.

To date, this patient demonstrates the longest reported response to interferon in idiopathic HES, bringing the number of successfully treated cases to five [20–23]. α-Interferon should be considered for patients who do not respond to hydroxyurea and prednisone with a reduction in peripheral blood eosinophilia and merits further investigation in larger clinical studies of the long term management of idiopathic hypereosinophilic syndrome.

REFERENCES

1. Parrillo JE, Fauci AS, Wolff SM: Therapy of the hypereosinophilic syndrome. Ann Intern Med 89:167, 1978.
2. Spry CJ: The hypereosinophilic syndrome: Clinical features, laboratory findings and treatment. Allergy 37:539, 1982.
3. Alfaham MA, Ferguson SD, Sihra B, Davies J: The idiopathic hypereosinophilic syndrome. Arch Dis Child 62:601, 1987.
4. Beaver PC, Danaraj TS: Pulmonary ascariasis resembling eosinophilic lung. Am J Trop Med Hygiene 7:100, 1958.
5. Winkelmann RK, Connolly SM, Quimby SR, Griffing LW, Lie JT: Histopathologic features of the L-tryptophan-related eosinophilia-myalgia (fasciitis) syndrome. Mayo Clin Proc 66:457, 1991.
6. Baumgarten E, Wegner RD, Fengler R, et al: Calla-positive acute leukaemia with t(5q;14q) translocation and hypereosinophilia-A unique entity? Acta Haematol 82:85, 1989.
7. Troxell ML, Mills GM, Allen RC: The hypereosinophilic syndrome in acute lymphocytic leukemia. Cancer 54:1058, 1984.
8. Goffman TE, Mulvihill JJ, Carney DN, Triche TJ, Whang-Peng J: Fatal hypereosinophilia with chromosome 15q− in a patient with multiple primary and familial neoplasms. Cancer Genet Cytogenet 8:197, 1983.
9. Flannery EP, Dillon DE, Freeman MVR, et al.: Eosinophilic leukemia with fibrosing endocarditis and short Y chromosome. Ann Intern Med 77:223, 1972.
10. Mitter NS, Weiskopf RW: Unusual chromosome 7 aberrations in a case of eosinophilic myeloproliferative syndrome. Cancer Genet Cytogenet 26:209, 1987.
11. Cofrancesco E, Cortellaro M, Pogliani E, et al.: Response to vincristine treatment in a case of idiopathic hypereosinophilic syndrome with multiple clinical manifestations. Acta Haematol 72:21, 1984.
12. Smit AJ, van Essen LH, de Vries EGE: Successful long-term control of idiopathic hypereosinophilic syndrome with etoposide. Cancer 67: 2826, 1991.
13. Marshall GM, White L: Effective therapy for a severe case of the idiopathic hypereosinophilic syndrome. Am J Pediatric Hematol Oncol 11:178, 1989.
14. Roberts WC, Liegler DG, Carbone PP: Endomyocardial disease and eosinophilia. Am J Med 46:28, 1969.
15. Hendren WG, Jones EL, Smith MD: Aortic and mitral valve replacement in idiopathic hypereosinophilic syndrome. Ann Thorac Surg 46: 570, 1988.
16. Blake DP, Palmer TE, Olinger GN: Mitral valve replacement in idiopathic hypereosinophilic syndrome. J Thorac Cardiovasc Surg 89:630, 1985.
17. Boustany CW, Murphy GW, Hicks GL: Mitral valve replacement in idiopathic hypereosinophilic syndrome. Ann Thorac Surg 51:1007, 1991.
18. Harley JB, McIntosh CL, Kirklin JJW, et al.: Atrioventricular valve replacement in the idiopathic hypereosinophilic syndrome. Am J Med 73:77, 1982.
19. Valerius T, Repp R, Kalden JR, Platzer E: Effects of IFN on human eosinophils in comparison with other cytokines. J Immunol 145:2950, 1990.
20. Busch FW, Schmidt H, Steinke B: Alpha-interferon for the hypereosinophilia syndrome. Ann Intern Med 114:338, 1991.
21. Zielinski RM, Lawrence WD: Interferon-α hypereosinophilia syndrome. Ann Intern Med 113:716, 1990.
22. Van Den Anker-Lugtenburg PJ, Van't Veer MB: Alpha-interferon in a case of hypereosinophilic syndrome. Br J Haematol 76:258, 1990.
23. Murphy PT, Fennelly DF, Stuart M, O'Donnell JR: Alfa-interferon in a case of hypereosinophilic syndrome. Br J Haematol 75:619, 1990.

American Journal of Hematology 45:252–257 (1994)

Pentosan Polysulfate-Induced Thrombocytopenia and Thrombosis

Brigitte Tardy-Poncet, Bernard Tardy, Françoise Grelac, Jacqueline Reynaud, Patrick Mismetti, Jean Claude Bertrand, and Denis Guyotat

Department of Hematology, CHU Hopital Nord, Saint-Etienne, France (B.T.-P., J.R., D.G.); Departments of Intensive Care (B.T., J.C.B.) and Clinical Pharmacology (P.M.), CHU Hopital Bellevue, Saint-Etienne, France; INSERM U348, Hopital Lariboisière, Paris, France (F.G.)

Pentosan polysulfate is a low-molecular-weight sulfated polysaccharide used as an antithrombotic drug. We present two patients who developed thrombocytopenia and venous thrombosis during treatment with pentosan polysulfate. The relationship between pentosan polysulfate and thrombocytopenia is supported by platelet aggregation and serotonin release tests. In the light of the literature and our two cases, it appears that pentosan polysulfate alone as standard heparin and low-molecular-weight heparin can induce thrombocytopenia and thrombosis. Platelet counts should therefore be periodically monitored during pentosan polysulfate treatment. In the case of pentosan polysulfate-induced thrombocytopenia, it seems that heparin or low-molecular-weight heparin should not be instituted during the acute phase even if platelet aggregation studies are negative, because of their low sensitivity. After remission of thrombocytopenia, whether or not glycoaminoglycans can be reinstituted, at least temporarily, after antibody had disappeared is still an open question.

Key words: pentosan polysulfate, thrombocytopenia, low-molecular-weight heparin, venous thrombosis

INTRODUCTION

Pentosan polysulfate (PPS), an analogue of heparin, is a low-molecular-weight sulfated polysaccharide [1] widely used in Europe as an antithrombotic drug. Recently PPS has proved to be a highly potent and selective inhibitor of human immunodeficiency virus type 1 replication in vitro [2–5]; therefore, several clinical trials with sulfated polysaccharides in the acquired immunodeficiency syndrome are underway. Furthermore, in the last few years, some cases of thrombocytopenia occurring during PPS treatment and mimicking the heparin-induced thrombocytopenia syndrome (HIT) have been reported, especially in the French literature. We describe two patients who developed thrombocytopenia with venous thrombosis 10–11 days after PPS treatment alone. In both cases the relationship between PPS and thrombocytopenia is supported by platelet aggregation and [^{14}C]serotonin release tests.

CASE REPORTS

Case 1

In August, 1991, a 50-year-old woman complained of blurred vision of the left eye. She had never been seriously ill before and was taking oral ethinyl estradiol for postmenopausal syndrome. Fluorescein angiography established the diagnosis of retinal venous thrombosis and ethinyl estradiol treatment was stopped. On November 1, 1991, the patient complained of persistence of visual disturbance and received intramuscular PPS, 200 mg/day for 10 days. Because of acute headache with vertigo, she was admitted to hospital on November 12, 1991. Examination revealed intracranial hypertension with left cerebellar incoordination and slight right hemiparesis. Brain CT scan showed an empty delta sign on the enhanced CT films, and cerebral angiography disclosed thrombosis of the superior sagittal sinus. The white-cell count was 8×10^9/liter, with a normal differential count. Platelet

Received for publication February 9, 1993; accepted August 18, 1993.

This work was presented in part at the 12th International Congress on Thrombosis (Florence, May 18–23, 1992). An abstract was published in *Thrombosis Research* [GS (Suppl 1):S115, 1992)].

Address reprint requests to Brigitte Tardy-Poncet, Department of Hematology, CHU Hopital Nord, Saint-Etienne, 42055 France.

count was 44 × 10^9/liter, with normal coagulation study results. Bone marrow examinations showed many megakaryocytes, indicating peripheral destruction. Heparinoid-induced thrombocytopenia was suspected, and consequently PPS treatment was stopped and acenocoumarol started. Four days later, platelet count increased to 176 × 10^9/liter. No infectious, neoplasic, or autoimmune diseases were found. Her subsequent course was uncomplicated, and the patient was discharged on November 29, 1991, with a platelet count of 236 × 10^9/liter and a stabilized dose of acenocoumarol (international normalized ratio 2.5).

Case 2

On November 18, 1991, an 86-year-old woman complained of posttraumatic left calf pain, and intramuscular PPS, 100 mg twice per day, was initiated for 11 days. Her history included hypertension and diabetes mellitus, and her treatment was lisinopril 5 mg/day and glicazide 8 mg/day. On December 2, 1991, she was admitted with progressive dyspnea and pleuretic chest pain. On examination she had tachypnoae at rest, tachycardia (120 bpm), with a blood pressure of 140/90 mm Hg, a loud pulmonary second sound, and high jugular venous pressure. Her PO_2 was 59 mm Hg on air, chest radiography was unremarkable, and the electrocardiogram showed right heart strain. A ventilation perfusion scan showed multiple bilateral defects, with normal ventilation, and venography revealed a left femoral vein thrombosis. Platelet count was 66 × 10^9/liter, with normal coagulation studies. Heparinoid-induced thrombocytopenia was suspected, so a vena cava filter (Greenfield filter) was placed and coumarin started. Five days later the platelet count increased to 156 × 10^9/liter. On December 17, 1991, the patient was discharged in good health, with a stable platelet count of 264 × 10^9/liter and stable coumarin dose (international normalized ratio 2).

MATERIALS AND METHODS

Materials

The following materials were used: standard heparin (calciparin; Choay Laboratories), PPS (hemoclar; Clin-Midy Laboratories), PK 10169 (Lovenox; Pharmuka Laboratories). 5-Hydroxy ^{14}C tryptamine (2,1 GBq/mmole) was purchased from Amersham Laboratories.

Preparation of Plasma

Plasma samples were obtained from healthy, nonthrombocytopenic individuals who had not taken any medication during the previous 10 days. For the platelet aggregometry assay (PPA), whole blood was collected on 0.1 vol of 110 mM trisodium citrate (9:1, vol:vol) and for the serotonin release test (SRT) on 0.1 vol of acide-citrate-dextrose (13 mM citric acid, 12,4 mM trisodium citrate, 11 mM glucose) (9:1, vol:vol). The platelet-rich plasma (PRP) was obtained from controls by centrifugation for 15 min at 100*g*. Platelet-poor plasma (PPP) was obtained from controls and patients by collecting blood into citrate anticoagulant, which was then centrifuged for 15 min at 1,000*g*. For some experiments, the PPP was used immediately for the PAA, while, for others, aliquots were stored at −80°C in view of the SRT.

Aggregation Studies

Aggregation studies were carried out on mixtures of patient's PPP (200 μl) and normal PRP (200 μl). Aggregation was monitored (Labintec aggregometer) for 15 min following the addition of each tested drug (10 μl). Saline- and arachidonic acid-induced aggregations were used as controls (of spontaneous aggregation and platelet function, respectively, on PPP-PRP mixtures). Results were expressed as percentage of aggregation: drug induced aggregation (%) and spontaneous (saline) aggregation (%). A positive result was defined as >20% [6]. PPS, heparin, and enoxaparin were tested at final concentrations of 10 g/ml, 1 IU/ml, and 1 IU/ml, respectively.

Serotonin Release Test (SRT)

The SRT was carried out as described for heparin [7], with minor modifications. PRP was labeled with [^{14}C]serotonin at a concentration of 0.5 μCi/10 ml of PRP, for 30 mn at room temperature. Platelets were washed once and resuspended in the reaction buffer. The final platelet count was adjusted to 300,000/μl. Twenty microliters of patient or control plasma was added to 75 μl [^{14}C]serotonin labeled platelets and mixed with 5 μl buffer or of one of two PPS concentrations (10 μg/ml or 5,000 μg/ml). The platelet suspension was gently mixed for 60 min at 22°C, at which time 100 μl 0.5% w/v EDTA in saline was added. Platelets were centrifuged for 5 min at 1,500*g* and 50 μl of the supernatant fluid was removed and counted in a liquid scintillation counter. All tests were expressed as the mean of a triplicate determination. Platelet release of serotonin was reported as a percentage of the total platelet radioactivity after correction for background radioactivity [8]. A positive test for PPS-induced thrombocytopenia has been defined as >20% release at 10 μl/ml PPS and <20% release at 5,000 μl/ml PPS. Positive controls included platelet serotonin release caused by thrombi alone at a final concentration of 0.02 U/ml. The absence of serotonin release by platelets in the presence of PPS alone was controlled. For the two patients, the SRT was performed on the sera collected during admission and also on the sera collected 4 and 5 months later, while the patients were nonthrombocytopenic and receiving only acenocoumarol treatment.

TABLE I. Effects of Patients Plasma on Platelet Aggregation and on Serotonin Release*

	Aggregation studies (lag time) (%)			Serotonine release test (%)		
	PPS (10 μg/ml)	Heparin (1U/ml)	PK 10169 (1 anti Xa U/ml)	PPS (10 μg/ml)	PPS (5000 μg/ml)	Saline buffer
Patient 1						
On admission	85 (3.30 min)	60 (9 min)	70 (11 min)	73	3	3
5 Months later	ND	ND	ND	2	2	2
Patient 2						
On admission	75 (4.30 min)	70 (10.30 min)	60 (9.30 min)	69	5	76
4 Months later	ND	ND	ND	2	2	2
Control				3	3	2

*PPS, pentosane polysulfate; ND, not done.

RESULTS

As expected, there was no spontaneous aggregation on the normal PRP-patient PPP mixtures. As is shown in Table I, the addition of PPS to the plasma obtained in the thrombocytopenic period from both patients induced strong platelet aggregation with a short lag time. Addition of standard heparin and of low-molecular-weight heparin (LMWH; enoxaparin) similarly induced platelet aggregation with both patient's plasma. During the thrombocytopenic period, the patients' plasma had PPS-dependent platelet serotonin release at pharmacological concentrations (10 μg/ml final) but not at high PPS concentration (5000 μg/ml final; Table I). For case 2, while there was no spontaneous aggregation, we noted a spontaneous serotonin release, which was inhibited by high concentrations of PPS. For the two patients, 4 and 5 weeks after PPS withdrawal, we noted the disappearance of the heparin-dependent antibody, as is commonly described.

DISCUSSION

Both patients in this study could be considered to have thrombocytopenia and thrombosis induced by PPS alone, since they fulfilled the following criteria: development of thrombocytopenia during PPS administration, exclusion of other causes of thrombocytopenia, and remission of thrombocytopenia after PPS withdrawal. These clinical criteria are similar to those currently used for the diagnosis of HIT [7]. This diagnosis is further supported by the positive results of aggregation studies with a cross-reaction between PPS, standard heparin, and LMWH. However the sensitivity and the specificity of this test are low [9]. In contrast, the serotonin release test is highly sensitive and specific [7]. It has been demonstrated that patients with heparin-induced thrombocytopenia have a unimodal curve of platelet release: Low concentrations of heparin trigger the release reaction, whereas high concentrations of heparin do not. This type of reaction is typical of immune complex binding to an Fc receptor, the complex being disrupted by the addition of increasing concentrations of antigen. The sensitivity of the serotonin release test is high because serotonin release is a more sensitive indicator of platelet activation than platelet aggregation. This test is also high specific (99%): Potential false-positive factors (antiplatelet autoantibodies, non-heparin-containing immune complexes) can be recognized because they result in platelet activation at both heparin concentrations [10]. Using a similar technique, we obtained in our case 1 the same results: [^{14}C]serotonin release occurred at low concentrations of PPS, and very high concentration of PPS inhibited the release reaction. For case 2, while the reaction was inhibited by high doses of PPS, [^{14}C]serotonin release was observed in the absence of added PPS. This has already been described for patients with HIT receiving heparin at the time the test was performed [7]. For case 2, the plasma was obtained 3 days after PPS withdrawal. This suggests the presence of small amounts of residual PPS or the presence of inactive antigenic PPS although no anti-X activity was detected using a chromogenic assay.

To our knowledge, there have been 25 case reports of thrombocytopenia in which the role of PPS has been discussed [11–24]. These 25 case reports can be separated into three different groups. In group 1, consisting of eight patients [11–17], the platelet count was normal during PPS treatment and thrombocytopenia occurred only during heparin relay after PPS withdrawal. For all these patients, heparin was introduced because of the occurrence of thrombotic events despite treatment or prophylaxis with PPS. For four patients [11,13,14,16], extensive or recurrent thrombosis was also observed during heparin treatment. Platelet aggregation studies, performed for all but one patient, were always positive in the presence of PPS. Positive cross-reaction between PPS and standard heparin was found in all cases and between PPS and LMWH in five cases [12–14,17]. The study of this group of patients indicates that PPS could be a factor of sensitization of heparin induced thrombocytopenia. In group 2, consisting of seven patients (Table II), throm

TABLE II. PPS Alone Induced Thrombocytopenia and Thrombosis*

		PPS				
No. [ref]	Age/sex	Indication	Route and dose (mg/24 hr)	Duration (days)	Platelet count (×10⁹/liter)	Complicating events
1	66/?	SVT	IM/100	10	<60	Myocardial infarct; death
2 [18]	70/?	SVT	IM/100	8	<60	Arterial thrombosis; death
3 [19]	73/F	Prophylaxis	IM/100	9	30	None
4 [20]	?/F	Prophylaxis	SC/100 and then	5		
			0/300 and then	15	33	Cutaneous hematoma
			SC/100	3		
5	66/F	SVT	IM/100	10	35	Myocardial infarct; PE; death
6 [15]	64/F	Vertigo	IM/50	8	41	Myocardial infarct; death
7 [17]	65/F	Prophylaxis	?/100	16	20	None

*SVT, superficial venous thrombosis; DVT, deep vein thrombosis; PE, pulmonary embolism; PPS, pentosane polysulfate; IM, intramuscular; SC, subcutaneous; O, oral.

TABLE III. Thrombocytopenia Occurring During PPS Treatment and Persisting During Heparin Relay*

		PPS			Heparin		
No. [ref]	Age/sex	Indication	Duration (days)	Complicating events	Route and dose (×10³ U/24 hr)	Duration (days)	Complicating events
1 [11]	67/F	Prophylaxis	21	Arterial thrombosis	IV/30	?	Three recurrent arterial thrombosis
2	60/F	SVT	8	PE	LMWH SC/5440UIAXA	>16	None after 8 days
3 [21]	48/F	SVT	8	Cerebral infarct	LMWH SC/5440UIAXA	6	PE, renal arterial thrombosis, sylvian arterial thrombosis; death
4 [22]	57/M	DVT	18	Arterial thrombosis	IV/40 and then	8	Two recurrent arterial thrombosis
					LMWH/?	2	One recurrent arterial thrombosis
5 [19]	52/F	Prophylaxis	8	Arterial thrombosis	IV/40	3	Progression of thrombosis
6 [23]	63/F	DVT	9	Myocardia infarct	IV/60	2	None
7 [15]	79/F	SVT	10	Myocardial infarct	IV/?	1	Cerebral infarct
8	50/F	Prophylaxis	8	Arterial thrombosis	?/10	2	Recurrent arterial thrombosis
9 [17]	50/F	SVT	10	Arterial thrombosis	?/25 and then	2	Recurrent arterial thrombosis
					LMWH ?/?	5	None
10 [24]	53/F	SVT	9	Myocardial infarct	SC/22	23	Extensive myocardial infarct biventricular thrombosis

*SVT, superficial venous thrombosis ; DVT, deep vein thrombosis; PE, pulmonary embolism; SC, subcutaneous; IV, intravenous; LMWH, low-molecular-weight heparin; PPS, pentosane polysulfate.

bocytopenia $<100 \times 10^9$/liter occurred during PPS treatment alone. In all cases in which thrombocytopenia was associated with thrombotic complications, death occurred (cases 1, 2, 5, 6). In all but one case (case 2), platelet aggregation studies were positive in the presence of PPS. Positive cross-reaction between PPS and heparin and between PPS and LMWH was demonstrated in four of six serum samples tested (cases 1, 3, 5, 6) and in one of two tested (case 3), respectively. In accordance with our two patients' results, the study of these seven cases led us to conclude that PPS alone as well as heparin may induce thrombocytopenia and thrombosis. In group 3, consisting of ten patients (Table III), thrombocytopenia $<100 \times 10^9$/liter occurred during PPS treatment and persisted after PPS withdrawal and heparin institution.

Thrombocytopenia was associated with thrombotic complications in all patients during PPS treatment. In these cases, the diagnosis of PPS-induced thrombocytopenia was not evoced, and, despite a platelet count $<100 \times 10^9$/liter, heparin was introduced as treatment for thrombosis. Extensive, recurrent thrombosis and thrombosis at other sites occurred in eight patients during heparin relay (cases 1, 3–5, 7–10). Whenever platelet aggregation in the presence of PPS was realized, the reaction was positive (cases 2, 3, 5–9). In the presence of heparin, the reaction was positive in six cases (cases 4–8,

10) and negative in two cases (cases 3, 9). In the presence of LMWH, the reaction was positive in three cases (cases 4, 5, 10) and negative in two cases (cases 2, 9). The evolution of thrombocytopenia and the recurrence of thrombosis led us to conclude that the immunologic cross-reactivity between PPS, heparin, and LMWH is not only an in vitro reaction but also an in vivo reaction and that heparin and LMWH are certainly not appropriate treatments for PPS-induced thrombocytopenia.

In light of our two cases and of the literature, it appears that PPS alone can induce thrombocytopenia and thrombosis as well as standard heparin and LMWH [25]. As well as heparin, PPS may induce thrombocytopenia whatever the route of administration (intramuscular or subcutaneous) or the dose (prophylactic or curative) may be. As in HIT syndrome, thrombocytopenia begins between 5 and 21 days after PPS institution, and the platelet count usually returns to baseline within 4 days of discontinuing PPS. As in HIT syndrome, the most common thrombotic events include lower limb arterial thrombosis, myocardial infarction, and lower extremity venous thrombosis, with or without thromboemboli. As in HIT syndrome, the treatment of PPS-induced thrombocytopenia is difficult, especially if ongoing antithrombotic therapy is required. However, we believe that, in light of the literature, heparin and LMWH should not be instituted during the acute phase of PPS-induced thrombocytopenia even if platelet aggregation studies are negative, because of their low sensitivity.

Finally we believe that PPS, as an antithrombotic agent, should be employed with great caution. Compared with that of standard heparin, the clinical efficacy of PPS in thromboembolic prophylaxis has never been demonstrated to be superior [26–28], and major sides effect are the same. Since PPS has been shown to exhibit significant anti-AIDS and antitumor activities in animals, clinical trials in AIDS patients using subcutaneous or continuous injection of PPS are underway [29,30]. We should alert clinicians that PPS may induce thrombocytopenia with arterial and venous thrombosis and that platelet count should be periodically monitored during PPS treatment.

ACKNOWLEDGMENTS

The authors thank Dr. S. Levy-Toledano for technical support of this work and Dr. J. Murphy for critical reading of the manuscript.

REFERENCES

1. Soria C, Soria J, Rickewaert JJ, Holmer E, Caen JP: Anticoagulant activities of a pentosane polysulphate: Comparison with standard heparin and a fraction of low molecular weight heparin. Thromb Res 19:455, 1980.
2. Mitsuya H, Looney DJ, Kuno S, Ueno R, Wong-Staal F, Broder S: Dextran sulfate suppression of viruses in the HIV family: inhibition of virion binding to $CD4^+$ cells. Science 240:646, 1988.
3. Baba M, Pauwels R, Balzarini J, Arnout J, Desmyter J, De Clercq E: Mechanism of inhibitory effect of dextran sulfate and heparin on replication of human immunodeficiency virus in vitro. Proc Natl Acad Sci USA 85:6132, 1988.
4. Baba M, Nakajima M, Schols D, Pauwels R, Balzarini J, De Clercq E: Pentosan polysulfate, a sulfated oligosaccharide, is a potent and selective anti-HIV agent in vitro. Antiviral Res 9:335, 1988.
5. Baba M, Schols D, Pauwels R, Nakajima H, De Clercq E: Sulfated polysaccharides as potent inhibitors of HIV-induced syncytium formation: A new strategy towards AIDS chemotherapy. J Acquired Immun Def Syndrome 3:493, 1990.
6. King DJ, Kelton JG: Heparin associated thrombocytopenia. Ann Intern Med 100:535, 1984.
7. Sheridan D, Carter C, Kelton JG: A diagnostic test for heparin induced thrombocytopenia. Blood 67:27, 1986.
8. Kelton JG, Sheridan D, Santos A, et al.: Heparin induced thrombocytopenia: laboratory studies. Blood 72:925, 1988.
9. Kelton JG, Sheridan D, Brain H, Powers PJ, Turpie AG, Carter CJ: Clinical usefulness of testing for a heparin-dependent platelet aggregation factor in patients with suspected heparin associated thrombocytopenia. J Lab Clin Med 103:606, 1984.
10. Warkentin TE, Kelton JG: Heparin induced thrombocytopenia. Progr Hemostas Thromb 10:1, 1991.
11. MaizaD, Derlon A, Khayat MC, Coulhon JP, Leporrier M: Rôle du polysulfate de pentosane dans le déclenchement de deux accidents thrombopéniques. Presse Med 14:1289, 1985.
12. Herpin D, Boinot C, Raynier P, Boutaud P, Amiel A: Thrombopénie lors d'un traitement séquentiel polysulfate de pentosane-héparine. Presse Med 16:309, 1987.
13. Allal J, Herpin D, Schnebert B, Elbaz C, Raynier P, Boinot C: Thrombopenias secondary to pentosane polysulfate. Ann Cardiol Angeol 36:85, 1987.
14. Paille F, Boccaccini A, De Korwin JD, et al.: Thrombopéniesous héparine de bas poids moléculaire après traitement par pentosane polysulfate. Therapie 43:322, 1988.
15. Meyer P, Couzi G, Bavle J, et al.: Disseminated coronary thrombosis and pentosane polysulfate-induced thrombocytopenia. Arch Mal Coeur 81:913, 1988.
16. Jacquin V, Salama J, Le Roux G, Delaporte P: Multiplex venous thrombosis and thrombocytopenia induced by pentosane polysulfate and impaired by heparin. Ann Med Interne 139:194, 1988.
17. Claisse JF, Andrejak M, Jarry G, Desablens B, Roussel B, Delobel J: Thrombocytopenia with or without thrombosis after pentosan polysulfate treatment. Therapie 45:514, 1990.
18. Bayle J, Chichmanian RM, Caramella A, et al.: Allergie thrombopenia with heparins or pentosane polysulfate. Therapie 41:339, 1986.
19. Follea G, Hamandjian I, Trzeciak MC, Nedey C, Striechenberger R, Dechavanne M: Pentosane polysulfate associated thrombocytopenia. Thromb Res 42:413, 1986.
20. Toque Y, Montpellier D, Roussel B, Lepointe F, Ossart M: Thrombopenie induite par le polysulfate de pentosane. Cah Anesthesiol 36: 243, 1988.
21. Bollaert PE, Laprevote-Heully MC, Maurizi M, Lambert H, Larcan A: Severe Thrombocytopaenia associated with pentosane polysulfate treatment. Ann Fr Anesth Reanim 5:539, 1986.
22. Papazian L, Alezia M, Levy G, François G: Thromboses artérielles et veineuses multiple associées à une thrombopénie: Rôle du polysulfate de pentosane et des héparines. Presse Med 15:1246, 1986.
23. Dalger J, Dussarat GV, Dumoulin M: Myocardial infarction complicating a thrombopenia induced by pentosane polysulfate. Ann Cardiol Angeol 37:191, 1988.
24. Leclerq C, De Place C, Rioux C, Mabo P, Paillard F, Daubert JC: Myocardial infarction and massive biventricular thrombosis in throm-

bocytopenia induced by pentosane polysulphate and heparin. Arch Mal Coeur 83:117, 1990.
25. Tardy B, Tardy-Poncet B, Zeni F, Comtet C, Reynaud J, Bertrand JC: Thrombocytopenia associated with low molecular weight heparin. Lancet 338:1217, 1991.
26. Joffe S: Drug prevention of postoperative deep vein thrombosis. A comparative study of calcium heparinate and sodium pentosan polysulfate. Arch Surg 111:37, 1976.
27. Bergqvist D, Efsing HO, Hallbook T, Lindblad B: Prevention of postoperative thromboembolic complications. Acta Chir Scand 146: 559, 1980.
28. Iribarnegaray M, Caudron D, Koumako J, Petit F: Etude comparative de l'emploi du polyester sulfurique de pentosane et de l'héparine calcique dans la prévention des accidents thrombo-emboliques. Artères Veines 5:51, 1986.
29. Newman ME: AIDS drug gets trial as cancer therapy. JNCI 82:1671, 1990.
30. Wellstein A, Zugmaier G, Califano III JA, Kern F, Paik S, Lippman ME: Tumor growth dependent on Kapoi's sarcoma-derived fibroblast growth factor inhibited by pentosan polysulfate. JNCI 83:716, 1991.

American Journal of Hematology 45:258–259 (1994)

Thrombocytopenia Following Acute Acetaminophen Overdose

Michael Fischereder and Jeffrry P. Jaffe

Department of Medicine, St. Paul-Ramsey Medical Center, St. Paul, and The University of Minnesota Medical School, Minneapolis, Minnesota

An unusual case of severe thrombocytopenia following acetaminophen overdose is presented along with a retrospective review of 174 patients with hospital admissions for acute acetaminophen toxicity. Thrombocytopenia occurred in 3.4% of these patients and strongly correlated with the degree of hepatotoxicity (as measured by peak AST values) but did not correlate with serum acetaminophen levels. The mechanism appears to be a transient direct toxic effect on platelets or megakaryocytes, and the finding of thrombocytopenia early in the course of acetaminophen overdose may identify a subset of patients at risk for significant hepatotoxicity.

Key words: hepatotoxicity, AST, megakaryocytes, platelets, drug toxicity

INTRODUCTION

Intentional or unintentional ingestion of toxic doses of acetaminophen is a frequently encountered problem. The clinical complications are primarily related to hepatotoxicity [1], although nephrotoxicity, pancreatitis, myocardial necrosis, hemolysis, neutropenia, and thrombocytopenia [2–9] have been observed. A case of severe thrombocytopenia following acetaminophen overdose prompted us to perform a retrospective analysis of 174 patients with hospital admissions for acute acetaminophen toxicity to determine the frequency and clinical significance of thrombocytopenia and to investigate its association with other clinical and laboratory findings.

CASE REPORT AND METHODS

A 37-year-old man was admitted 8 hr after the intentional ingestion of 25 g acetaminophen, preceded by the ingestion of 10 g acetaminophen 2 days earlier. No other drugs or alcohol were ingested during this period, although he admitted to drinking approximately 12 beers per week prior to this. Physical examination revealed mild icterus, mild diffuse abdominal tenderness, and a liver span of 13 cm. There were no petechiae, purpura, ecchymoses, melena, or splenomegaly. Admission laboratory tests showed hemoglobin 15.3 g/dl, WBC 5.1×10^9/liter, platelets 9×10^9/liter, PT 18.7 sec, TT 16.7 sec, APTT 31.9 sec, AST 1,119 IU/liter, total bilirubin 2.6 mg/dl, acetaminophen level 146 μg/ml, fibrinogen 232 μg/dl, fibrinogen-fibrin degradation products undetectable, and drug-dependent serum antiplatelet antibody studies using acetaminophen were negative. The patient was admitted to the intensive care unit, received N-acetylcysteine, and was transfused with 6 units multidonor platelets with a 1 hr postinfusion platelet count of 44×10^9/liter. The patient's platelet count continually increased to normal by day 8, and, except for transient petechiae, no bleeding occurred. The AST peaked at 12,474 IU/liter on day 3, with a PT of 36.1 sec on that day, but gradually normalized, and the patient recovered and was discharged on day 8.

We subsequently reviewed the medical records of 174 previous admissions for acute acetaminophen toxicity, recording nadir platelet counts, peak AST values, acetaminophen levels (measured within 4–10 hr of ingestion in 91% of cases), age, gender, and subsequent clinical outcome. The data were analyzed using the Wilcoxon test, and correlation coefficients were calculated.

RESULTS

There were six of 174 patients (3.4%) with a nadir platelet count $<100 \times 10^9$/liter. The mean peak AST

Received for publication May 26, 1993; accepted June 30, 1993.

Address reprint requests to Jeffrry P. Jaffe, MD, Department of Medicine, St. Paul-Ramsey Medical Center, 640 Jackson Street, St. Paul, MN 55101.

level for these six patients was significantly higher than the mean AST level of patients with a nadir platelet count $>100 \times 10^9$/liter (8,145 IU/liter vs. 453 IU/liter, $P < 10^{-4}$), but the acetaminophen levels did not differ significantly between these two groups. Conversely, 21 patients with a peak AST level >1,000 IU/liter had a significantly lower mean platelet nadir than 153 patients with a peak AST level <1,000 IU/liter (178×10^9/liter vs. 300×10^9/liter; $P < 10^{-4}$). Again, acetaminophen levels did not differ significantly between these two AST groups.

There was a highly significant correlation between peak AST values and nadir platelet counts ($R = -0.43$, $P < 10^{-8}$) but no significant correlation between acetaminophen levels and nadir platelet counts ($R = 0.08$, $P = 0.36$) or between acetaminophen levels and peak AST values ($R = 0.01$, $P = 0.87$). In all patients, the thrombocytopenia was transient, and there were no deaths or major bleeding episodes in this series.

DISCUSSION

This case typifies acute hepatotoxicity from acetaminophen overdose with the exception of the severe thrombocytopenia on presentation. The absence of laboratory evidence for disseminated intravascular coagulation (DIC), the absence of serum drug-dependent antiplatelet antibodies during the acute thrombocytopenia, and the immediate and prolonged response to a single 6 unit platelet transfusion all suggest a transient direct toxic effect on megakaryocytes (or circulating platelets) rather than a platelet-consumption process, either thrombotic or immune.

Thrombocytopenia related to chronic low-dose acetaminophen ingestion has been described [2–6], presumably mediated by an immune mechanism as suggested by the presence of drug-dependent antibodies to acetaminophen or a metabolite [2,3], clinical response to drug discontinuation with or without steroid treatment [4,5] or recurrence of thrombocytopenia on rechallenge with the drug [6]. In none of these cases was significant hepatic toxicity reported.

Thrombocytopenia secondary to acute acetaminophen overdose has been uncommonly reported in the literature [7,8] although thrombocytopenia is a common finding in hepatic failure from any cause [9]. In general, this has been attributed to the presence of DIC, a consistent finding in previous reports [7,9] but not present in this case.

Statistical evaluation of our data documented a highly significant correlation between serum AST levels and nadir platelet counts, suggesting a direct association of hepatotoxicity and thrombocytopenia. This may represent a direct toxic effect on platelets (or megakaryocytes), although the lack of correlation between platelet counts and acetaminophen levels suggests that this may be mediated through a toxic metabolite such as N-acetyl-p-benzoquinone (NAPQI), the primary toxic metabolite causing hepatocellular necrosis in susceptible individuals [1].

We conclude that thrombocytopenia occurring early in the course of acetaminophen overdose is not an infrequent finding and may identify a subset of patients at risk for significant hepatotoxicity. The mechanism appears to be a transient direct toxic effect on platelets (or megakaryocytes), possibly mediated through NAPQI or other toxic metabolites of acetaminophen.

ACKNOWLEDGMENTS

We thank George Logan, MD, for performing the statistical analysis of our data; Samuel Hall, MD, for his toxicologic input; and Ms. Helen Finch for help in manuscript preparation.

REFERENCES

1. Black M: Acetaminophen hepatotoxicity. Gastroenterology 78:382–392, 1980.
2. Eisner EV, Shahidi NT: Immune thrombocytopenia due to a drug metabolite. N Engl J Med 287:376–381, 1972.
3. Shoenfeld Y, Shaklai M, Livni E, Pinkhas J: Thrombocytopenia from acetaminophen. N Engl J Med 303:47, 1980.
4. Skokan JD, Hewlett JS, Hoffman GC: Thrombocytopenic purpura associated with ingestion of acetaminophen (Tylenol). Cleveland Clin Q 40:89–91, 1973.
5. Scheinberg IH: Thrombocytopenic reaction to aspirin and acetaminophen. N Engl J Med 300:678, 1979.
6. Kornberg A, Polliack A: Paracetamol-induced thrombocytopenia and haemolytic anemia. Lancet ii:1159, 1978.
7. Thornton JR, Losowsky MS: Severe thrombocytopenia after paracetamol overdose. Gut 31:1159–1160, 1990.
8. Gazzard BG, Clark R, Borirakchanyavat V, Williams R: A controlled trial of heparin therapy in the coagulation defect of paracetamol-induced hepatic necrosis. Gut 15:89–93, 1974.
9. Hillenbrand P, Parbhoo SP, Jedrychowski A, Sherlock S: Significance of intravascular coagulation and fibrinolysis in acute hepatic failure. Gut 15:83–88, 1974.

American Journal of Hematology 45:260–261 (1994)

Hereditary Hemochromatosis and Red Cell Aplasia

Paul C. Adams
Department of Medicine, University of Western Ontario, University Hospital, London, Ontario, Canada

A 63-year-old white man with myasthenia gravis and red cell aplasia was found to have hepatic iron overload. The differential diagnosis included hereditary hemochromatosis and secondary iron overload related to red cell aplasia. Family studies of siblings, including HLA typing, initially suggested a diagnosis of secondary iron overload. The investigation of a remote sibling led to the final diagnosis of hereditary hemochromatosis. The case illustrates the importance of complete family investigations in the differentiation between hereditary hemochromatosis and secondary iron overload and the potential hazard of using HLA typing as an indirect genetic test for hereditary hemochromatosis.

Key words: Iron, secondary iron overload, HLA typing

CASE HISTORY

The diagnosis of myasthenia gravis was established in 1972 with clinical symptoms of muscular weakness affecting respiratory and extraocular muscles. Acetylcholine receptor antibodies were elevated at 13.1 nm/liter (normal <1 nm/liter). A thymoma was detected by CT scan and was treated with thymic irradiation. The patient was treated with prednisone and pyridostigmine. In 1992, he presented with anemia (hemoglobin 8.4 g/dl, MCV 89, WBC 4600, platelets 354,000). Bone marrow biopsy confirmed a diagnosis of red cell aplasia. Biochemical iron studies showed a marked elevation in serum ferritin at 2,176 μg/liter (normal 15–300 μg/liter) and transferrin saturation at 91% (normal 20–55%). There was no history of transfusions, alcohol abuse, or oral iron ingestion or known family history of hereditary hemochromatosis. A percutaneous liver biopsy was performed, which showed marked parenchymal iron deposition and mild portal fibrosis. Hepatic iron concentration was elevated at 171 μmol/g (9,542 μg/g; dry weight, normal 0–40 μmol/g), with a hepatic iron index of 2.7 [1]. Initially, two HLA-identical siblings were evaluated and found to have no clinical evidence of hemochromatosis and a normal serum ferritin and transferrin saturation (Fig. 1). HLA typing has been used as an indirect genetic test for hemochromatosis because of the well documented close linkage between the HLA-A locus and the putative hemochromatosis gene [2]. Therefore, a tentative diagnosis of secondary iron overload related to the red cell aplasia was considered. Treatment for the red cell aplasia included trials of antithymocyte globulin (ATGAM), intravenous immune globulin, plasmapheresis, and cyclosporin, with no demonstrable benefit. Because of the patient's anemia, venesection therapy was not possible. Chelation therapy with deferoxamine was discussed with the patient and was refused. A 61-year-old brother returned from overseas and was found to have arthropathy of the hands and abnormal iron studies (serum ferritin 1,200 μg/liter, transferrin saturation 84%). HLA typing showed that he was also HLA identical to his affected brother. Percutaneous liver biopsy showed parenchymal iron overload, with a hepatic iron concentration of 149 μmol/g (8,314 μg/g) and hepatic iron index 2.44. He underwent 32 venesections of 500 ml until his serum ferritin was 33 μg/liter.

DISCUSSION

Hereditary hemochromatosis is a common autosomal recessive disorder, with a prevalence of approximately 1 in 300 in whites. The differential diagnosis of hereditary hemochromatosis includes secondary iron overload associated with alcoholic liver disease and iron loading anemias. The most common anemias associated with iron

Received for publication July 9, 1993; accepted July 21, 1993.

Address reprint requests to Paul C. Adams, Department of Medicine, University of Western Ontario, University Hospital, London, Ontario, Canada N6A 5A5.

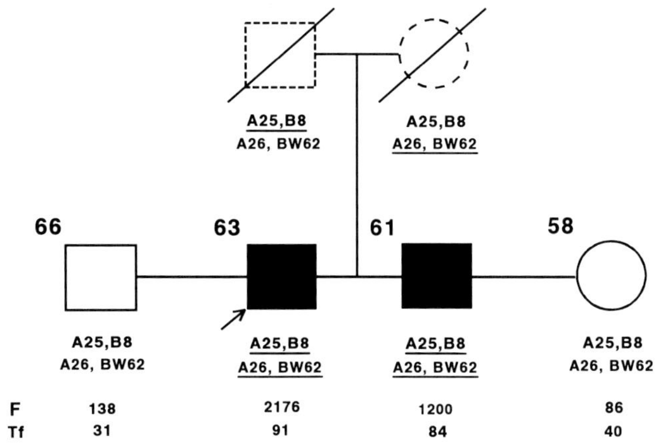

Fig. 1 Family study of 4 HLA-identical siblings. The proband and his younger brother had phenotypic evidence of hemochromatosis. The older brother and younger sister had no biochemical evidence of iron overload. A possible HLA typing pattern of the deceased parents is illustrated. HLA haplotypes carrying the putative hemochromatosis gene are underscored. The serum ferritin (F;normal range 15–300 μg/liter) and transferrin saturation (Tf; normal range 20–55%) are given for each sibling.

overload have been thalassemia and sideroblastic anemia [3]. These conditions are associated with increased intestinal iron absorption, and the problem of iron overload is also exacerbated by transfusions. Red cell aplasia is an uncommon disorder that could theoretically lead to enhanced iron absorption and secondary iron overload.

In this study, further family investigations were undertaken to search for evidence of hereditary hemochromatosis. The initial studies on the two HLA-identical siblings did not support a diagnosis of hereditary hemochromatosis. Previous studies have demonstrated the high predictive value of HLA typing in the identification of homozygotes among siblings of the proband case [4]. However, the later discovery of hereditary hemochromatosis in a third HLA-identical sibling provided strong evidence in favor of a familial iron loading disorder. A possible HLA pattern of the parents is illustrated in Figure 1. The role of HLA typing in the evaluation of siblings, including the costs of the test, has recently been reviewed [5]. The shortcomings of using HLA typing as a genetic test are demonstrated in this case study. In this instance, complete evaluation of all siblings for the phenotypic expression of the disease (serum ferritin, transferrin saturation, hepatic iron concentration) would have provided less confusing information than the combination of phenotypic and surrogate genotypic information. Genetic studies in hemochromatosis using new molecular probes on chromosome 6 and linkage analysis to the HLA locus must include a full phenotypic evaluation of all siblings to avoid an erroneous assumption of a genetic recombination based on HLA typing.

ACKNOWLEDGMENTS

The author acknowledges the advice and assistance of Dr. Moira Cruickshank and Dr. George Ebers.

REFERENCES

1. Bassett ML, Halliday JW, Powell LM: Value of hepatic iron measurements in early hemochromatosis and determination of the critical iron level associated with fibrosis. Hepatology 6:24–29, 1986.
2. Simon M, Bourel M, Genetet B, Fauchet R: Idiopathic hemochromatosis: Demonstration of recessive transmission and early detection by HLA typing. N Engl J Med 297:1017–1021, 1977.
3. Adams PC, Halliday JW, Powell LW: Early diagnosis and screening for hemochromatosis. Adv Intern Med 34:111–126, 1989.
4. Powell LW, Summers KM, Board PG, Axelsen E, Webb S, Halliday JW: Expression of hemochromatosis in homozygous subjects: Implications for early diagnosis and treatment. Gastroenterology 98:1625–1632, 1990.
5. Adams PC, Kertesz AE: Human leucocyte antigen typing in siblings in hemochromatosis: A cost model. Hepatology 15:263–268, 1992.

American Journal of Hematology 45:262–264 (1994)

IgE Plasma Cell Leukemia Successfully Treated With Combination VAD (Vincristine, Doxorubicin, Dexamethasone) and MP (Melphalan, Prednisolone) Followed by Interferon-α

Noboru Yamagata, Chihiro Shimazaki, Hideo Goto, Toshiyuki Hirata, Eishi Ashihara, Naritoshi Oku, Tohru Inaba, Naohisa Fujita, and Masao Nakagawa

Second Department of Medicine (N.Y., C.S., H.G., T.H., E.A., N.O., T.I., M.N.), and Department of Laboratory Medicine (N.F.), Kyoto Prefectural University of Medicine, Kyoto, Japan

A 69-year-old woman with IgE/κ plasma cell leukemia (PCL) was treated with a sequential combination of VAD (vincristine, doxorubicin, dexamethasone) and MP (melphalan, prednisolone) followed by interferon-α (IFNα). A complete remission was achieved for 14 months. Maintenance therapy with IFNα has continued for an additional 10 months. IgE PCL is extremely rare. The biological characteristics of the myeloma cells, including surface marker, adhesion molecule, karyotype, DNA analysis, and the response to various cytokines, are presented.

Key words: IgE plasma cell leukemia, sequential VAD-MP chemotherapy, interferon-α, adhesion molecule

INTRODUCTION

IgE multiple myeloma is rare, with a poor prognosis, and thus far fewer than ten cases of IgE plasma cell leukemia (PCL) have been reported [1]. We present a patient with IgE PCL who achieved a complete response (CR) and long-term survival with sequential combination therapy of VAD (vincristine, doxorubicin, dexamethason) and MP (melphalan, prednisolone) followed by interferon-α (IFNα) and demonstrate the biological characteristics of myeloma cells, including surface marker, adhesion molecule, karyotype, DNA analysis, and the response to various cytokines.

CASE REPORT

A 69-year-old woman was admitted to our hospital in December, 1990, with fever and general malaise. Physical examination revealed pale, anemic conjunctiva. Hematological data revealed the following: RBC 3.15×10^{12}/liter, hemoglobin 9.7 g/dl, platelets 11.9×10^9/liter, and WBC 20.7×10^9/liter with 44% myeloma cells, which showed mature plasma cell morphology. Bone marrow examination revealed a hypercellular marrow, with 72.4% plasma cells. Other laboratory data were as follows: total serum protein 8.5 g/dl, lactate dehydrogenase 588 IU/liter (normal range 234–471), alkaline phosphatase 271 IU/liter (normal range 81–266), creatinine 1.1 mg/dl, blood urea nitrogen 8.4 mg/dl, and calcium 9.6 mg/dl. Serum interleukin-6 (IL-6) level was <10.0 pg/ml. The β_2-microglobulin level was 8.9 mg/liter (normal range 0.6–2.1) in serum and 16,000 μg/liter (normal <370) in urine. Fractional quantitation of serum immunoglobulins revealed IgG 375 mg/dl, IgA <14 mg/dl, IgM <15 mg/dl, and IgE $1{,}177 \times 10^4$ U/ml (normal <400). Immunoelectrophoresis showed IgE/κ M-protein in serum and Bence Jones κ protein in urine. Karyotypic analysis of peripheral leukemic cells revealed 47, X, −X, +7, +9, −12, −14, −20, +der(X)t(X;1)(q28;q21), der(16)t(16;?)(p13;?), +marl, +mar2. Analysis of immunoglobulin gene revealed the presence of both heavy and κ light chain rearrangements, but the TCR-β and bcl-2 genes remained in germ line configuration. Surface markers of leukemic cells analyzed as previously described [2] revealed that CD38 and adhesion molecules such as CD11a, CD11b, CD11c, CD44 and

Received for publication July 9, 1993; accepted July 21, 1993.

Address reprint requests to Noboru Yamagata, MD, Second Department of Medicine, Kyoto Prefectural University of Medicine, 465 Kawaramachi-Hirokoji, Kamigyoku, Kyoto 602, Japan.

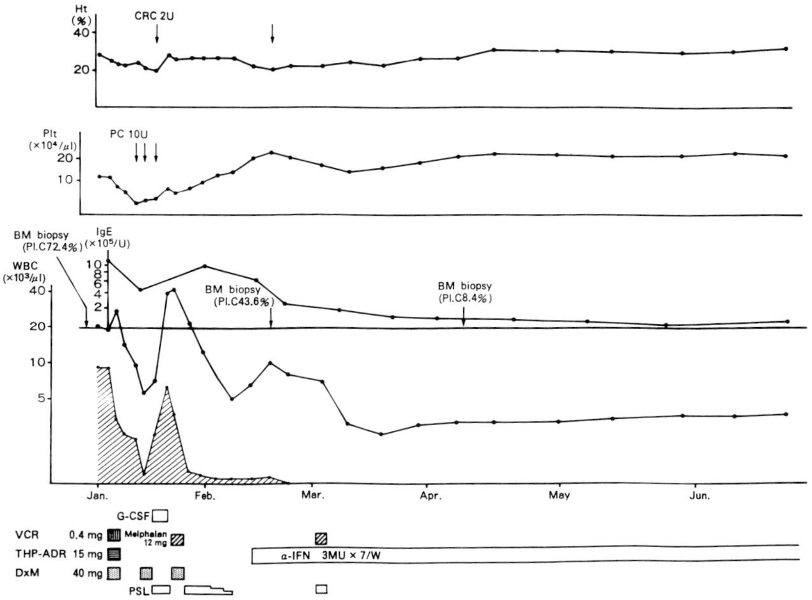

Fig. 1. Summary of clinical course. PCL, plasma cell leukemia; Ht, hematocrit; CRC, concentrated red cells; U, unit; Plt, platelet; PC, platelet concentrate; BM biopsy, bone marrow biopsy; WBC, white blood cells, P1.C (shaded), plasma cell; G-CSF, granulocyte colony-stimulating factor; VCR, vincristine,; THP-ADR, pirarubicin; DXM, dexamethasone; PSL, prednisolone; α-IFN, interferon-α

CD54 were positive. We also evaluated the response of the leukemic cells to various cytokines by the ^{3}H-thymidine uptake method [3]. However, none of the cytokines, including granulocyte colony-stimulating factor (G-CSF), granulocyte-macrophage colony-stimulating factor (GM-CSF), interleukin 3 (IL-3), and IL-6 stimulated the proliferation of leukemic cells. X-rays revealed the presence of diffuse osteoporosis throughout the skeleton.

A diagnosis of primary PCL (IgE/κ type, stage IIIa) was made using the clinical staging system proposed by Durie and Salmon [4]. The patient's clinical course during treatment is summarized in Figure 1. Combination chemotherapy with VAD and MP followed by IFNα cleared the leukemic cells from the peripheral blood. Serum IgE level decreased to 38,000 U/Ml and the other classes of immunoglobulins returned to the normal level. Serum β_2-microglobulin level decreased to the normal range, and Bence-Jones protein disappeared from urine. The patient obtained a CR according to the criteria proposed by Bernasconi et al. [5] (CR was defined as a complete disappearance of circulating plasma cells and a decrease of >50% in either the serum or the urine M-protein level.). CR was maintained for 14 months. The patient has survived for 2 years by continuing to receive IFNα.

DISCUSSION

The mean survival of patients with PCL is about 2–6 months. Even with intensive therapy, a CR is rarely obtained [6], and a successful therapeutic regimen has not been established. Dexamethasone is thought to be more effective against differentiated myeloma cells, which have a long cell cycle, while melphalan and IFNα are more effective against clonogenic myeloma cells [7]. We therefore used the VAD regimen to reduce the massive number of differentiated leukemic plasma cells and then administered melphalan and IFNα to reduce the number of clonogenic myeloma cells, which led to CR.

Some cytokines have recently been reported to stimulate myeloma cell growth, with IL-6 thought to be the major one [8]. Bataille et al. [9] reported that the serum IL-6 level reflects disease severity in plasma cell dyscrasias; the best in vitro response of myeloma cells to IL-6 is often observed in PCL [8]. In our patient, the serum level of IL-6 was low, and the leukemic cells did not respond to IL-6, suggesting that the growth of myeloma cells in this case was not dependent on IL-6. Interestingly, the myeloma cells of this patient expressed several adhesion molecules. It was recently reported that cellular interactions of several adhesion molecules correlated with the proliferation of myeloma cells [10]. Little is known about the expression of adhesion molecules in PCL. Further investigation of the biological characteristics of PCL is warranted.

REFERENCES

1. Invermizzi F, Monti G, Caviglia AG, et al.: A new case of IgE myeloma. Acta Haematol 85:41–44, 1991.

2. Shimazaki C, Goto H, Ashihara E, et al.: Immunophenotype and DNA content of myeloma cells in primary plasma cell leukemia. Am J Hematol 39:159–162, 1992.
3. Goto H, Shimazaki C, Ashihara E, et al.: Effects of interleukin-3 and interleukin-6 on peripheral blood cells from multiple myeloma patients and their clinical significance. Acta Haematol 88:129–135, 1992.
4. Durie BGM, Salmon SE: A clinical staging system for multiple myeloma. Cancer 36:842–854, 1975.
5. Bernasconi C, Castelli G, Pagnucco G, et al.: Plasma cell leukemia: a report on 15 patients. Eur J Haematol 43:76–83, 1989.
6. Malhotra H, Dhabhar BN, Saikia TK, et al.: Ifosfamide in plasma cell leukemia. Am J Hematol 40:226–228, 1992.
7. Barlogie B, Epstein J, Peter S, et al.: Plasma cell myeloma. New biological insights and advances in therapy. Blood 73:865–879, 1989.
8. Zhang XG, Klein B, Batille R: Interleukin-6 is a potent myeloma-cell growth factor in patients with aggressive multiple myeloma. Blood 74:11–13, 1989.
9. Bataille R, Jourdan M, Zhang XG, et al.: Serum levels of interleukin 6, a potent myeloma cell growth factor, as a reflect of disease severity in plasma cell dyscrasias. J Clin Invest 84:2008–2011, 1989.
10. Ahsmann EJM, Lokhorst HM, Dekker AW, et al.: Lymphocyte function-associated antigen-1 expression on plasma cells correlates with tumor growth in multiple myeloma. Blood 79:2068–2075, 1992.

American Journal of Hematology 45:265–267 (1994)

Mild β^+(−87)-Thalassemia CACCC Box Mutation Is Associated With Elevated Fetal Hemoglobin Expression in Cis

John G. Gilman, Laura Manca, Laura Frogheri, Paola Pistidda, Luciana Guiso, Maurizio Longinotti, and Bruno Masala

Division of Hematology, Albert Einstein College of Medicine/Montefiore Medical Center, Bronx, New York (J.G.G.); Instituto di Fisiologia Generale e Chimica Biologica, (L.M., B.M.); Instituto di Ematologia, (M.L.); Università di Sassari, Sessari, Italy; Instituto CNR per lo Studio della Patologia del Sangue e degli Organi Emopoietici, Sassari, Italy (L.F., M.L.); Instituto CNR per lo Studio delle Talassemie ed Anemie Mediterranee, Sassari, Italy (P.P., L.G.)

The β°-thalassemia codon 39 nonsense mutation predominant in Sardinia is severe, and homozygotes are transfusion dependent. Two-thirds of β° 39 alleles are linked to $^A\gamma^T$ (haplotype II). One-fourth are linked to $^A\gamma^I$ (haplotypes I and IX), as is the mild β^+-thalassemia −87 C→G mutation (haplotype VIII). β^+/β°-Thalassemia VIII/II compound heterozygotes have significantly higher $^A\gamma^I$:$^A\gamma^T$ (23:7) than β°-thalassemia I/II (24:20) or IX/II (16:17) cases. This suggests that the β^+ −87 mutation is associated with elevated γ expression in cis, which may contribute to the lack of transfusion-dependence in β^+/β° cases.

Key words: thalassemia, β-thalassemia, $^A\gamma^T$

INTRODUCTION

In northern Sardinia, β°-thalassemia is due almost exclusively to the nonsense mutation at codon 39 of the β-globin gene. Two β-globin gene cluster haplotypes, I and II, account for one-fourth and two-thirds of these cases, respectively [1,2]. While haplotype I carries the normal fetal $^A\gamma$ gene ($^A\gamma^I$:isoleucine at codon 75), haplotype II carries the $^A\gamma^T$ variant (threonine at 75) [3,4]. The latter is linked to a 4 bp deletion at −225 to −222 of the $^A\gamma$ promoter, which is associated with decreased $^A\gamma^T$ gene expression: In I/II β°-thalassemia cases, $^A\gamma^I$ is about 25% higher than $^A\gamma^T$ [4]. It was previously reported that thalassemia intermedia in β^+/β° cases resulted from the mild haplotype VIII β^+ thalassemia C → G CACCC box mutation at −87 of the β-globin gene promoter, which yielded 30–70% β in peripheral blood [5]. We now report that β^+/β° compound heterozygotes with haplotypes VIII ($^A\gamma^I$) and II ($^A\gamma^T$) have significantly higher $^A\gamma^I$:$^A\gamma^T$ ratios than β°-thalassemia I/II cases. This suggests that expression of $^A\gamma^I$ linked to β^+ −87 is significantly higher than that of $^A\gamma^T$ linked to β° 39, and that the elevated γ expression associated with β^+ −87 could also contribute to the mild clinical course in these β^+/β° patients.

MATERIALS AND METHODS

Blood was taken from patients, DNA was isolated from white cells, and $^G\gamma$:$^A\gamma$ ratios were determined by HPLC as previously described [4]. For some of these cases, haplotypes and the presence of the β^+ −87 C → G mutation were determined previously [5]. For the others, haplotypes were determined for seven sites 3′ of the ϵ-globin gene including XmnI [6], by blot hybridization [4]. The presence or absence of the β^+ −87 mutation was determined using β promoter DNA generated by PCR: The 5′ primer sequence was at −674 to −655 of the β promoter (CTAATGCACAGAGCACATTG), while the 3′ primer was at +27 to +47 (GTCTGTTTGAGGTTGCTAGTG). PCR DNA was slot blotted to a nylon filter and then hybridized to normal and mutant 19-mer oligos centered at −87, with procedures described by Manca et

Received for publication August 4, 1993; accepted August 18, 1993.

Address reprint requests to John G. Gilman, PhD, Division of Hematology, Department of Medicine, Montefiore Medical Center, 111 E. 210th St., Bronx, NY 10467.

TABLE I. β-Thalassemia Intermedia (β°/β⁺) Patients With the Rare β⁺ −87 Mutation

Patient	β-Thal	Haplotype	α	$^G\gamma$:$^A\gamma^I$:$^A\gamma^T$	HbA_2	HbF	Hb	Age (years)
R.F.	$\beta°/\beta^+$ (−87)	I/VIII	−α/αα	69:31:0	5.5	63.8	8.9	40
R.V.	$\beta°/\beta^+$ (−87)	I/VIII	N.D.	68:32:0	5.5	63	4.6	35
C.A.	$\beta°/\beta^+$ (−87)	I/VIII	−α/−α	65:35:0	5.2	67.6	8.2	35
P.C.	$\beta°/\beta^+$ (−87)	I/VIII	αα/αα	66:34:0	4.2	71.6	11.3	30
R.G.M.	$\beta°/\beta^+$ (−87)	II/VIII	αα/αα	68:22:10	3.4	35.6	10.3	30
S.R.	$\beta°/\beta^+$ (−87)	II/VIII	−α/αα	68:24:8	4.4	65.6	7.4	29
C.M.	$\beta°/\beta^+$ (−87)	II/VIII	−α/−α	73:22:5	12.6	36.4	8.3	76
P.A.	$\beta°/\beta^+$ (−87)	II/VIII	N.D.	69:22:8	6.4	62.4	13.0	34
C.G.	$\beta°/\beta^+$ (−87)	II/VIII	−α/−α	69:26:5	8.8	51	9.5	25

al. [4] (final wash at 60°C): normal, GAGCCACACCCTAGGGTTG; mutant, GAGCCACACGCTAGGGTTG.

RESULTS

Table I shows $^G\gamma$:$^A\gamma^I$:$^A\gamma^T$ values for nine $\beta^+/\beta°$-thalassemia haplotype VIII/I and VIII/II compound heterozygotes. These all have the rare C → G CACCC box mutation at −87 of the β promoter on the haplotype VIII chromosome and the common β° codon 39 nonsense mutation on the other. None is transfusion dependent, and four (R.V., C.M., P.A., and C.G.) have never been transfused.

These $\beta^+/\beta°$-thalassemia haplotype VIII/(I or II) cases were all +/− for the XmnI site 5′ of $^G\gamma$, which is associated with elevated $^G\gamma$ levels [6]. The XmnI site is on haplotype VIII, since haplotypes I and II are negative for XmnI [2]. For comparison, the few β°-thalassemia XmnI-positive haplotype IX [2] patients found during routine screening were analyzed for $^G\gamma$:$^A\gamma^I$:$^A\gamma^T$ values: Four IX/II had 70:16:14, 67:17:16, 67:15:18, and 68:14:18, while one IX/I had 65:35:0. It is clear that cases with haplotypes VIII or IX have elevated $\%^G\gamma$, as expected: For VIII/II and IX/II cases, mean ± S.D. for $\%^G\gamma$ was 69.4% ± 2.1% and 68% ± 1.4%, respectively, compared to 56% ± 3.2% that we found for haplotype I/II [4].

$\beta^+/\beta°$-Thalassemia haplotype VIII/II cases had significantly lower $^A\gamma^T$ than β°-thalassemia I/II, 7.2% ± 2.1% (mean value in Table I) vs. 19.6% ± 2.5% [data from 4], respectively ($P < 0.01$). $^A\gamma^I$ values did not differ between VIII/II and I/II, 23.2% ± 1.7% (Table I) vs. 24.4% ± 2.9% (4), respectively, but $^A\gamma^I$ was less for β°-thalassemia haplotype IX/II (15.5% ± 1.3%). While $^A\gamma^T$ of IX/II cases (16.5% ± 1.9%) was slightly lower than that of I/II cases, the difference was not significant.

DISCUSSION

Previous data have shown a strong correlation of the 4 bp deletion at −225 to −222 of the $^A\gamma^T$ globin gene promoter with decreased expression of $^A\gamma^T$ [4,7]. We have shown this in haplotype I/II β°-thalassemia patients, all transfusion dependent and homozygous for the β° 39 nonsense mutation, who have the 4 bp deletion and $^A\gamma^T$ on haplotype II and the normal promoter and $^A\gamma^I$ on haplotype I [4].

Table I presents new data for nontransfusion-dependent β-thalassemia intermedia cases who are double heterozygotes for the β° 39 mutation (haplotypes I or II) and the haplotype VIII β^+-thalassemia CACCC box mutation at −87 of the β promoter. The association of haplotype VIII with $^A\gamma^I$ and haplotype II with $^A\gamma^T$ permits the determination of relative quantities of $^A\gamma$ globin produced by the β^+ chromosome and the β° chromosome in haplotype VIII/II ($^A\gamma^I/^A\gamma^T$) heterozygotes. The VIII/II $\beta^+/\beta°$-thalassemia cases had significantly higher $^A\gamma^I$:$^A\gamma^T$ than I/II β°-thalassemia cases: 23.2:7.2 (mean values in Table I) compared to 24.4:19.6 [4], respectively. This suggests that production of $^A\gamma^I$ by the β^+ chromosome is considerably higher than that of $^A\gamma^T$ by the β° chromosome.

Haplotypes VIII and IX are both linked to the $^G\gamma$ −158 T mutation (XmnI positive 5′ of the $^G\gamma$ gene), which is associated with elevated $^G\gamma$ levels [6]. Comparing $^G\gamma$:$^A\gamma^I$:$^A\gamma^T$ values of $\beta^+/\beta°$-thalassemia VIII/II and β°-thalassemia IX/II, the latter had % $^A\gamma^T$ similar to β°-thalassemia I/II cases ($^G\gamma$ −158 C, XmnI negative), which suggests that it is indeed the β^+ −87 mutation and not the $^G\gamma$ −158 T mutation that correlates with the increased $^A\gamma^I$ of haplotype VIII. We have performed a nonlinear least-squares fit of the data for I/II, IX/II, and VIII/II cases to a simple model in which the β^+ −87 mutation is associated with the same increase in $^G\gamma$ and $^A\gamma^I$ expression, while the $^G\gamma$ −158 C → T mutation affects only $^G\gamma$ expression. This analysis suggested a 2.7-fold increase in $^G\gamma$ and $^A\gamma^I$ linked to β^+ −87 and a 1.8-fold increase in $^G\gamma$ due to T at −158.

The molecular basis for the increase in γ expression in association with the β^+ −87 mutation is unclear. However, analogous increases have been observed for β°-thalassemia cases with deletions of the β-globin promoter, while a deletion of part of the β gene not affecting the promoter did not cause increased γ expression [8]. One may propose that mutations or deletions in the β-globin promoter that reduce β transcription may inhibit the β promoter from interacting with the LCR, giving the γ genes the opportunity to interact with the LCR and be expressed under conditions of anemic stress.

While the simple lack of the β-globin gene did not activate γ in transgenic mice [9], the mild to severe anemia associated with deficiencies in β expression may remove some of the blockage of γ-globin gene transcription in adult erythroid cells, making it possible for the γ gene to compete with β for the LCR. This may be especially true when the β promoter is weakened by mutations such as β^+ −87 C → G. Such an effect is suggested by data showing that mutations in the LCR site 2 are associated with increased levels of fetal hemoglobin in sickle cell anemia cases and in a β^+-thalassemia case with the CACCC box β^+ −88 C → T mutation [10]. Hence it is likely that studies in nonanemic transgenic mice [9] may not adequately mirror effects seen in anemic humans and that human erythroid cells programmed in the course of anemia may be capable of producing elevated levels of fetal hemoglobin when the β promoter CACCC box is mutated or the β promoter is deleted.

ACKNOWLEDGMENTS

This work was supported by CNR grants 92.02264.14 to B.M. and 90.04186.MZ77 to M.L. and by NIH grant HL38655.

REFERENCES

1. Pirastu M, Galanello R, Doherty MA, Tuveri T, Cao A, Kan YW: The same β-globin gene mutation is present on nine different β-thalassemia chromosomes in a Sardinian population. Proc Natl Acad Sci USA 84:2882–2885, 1987.
2. Masala B, Manca L, Gallisai D, Stangoni A, Lanclos KD, Kutlar F, Yang KG, Huisman THJ: Biochemical and molecular aspects of β°-thalassemia types in northern Sardinia. Hemoglobin 12:661–671, 1988.
3. Huisman THJ, Kutlar F, Nakatsuji T, Bruce-Tagoe A, Kilinc Y, Cauchi MN, Romero Garcia C: The frequency of the γ chain variant $^A\gamma^T$ in different populations, and its use in evaluating γ gene expression in association with thalassemia. Hum Genet 71:127–133, 1985.
4. Manca L, Cocco E, Gallisai D, Masala B, Gilman JG: Diminished $^A\gamma^T$ fetal globin levels in Sardinian haplotype II β°-thalassemia patients are associated with the four base pair deletion in the $^A\gamma^T$ promoter. Br J Haematol 78:105–107, 1991.
5. Rosatelli MC, Oggiano L, Leoni GB, Tuveri T, Di Tucci A, Scalas MT, Dore F, Pistidda P, Massa A, Longinotti M, Cao A: Thalassemia intermedia resulting from a mild β-thalassemia mutation. Blood 73: 601–605, 1989.
6. Gilman JG, Huisman THJ: DNA sequence variation associated with elevated fetal $^G\gamma$ globin production. Blood 66:783–787, 1985.
7. Beldjord C, Ducrocq R, Nadifi S, Lapoumeroulie C, Elion J, Labie D: A haplotype-linked four base pair deletion upstream of the $^A\gamma$ globin gene coincides with decreased gene expression. Hum Genet 89:625–628, 1992.
8. Anand R, Boehm CD, Kazazian HH Jr, Vanin EF: Molecular characterization of a β°-thalassemia resulting from a 1.4 kilobase deletion. Blood 72:636–641, 1988.
9. Strouboulis J, Dillon N, Grosveld F: Developmental regulation of a complete 70-kb human β-globin locus in transgenic mice. Genes Dev 6:1857–1864, 1992.
10. Beris P, Kitundu MN, Baysal E, Oner C, Lanclos KD, Dimovski AJ, Kutlar F, Huisman THJ: Black β-thalassemia homozygotes with specific sequence variations in the 5′ hypersensitive site-2 of the locus control region have high levels of fetal hemoglobin. Am J Hematol 41:97–101, 1992.

American Journal of Hematology 45:268–276 (1994)

LETTERS AND CORRESPONDENCE

Letters and correspondence submitted for possible publication must be identified as such. Text length must not exceed 500 words and five bibliographic references. A single concise figure or table may be included if it is essential to support the communication. Letters not typed double-spaced will not be considered for publication. Letters not meeting these specifications will not be returned to authors. Letters to the Editor *are utilized to communicate a single novel observation or finding.* Correspondence *is to be used to supplement or constructively comment on the contents of a publication in the journal and cannot exceed the restrictions for Letters to the Editor. The Editor reserves the right to shorten text, delete objectional comments and make other changes to comply with the style of the journal. Permission for publication must be appended as a postscript. Submissions must be sent to Marcel E. Conrad, M.D., Associate Editor, American Journal of Hematology, USA Cancer Center, Mobile, Alabama 36688 to permit rapid consideration for publication.*

Lung Perfusion Scaning in Two Patients With Malignant Histiocytosis

To the Editor: In 1966, Rappaport [1] introduced the term *malignant histiocytosis* for a malignant process that he believed to be an invasive, progressive proliferation of neoplastic histiocytes. Malignant histiocytosis is characterized by fever, lymphadenopathy, hepatosplenomegaly, and pancytopenia [2]. Pulmonary involvement has also been demonstrated by roentgenograms, open lung biopsy, bronchoalveolar lavage (BAL), or autopsy [3–5]. Here we describe two patients with malignant histiocytosis, in whom ^{99m}Tc-MAA lung perfusion scaning showed multiple defects in the lung fields.

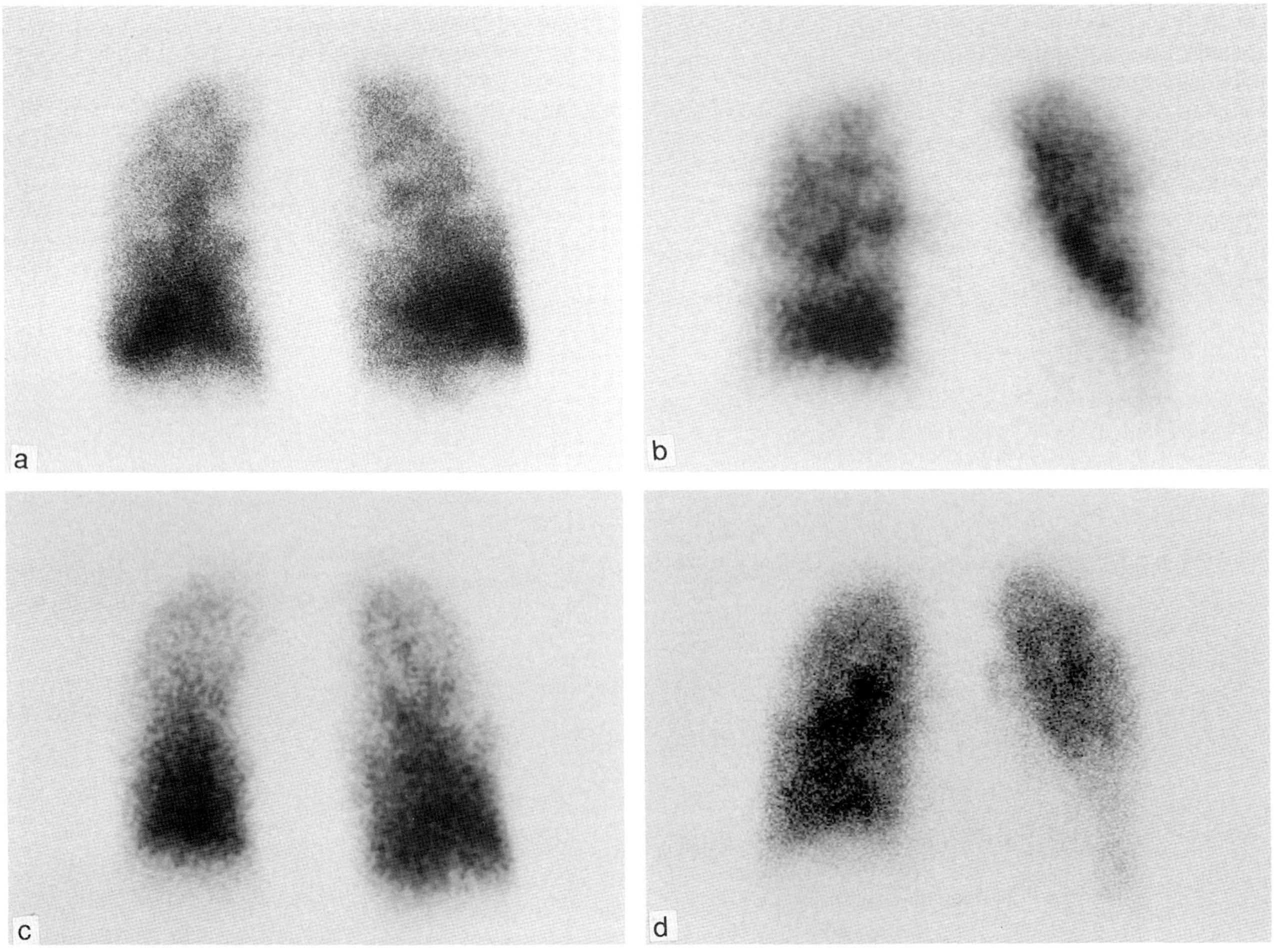

Fig. 1. Lung perfusion scaning showed multiple defects (a,b), which disappeared after chemotherapy (c,d). a,c; Case 1; b, d; case 2.

Case 1

On January 5, 1993, a 69-year-old man was admitted for evaluation of dyspnea and fever. Physical examination detected pallor and hepatosplenomegaly. Hematological parameters were as follows: hemoglobin, 7.1 g/dl; white cell count, 1,600/μl; and platelet count, 38,000/μl. Bone marrow aspiration revealed 1.6% neoplastic histiocytes. Laboratory investigations showed a serum LDH level of 1,224 U/liter, total protein (TP) of 5.8 g/dl, albumin of 2.4 g/dl, and total bilirubin (TB) of 2.1 mg/dl. Blood gas analysis revealed a pH of 7.4, PCO_2 of 19.8 mm Hg, and PO_2 of 56.5 mm Hg. Coagulation studies showed the following: fibrinogen 397 mg/dl, fibrin degradation products (FDP) 1,021 ng/ml, and antithrombin III (AT III) 48%. The chest X-ray film showed diffuse interstitial pneumonia.

Case 2

On February 2, 1993, a 70-year-old woman was admitted for evaluation of fatigue and fever. Physical examination detected pallor, but no lymphadenopathy or hepatosplenomegaly. Hematological tests revealed the following: hemoglobin 7.6 g/dl; white cell count 5,200 μl, with 3% neoplastic histiocytes; and platelet count 25,000/μl. Bone marrow aspiration revealed 32% neoplastic histiocytes. Laboratory investigations showed a serum LDH level of 1,423 U/liter, a TP of 4.9 g/dl, an albumin of 2.0 g/dl, and a TB of 1.3 mg/dl. Blood gas analysis revealed a pH of 7.5, PCO_2 of 30.4 mm Hg, and PO_2 of 52.3 mm Hg. Coagulation studies showed the following: fibrinogen 169 mg/dl, FDP 1,132 ng/ml, and AT III 66%. The chest X-ray film was normal.

These two patients were diagnosed as having malignant histiocytosis from the results of peripheral blood and bone marrow examination. ^{99m}Tc-MAA lung perfusion scaning showed multiple defects in the bilateral lung field in both patients (Fig. 1). They were treated with vindesine sulfate, etoposide, and dexamethasone. All evidence of malignant histiocytosis disappeared, including the multiple defects on lung perfusion scans. Both BAL and open lung biopsy are difficult to perform in patients with a bleeding tendeny and acute respiratory failure, often making antemortem diagnosis impossible. Lung perfusion scaning proved to be very helpful in the present patients, both for initial diagnosis and for follow-up.

Hideyo Natori
Ken Tanaka
Kaori Shiraishi
Seishi Osabe
Hiroto Jojima
Kotaro Oizumi
First Department of Internal Medicine, Kurume University School of Medicine, Fukuoka, Japan
Masatoshi Ishibashi
Department of Radiology, Kurume University School of Medicine, Fukuoka, Japan

References

1. Rappaport H: Tumors of the hematopoietic system. In: "Atlas of Tumor Pathology." Washington, DC: Armed Forces Institute of Pathology: 49, 1966.
2. Ducatman BS, Wick MR, Morgan TW, Banks PM, Pierre RV: Malignant histiocytosis: A clinical histologic and immunohistochemical study of 20 cases. Hum Pathol 15:368, 1984.
3. Dunnick NR, Parker BR, Warnke RA: Radiographic manifestations of malignant histiocytosis. Am J Roentgenol 127:611, 1976.
4. Colby TV, Carrington CB, Mark GJ. Pulmonary involvement in malignant histiocytosis. Am J Surg Pathol 5:61, 1981.

Good Response to High-Dose Intravenous Immunoglobulin in Patients With Alveolar Hemorrhage Refractory to Platelet Transfusion

To the Editor: Intravenous immunoglobulin (IVIG) has been used to treat patients with autoimmune cytopenias with varying degrees of success [1,2]. However, optimal dose and timing of therapy are unclear. Recently it has been suggested that the beneficial effects of IVIG therapy may be related to IgG levels achieved or maintained [3,4], and individualization of dosage or frequency of dosing may be required to obtain a specific IgG level [5,6]. We have used prolonged IVIG therapy in three patients with alveolar hemorrhage requiring mechanical ventilation in the intensive care unit (ICU). All three were refractory to platelet transfusions after standard doses of IVIG. IgG levels achieved and maintained were monitored. All three patients showed improved response to platelet transfusion and ceasation of hemorrhage after their IgG levels reached 2,000 mg/dl.

Patient 1

Patient 1 was a 26-year-old woman with acute myeloblastic leukemia. On ICU admission she was febrile and on broad-spectrum antibiotics, with no pathogen cultured, a platelet count of 24,000/mm^3, normal-sized spleen, normal coagulation profile, and multispecific HLA antibodies. She failed to respond to transfusions of HLA-matched or compatible platelets. On ICU day 4, IVIG therapy was started (Sandoglobulin, Sandoz, Hanover, NJ) at 400 mg/kg/day × 9 days (baseline IgG level 950 mg/dl). By ICU day 5 she was afebrile except when receiving amphotericin B. By ICU day 11, good increments to HLA-compatible platelets were evident. Serum IgG at the end of IVIG therapy was 2,640 mg/dl. No evidence of marrow recovery was seen during this period (Fig. 1).

Patient 2

Patient 2 was a 79-year-old man with idiopathic severe aplastic anemia. On ICU admission he was afebrile and on no antibiotics, with a platelet count of 18,000/mm^3, normal-sized spleen, and normal coagulation profile. Testing showed lymphocytotoxic HLA antibodies of limited specificity on ICU day 3. Use of HLA-matched platelets did not improve response to transfusion. He received IVIG at 400 mg/kg/day × 9 days (baseline IgG 1,580 mg/dl). At the end of IVIG therapy, serum IgG was 3,180 mg/dl, and good response to platelets was evident. No evidence of marrow recovery was noted.

Patient 3

Patient 3 was a 46-year-old man 10 days postautologous marrow transplantation. On ICU admission, he was febrile and on broad spectrum antibiot-

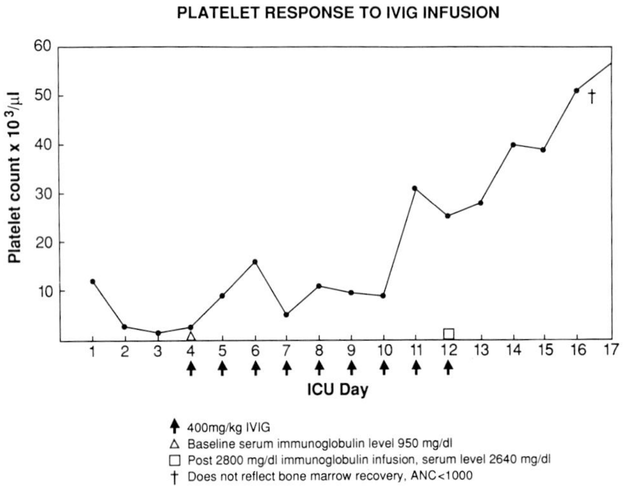

Fig. 1. Platelet counts during IVIG therapy in patient 1. Platelet transfusions were given daily. The patient showed no sign of recovering neutrophil or erythrocyte counts by ICU day 17.

ics, with a platelet count of 60,000/mm^3, normal coagulation profile, and normal-sized spleen. He soon became unresponsive to platelet transfusions, without HLA antibodies. IVIG at 400 mg/kg/day × 8 days was given (baseline IgG 293 mg/dl). Serum IgG at the end of IVIG therapy was 2,100 mg/dl, at which time he responded well to platelet transfusion. No evidence of marrow reconstitution was seen.

Multiple potential mechanisms of action for IVIG [1,7,8] and the fact that not all patients respond to the same dose [9] suggest that a dose-response curve may exist. A previous study looking at IgG levels and their relationship to platelet refractoriness in alloimmunized patients reported no benefit from achieving levels >2,000 mg/dl [10]. However, at least two patients in that study lost their lymphocytotoxic antibodies after IVIG therapy and became responsive to pooled random donor platelets. We suggest that, if IVIG is given to patients refractory to platelet transfusion, it would be useful to evaluate response to therapy as a function of IgG levels achieved and maintained.

M.E. Purucker
M. Cottler-Fox

Critical Care Medical Department and Department of Transfusion Medicine, Warren G. Magnuson Clinical Center, National Institutes of Health, Bethesda, Maryland

References

1. Dwyer JM: Manipulating the immune system with immune globulin. N Engl J Med 326:107–116, 1992.
2. Hesseling PB: High-dose immunoglobulin therapy in four patients with onyalai. Trans R Soc Trop Med Hygiene 85:131–132, 1991.
3. Cottler-Fox M, Lynch M, Pickle LW, Cahill R, Spitzer TR, Deeg HJ: Some but not all benefits of intravenous immunoglobulin therapy after bone marrow transplantation appear to correlate with IgG trough levels. Bone Marrow Transplant 8:27–33, 1991.
4. Baker CJ, Melish ME, Hall RT, et al.: Intravenous immune globulin for the prevention of nosocomial infection in low birth-weight neonates. N Engl J Med 327:213–219, 1992.
5. Leen CLS, Yap PL, McClelland DBL: Increase of serum immunoglobulin level into the normal range in primary hypogammaglobulinaemia by dosage individualization of intravenous immunoglobulin. Vox Sang 51:278–286, 1986.
6. Schiff RI: Individualizing the dose of intravenous immune serum globulin for therapy of patients with primary humoral immunodeficiency. Vox Sang 49(Suppl 1):15–24, 1985.
7. Grosse-Wilde H, Blasczyk R, Westhoff U: Soluble HLA class I and class II concentrations in commercial immunoglobulin preparations. Tissue Antigens 39: 74–77, 1992.
8. Blasczyk R, Westhoff U, Grosse-Wilde H: Soluble CD4, CD8, and HLA molecules in commercial immunoglobulin preparations. Lancet 341:789–790, 1993.
9. Ziegler ZR, Shadduck RK, Rosenfeld CS, et al.: High dose intravenous gamma globulin improves responses to single donor platelets in patients refractory to platelet transfusion. Am J Hematol 138:15–23, 1991.
10. Lee EJ, Norris D, Schiffer CA: Intravenous immune globulin for patients alloimmunized to random donor platelet transfusion. Transfusion 27:245–247, 1987.

Normal Pregnancy and Delivery in Essential Thrombocythemia Even Without Interferon Therapy

To the Editor: We read with interest the letter by Petit et al. [1] on a normal pregnancy in a patient with essential thrombocythemia (ET) treated with α_2- interferon. It is surprising to note that the platelet counts shown by the proposita during pregnancy and at delivery are not reported. It is well known that the beneficial effect of interferon is often fleeting, where in a few weeks basal levels are again attained. This appears to be true even in CML [2]. In ET patients it is known that, after cessation of treatment with interferon, the platelet number may return to the basal levels in a few weeks [3,4].

Therefore, it is likely that platelet number at the time of delivery was as high as in the pretreatment period. As a consequence, it could be surmised that a normal pregnancy was carried through in spite of a high platelet count. This is in agreement with other cases reported in the literature [5,6] and with our experience.

In 1980–1981, we had the opportunity to evaluate two women, aged 18 and 21 years, in whom a diagnosis of essential thrombocythemia was made, for both during the third month of pregnancy. At that time we did not have interferon available, and we obviously did not use any alkylating agent. Both women delivered normal, full-term babies without any complication. A follow-up study after 5 and 3 years, respectively, was uneventful. Moreover, in 1990, we studied two additional women, aged 30 and 45 years, who we saw after a diagnosis of ET had been made in another hospital 2 or 3 years before they became pregnant. Pregnancy in both instances was uneventful, and two normal babies were born without complications. It is likely therefore that the normal pregnancy observed by Petit et al. was not due to the previous interferon treatment, since even untreated women with ET may have a normal pregnancy and delivery.

Maria Luigia Randi
Ersilia Barbone
Antonio Girolami

Institute of Medical Semeiotics, and IV Chair of Internal Medicine,ql University of Padua Medical School, Padua, Italy

References

1. Petit JJ, Callis M, Fernandez de Sevilla A: Normal pregnancy in a patient with essential thrombocythemia treated with Interferon alpha-2b. Am J Hematol 40:80, 1992.
2. Talpaz M, Kantarjian HM, Mc Credie KB, et al.: Clinical investigation of human alpha interferon in chronic myelogenus leukemia. Blood 69:1280–1288, 1987.
3. Kasparu H, Barnhart M, Krieger O, Lutz D: Remission may continue after termination of rIFN alpha-2b treatment for essential thrombocythemia. Eur J Hematol 48:333–362, 1992.
4. Gisslinger H, Ludwig H, Linkesch W, Chott A, Fritz E, Radaszkiewicz T: Long-term therapy for thrombocytosis in myeloproliferative diseases. Lancet ii:634–637, 1989.
5. Linares M, Pastor E, Jarque I, Sanz G, Sanz M: Essential thrombocythemia and pregnancy. Am J Hematol 28:66, 1988.

6. Beard J, Hillman P, Anderson CC, Lewis SM, Pearson TC: Primary thrombocythemia in pregnancy. Br J Haematol 77:371–374, 1994.

Author's Reply

To the Editor: The letter by Dr. Randi points out two well known facts: first, that the effect of interferons on platelet count disappears after the drug is stopped; second, that many patients, but obviously not all, with essential thrombocythemia who become pregnant do not show complications during pregnancy and deliver normal infants.

Our report was focused on interferon and fertility. We never said, nor even suggested, that the normality of the pregnancy and of the delivery was due to the interferon that our patient was receiving when she became pregnant.

José Petit
Servicio de Hematología Clínica, Hospital Duran i Reynals, Barcelona, Spain

Common Acute Lymphoblastic Leukemia Antigen (CD10)-Positive Sézary's Syndrome

To the Editor: Expression of CD10/NEP (cell surface-neutral endopeptidase) in postthymic T-cell malignancies is extremely rare [1]: To our knowledge, there have been no reports concerning the expression of CD10 antigen in cutaneous T-cell lymphoma (CTCL). We report a patient with Sézary's syndrome, a leukemic variant of CTCL, in which neoplastic T cells in the blood showed a unique phenotype coexpressing CD4 and CD10 antigens on a single cell.

A 69-year-old woman was admitted to our hospital in November, 1992, because of a generalized erythrodermia. The patient had a 10 year history of recurrent eczematous rash. Physical examination on admission showed a generalized erythrodermia and slightly enlarged axillary and inguinal lymph nodes. The leukocyte count was 7.4×10^9/liter, with 38% neutrophils, 1% eosinophils, 6% monocytes, and 47% atypical lymphocytes with cleft or dumbbell-shaped nuclei. Hemoglobin was 11.5 g/dl, and the platelet count was 182×10^9/liter. Antibody for human T-lymphotropic virus type I was negative. The skin biopsy specimen disclosed a band-like superficial dermal infiltrate, with a predominance of atypical lymphoid cells, which showed highly irregular nuclear convolutions with peripheral condensation of chromatin by electron microscopic analysis. Immunophenotyping of peripheral blood mononuclear cells using flow cytometry was as follows: CD2 87%, CD3 82%, CD4 79%, CD5 87%, CD7 12%, CD10 37%, CD29 81%, and HLA-DR 16%. Two-color flow cytometry confirmed the biphenotypic expression of both CD4 and CD10 antigens on nearly one-half of the tumor cells (Fig. 1).

Immunogenotypic studies of peripheral blood cells showed rearrangements of both T-cell receptor β and γ genes and germline configuration of J_H gene. Accordingly, the patient was diagnosed as having Sézary's syndrome and was treated with oral chlorambucil, 2 mg daily, which resulted in an improvement of generalized erythrodermia.

CD10 has recently been identified as the cell surface NEP that cleaves peptide bonds on the amino side of hydrophobic amino acids and inactivates a variety of peptide hormones, including substance P, endothelin, and interleukin-1 [2,3]. Although CD10/NEP is expressed both on immature lymphoid progenitors and on follicular center cells among normal lymphoid lineage, CD10-positive mature T cells have not been immunophenotypically identified [1]. There are several possible explanations for the significance of CD10 expression by CTCL cells in the present case. First, CD10-positive CTCL is considered as a neoplasm derived from a not yet identified CD10-positive, mature T-cell subpopulation, which may preferentially reside in the skin and have an important role in cutaneous immune response. Second, high levels of CD10 expression may not imply the existence of a specialized subset of T cells but simply reflect a functional state of CTCL cells showing enhanced cell-surface NEP activity, which has recently been detected using enzymatic assays in both mature B- and T-cell lineage, albeit at lower levels [3]. Alternatively, an initial oncogenic event has occurred at an early stage of CD10-positive precursor T-cell level [4], and CD10 expression has been preserved even after the differentiation of the original clone to the mature T cells.

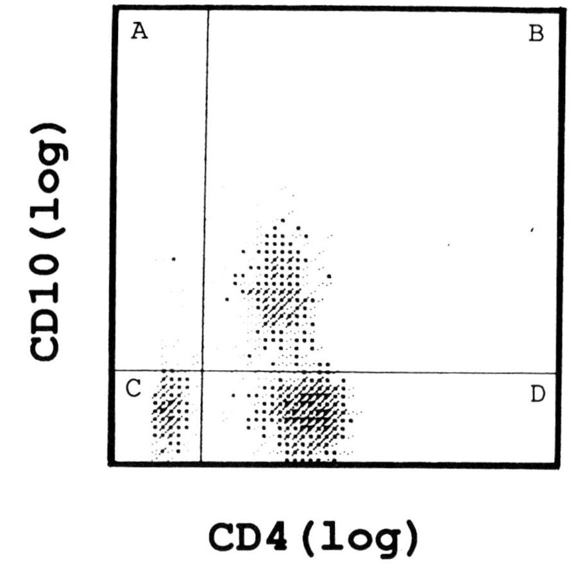

Fig. 1. Two-color flow cytometric analysis of peripheral blood mononuclear cells shows that >40% of CD4-positive cells coexpress CD10 antigen simultaneously. CD10: J5-RD1 (Coulter Immunology, Hialeah, FL) CD4: Leu3a-FITC (Becton Dickinson, Mountain View, CA). A: 3.2%. **B:** 34.7%. **C:** 16.1%. **D:** 46.0%.

Akihiko Chubachi
Takako Ishino
Noriko Satoh
Akira B. Miura
Third Department of Internal Medicine and Department of Dermatology, Akita University School of Medicine, Akita, Japan

References

1. LeBien TW, McCormack RT: The common acute lymphoblastic leukemia antigen (CD10): Emancipation from a functional enigma. Blood 73:625–635, 1989.
2. Pierart ME, Najdovski T, Appelboom TE, Deschodt-Lanckman MM: Effect of human endopeptidase 24.11 ("enkephalinase") on IL-1-induced thymocyte proliferation activity. J Immunol 140:3808–3811, 1988.
3. Beaumont A, Brouet JC, Roques BP: Neutral endopeptidase 24.11 and angiotensin-converting enzyme like activity in calla positive and calla negative lymphoid cells. Biochem Biophys Res Commun 160:1323–1329, 1989.

4. Hokland P, Hokland M, Daley J, Ritz J: Identification and cloning of a prethymic precursor T lymphocyte from a population of common acute lymphoblastic leukemia antigen (calla)-positive fetal bone marrow cells. J Exp Med 165:1749–1754, 1987.

Acquired Platelet Storage Pool Deficiency Due to Severe Valvular Disease Corrected by Prosthetic Valve Replacement

To the Editor: Acquired platelet storage pool deficiency is a platelet function disorder associated with a variety of conditions, including autoimmune diseases, disseminated intravascular coagulation, myeloproliferative diseases, and cardiopulmonary bypass [1]. Valvular heart disease has previously been associated with this condition [2], although platelet ultrastructure and the effect of valve replacement were not reported. We describe a patient with severe valvular disease and platelet dense granule depletion, which were corrected with valve replacement.

A 39-year-old man with symptomatic, severe aortic stenosis and insufficiency was referred for hematologic study due to a prolonged preoperative template bleeding time (20 min). There was no history of lifelong excessive bleeding or easy bruising. Six months earlier, while not taking aspirin, he had unexplained epistaxis lasting for approximately 1 month. The patient had diabetes mellitus, and his medications included insulin, aspirin, digoxin, furosemide, captopril, and isosorbide dinitrate. Physical examination was remarkable only for an aortic insufficiency and stenosis murmur. There was no cutaneous or mucosal bleeding. Complete blood count and peripheral blood smear were normal. Platelet count was 306,000/mm^3. Chemistries were normal except for mild azotemia: creatinine 132.6 μmol/liter (1.5 mg/dl) and blood urea nitrogen 12.14 μmol/liter (34 mg/dl). Echocardiogram revealed an aortic valve area of 0.7 cm^2 and transvalvular gradient of 44 mm Hg.

Aspirin was discontinued and the bleeding time 14 days later was 20 min (normal <8 min). Fibrinogen, factor VIII levels, von Willebrand factor antigen, ristocetin cofactor activity, and prothrombin, partial thormboplastin, and thrombin times were normal. Platelet aggregation tests revealed an absent secondary aggregation wave to ADP (2.5 μM), with normal aggregation to epinephrine (5.5 μM), ristocetin (1.5 mg/ml), and collagen (0.8 μg/ml), consistent with a platelet secretion defect. Platelet electron microscopy was performed on peripheral blood.

Following platelet and cryoprecipitate transfusions, a St. Jude's valve was placed uneventfully. Aortic valve pathology revealed calcific changes; warfarin was begun postoperatively. Three weeks later, platelet aggregation tests and electron microscopy were repeated. A selective depletion of platelet dense granules and marked platelet polymorphism were evident preoperatively. Postoperatively, platelet morphology and aggregation tests were normal (Fig. 1).

The present case illustrates an acquired platelet storage pool deficiency in a patient with severe aortic valve disease. Abnormal aggregation to ADP correlated with morphologic evidence of platelet dense granule depletion. The correction of morphologic and functional platelet abnormalities with prosthetic valve replacement is evidence that the valvular disease caused this abnormality. The cause of platelet dysfunction under these conditions is unclear, although an in vivo exposure of platelets to inducers of activa-

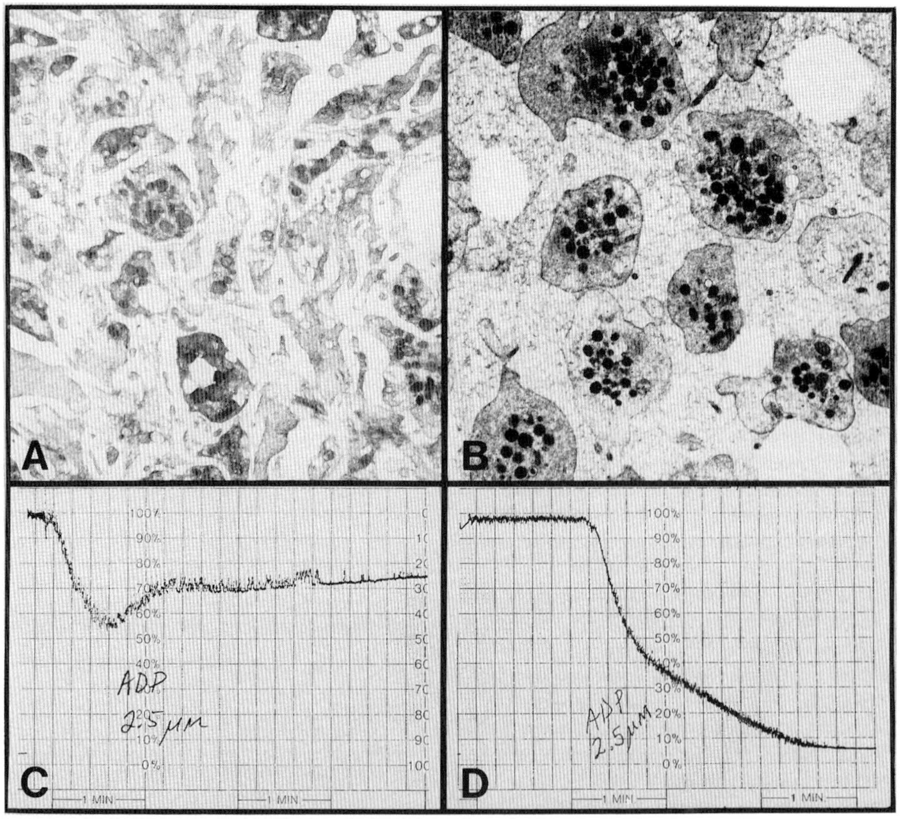

Fig. 1. A: Preoperative platelet electron microscopy revealing marked polymorphism and dense granule depletion. ×14,250. B: Postoperative platelet electron microscopy revealing normal platelet morphology. ×14,250. C: Preoperative platelet aggregation to ADP, with absent secondary wave of aggregation. D: Postoperative platelet aggregation to ADP normal.

tion has been suggested [3]. Turbulent flow-related shear stresses [4] created by the severe valvular abnormality, possibly in conjunction with endothelial cell injury, may have contributed to platelet activation, causing granule release and circulation of hypofunctional platelets.

The prevalence and clinical significance of acquired platelet storage pool disease in patients with valvular heart disease is at present unknown. This entity should be considered in the evaluation of such patients with bleeding manifestations and/or a prolonged bleeding time. In such cases, replacement of the abnormal valve may benefit the patient both hemodynamically and hemostatically.

Rolando E. Rumbaut
Michael H. Kroll
Ferenc Gyorkey
Andrew I. Schafer
Departments of Medicine and Pathology, Baylor College of Medicine and Houston V.A. Medical Center, Houston, Texas

References

1. Nieuwenhuis HK, Akkerman JN, Sixma JJ: Patients with a prolonged bleeding time and normal aggregation tests may have storage pool deficiency: studies on one hundred six patients. Blood 70:620–623, 1987.
2. Beurling-Harbury C, Galvan CA: Acquired decrease in platelet secretory ADP associated with increased postoperative bleeding in post-cardiopulmonary bypass patients and in patients with severe valvular heart disease. Blood 52:13–23, 1978.
3. Pareti FI, Capitanio A, Mannucci L, Ponticelli C, Mannucci PM: Acquired dysfunction due to circulation of "exhausted" platelets. Am J Med 69:235–40, 1980.
4. Chow TW, Hellums JD, Moake JL, Kroll MH: Shear stress-induced von Willebrand factor binding to platelet glycoprotein Ib initiates calcium influx associated with aggregation. Blood 80:113–20, 1992.

Detection of Human T Lymphotropic Virus Type I Proviral DNA in Fresh Cells From Ascitic Fluid in a Patient With Adult T-Cell Leukemia

To the Editor: Since Kagoshima district in Japan is highly endemic for human lymphotropic virus type I (HTLV-I), it is difficult to distinguish atypical adult T-cell leukemia (ATL) from other lymphoproliferative disorders [1–3]. We report a patient with ATL who showed monoclonal integration of HTLV-I proviral DNA in fresh cells from ascitic fluid.

A 64-year-old woman was admitted to National Kirishima Hospital in the Kagoshima district because of general malaise and ascites. This patient suffered from hepatomegaly along with ascites. Systemic lymphadenopathy was not observed, except for paraaortic lymph nodes. The leukocyte count was 7.1×10^9/liter, with a differential count of 2% abnormal lymphocyte. Coagulation studies showed a characteristic of disseminated intravascular coagulopathy (DIC). Next, it was important to examine the cytology, virology, and surface phenotype of the cells from ascitic fluid. The ascitic fluid contained abnormal lymphocytes and multinuclear giant cells; 95.8% of the cells, including most of the abnormal lymphocytes, were found to be CD2 positive. With these cells, HTLV-I proviral DNA was examined. The methods of DNA extraction, Southern blotting analysis, and molecularly cloned HTLV-I probe analysis have been reported [3–5]. The fresh cells from ascitic fluid contained HTLV-I proviruses with discrete band (Fig. 1). From these data, this patient was diagnosed as ATL. In this case, not associated with leukocytosis, skin lesions or peripheral lymphadenopathy, the detection of HTLV-I provial DNA in cells from ascites was useful for diagnosis of ATL. We could directly verify abnormal lymphocytes in ascitic fluid were leukemic cells.

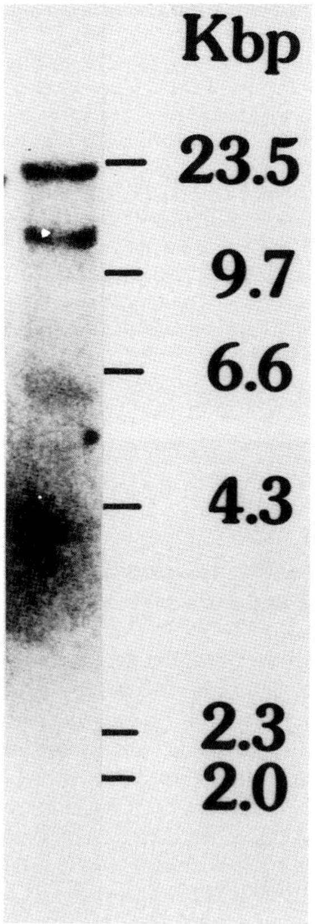

Fig. 1. Monoclonal integration of HTLV-I proviral DNA into cellular DNA in fresh cells from the patients ascitic fluid. DNA from fresh cells from ascitic fluid (5 μg) was digested completely with EcoRI and after gel electrophoresis through 0.8% agar, and a Southern blotting experiment with a ^{32}P nick-labeled HTLV probe was performed. The fresh cells contained HTLV-I provirus, with discrete bands. This patient retained two copies.

Masahito Iwahashi
The Second Department of Internal Medicine, Oita Medical University, Oita, Japan
Maki Otsuka
Makoto Matsumoto
Kagoshima Tishin Hosptial for the Ministry of Posts and Telecommunications, Kagoshima, Japan
Shigemi Shimotakahara
National Kirishima Hospital, Kagoshima, Japan
Nobuyuki Kobayashi
Department of Virology and Parasitology, Yamaguchi University, School of Medicine, Yamaguchi, Japan

References

1. Hanada S, Uematsu T, Iwahashi M, Nomura K, Utsunomiya A, Kodama M, Ishibashi K, Terada A, Saito T, Makino T, Uozumi K, Kuwazuru Y, Otsuka M, Harada R, Hashimoto S, Sakurami T: The prevalence of human T-cell leukemia virus type-I infection in patients with hematologic and nonhematologic disease in adult T-cell leukemia-endemic area of Japan. Cancer 64:1290–1295, 1989.
2. Matsumoto T, Matsumoto M, Yunoki K, Hanada S, Iwahashi M, Utsunomiya A, Kato Y, Kodama M, Fukuda T, Nishioka K, Nomura K, Hashimoto S, Hinuma Y:

Hodgkin's disease in the endemic area of adult T-cell leukemia (ATL). Jpn J Clin Oncol 13(Suppl 2):301–308. 1983.
3. Iwahashi M, Hanada S, Nomura K, Hashimoto S, Matsumoto T, Younoki K, Kobayashi N, Konishi H, Hatanaka M: Clinical significance of adult T-cell leukemia (ATL) associated antigen (ATLA), anti-ATLA antibody and adult T-cell leukemia virus (ATLV)/human T-cell leukemia virus type-I (HTLV-I) proviral DNA in ATL, adult T-cell malignant lymphoma (AT-ML) and Hodgkin's disease in Kagoshima district. Rinsho Ketsueki 27:1603–1610, 1986.
4. Kobayashi M, Yamamoto N, Koyanagi Y, Schneider J, Hansmann G, Hatanaka M: Translation of HTLV (human T-cell leukemia virus) RNA in a nuclease-treated rabit reticulocyte system. EMBO J 3:321–325, 1984.
5. Kobayashi N, Konishi H, Sabe H, Shigesada K, Noma T, Hajis S, Hatanak M: Genomic structure of HTLV:detection of defective genome and its amplification in MT-2 cells. EMBO J 3:1339–1343, 1984.

Parvovirus B19 Infection Causing Severe Peripheral Blood Thrombocytopenia and Persistent Viremia

To the Editor: Parvovirus B19 infection causes red cell aplasia in the patients with chronic hemolytic anemia and short red cell life span [1]. The virus infects primarily the erythorid progenitors and propagates, causing direct cytotoxicity [1]. The infection sometimes accompanies mild neutropenia and thrombocytopenia [1]. The anemia improves and the viral antigen disappears soon after the appearance of antibodies to the virus [1]. We recently experienced an extremely rare case of severe thrombocytopenia complicating severe hemorrhagic episodes due to parvovirus B19 infection.

A 73-year-old previously healthy women suffered from fever, arthralgia, and diarrhea on December 3, 1992 (Fig. 1).On the next day, the patient noticed petechiae of the legs. Two days later, the hemorrhagic symptoms aggravated, and epistaxisis, bloody sputum, and hematoma of the oral cavity appeared. Peipheral blood cell counts revealed RBC 484 $\times$ $10^4/\mu l$, Ht 46.5%, Hb 15.5 g/dl, reticulocytes 1%, WBC 6,400/μl (neutrophils 40%, lymphocytes 50%, atypical lymphocytes 5%, monocytes 5%), and platelets 1 $\times$ $10^4/\mu l$. The bone marrow aspiration smear revealed increased numbers of megakaryocytes and their naked forms, and erythroid and myeloid series were normally present and were morphologically normal. Bone marrow necrosis was not observed on a biopsy specimen. The patient had normal serum immunolglobulin levels and T cells normal in both number and subsets. With the initial diagnosis of idiopathic thrombocytopenic purpura, prednisolone and then commercially available immunoglobulin were administered. Subsequently, danazol was administered, but it was stopped because of the side effect of liver damage. An increase in the platelet count began 1 month after admission, and the platelet count was normal thereafter.

Parvovirus B19 DNA in the serum was extracted and was amplified with 35 cycles of polymerase chain reaction (PCR). Amplified DNA was electrophoresed and then was hybridized with the synthetic oligonucleotide probes coding the nonstructural protein (NSP) and was detected as 171 base pair bands. The viral DNA was detected in the serum at diagnosis and for more than 6 months thereafter except for on December 26, 1992. The antibodies to parvovirus B19 were measured using parvovirus antibody ELISA kits for viral capsid protein: IgG to VP-1 and IgM to VP-2 (Immunological Laboratories, Hamburg, Germany). IgM antibodies were not detected in the serum throughout the observation period, and IgG antibody was positive only on December 10, 1992, and was weakly positive on May 6, 1993, but was otherwise negative. The recovery of platelets may be due to the intial increase of IgG antibodies as well as to the administration of immunoglobulin.

There was in vitro evidence of involvement of myeloid and megakaryocytic series by paravovirus B19 infection. The viral DNA was detected in the granulocytes [2] along with viral RNA in the megakaryocytes [3]. The infected serum inhibited the growth of myeloid and megakaryocytic as well as erythroid progenitors in vitro [4].

Chronic or recurrent bone marrow failure in the combined immunodeficiency with immunoglobulins (Nezelof's syndrome), pure red cell aplasia in acquired immunodeficieny syndrome, severe anemia in acute lymphocytic leukemia during chemotherapy, and granulocytic aplasia in subtle immunodeficiency had been reported with persistent viremia [1]. Parovovirus B19 infection also caused bone marrow necrosis in sickle cell disorders [5]. Why the present patient had persistent parvovirus B19 viremia and

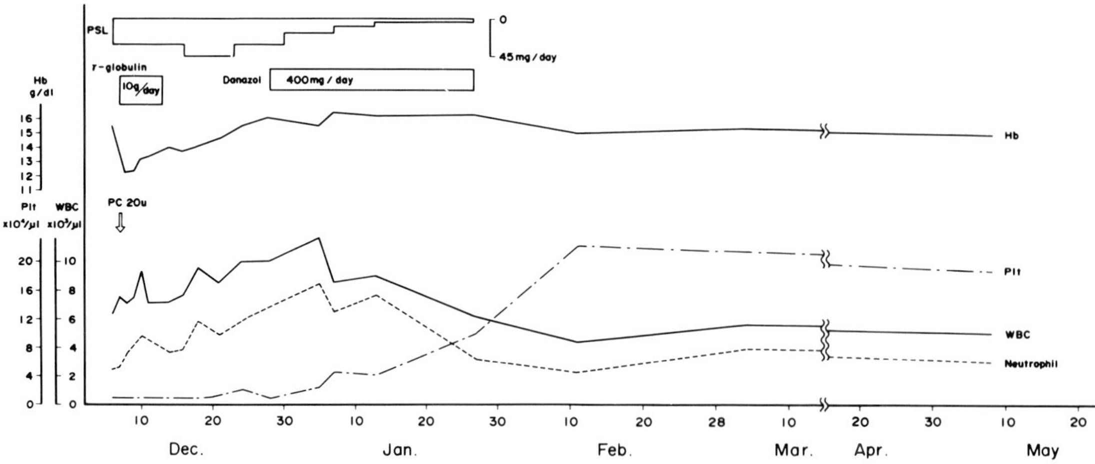

B19	DNA	(+)	(−)	(+)	(+)	(+)
	IgM	< 1.0	< 1.0	< 1.0	< 1.0	< 1.0
	IgG	2.37	< 1.0	< 1.0	< 1.0	1.0

Fig. 1. Clinical course of the patient. PSL, prednisolone, PC: platelet concentrate. The normal values of parvovirus B19 antibodies were <1.0 for IgM and IgG antibodies.

poor response of antibody production despite normal immunological function remains unknown. The method of direction of viral antigen has improved such that even a minimal amount of viral DNA can be detected by amplification.

EIICHI OEDA
KENJI SHINOHARA
HIROFUMI INOUE
JUN NOMIYAMA
Division of Hematology, Department of Medicine, Yamaguchi Prefecture Central Hospital, Hofu, Japan

REFERENCES

1. Harris JW: Parvovirus B19 for the hematologist. Am J Hematol 39:119–130, 1992.
2. Kutzman GJ, Gascon P, Caras M, Cohen B, Young NS: B19 parvovirus replicates in circulating cells of acutely infected patients. Blood 71: 1448–1454, 1988.
3. Srivastava A, Bruno E, Briddell R, Copper R, Srivastava C, Besien K, Hoffman R: Parvovirus B-19 induced perturbation of human megakaryopoiesis in vitro. Blood 76:1997–2004, 1990.
4. Hanada T, Koike K, Takeya T, Nagasawa T, Matsunaga Y, Takita H: Human parvovirus B-19 induced transient pancytopenia in a child with hereditary spherocytosis. Br J Haematol 70:113–115, 1988.
5. Conrad ME, Studdard H, Anderson LJ: Case report: Aplastic crisis in sickle cell disorders: Bone marrow necrosis and human parvovirus infection. Am J Med Sci 295:212–215, 1988.

Leishman's Stain, A Romanowsky Stain Suboptimal for Demonstration of Auer Rods

To the Editor: In patients with acquired immunodeficiency syndrome, detection of negatively stained cytoplasmic inclusions on examination of Giemsa-stained blood smear permits a rapid diagnosis of mycobacterial infection to be made [1]. In an index case of acute promyelocytic leukemia (APL) stained with Leishman's stain (a Romanowksy dye used for quick stain), similar negatively stained rod-shaped inclusions were observed. They were subsequently shown to be Auer rods on staining with May-Grünwald Giemsa. This study was therefore performed to determine if Leishman's stain was inferior to Giemsa stain for demonstration of Auer rods.

The index case was a 17-year-old man hospitalized because of sudden collapse and subsequently found to have intracerebral hemorrhage and pancytopenia. Examination of a Leishman-stained blood smear showed many heavily granulated and often bilobed immature cells, yielding a diagnosis of APL [2]. Auer rods were not identified. However, some cells contained negatively stained rod-shaped inclusions, giving a crisscross pattern in the cytoplasm and sometimes slit-like spaces in the nuclei (Fig. 1A). Staining for microorganisms including mycobacteria was negative. A May-Grünwald Giemsa stain performed subsequently showed many *faggot* cells (Fig. 1), which proved that the negative images as seen in the Leishman's stain in fact represented Auer rods.

Marrow blood smears from seven APL cases, which had been stored at −70°C, were retrieved from the archival hematology files. They were

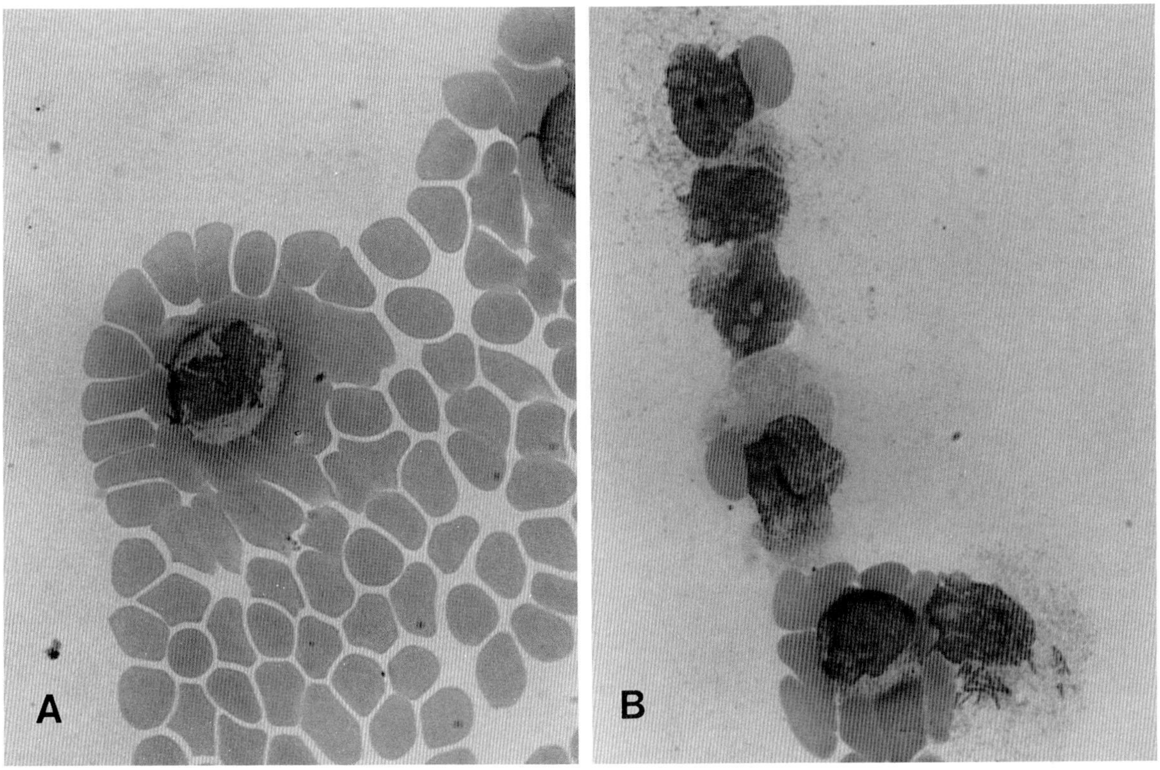

Fig. 1. A: Leukemic promyelocyte containing negatively stained rod-like inclusions, with a superficial resemblance to mycobacterium-infected cells. Leishman stain ×750. B: Promyelocytes from the same patient, showing many Auer rods in the ctyoplasm. Giemsa stain. ×750. erythrocyte counts by ICU day 17.

stained with both Leishman's and May-Grünwald Giemsa stains according to standard methods [3]. Five hundred abnormal promyelocytes or myeloblasts were examined under 100× oil immersion field. Cells with negatively stained rod-shaped cytoplasmic inclusions were identified in five cases and only in the Leishman's preparation. They corresponded to those cases with abundant *faggot* cells detectable by the Giemsa stain. Auer rod-containing cells were demonstrable in the Leishman's-stained smears in only one case, whereas they were found in all cases in the Giemsa-stained smears.

Examination of Romanowsky-stained blood or marrow smear is an important part in the investigation of hematologic disorders. A number of Romanowsky stains are available. Among them, Leishman's stain has the advantage of being a quick procedure that requires only about 10 min to complete [3]. However, fixation artefacts such as vacuolation of red cells may occur if the stain is contaminated by water [3]. Another problem with this stain is the failure to demonstrate Auer rods in APL, as shown in the present study. Similar results were also observed in acute myeloid leukemia of M1 or M2 subtype (FAB classification) [2]. Among 18 cases studied (data not shown), Auer rods were readily detected in six cases in the Giemsa-stained smears but were only barely recognizable in one of the Leishman's preparations. Failure to demonstrate Auer rods and, in particular, *faggot* cells in the microgranular form of APL [4] may lead to misclassification of the leukemia and thus deny the patient effective all-trans-retinoic acid treatment. Furthermore, the detection of negatively stained inclusions (Auer rods) in the leukemic cells may lead to an unnecessary search for mycobacterial infection and delay in the treatment of the leukemia. Hence caution has to be exericsed when Leishman's stain is used for the initial investigation of patients with acute leukemia.

K.F. Wong
S.K. Ma
J.K.C. Chan
J.S.L. Chung

Department of Pathology, Queen Elizabeth Hospital, Hong Kong

REFERENCES

1. Godwin JH, Stopeck A, Chang VT, Godwin TA: Mycobacteremia in acquired immune deficiency syndorme: Rapid diagnosis based on inclusions in the peripheral blood smear. Am J Clin Pathol 95:369–375, 1991.
2. Bennett JM, Catovsky D, Daniel M, Flandrin G, Galton DAG, Gralnick HR, Sultan C: Proposals for the classification of the acute leukemias: French-American-British (FAB) co-operative group. Br J Haematol 33:451–458, 1976.
3. Chanarin I (ed): "Laboratory Haematology: An Account of Laboratory Techniques." Edinburgh: Churchill Livingstone, 1989.
4. Bennett JM, Catovsky D, Daniel M, Flandrin G, Galton DAG, Gralnick HR, Sultan C: A variant form of hypergranular promyelocytic leukaemia (M3) (letter). Br J Haematol 44:169–170, 1980.

American Journal of Hematology 45:279–282 (1994)

Alpha Thalassemia and Stroke Risk in Sickle Cell Anemia

Robert J. Adams, Abdullah Kutlar, Virgil McKie, Elizabeth Carl, Fenwick T. Nichols, Jin Cai Liu, Kathleen McKie, and Anthony Clary

Departments of Neurology (R.J.A., E.C., F.T.N., A.C.), Biochemistry and Molecular Biology (A.K., J.C.L.), Pediatric Hematology/Oncology (V.M., K.M.), and Medicine (A.K.), Medical College of Georgia, Augusta

In an effort to identify possible risk factors for stroke in Sickle Cell Anemia (Hb SS), we analyzed the distribution of alpha-globin gene deletions in a group of Hb SS patients with and without stroke. The group with stroke consisted of 44 patients, (27 male, 17 female) with a mean of 7.5 years at time of stroke. The control group (non-stroke) had 256 Hb SS patients (126 male, 130 female) with a mean age of 7.7 years. There were 9 patients with heterozygous α-thalassemia in the stroke group (20.5%). In the control group, there were 93 patients with heterozygous α-thalassemia and 5 with homozygous α-thalassemia. The incidence of α-thalassemia in Hb SS patients without stroke (38%) was comparable to that reported for the African-American population in general. The incidence in the stroke population (20.5%) was significantly lower (*P* = 0.02) These results indicate that α-thalassemia is associated with a lower risk of stroke in Hb SS. This observation should be confirmed in studies involving larger numbers of patients. Possible protective effects of α-thalassemia are unknown but may be related to decreased hemolysis and more favorable rheologic properties of red blood cells.

Key words: stroke, sickle cell disease, thalassemia

INTRODUCTION

Stroke occurs in approximately 6–9% of children with sickle cell disease (Hb SS) [1]. Ischemic stroke is caused primarily by an occlusive vasculopathy involving the distal intracranial segments of the internal carotid artery, and proximal middle and anterior cerebral arteries [2]. It is clinically associated with significant morbidity and mortality in Hb SS children, often necessitating prolonged transfusion therapy to prevent recurrences.

The clinical course of Hb SS can be modified by certain genetic factors. Among these are α-thalassemia and the "high F" determinants which may or may not be linked to β-gene cluster haplotypes [3,4]. α-thalassemia is known to occur in approximately 30% of African-Americans [5] and co-inheritance of α-thalassemia (gene deletions) with Hb SS does have distinct effects on hematologic parameters. α-thalassemia decreases the rate of hemolysis by decreasing the MCHC, thereby resulting in higher Hb, HCT, and RBC values, and lower reticulocyte counts [6,7]. The clinical consequences of this interaction, however, are variable. While it is believed to decrease complications such as leg ulcers and kidney damage, it increases the likelihood of osteonecrosis and retinopathy. The effect of concomitant α-thalassemia on the overall survival of sickle cell patients is favorable, resulting in a higher frequency (up to 50%) of α-thalassemia in older patients [3,22,24].

Two reports have addressed the issue of α-thalassemia and its effect on stroke risk in Hb SS. Piomelli et al. [8] concluded that α-thalassemia was protective against early stroke, while Miller et al. [9] found no difference in the frequency of α-thalassemia in a small group of patients with Hb SS and stroke compared to the general African-American population.

Our goal was to study our pediatric Hb SS population with α-thalassemia for correlation with the prevalence of stroke.

METHODS

Three hundred patients with Hb SS attending the Pediatric Sickle Cell Clinic at the Medical College of Georgia

Received for publication July 7, 1992; accepted June 30, 1993.

Address reprint requests to Dr. Robert J. Adams, Department of Neurology, HB-2060, Medical College of Georgia, Augusta, Georgia 30912.

TABLE I. Hb SS Patients With and Without Stroke*

	Stroke (n = 44)	No stroke (n = 256)	*P*
Age: Mean ± SD	7.5 ± 3.8	7.7 ± 4.7	0.96
Range	1–18 years	6 mo–19 years	—
Sex: Male	27	126	—
Female	17	130	—
RBC ($\times 10^{12}$/L)	2.48 ± 0.40	2.78 ± 0.55	0.001
Hb (g/dl)	7.7 ± 1.1	7.9 ± 1.2	0.2
Hct (%)	21.7 ± 3.0	23.7 ± 3.7	0.001
MCV (fl)	88 ± 5.7	85.9 ± 9.3	0.1
MCH (pg)	31.1 ± 2.2	28.3 ± 3.5	<0.001
MCHC (g/dl)	35.0 ± 2.3	32.9 ± 2.2	<0.001
reticulocytes (%)	12.8 ± 4.5	10.9 ± 5.6	0.01
α-thalassemia	9/44 (20.5%)	98/256 (35%)	0.02
Hb F	6.3 ± 3.9	12.4 ± 9.8	<0.001

*Hb, hemoglobin; Hb F, fetal hemoglobin; Hct, Hematocrit; MCH, mean corpuscular hemoglobin; MCHC, mean corpuscular hemoglobin concentration; MCV, mean corpuscular volume; RBC, red blood cells.

formed the subjects of this study. The subjects all had α-globin gene numbers determined as part of their clinical diagnosis. Informed consent was obtained for all who participated in this study; 44 had a history of stroke documented by clinical and neurodiagnostic evaluations.

Hematologic data were obtained on a Sysmex K-1000 electronic cell counter (TOA Medical Electronics, Kobe, Japan) from venous blood collected in vacutainers containing EDTA as anticoagulant. Reticulocyte counts were performed manually on new methylene blue stained peripheral blood smears. Hemoglobin analyses and quantitations (IEF, citrate agar electrophoresis, and HPLC) were performed according to previously described methods [10,11].

DNA was isolated from peripheral blood WBC as described by Poncz et al. [12]. Five micrograms of genomic DNA from each patient was digested with restriction enzymes Bam HI and Bgl II, electrophoresed on agarose, transferred to a nitrocellulose membrane, and hybridized with an α-globin gene probe (PBR-α) to detect α-globin gene specific fragments, as described earlier by Fei et al. [13]. Descriptive statistics of the hematologic measurements were computed for the stroke and non-stroke groups. Owing to non-normality of the distributions of these variables, comparisons between the two groups were made using Wilcoxon's rank sum statistic.

The association of α-thalassemia status and stroke during the study period was evaluated by means of a contingency table, using the odds ratio as an estimate of the relative risk of stroke, given α-thalassemia status. Statistical significance was determined using the chi-square statistic. A 95% confidence interval was calculated for the odds ratio. Further analysis of this association used logistic regression to control for possible confounding by age and fetal hemoglobin levels of the study subjects. The odds ratio and its associated 95% confidence limits were calculated. In both methods, positive α-thalassemia status was considered the reference, or lower-risk, level.

RESULTS

The age, sex, hematologic data, and the frequency of α-thalassemia in 44 Hb SS patients with stroke compared with 256 Hb SS patients without stroke (SSNS) are presented in Table I. Of the 44 stroke patients, 42 had cerebral infarction and 2 had intracranial hemorrhage.

Mean age at the time of stroke was 7.5 years with a SD of ± 3.5. Mean age of the SSNS group was 7.7, with a SD of ± 4.7. Of the hematologic parameters shown in Table 1, RBC and hematocrit were significantly higher (2.78 ± 0.55 vs. 2.48 ± 0.40; $P = 0.001$, and 23.7 ± 3.7 vs. 21.7 ± 3.0; $P = 0.001$, respectively), and MCH and MCHC significantly lower (28.3 ± 3.5 vs. 31.1 ± 2.2; $P < 0.001$, respectively) in the SSNS group. Although MCV was lower in the SSNS group (85.9 ± 9.3 vs. 88.0 ± 5.7), the difference did not reach statistical significance ($P = 0.1$). Steady-state reticulocyte counts also differed significantly between the two groups (12.8 ± 4.5 vs. 10.9 ± 5.6%; $P = 0.01$) with higher values in the stroke group.

The difference in Hb F levels between the two groups was highly significant (6.5 ± 4.7 in the stroke group vs. 12.4 ± 9.7 in the SSNS group, $P < 0.001$).

The frequency of α-thalassemia in the stroke group was 20.5% (9/44 patients) compared to 38% (98/256 patients) in the SSNS group. All nine patients in the stroke group had heterozygous α-thalassemia (−α/αα). In the SSNS group, 93 patients were heterozygous (−α/αα) and 5 were homozygous (−α/−α) for α-thalassemia. All α-thalassemia deletions observed were of the $-\alpha^{3.7}$ type. The difference between the two groups was statistically significant (chi-square = 5.2; P =

0.023), with a crude odds ratio of 2.4 (95% confidence limits: 1.1–5.2). Using a logistic regression model including age and fetal hemoglobin levels, α-thalassemia was found to be associated with an odd ratio of 5.040 (95% confidence limits: (1.8–14). The absence of α-thalassemia was thus significantly associated with stroke after controlling for age and Hb F level.

DISCUSSION

The results of this study indicate that Hb SS children who develop stroke have a significantly lower frequency of α-thalassemia compared to those who do not develop stroke. The overall frequency of α-thalassemia in this cohort (38%) is comparable to that reported for pediatric Hb SS patients [14,15]. However, α-thalassemia is less prevalent in the stroke group (20% vs. 38%) with the difference between the two groups reaching statistical significance ($P = 0.02$). This study suggests that α-thalassemia exerts a protective effect against stroke in children with Hb SS.

Our results confirm and extend the observations of Piomelli et al. [8], who found only 4 patients with heterozygous α-thalassemia among 16 patients with stroke (25%), out of a total of 78 Hb SS patients with an overall frequency of 36% with α-thalassemia. Furthermore, among 11 patients who developed "early" stroke, none had α-thalassemia. The authors concluded that α-thalassemia protected against stroke occurring at early ages in Hb SS children.

In a more recent report, Miller et al. [9] found 5 of 20 Hb SS stroke patients to have heterozygous α-thalassemia (25%) and, comparing this to the approximate 30% frequency reported in the literature for the African-American population, concluded that single gene deletion (heterozygous α-thalassemia) did not protect from stroke in Hb SS. This study did not have a control population of Hb SS patients for comparison. Our results show a lower frequency of α-thalassemia in Hb SS stroke patients compared to controls without stroke suggesting that some degree of protection is associated with α-thalassemia.

The mechanisms responsible for this apparent protective effect of α-thalassemia against stroke in Hb SS are unknown. It is well established that α-thalassemia has marked effects on the hematology of Hb SS. These are mediated primarily through decreased intraerythrocytic Hb S concentration reflected in lower MCHC, leading to a decrease in deoxy Hb S polymerization (sickling), lower numbers of irreversibly sickled cells, and consequently reduced rate of hemolysis. This accounts for higher Hb, HCT, and RBC values, and lower reticulocyte counts [6,7,24]. These changes are more pronounced in Hb SS patients who are also homozygous for α-thalassemia (−α/−α), while those who have heterozygous α-thalassemia (−α/αα) are intermediate between the homozygotes and those who have normal α-globin genes (αα/αα).

Longitudinal study of developmental hematologic changes in Hb SS children has shown that differences in some hematologic parameters (MCHC, Hb, and % Hb F) between patients with four and three α-globin genes do not become apparent until age 7–8 years [14,16]. On the other hand, some other characteristics of α-thalassemia (decreased MCV and MCH, and lower reticulocyte counts) become evident as early as a few months after birth [16].

Another important consequence of concomitant α-thalassemia on the sickle RBC is its effect on red cell density distribution. Studies utilizing phthalate ester or stractan density gradient separation of RBCs have shown that, in addition to a significant decrease in the ISC or irreversibly sickled cells fraction, patients with α-thalassemia also show a reduction in cell heterogeneity, and a decrease in the proportion of dense cells [17–21]. Additionally, α-thalassemia improves RBC deformability in Hb SS [20]. The impact of these hematologic changes on the clinical manifestations is variable. Beneficial effects include prolonged survival, a decrease in chronic leg ulcers, and possibly kidney disease [3,19,21–23]. The severity and frequency of painful crises is not affected; skeletal complications such as the aseptic necrosis of femur and humerus, and retinopathy are increased, presumably as a result of the deleterious effect of a high hematocrit on blood viscosity [3,19,22–24].

The statistically significant differences in some hematologic parameters between Hb SS patients with and without stroke in our series (higher RBC and lower MCH and MCHC in the SSNS group) reflects a higher frequency of α-thalassemia in the non-stroke group (38%).

The difference in Hb F levels between the two groups are of interest since Hb F may also impact on stroke risk. Whether this difference in Hb F levels reflects a difference in the distribution of β globin gene cluster haplotypes between the two groups is currently under study. However, despite this highly significant difference in Hb F levels, logistic regression analyses controlling for fetal hemoglobin, age, and gender, still show that α-thalassemia is associated with a lower stroke risk.

It is conceivable that a decrease in the dense cell population, which includes the layer shown to be most adherent to endothelial cells ("deformable discocytes"), is associated with less damage to vascular endothelium and less severe vasculopathy involving major cerebral arteries.

An alternative pathogenetic mechanism may involve plasma hemoglobin. It has been speculated that direct contact with the Hb molecule may have a deleterious effect on endothelial cell function, presumably by inhibiting the synthesis of EDRF, and/or increasing the expression of Endothelin-1, thereby leading to vasoconstriction [25]. This mechanism has been incriminated in the pathogenesis of vasospasm after subarachnoid hemorrhage but has not been investigated in Hb SS related cerebrovascular disease. α-thalassemia may exert a beneficial effect by decreasing plasma hemoglobin concentration as a consequence of decreased hemolysis. Further studies are required to determine the mechanism of risk reduction for stroke in Hb SS with α-thalassemia.

ACKNOWLEDGMENTS

This work was supported in part by NIH-NHLBI grant HL-41544, T.H. J. Huisman, principal investigator. The contribution of Pam Lewis to the production of the manuscript and the cooperation of the patients and their families is gratefully acknowledged.

REFERENCES

1. Ohene-Frempong, K: Stroke in sickle cell disease: Demographic, clinical, and therapeutic considerations. Seminar Hematol 28:213, 1991.
2. Adams RJ, McKie V, Nichols FT, Carl EM, Zhang DL, McKie K, Figueroa R, Litaker M, Thompson WO, Hess DC: The use of transcranial ultrasonography to predict stroke in sickle cell disease. NEJM 326:605, 1992.
3. Nagel RL: Severity, pathobiology, epistatic effects and genetic markers in sickle cell anemia. Seminar Hematol 28:108, 1991.
4. Powars DR: Sickle cell anemia: β^s-gene cluster haplotypes as prognostic indicators of vital organ failure. Seminar Hematiol 28:202, 1991.
5. Dozy AM, Kan YW, Embury SH, et al.: α-globin gene organization in blacks precludes the severe form of α-thalassemia. Nature 280:605, 1979.
6. Embury SH, Dozy AM, Miller J, et al.: Concurrent sickle cell anemia and α-thalassemia: Effect on severity of anemia. NEJM 306:270, 1982.
7. Higgs DR, Aldridge BE, Lamb J, et al.: The interaction of α-thalassemia and homozygous sickle cell disease. NEJM 306:1441, 1982.
8. Piomelli S, Seaman C, Cirella B, et al.: Does α-thalassemia protect from early stroke in sickle cell anemia? Pediatr Res 10:285A, 1986.
9. Miller ST, Rieder RF, Rao SP, Brown AK: Cerebrovascular accidents in children with sickle cell disease and α-thalassemia. J Pediatr 113: 847, 1988.
10. Kutlar A, Huisman THJ: The detection of hemoglobinopathies. In F. Hommes (ed): "Techniques in Diagnostic Human Genetics." New York: Wiley-Liss, 1990, pp 519–560.
11. Wilson JB, Headlee ME, Huisman THJ: A new high performance liquid chromatographic procedure for the separation and quantification of various hemoglobin variants in adults and newborn babies. J Lab Clin Med 102:174, 1983.
12. Poncz M, Solowiejczyk D, Harpel B, Mory Y, Schwartz E, Surrey S: Construction of human gene libraries from small amounts of peripheral blood: Analysis of β-like globin genes. Hemoglobin 6:27, 1982.
13. Fei YJ, Kutlar F, Harris HF, Wilson MM, Milana A, Sciacca P, Schiliro G, Masala B, Manca L, Altay C, Gurgey A, de Pablos JM, Villegas A, Huisman THJ: A search for the anomalies in the ζ, α, β, and γ globin gene arrangements in normal Black, Italian, Turkish and Spanish newborns. Hemoglobin 13:45, 1989.
14. Felice AE, McKie KM, Cleek MP, Marino EM, Kutlar A, McKie VC: Effects of α-thalassemia-2 on the developmental changes of hematological values in children with sickle cell disease from Georgia. Am J Hematol 25:389, 1987.
15. Schroeder WA, Powars DR, Kay LM, Chan LS, Huynh V, Shelton JB, Shelton JR: β-cluster haplotypes, α-gene status and hematological data from SS, SC and S-β-thalassemia patients from Southern California. Hemoglobin 13:325, 1989.
16. Stevens MCG, Maude GH, Beckford M, Grandison Y, Mason K, Taylor B, Serjeant BE, Higgs DR, Teal H, Weatherall DJ, Serjeant GR: α-thalassemia and the hematology of homozygous sickle cell disease in childhood. Blood 67:411, 1986.
17. Rodgers GP, Schechter AN, Noguchi CT: Cell heterogeneity in sickle cell disease: Quantitation of the erythrocyte density profile. J Lab Clin Med 106:30, 1985.
18. Noguchi CT, Dover GJ, Rodgers GP, Serjeant GR, Antonarakis S, Anagnou NP, Higgs DR, Weatherall DJ, Schechter AN: α-thalassemia changes erythrocyte heterogeneity in sickle cell disease. J Clin Invest 75:1632, 1985.
19. Nagel RL, Fabry ME: The many pathophysiologies of sickle cell anemia. Am J Hematol 20:195, 1985.
20. Embury SH, Clark MR, Monroy G, Mohandas N: Concurrent sickle cell anemia and α-thalassemia: Effect on pathologic properties of sickle erythrocytes. J Clin Invest 73:116, 1984.
21. Fabry ME, Mears JG, Patel P, Schaefer-Rego K, Carmichael LD, Martinez G, Nagel RL: Dense cells in sickle cell anemia: The effects of gene interaction. Blood 64:1042, 1984.
22. Mears JG, Lachman HM, Labie D, Nagel RL: α-thalassemia is related to prolonged survival in sickle cell anemia. Blood 62:286, 1983.
23. Powars DR, Chan L, Schroeder WA: β^S-gene cluster haplotypes in sickle cell anemia: Clinical implications. Am J Ped Hemat/Oncol 12: 367, 1990.
24. Steinberg MH, Rosenstock W, Coleman MB, et al.: Effects of thalassemia and microcytosis on the hematologic and vasoocclusive severity of sickle cell anemia. Blood 63:1353, 1984.
25. Rybicki AC, Musto S, Swinson GI, Benjamin LJ, Nagel R, Schwartz RS: Increased levels of endothelin-1 in plasma of sickle cell anemia patients. Blood 78:202A, 1991.

American Journal of Hematology 45:283–287 (1994)

Autologous Peripheral Stem Cell Transplantation of the Blastic Phase of Chronic Myeloid Leukemia Following Sequential High-Dose Cytosine Arabinoside and Melphalan

Ursula A. Matulonis, James D. Griffin, and George P. Canellos
Divisions of Medical Oncology and Hematologic Malignancies, Dana-Farber Cancer Institute, Boston, Massachusetts

Blast-phase chronic myelogenous leukemia (CML) is the terminal phase in CML and is uniformly fatal. We treated 12 patients with blast-phase CML with a program of high-dose cytarabine 3.0 g/m^2 and melphalan 140 mg/m^2, followed by reinfusion of stem cells obtained from peripheral blood during the chronic phase.

Seven patients achieved either a partial or complete hematologic remission, while five patients showed no response to therapy. One patient returned to chronic phase features with loss of a chromosomal abnormality acquired at blast phase, restoration of hematopoiesis, and a decrease in the amount of bone marrow blasts to less than 10%. Six patients cleared their peripheral blasts and showed recovery of their myeloid and platelet lineages, but all six required treatment for acceleration within 3 months. Of the five nonresponding patients, three died with aplastic bone marrow, one patient never cleared peripheral blasts after chemotherapy, and one patient had evidence of peripheral blasts 3 weeks after the autologous stem cell reinfusion. None of the patients returned to a normal karyotype. The ablative regimen was effective in eradicating bone marrow blasts to <10% in 8 of 10 patients in whom interpretable bone marrow samples were performed following chemotherapy. Overall, the median survival for all patients from the time of stem cell reinfusion was 5.5 months.

We conclude that autotransplants with peripheral blood can successfully be used to support hematopoiesis during high-dose therapy for CML blast crisis, however, has no role by itself in the curative therapy of blast crisis CML. A small number of patients can be restored to chronic phase features, and this may provide an opportunity to administer subsequent alternative treatments designed to eradicate the malignant stem cell population. Autotransplants with stem cells may also be used as therapy for patients without a histocompatible marrow donor. However, the autotransplant may be more effective when used during the chronic phase of CML, with the use of hematopoietic growth factors, and with reinfusion of stem cells depleted of the malignant Philadelphia chromosome-positive clone.

Key words: CML, autotransplants, blast crisis, stem cells

INTRODUCTION

Chronic myelogenous leukemia (CML) is a clonal stem cell disorder characterized by a translocation of the long arms of chromosomes 9 and 22 forming the Philadelphia (Ph) chromosome. Clinically, CML is divided into three sequential phases: the chronic or stable phase, the accelerated phase, and the terminal blast phase.

Although patients in the chronic phase usually respond well to chemotherapy, results with cytotoxic chemotherapy during the blast phase are poor [1]. Results with allogeneic transplantation have varied according to the clinical phase of CML at the time of transplantation and the degree of histocompatibility between the donor and

Received for publication September 29, 1992; accepted September 22, 1993.

Address reprint requests to Dr. George P. Canellos, Division of Medical Oncology, Dana-Farber Cancer Institute, 44 Binney Street, Boston, MA 02115.

TABLE I. Patient Characteristics*

Pt. no.	Sex	Interval from diag. to PSCT	Age at PSCT	Type of blast crisis	Interval from PSCT to death
1	M	62 mo	30	My	7 mo
2	F	31 mo	43	My	53 days
3	M	100 mo	41	My	50 days
4	F	88 mo	43	L	43 days
5	M	34 mo	33	My	3 mo
6	M	43 mo	35	My	6 mo
7	F	50 mo	42	My	5 mo
8	M	82 mo	50	My	7 mo
9	M	42 mo	39	My	5 mo
10	M	46 mo	43	My	7 mo
11	F	13 mo	42	L	8 mo
12	M	24 mo	33	My	10 mo

*My, myeloid; L, lymphoid, PSCT, peripheral blood stem cell transplant.

the recipient [2,3]. Complications including leukemic relapse, graft-versus-host disease, interstitial pneumonitis, and graft failure contribute to morbidity and mortality. In addition, allogeneic transplantation excludes older patients and those not possessing a histocompatible donor.

Autologous stem cell reinfusion following systemic chemotherapy is a technique that allows patients to be treated with high-dose ablative chemotherapy and avoids the complications unique to allogeneic transplantation. Due to the unique situation in chronic-phase CML, during which the peripheral blood pool of hematopoietic stem cells is massively expanded, stem cells can be harvested and collected from these patients via the peripheral blood [6]. Our previous experience using autologous stem cells and four days of continuous conventional dose ara-c at 200 mg/m^2, followed by intravenous BCNU 600 mg/m^2, was successful in five of six patients, but all patients eventually relapsed and nonhematologic organ toxicity was excessive.

Cytarabine (ara-C), an S-phase specific agent, has efficacy in the treatment of CML blast crisis [4]. Kufe et al. [5] demonstrated that ara-C incorporation into the DNA results in loss of clonogenic survival. The incorporated ara-CTP is vulnerable to alkali degradation and leads to increased susceptibility to alkylating agents. These observations led to the suggestion that combining ara-C and alkylating agents may have a synergistic effect on leukemia cells.

We report here the results of a phase I regimen for the treatment of blast crisis CML consisting of high-dose ara-C and standard-dose melphalan as ablative chemotherapeutic agents followed by reinfusion of autologous stem cells collected during the chronic phase. Our goals were to assess clinical efficacy and define toxicity.

METHODS

Twelve patients with chronic phase CML underwent peripheral stem cell harvesting between 1978 and 1986. When patients were confirmed to be in the blast phase of CML, chemotherapy was initiated, followed by reinfusion of the autologous stem cells. Informed, written consent was obtained from all patients. Clinical and laboratory data are shown for these patients in Table I. All patients were Ph-positive by chromosomal analysis at the time of diagnosis. Ten patients had a myeloid blast crisis, and two had a lymphoid blast crisis determined by immunophenotyping.

Eligibility requirements included (1) documentation of patients in the blast phase of CML as defined by 30% blasts or promyelocytes in the bone marrow; (2) age <50 years; (3) previous leukopheresis and cryopreservation of peripheral chronic phase cells; (4) performance status of 0–2 (ECOG scale); (5) normal renal and hepatic function as defined by bilirubin <1.5 mg%, SGOT <60 IU, creatinine <1.5 mg/dl, and BUN <25 mg/dl; and (6) absence of active infection.

Seven of 12 patients underwent peripheral stem cell harvest at diagnosis or within 3 months of diagnosis. The remaining five patients underwent harvesting at 10 months, 1 year, 2.5 years, 3 years, and 4.5 years following diagnosis. Stem cells were collected peripherally during the chronic phase by means of a continuous-flow blood cell separator [6]. The cells were stored in 10% DMSO and frozen in liquid nitrogen (−196°C). Stem cells were stored for a median of 3 years (range 8 months to 6 years).

Patients were eligible to start systemic chemotherapy and stem cell reinfusion, once they were confirmed to be in blast phase. Following admission to the Dana-Farber Cancer Institute, patients were hydrated with 12 hr of intravenous saline (rate of 125 ml/hr) prior to chemotherapy, throughout chemotherapy, and for 24 hr after the last dose. Allopurinol 100 mg PO TID was begun 24 hr before therapy and continued throughout therapy. Cytosine arabinoside 3.0 g/m^2 was given intravenously over 3 hr for four doses at 0, 11, 24, and 36 hr. Melphalan 140 mg/m^2 was given intravenously over 60 min 12 hr after

TABLE II. Stem Cell Characteristics and Hematopoietic Reconstitution*

Patient no.	Amount of PB stem cells infused; viability[a]	Interval from SC collect. to reinfusion	No. of days to PMN recovery	No. of days to PLT recovery	No. of days to RBC recovery
1	13.2×10^{10}	5 yr	17	13	12
2	1) 3.4×10^{10} (88%)	2.5 yr	Never	Never	Never
	2) 3.7×10^{10} (86%)				
3	N/A	N/A	Never	Never	Never
	(1) 3.6×10^{9} (90%)	3 yr			
4	(2) 2.4×10^{9} (89%)		Never	Never	Never
	(3) 2.2×10^{10}				
5	1.34×10^{11} (91%)	3 yr	Never	11	13
6	2.7×10^{8} (66%)	8 mo	21	Never	Never
7	6.39×10^{10} (85%)	4 yr	19	13	16
8	2.25×10^{10} (91%)	6 yr	28	38	43
9	6.1×10^{10} (88%)	2.5 yr	13	11	19
10	3×10^{10} (68%)	4 yr	18	26	27
11	3.4×10^{9} (95%)	10 mo	18	25	26
12	5.9×10^{10}	2 yr	13	13	14

*PB, peripheral blood; SC, stem cell; PMN, neutrophils; PLT, platelets; RBC, red blood cells; PSCT, peripheral blood stem cell transplant.

[a]Percentage viability is given in parentheses.

the start of the initial cytosine arabinoside dose. Autologous stem cells were reinfused 60 hr following the start of the first dose of ara-C.

Bone marrow biopsies and aspirates were performed to document blast crisis prior to chemotherapy and stem cell reinfusion and post-stem cell infusion when clinically indicated. Cytogenetics pre- and post-stem cell reinfusion are listed in Table II.

Responses were scored as follows: a *complete response* was defined as restoration of chronic phase features, loss of acquired chromosomal abnormalities, and decrease in the number of bone marrow blasts to <10%, a *partial response* was defined as clearance of peripheral blasts and recovery of platelet and myeloid lines (plts > or = 20,000/mm^3 and absolute neutrophil count (ANC) >500 cells/mm^3), and *no response* was defined as failure to recover adequate hematopoiesis after transplant and/or failure to clear peripheral blasts.

RESULTS

All patients were evaluable for response to therapy. Patient No. 1 achieved a complete response, lost the acquired chromosomal abnormality t (16;16) (p13;q23) and showed a decrease in number of bone marrow blasts to <10%. This patient also recovered platelets to >100,000/mm^3 and Hgb >10g/dl. The patient remained in stable phase until dying of complications from a subsequent allogeneic bone marrow transplant.

Six patients (Nos. 7–12) showed a partial response to therapy with clearance of peripheral blasts and recovery of their platelet and myeloid lines (plts ≥20,000/mm^3 and absolute neutrophil count (ANC) > 500 cells/mm^3). All six patients required additional chemotherapy for acceleration within 3 months after return of their peripheral blood counts.

Five patients were scored as nonresponders. Three patients died without evidence of hematopoietic reconstitution. Patient No. 2 received a second stem cell reinfusion on day 42 because of failure to engraft and died of an intracranial hemorrhage on day 53. Patient No. 3 showed slow and incomplete myeloid recovery, no platelet recovery, and died of an intracranial hemorrhage on day 50 following the transplant. Patient No. 4 received two additional stem cell reinfusions for persistent aplasia on days 26 and 40. This patient died of sepsis on day 43 with no marrow recovery.

Patient No. 5 showed megakaryocytic recovery but remained in continuous CML blast relapse with the presence of peripheral blood blasts and bone marrow aspirates consistent with 20–30% blasts. He died 3 months after transplantation. Patient No. 6 relapsed with blasts in the peripheral blood as the peripheral counts returned on day 21 and was platelet and RBC transfusion dependent until he died 6 months after transplant.

The ablative regimen cleared bone marrow blasts to <10% in 8 of 10 patients with interpretable bone marrow biopsies. One patient (No. 3) had no bone marrow examination following chemotherapy, and pt. No 8 had 50% necrotic versus leukemic cells in the marrow when a biopsy was performed 1 month after chemotherapy.

Cytogenetics before and after chemotherapy and stem cell transplant are listed in Table III.. Patient Nos. 1, 6, 7, and 11 had partial loss of acquired chromosomal aberrations, but none reverted to a normal karyotype.

Toxicities with this regimen included eight episodes of bacteremia in six patients. The organisms involved were *Klebsiella* in two, *Staphylococcus aureus* in three, *Sta-*

TABLE III. Cytogenetics Before and After Stem Cell Transplantation*

Patient no.	Cytogenetics	
	Pretreatment	Post-treatment
1	Ph+ duplication t(16;16)(p13;q23)	Ph+ only
2	Ph+	No change
3	Ph+	N/A
4	Ph+	N/A
5	Ph+ isochromosome 17q	No change
6	Ph+ duplication duplication 17(q21-qter)	Ph+
7	Ph+ duplication isochromosome 17q trisomy 21	Ph+ isochromosome 17q
8	Ph+	N/A
9	Ph+ duplication ring chromosome 17 trisomy 8, 16, 19	N/A
10	Ph+ trisomy 8 extra Y chromosome	No change
11	Ph+ monosomy 7 t(9;9)(p11;p24)	Ph+
12	Ph+	N/A

*Ph, Philadelphia chromosome; N/A, not available.

phylococcus epidermidis in two, and *Escherichia coli* in one. Liver function tests were elevated in two patients, and four patients had oral herpes simplex viral infections. Two patients had tumor lysis syndromes after receiving the ara-C and melphalan. One patient (No. 8) experienced transient hypoxia and a fever after the stem cell reinfusion with transient hypoxia and a fever. One patient (No. 10) had a generalized tonic clonic seizure of unknown cause treated successfully with anticonvulsants.

Overall, the median survival for all patients from the time of stem cell reinfusion was 5.5 months, with a mean of 5.5 months. The survival curve is shown in Figure 1.

DISCUSSION

We treated twelve patients in the blast phase of CML with high-dose ara-C and melphalan followed by reinfusion of peripheral blood stem cells collected during the chronic phase of CML. Seven patients had full recovery of their myeloid and platelet lines, while five patients had partial or no recovery of hematopoiesis. Of these five, three patients displayed failure to engraft, and two had early relapse of CML.

Autologous transplantations for CML in blast crisis have been attempted by several groups [7–10] with generally poor long-term results. Median survival for blast crisis in these studies following stem cell reinfusion ranged from 4.5 to 11 months, similar to our observed median survival of 5.5 months.

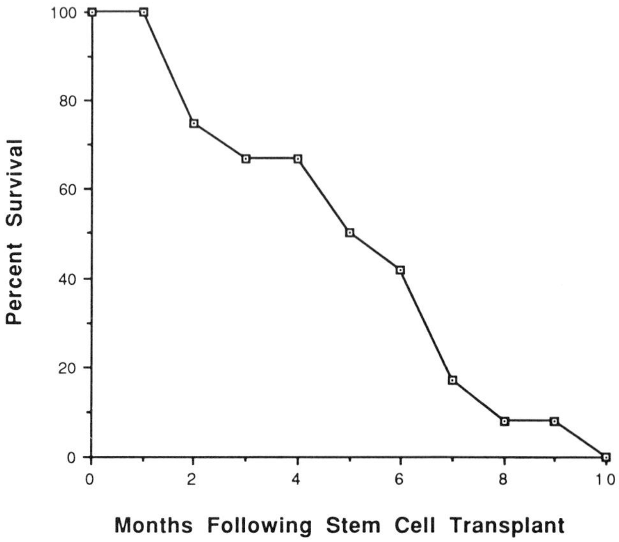

Fig. 1. Survival following peripheral stem cell autotransplantation for blast crisis CML.

Failure to undergo hematopoietic reconstitution was a significant problem in this study, with three patients dying in aplasia and two other patients failing to recover hematopoiesis, possibly due to leukemic relapse (Nos. 5 and 6). The patients who exhibited graft failure all had splenomegaly, but none showed evidence of bone marrow fibrosis (bone marrow data are not available for patient No. 3). The content of progenitor cells was not measured in the leukopheresis samples, but may have been inadequate in some cases. Also, stem cells were stored for up to 6 years, and the potential for loss of stem cells over long-term storage of CML cells is unknown.

The chemotherapeutic regimen of high-dose ara-C and melphalan was effective and cleared bone marrow blasts in 8 of 10 patients who had interpretable bone marrow examinations performed following chemotherapy. However, the ablative effects were short-lived and, as in previous studies, leukemia relapse occurred rapidly. Only one patient returned to stable phase, and 50% of patients failed to clear bone marrow blasts for more than 2 months. Thus, despite the apparent successful hematopoietic support of the stem cell autograft in the majority of patients in this study, resistant disease severely limited the success of this approach.

Methods of improving autologous transplantation results should focus on improving ablative chemotherapy regimens and using transplantation earlier in the disease. Efforts should also be made to improve engraftment, and the use of hematopoietic growth factors may be beneficial. Bone marrow from patients with CML grown in liquid culture with no added hematopoietic growth factors can spontaneously become depleted of Ph-positive cells [11]. This observation has been used clinically with uncertain early results [12,13] and may in the future improve the results of autologous transplants. Also, other techniques to purge Ph-positive cells from CML autografts have been explored, including mafosfamide purging and enrichment of CD34 + DR− stem cells [14].

Clearly, the therapeutic opportunity to obliterate the Ph-positive stem cell population lay in the chronic phase, since ablative chemotherapeutic regimens with or without radiation therapy have been unable to achieve effective eradication of the blast cells of the transformed phase.

REFERENCES

1. Coleman M: Combination chemotherapy for terminal-phase chronic granulocytic leukemia. Cancer and Leukemia Group B studies. Blood 55:29, 1980.
2. Goldman JM: Bone marrow transplantation for chronic myelogenous leukemia in chronic phase. Ann Inter Med 108:806, 1988.
3. Thomas ED: Indications for marrow transplantation in chronic myelogenous leukemia. Blood 73:861, 1989.
4. Iacoboni SJ: High-dose cytosine arabinoside: Treatment and cellular pharmacology of chronic myelogenous leukemia blast crisis. J Clin Oncol 4:1079, 1986.
5. Kufe DW: Correlation of cytotoxicity with incorporation of ara-C into DNA. J Biol Chem 255:8997, 1980.
6. Parker LM: Modifications of techniques for storage and reinfusion of chronic granulocytic leukemia (CGL) peripheral blood stem cells (PBSC). Proc AACR 22:172, 1981 (abst).
7. Butturini A: Autotransplants in chronic myelogenous leukemia: Strategies and results. Lancet 335:1255, 1990.
8. Reiffers J: Autografting for chronic granulocytic leukemia in transformation. J Natl Cancer Inst 76:1307, 1986.
9. Karp DD: Treatment of the blastic transformation of chronic granulocytic leukemia using high-dose BCNU chemotherapy and cryopreserved autologous peripheral blood stem cells. Am J Hematol 18:243, 1985.
10. Vellekoop L: Piperazinedione, total body irradiation, and autologous bone marrow transplantation in chronic myelogenous leukemia. J Clin Oncol 4:906, 1986.
11. Coulombel L: Long-term marrow culture reveals chromosomally normal hematopoietic progenitor cells in patients with Philadelphia chromosome-positive chronic myelogenous leukemia. N Engl J Med 308: 1493, 1983.
12. Barnett MJ: Successful autografting in chronic myeloid leukemia after maintenance of marrow in culture. Bone Marrow Transplant 4:345, 1989.
13. Barnett MJ: Autografting in chronic myeloid leukemia with cultured marrow. Leukemia 6(Suppl 4):118, 1992.
14. Carlo-Stella C: In vitro marrow purging in chronic myelogenous leukemia: Effect of mafosfamide and recombinant granulocyte-macrophage colony stimulating factor. Bone Marrow Transplant 8(4):265–273, 1991.

American Journal of Hematology 45:288–292 (1994

Serum Transferrin Receptor in Hereditary Hemochromatosis and African Siderosis

Roy D. Baynes, James D. Cook, Thomas H. Bothwell, Brian M. Friedman, and Theo E. Meyer

Divisions of Hematology (R.D.B., J.D.C.) and Cardiology (B.M.F.), Department of Medicine, Kansas University Medical Center, Kansas City, Kansas; and MRC Iron and Red Cell Metabolism Unit, Department of Medicine, University of the Witwatersrand, Medical School, Johannesburg, South Africa (T.H.B., T.E.M.)

The present investigation evaluated the serum transferrin receptor concentration in subjects with nontransfusional iron overload who were identified in two separate studies on the basis of a serum ferritin level above 400 μg/L. Subjects with preclinical hereditary hemochromatosis were evaluated in the first study and those with the African form of iron overload in the second. In the first study, hereditary hemochromatosis was identified in 14 white men on the basis of a persistent elevation in transferrin saturation above 55%. The serum receptor concentration was elevated above the upper cut-off of 8.5 mg/L in two of the subjects, but the mean receptor of 6.1 ± 1.4 mg/L (mean ± 2 SE) did not differ significantly from the normal mean for this assay of 5.6 ± 0.3 mg/L. In the same study, 60 control subjects with secondary iron overload were identified on the basis of a serum ferritin persistently above 400 μg/L, with a normal serum C-reactive protein concentration but with a transferrin saturation <55%. Three of these subjects had an elevated serum receptor concentration but the mean value of 5.5 ± 0.4 mg/L did not differ from normals nor from subjects with hemochromatosis. In the second study, 49 black Africans with iron overload were divided into those with or without an elevated transferrin saturation. The mean serum receptor concentration of 5.0 ± 0.8 mg/L and 4.5 ± 0.4 mg/L, respectively, did not differ statistically. It was concluded that there is no evidence of generalized dysregulation of the transferrin receptor in hemochromatosis or African siderosis.

Key words: serum transferrin receptor, hemochromatosis, African siderosis

INTRODUCTION

Hereditary hemochromatosis is an HLA-linked genetic disorder characterized by a limited but persistent, excess of dietary absorption relative to body iron stores [1,2]. The homozygous state for this common iron-loading disease is recognized in the laboratory by an elevation in plasma transferrin saturation prior to the development of clinical manifestations. The nature of the metabolic abnormality is not known. Many investigators believe that the disease results from an abnormality in the uptake, storage, or transport of iron by the gastrointestinal mucosal cell. This theory is in keeping with evidence that the mucosal cell in hereditary hemochromatosis is iron deficient relative to body iron stores [3–6]. An alternative explanation for the excessive absorption in these individuals is an abnormaly in the regulatory control of iron absorption by the intestinal tract. It is known that iron absorption is influenced by iron status and erythropoietic activity [7,8], but the precise mechanism for regulating iron absorption has not been identified.

The African form of iron overload is believed to result from an excessive intake of dietary iron in a highly bioavailable form [9] rather than a genetic abnormality of the host. However, recent family studies in black Africans with iron overload suggest that this condition may also be genetically determined and thereby result from the combined effect of environmental and host factors. The genetic basis of this African form of the disease is not associated with the HLA locus [10].

Received for publication March 13, 1993; accepted September 22, 1993.

Address reprint requests to Roy D. Baynes, Division of Hematology, Kansas University Medical Center, 3901 Rainbow Blvd., Kansas City, Kansas 66160-7402.

The transferrin receptor is a key iron-related protein that controls the uptake of iron from the circulation. A soluble form of the transferrin receptor has recently been identified in human serum [11–13], the concentration of which reflects the total body mass of tissue receptor [14]. Variations in the concentration of serum and tissue receptor are closely linked to iron absorption [15], with both increasing when there is iron deficiency or enhanced red cell production. This association raises the possibility that the serum receptor or its tissue form play a part in the regulation of iron absorption and are thereby linked to the absorptive defect in patients with hereditary hemochromatosis and/or African siderosis. While hereditary hemochromatosis is linked to chromosome 6 and the receptor coded on chromosome 3, the cis- and trans-acting regulatory factors and their chromosomal localizations are incompletely defined. In the present investigation, serum receptor measurements were performed in subjects with hemochromatosis and in subjects with iron overload from other causes. The objective was to evaluate the influence of iron overload on serum receptor levels and to search for a quantitative abnormality in serum receptor levels that might indicate a role for the transferrin receptor in the pathogenesis or as a marker of disordered cellular regulation of iron metabolism in the genetic disorder.

MATERIALS AND METHODS

Two independent studies were performed in men over 40 years of age to detect iron overload. In the first study, serum ferritin and transferrin saturation measurements were performed on normal white Afrikaner males participating in a coronary artery risk study, as previously described [2]. Iron overload was defined as a persistent serum ferritin concentration of >400 μg/L. Measurements of serum C-reactive protein were obtained as an index of inflammation and serum γ-glutamyl transpeptidase as an index of alcohol abuse. Normal values for these two measurements are <12 mg/L and 60 U/L, respectively. Subjects were further divided, on the basis of a transferrin saturation [2], into those with HLA-linked hemochromatosis (>55%) and secondary iron overload (<55%). Serum receptor measurements were performed in 74 out of 79 patients who were identified as having iron overload in the original survey.

A second study involved normal black males living in rural South Africa and at risk of nutritional iron overload on the basis of their geographic location, dietary intake, and their cooking and brewing practices [16]. Iron overload in this population occurs commonly as the result of ingesting large amounts of iron contained in local beverages fermented in iron cooking utensils. Recent studies have also raised the possibility that a portion of this population may suffer from a genetic defect in regulating iron absorption that is independent of the HLA-linked genetic disorder in populations of Northern European descent [10]. Forty-nine subjects were identified as having iron overload based on a serum ferritin of >400 μg/L, with 17 possibly having a genetic abnormality based on a transferrin saturation of >55%.

The serum iron and UIBC were determined using the methods of the Iron Panel of the International Committee for Standardization in Hematology [17,18]. Serum ferritin concentrations were assayed by an enzyme-linked immunosorbent assay (ELISA) technique [19]. The serum γ-glutamyl transpeptidase was measured as described by Persijn and van der Silk [20]. C-reactive protein was measured by an immunoturbidometric method after Melamies [21]. HLA-A, -B, and -C typing of T lymphocytes was performed by the method of Terasaki et al. [22]. The serum transferrin receptor was measured by ELISA established with monoclonal antibodies against purified human placental receptor and standardized in relation to intact transferrin receptor (13). Sera were stored at −20°C until the day of the assay.

Mean values for the various laboratory measurements were compared by unpaired t-tests to examine differences between individual groups within each study. Relationships between parameters were evaluated by the Pearson coefficient of correlation.

TABLE I. Laboratory Measurements in the Hemochromatosis Study

	Idiopathic hemochromatosis	Secondary iron overload
Number	14	60
Age (yr)	51.4 (4.8)[a]	52.6 (1.6)
HLA-A_3 frequency	0.64*	0.27
Hemoglobin concentration (g/L)	153 (8)	153 (4)
Transferrin saturation (%)	62.7 (3.6)	36.7 (2.2)
Serum ferritin (μg/L)	752* (557–1,016)	590 (541–644)
C-reactive protein (mg/L)	5.6 (2.1)	5.3 (1.2)
γ-Glutamyl transpeptidase (U/L)	88.6 (68.8)	62.3 (19.4)
Serum transferrin receptor (mg/L)	6.1 (1.4)	5.5 (0.4)

[a]Mean ± 2 SE.
*$P < 0.05$.

RESULTS

In the first study, the geometric mean serum ferritin in subjects diagnosed as being homozygous for hereditary hemochromatosis was 752 μg/L, which is significantly higher than the mean of 590 μg/L in subjects with secondary iron overload ($P < 0.05$) (Table I). The mean γ-glutamyl transpeptidase was also slightly higher in the hemochromatosis group but the difference was not statistically significant.

The serum transferrin receptor was elevated above normal in 2 out of 14 subjects with hereditary hemochroma-

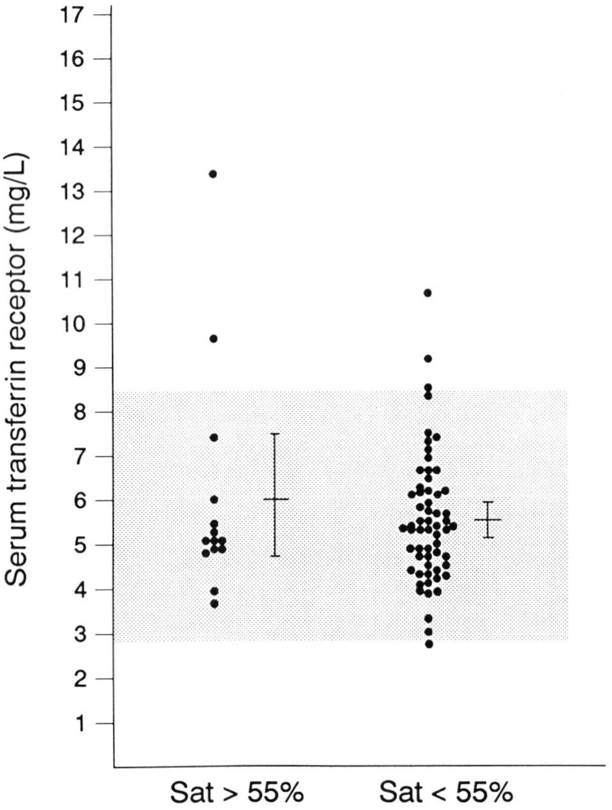

Fig. 1. Serum transferrin receptor concentrations in the hemochromatosis study. Mean ± SE values are represented. The shaded area represents the normal range.

tosis and in 3 out of 60 individuals with secondary iron excess (Fig. 1). The mean serum receptor of 6.1 mg/L in hereditary hemochromatotic subjects was nearly identical to the mean of 5.6 ± 0.3 mg/L previously observed in normal subjects. The mean serum transferrin receptor concentrations of 5.5 mg/L in subjects with secondary iron overload was also very close to the normal mean and did not differ significantly from subjects with hereditary hemochromatosis. Correlations among serum transferrin receptor concentration, transferrin saturation, and serum ferritin concentration were evaluated in order to assess whether iron overload was associated with a down-regulation of receptor below normal. None of the correlations were statistically significant when examined separately in the two subgroups or in the total group of 74 subjects.

In the African siderosis study, there were 17 males with a transferrin saturation >55% who were suspected of having a genetic component to their disease and 32 males with a transferrin saturation <55% and secondary iron overload (Table II). The group with a suspected genetic component, had a significantly higher geometric mean serum ferritin (2,132 μg/L) than those with secondary iron overload (841 μg/L; $P < 0.0001$). In neither group was the serum transferrin receptor elevated above the normal range, and in only one of the subjects was the value below the lower cut-off of 2.8 mg/L (Fig. 2). There was no difference between the mean serum transferrin receptor concentration in those with an elevated transferrin saturation as compared with those with a normal transferrin saturation (5.0 mg/L and 4.5 mg/L, respectively).

TABLE II. Laboratory Measurements in the African Siderosis Study

	Elevated transferrin saturation	Normal transferrin saturation
Number	17	32
Age (yrs)	56.4 (6.6)[a]	53.6 (4.6)
Hemoglobin concentration (g/L)	120 (13)	129 (11)
Transferrin saturation (%)	74.4 (7.4)	38.6 (3.4)
Serum ferritin (μg/L)	2132* (1,454–3,125)	841 (691–1,024)
C-reactive protein (mg/L)	3.6 (2.6)	5.0 (3.0)
γ-Glutamyl transpeptidase (U/L)	151.2 (84.8)	80.7 (35.2)
Serum transferrin receptor (mg/L)	5.0 (0.8)	4.5 (0.4)

[a]Mean ± 2 SE.
*$P < 0.05$.

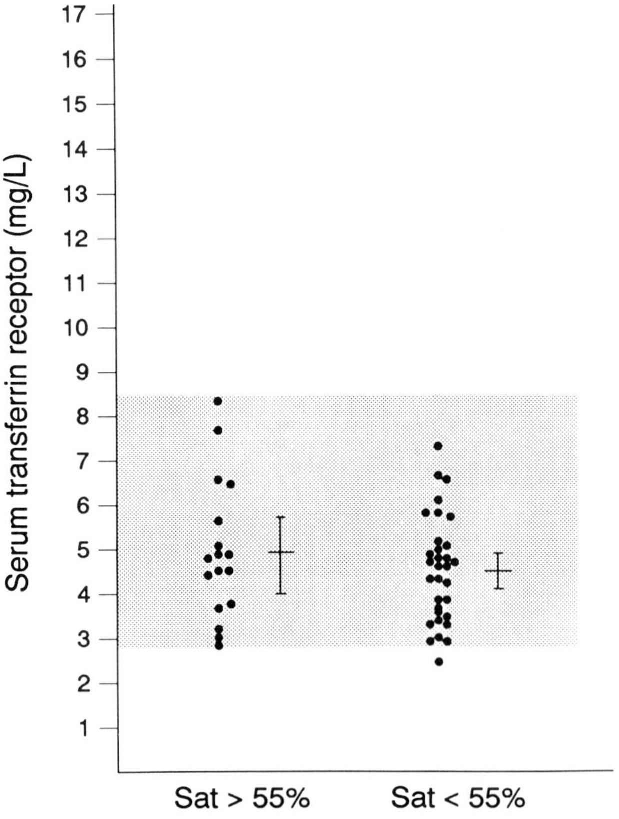

Fig. 2. Serum transferrin receptor concentrations in the African siderosis study. Mean ± SE values are represented. The shaded area represents the normal range.

No significant correlation was noted among serum receptor, serum ferritin, or transferrin saturation, either in the total group or in those with a transferrin saturation <55%.

DISCUSSION

The ability to measure the concentration of transferrin receptors in the serum has afforded an opportunity to explore more precisely the relationship between iron absorption and tissue iron uptake. It is possible to do so, since the main determinant of this new iron-related measurement is the total body mass of tissue receptors. The serum transferrin receptor has been shown to correlate with iron absorption in normal subjects [15] with both the serum receptor and iron absorption being increased in iron deficiency. Apart from iron status, the other major determinant of iron absorption is the rate of erythropoiesis. When erythropoiesis is enhanced, there is an increase both in iron absorption and serum transferrin receptor measurements as recently demonstrated in normal subjects given recombinant erythropoietin [8]. An increase in tissue receptor, as reflected in the serum receptor level, may also explain the dramatically higher absorption in patients with ineffective erythropoiesis as compared to those with hemolytic anemia and effective red cell production. In a recent study, it was shown that the elevation in serum receptor is significantly higher in patients with ineffective erythropoiesis due to hemoglobin E-thalassemia than in patients with hemolytic anemia [14].

The association in various clinical disorders between serum receptor concentration and iron absorption prompted the present study to evaluate serum transferrin receptor concentrations in two different forms of non-transfusional iron overload, namely hereditary hemochromatosis and African siderosis. The first is due to an inherited genetic defect located close to the HLA region on chromosome 6, while the latter results from an excess of dietary iron together with a possible genetic defect different from that responsible for hereditary hemochromatosis. Theoretically, either of these forms of iron overload could be the results of inappropriately raised levels of tissue transferrin receptor. The fact that the transferrin receptor is located on chromosome 3 and the hereditary hemochromatosis gene on chromosome 6 makes it unlikely that the receptor gene is directly responsible. However, the factors regulating receptor expression and their chromosomal origins are as yet incompletely established.

No evidence was found in the present study of inappropriately high serum transferrin receptor concentrations in untreated patients with preclinical hereditary hemochromatosis. This was true when the levels were compared with normal subjects and controls with a comparable degree of tissue iron excess. Our findings are in keeping with a prior report of serum transferrin receptor measurements using a polyclonal antibody assay in seven patients with treated hemochromatosis [14]. Although other iron measurements were not reported, the mean transferrin receptor was 9.50 mg/L whole blood as compared to 8.30 mg/L in normal subjects, which is similar to the findings in the present study. In neither study were the differences statistically significant. These results suggest that the HLA-linked iron-loading disorder is not the result of a generalized abnormality in transferrin receptor expression. If there is a regulatory abnormality affecting both ferritin and transferrin receptor, it would appear to be either localized to the gut or too subtle to be reflected in serum measurements.

The second major form of non-transfusional iron overload is African siderosis [9]. This condition results from the ingestion of increased dietary iron in a highly bioavailable form which is derived from the iron utensils used for the prepartion of fermented alcoholic beverages. A recent genetic study has raised the possibility that there may, in addition, be a non-HLA-linked hereditary component to African siderosis [10]. On the assumption that such a defect would lead to a raised transferrin saturation, as is the case in hereditary hemochromatosis, values above 55% were used to identify those patients who might have both a genetic abnormality and excessive intake of dietary iron. This approach had been used in the previously cited African siderosis study [10]. Serum transferrin receptor concentrations were, however, within the normal range in both those with a normal and elevated transferrin saturation, which suggests that any putative absorptive defect in the disorder is unrelated to an abnormality in transferrin receptor synthesis or expression. It should be noted that the subjects with African siderosis and an elevated transferrin saturation had a significantly greater degree of iron overload, as measured by the serum ferritin concentration, and this iron excess, rather than a genetic abnormality, may have accounted for their higher transferrin saturation.

ACKNOWLEDGMENT

This work was supported by NIH grant DK39246.

REFERENCES

1. Bothwell TH, Charlton RW, Motulsky A: Hemochromatosis. In Scriver CR, Beaudet AL, Sly WS, et al. (eds): "The Metabolic Basis of Inherited Disease." New York: McGraw-Hill, 1989, p 1433.
2. Meyer T, Baynes R, Bothwell T, Jenkins T, Jooste P, Du Toit E, Martell R, Jacobs P: Phenotypic expression of the HLA linked iron-loading gene in males over the age of 40 years: A population study using serial serum ferritin estimations. J Intern Med 227:397, 1990.
3. Valberg LS, Simon JB, Manley PN, Corbett WE, Ludwig J: Distribution of storage iron as body stores expand in patients with hemochromatosis. J Lab Clin Med 86:479, 1975.

4. Whittaker P, Skikne BS, Covell AM, Flowers C, Cooke A, Lynch SR, Cook JD: Duodenal iron proteins in idiopathic hemochromatosis. J Clin Invest 83:261, 1989.
5. Francanzani AL, Fargion S, Romano R, Piperno A, Arosio P, Ruggeri G, Ronchi G, Fiorelli G: Immunohistochemical evidence for a lack of ferritin in duodenal absorptive epithelial cells in idiopathic hemochromatosis. Gastroenterology 96:1071, 1989.
6. Pietrangelo A, Rocchi E, Casalgrandi G, Rigo G, Ferrari A, Perini M, Ventura E, Cairo G: Regulation of transferrin, transferrin receptor, and ferritin genes in human duodenum. Gastroenterology 102:802, 1992.
7. Bothwell TH, Pirzio-Biroli G, Finch CA: Iron absorption. I. Factors influencing absorption. J Lab Clin Med 51:24, 1958.
8. Skikne BS, Cook JD: Effect of enhanced erythropoiesis on iron absorption. J Lab Clin Med 120:746, 1992.
9. Bothwell TH, Charlton RW, Cook JD, Finch CA: "Iron Metabolism in Man." Oxford: Blackwell Scientific, 1979, pp 1–576
10. Gordeuk V, Mukiibi J, Hasstedt SJ, Somowitz W, Edwards CQ, West G, Ndambire S, Emmanual J, Nkanza N, Chapanduka Z, Randall M, Boone P, Romano P, Martell RW, Yamashita T, Effler P, Brittenham G: Iron overload in Africa. Interaction between a gene and dietary iron intake. N Engl J Med 326:95, 1992.
11. Kohgo Y, Nishisato T, Kondo H, Tsushima N, Niitsu Y, Urushizaki I: Circulating transferrin receptor in human serum. Br J Haematol 64: 277, 1986.
12. Kohgo Y, Niitsu Y, Kondo H, Kato J, Tsushima N, Sasaki K, Hirayama M, Numata T, Nishisato T, Urushizaki I: Serum transferrin receptor as a new index of erythropoiesis. Blood 70:1955, 1987.
13. Flowers CH, Skikne BS, Covell AM, Cook JD: The clinical measurement of serum transferrin receptor. J Lab Clin Med 114:368, 1989.
14. Huebers HA, Beguin Y, Pootrakul P, Einspahr D, Finch CA: Intact transferrin receptors in human plasma and their relation to erythropoiesis. Blood 75:102, 1990.
15. Cook JD, Dassenko S, Skikne BS: Serum transferrin receptor as an index of iron absorption. Br J Haematol 75:603, 1990.
16. Friedman BM, Baynes RD, Bothwell TH, Gordeuk VR, MacFarlane BJ, Lamparelli RD, Robinson EJ, Sher R, Hamberg S: Dietary iron overload in southern African rural blacks. S Afr Med J 78:301, 1990.
17. International Committee for Standardization in Haematology: Recommendations for measurement of serum iron in human blood. Br J Haematol 38:291, 1978.
18. International Committee for Standardization in Haematology: The measurement of total and unsaturated iron-binding capacity in serum. Br J Haematol 38:281, 1978.
19. Conradie JD, Mbhele BE: Quantitation of serum ferritin by enzyme-linked immunosorbent assay (ELISA). S Afr Med J 57:282, 1980.
20. Persijn J, van der Silk N: A new method of the determination of gamma-glutamyl transferase in serum. J Clin Chem Clin Biochem 11:421, 1976.
21. Melamies L: Rapid quantification of C-reactive protein by centrifugal analyses. Clin Chem 29:696, 1983.
22. Terasaki P, McClelland J, Park MS, McCurdy B: Microdroplet lymphocyte cytotoxicity test. In "Manual of Tissue Typing Techniques." Bethesda: National Institutes of Health, 1974, pp 67–72.

American Journal of Hematology 45:293–297 (1994)

Molecular Basis and Hematological Characterization of Hb H Disease in Southeast Asia

Ta-Chih Liu, Shyh-Shin Chiou, Sheng-Fung Lin, Tyen-Po Chen, Wen-Ping Tseng, Pao-Huei Chen, and Jan-Gowth Chang

Department of Internal Medicine and Pediatrics, Kaohsiung Medical College, Kaohsiung, Taiwan (T-C.L., S-S.C., S-F.L., T-P.C.); Department of Molecular Medicine and Clinical Pathology, Taipei Municipal Jen-Ai Hospital and Taipei Institute of Pathology, Taipei, Taiwan (W-P.T., P-H.C., J-G.C.)

We molecularly characterized sixty-seven cases of Hb H disease by the polymerase chain reaction. The strategy depends on amplifying the α-thalassemia-1 (α-thal-1) gene by primers flanking the breakpoint and sequence differences of the 3′ end of the α-globin gene and the nonhomologous elements I, II, and III among different types of α-thala-2. In the 67 cases studied, all involved α-thal-1 of the Southeast Asia type (SEA) in combination with deletional or nondeletional α-thal-2. Thirty-two cases were of the deletion form and 35 cases were of the nondeletion form. In 32 cases of the deletion form, 29 cases were rightward deletion ($-\alpha^{3.7}$), and three cases were leftward deletion ($-\alpha^{4.2}$). We found that all of the nondeletion forms were α-thal-1 of SEA type with Hb CS. After the subtyping of Hb H with $-\alpha^{3.7}$, 26 out of 29 were type I deletion and 3 out of 29 were type II deletion. Comparisons of clinical data of deletion forms and the nondeletion form showed that there were earlier occurrence of anemic symptoms and a larger erythrocyte volume in the nondeletion form group ($P < 0.005$).

Key words: Hb H disease, Southeast Asia, PCR, restriction enzyme digestion

INTRODUCTION

The α-thalassemia (thal) syndromes represent a common genetic disorder due to an absence or diminished synthesis of α globin chain of the hemoglobin [1,2]. The human globin gene cluster is located on chromosome 16p13.3-pter [3,4]. This cluster contains three functional genes (ζ2, α2, α1), three pseudogenes (ψζ1, ψα2, ψα1), and one gene of undetermined function (θ1) arranged in the order of telomere-ζ2-ψζ1-ψα2-ψα1-α2-α1-θ1-centrome within a 40-kb segment [5–7]. α-Thalassemia frequently results from deletions involving one (−α) or both (- -) α-globin genes; it is less frequently a result from nondeletional mutations involving one or a few nucleotides within the structural gene ($\alpha^T\alpha$ or $\alpha\alpha^T$) [8].

Individuals with α-thalassemia traits have mild microcytic hypochromic anemia, which is usually caused by a deletion of one (−α/αα) or two (- -/αα or −α/−α) α-genes. The patients with Hb H disease (- -/−α) have a moderately severe hemolytic anemia with a variable clinical course. In cases of hydrops fetalis with Hb Bart's (--/--), severe intrauterine anemia develops and results in fetal death at or around the time of birth [8].

Population studies have indicated that the types and frequencies of the different α-thalassemia defects vary among different ethnic groups [8]. In China and Southeast Asia, the most common α-thal-1 defect is the Southeast Asia (SEA) type deletion, which loses nearly 20 kb DNA of the α-globin gene cluster. The most common defect of α-thal-2 is the rightward deletion ($-\alpha^{3.7}$), followed by the leftward deletion ($-\alpha^{4.2}$) [9–11]. Hb H disease results from co-inheritance of the α-thal-1 of SEA type and α-thal-2 (deletion or nondeletion form) [12,13]. The most common nondeletional form is Hb Constant Spring (Hb CS). The molecular characterization of Hb H disease mentioned in previous reports was performed by restriction enzyme mapping of the Southern blot hybridization. In this study, we present a rapid, simple, and

Received for publication March 22, 1993; accepted September 22, 1993.

Address reprint requests to Dr. Jan-Gowth Chang, Department of Molecular Medicine and Clinical Pathology, Taipei Municipal Jen-Ai Hospital, 10, Section 4, Jen-Ai Road, Taipei, Taiwan.

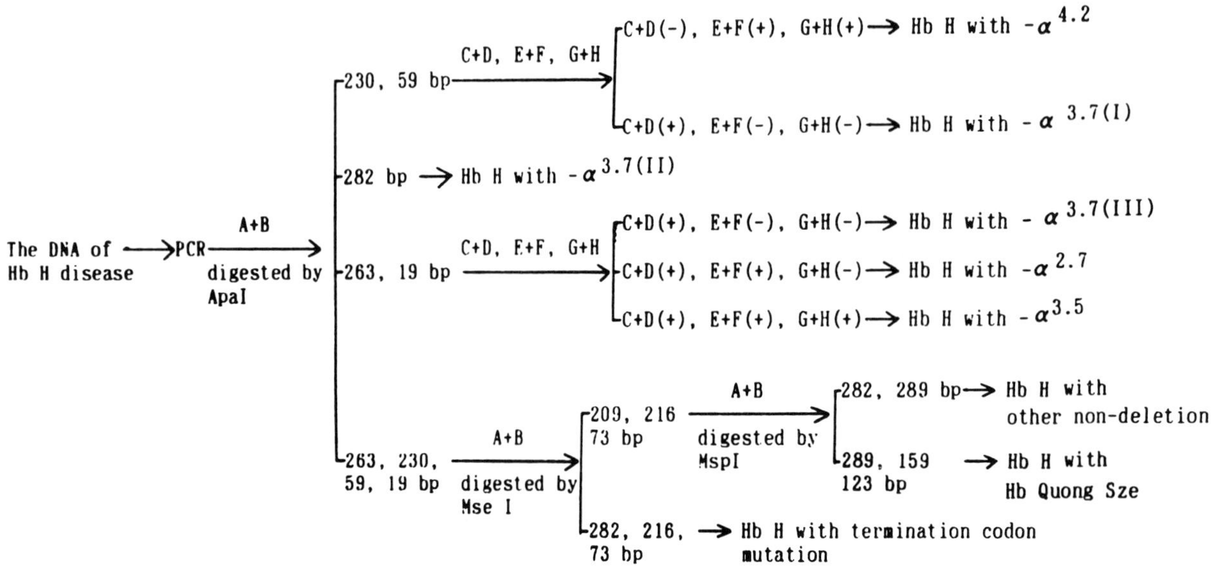

Fig. 1. Strategy for diagnosis of Hb H disease by PCR and restriction enzyme digestion. The fragments amplified by primers A+B and digestion by *Apa*I were used to differentiate between the deletion and nondeletion forms. The PCR products of primers C+D, E+F, and G+H were used to distinguish the subtypes of the deletion forms. The nondeletion form of Hb H was further divided to terminate codon mutation. Hb Quong Sze, and other nondeletion forms by PCR of primers A+B and digested by *Mse*I and *Msp*I, respectively. A+B, C+D, E+F, and G+H denote primer pairs, which are shown in Fig. 2.

accurate method for molecular diagnosis of Hb H disease in Southeast Asians.

MATERIALS AND METHODS

Patient Selection

Sixty-seven cases of Hb H disease of different families were collected from Kaohsiung Medical College Hospital, Taipei Jen-Ai Hospital and Taipei Institute of Pathology from July 1987 to June 1992. Hematological data were obtained by standard methods. DNA was extracted from peripheral blood by phenol and chloroform as described [14]. Eleven cases previously analyzed by Southern blot hybridization method were used as positive controls. Several cases of hydrops fetalis and normal subjects were used as positive and negative controls for the α-thal-1 gene of the SEA type, respectively [15].

Strategy for Hb H Disease Diagnosis

The strategy of diagnosis of Hb H disease in this study is shown in Figure 1. It is based on the three important aspects of Hb H disease in Southeast Asia. First, the α-thal-1 gene of Hb H disease in this area is mostly due to the SEA type, but rarely of Philippine or Thailand type. The deletions of these types involved almost all of the α-globin gene cluster (at least ψα2, ψα1, α2, α1) [15–17]. Second, the deletional types of α-thal-2 involved different portions of the nonhomologous region of the α-globin gene cluster. For the $-\alpha^{3.7}$ deletion, nonhomologous II and III are deleted, but region I remains intact. $-\alpha^{4.2}$ deletes nonhomologous I, but regions II and III remain intact. However, all the nonhomologous regions are intact in the non-deletional form of α-thal-2 [8,9,18–21]. Finally, the fragments were different between the deletion form and nondeletion form after restriction enzyme *Apa*I digestion of the PCR products for 3′ end of α-globin gene [18].

The Primers and PCR Procedure

The primers used to detect α-thal-1 gene were the same as in our previous reports [15,16]. The experimentally designed primers for α-thal-2 gene are shown in Figure 2. For distinguishing between the deletion form and nondeletion form Hb H disease, PCR products of primers A+B were digested by ApaI. The PCR products of primers C+D, E+F, and G+H for nonhomologous regions I, II, and III were used to distinguish further the types of deletion. To characterize the nondeletional form α-thal-2, the PCR products of primers A+B were digested by *Mse*I and *Msp*I to detect termination codon mutation and Hb Quong Sze, respectively [2,22]. For further differentiation of $\alpha^{cs}\alpha$ from other termination codon mutations, two pairs of mutagenesis primers were used as described [23]. PCR was performed as described [24], and the program was determined by the length and Tm of the primers. The PCR products were analyzed by electrophoresis in 3% agarose gel, stained with ethidium bromide.

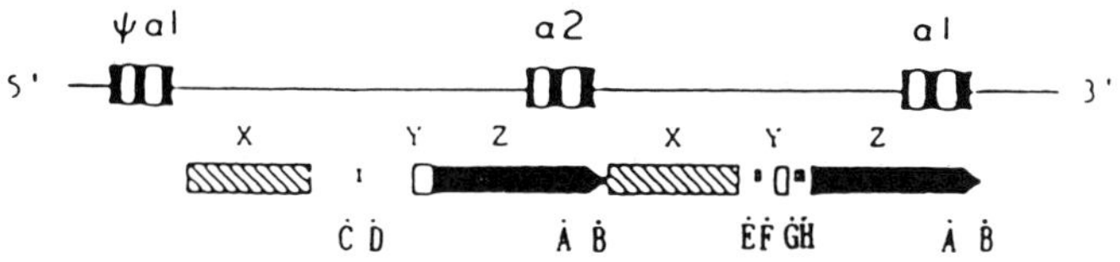

Primer sequence	Position
A = 5'-GCAGAGGATCACGCTGGTTG-3'	nt 60 to 80 downstream to the 3' end of the exon 2
B = 5'-GGTGCAAGAAGGGGAGGAG-3'	nt 51 to 70 downstream to the termination codon
C = 5'-GTGTTACTAAAGTAGGAGAGTGTC-3'	nt -2000 to -1977 upstream to the α 2
D = 5'-TAATCAGTGAGACTGTGGAATGG-3'	nt -1717 to -1739 upstream to the α 2
E = 5'-GAAGCATTGCTAAGCTGGTCG-3'	nt -1533 to -1513 upstream to the α 1
F = 5'-CAGCCTGAGAAATCACTGATAAG-3'	nt -1325 to -1347 upstream to the α 1
G = 5'-CAGGAAGCCCTCAGACTAACC-3'	nt -1051 to -1031 upstream to the α 1
H = 5'-CAATAGCTGGAACCGGCTGGA-3'	nt -885 to -905 upstream to the α 1

Fig. 2. Schematic diagram of a portion of α-globin gene cluster and the location of primer pairs in relation to the gene cluster. The duplicated XYZ boxes and nonhomologous regions I, II, and III are also shown. The sequences and position of primers are shown below the diagram.

RESULTS

All our cases had an α-thal-1 allele of SEA type (data not shown) and an α-thal-2 allele of different types. The results of the different types of α-thal-2 are shown in Figure 3. For Hb H disease with $-\alpha^{3.7(I)}$, there was an *Apa*I restriction site at the 3′ end of the remaining α-globin gene; a 230-base pair (bp) fragment was found after *Apa*I digestion of PCR products of primers A+B (Fig. 3A,E). In the Hb H with $-\alpha^{3.7(II)}$, a 282-bp fragment was noted after *Apa*I digestion, because there was no *Apa*I site in the remaining α-globin gene (Fig. 3B,E). The 230-bp fragment was also noted in Hb H with $-\alpha^{4.2}$ (Fig. 3C). To discriminate $-\alpha^{3.7}$ and $-\alpha^{4.2}$ further, PCR was performed with the primers C+D, E+F, and G+H. The PCR products of primers C+D (284 bp), but not E+F (209 bp) or G + H (167 bp), were found in HB H with $-\alpha^{3.7}$ (Fig. 3A,B). However, the PCR products of E+F and G+H, but not C+D, were noted in $-\alpha^{4.2}$ (Fig. 3C). For Hb H with Hb CS, which has two α-globin genes, the 282-bp and 230-bp fragments were noted after digestion of PCR products of primers A+B. The PCR products of C+D, E+F, and G+H were also found (Fig. 3D). To differentiate termination codon mutation from other nondeletion forms, the PCR products of primers A+B were digested by *Mse*I. There is a *Mse*I site at the 3′ end of the normal α1- and α2-genes, but the restriction site was abolished in the α2-gene of the termination codon mutation (Fig. 3D). The results showed that 35 cases were Hb CS, 29 cases were $-\alpha^{3.7}$, and three cases were $-\alpha^{4.2}$. Of 29 $-\alpha^{3.7}$ deletion, 26 cases were type I deletion and 3 cases were type II deletion.

The clinical data are shown in Table I. There are significant differences in ages for the patient's first time to be examined by a doctor due to anemic symptoms or signs (exertional dyspnea, palpitation, headache, dizziness, or pale face), and there was also a significant difference of mean corpuscular volume (MCV) between the deletion and nondeletion forms of Hb H disease. We found that the patients of Hb H with Hb CS had an earlier occurrence of anemic symptoms or signs (9.9 ± 7.6 years of age) and higher MCV (71.0 ± 7.5 fl) as compared to the deletion form Hb H disease (33.1 ± 16.9 years of age for the occurrence of symptoms or signs and 65.4 ± 6.7 fl for MCV). There were no other differences between the hematologic data of these two groups.

DISCUSSION

We have developed a simple and rapid method to molecularly characterize the Hb H disease. The method could be used in regions that have cases of α-thal-1 with a long deletion of α-globin gene cluster (delete ψα, α2, α1 gene), such as -- MC type, -- CL type, -- Brit type, -- SA type, $-(\alpha)^{20.5}$, -- MED type, -- SEA type, -- THAI type, and -- FIL type. However, this method cannot be used to detect $\alpha\alpha^{RA}$ type and $-(\alpha)^{5.2}$ type [8].

In addition to the $-\alpha^{3.7}$ and $-\alpha^{4.2}$ α-thal-2 deletions, three other types of α-thal-2 have been reported ($-\alpha^{3.5}$,

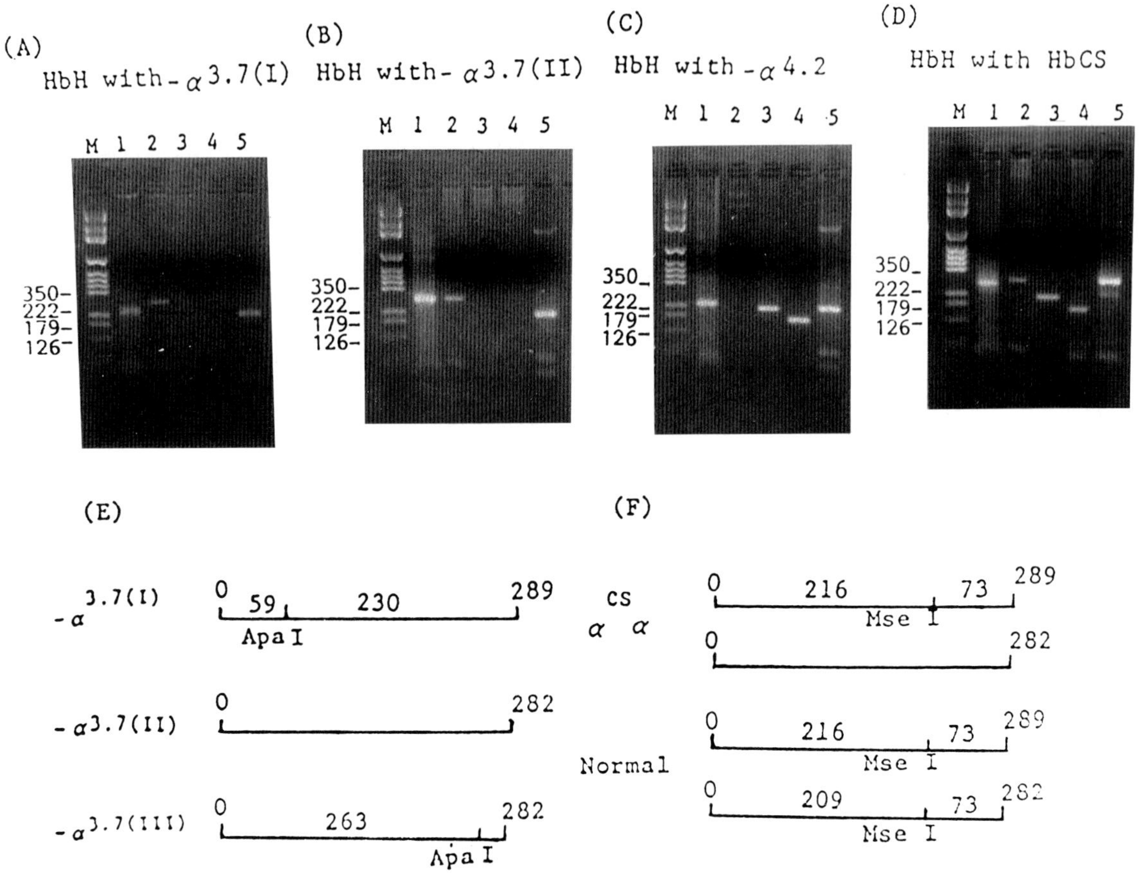

Fig. 3. The results of PCR products and restriction enzyme digestion. The amplified products of primers A+B are 289 bp (α1) and 282 bp (α2). The PCR products were digested by *ApaI* (lane 1) or *MseI* (lane 5). The PCR products of primers C+D (lane 2) is 284 bp, primers E+F (lane 3) is 209 bp, and primers G+H (lane 4) is 167 bp. A: The result of Hb H with $-\alpha^{3.7(I)}$. B: The result of Hb H with $-\alpha^{3.7(II)}$. C: The result of Hb H with $-\alpha^{4.2}$. D: The result of Hb H with Hb CS. E,F: Length and restriction sites (*ApaI*, *MseI*) of the products amplified by primers A+B. M represents the pGem marker.

TABLE I. The Hematological Parameters of Hb H Disease†

Parameters	Nondeletion form (n = 35)	Deletion form (n = 32)
Age (y/o)*	9.9 ± 7.6	33.1 ± 16.9
RBC × 10^4 (μl)	456 ± 77	487 ± 66
Hb (g/dl)	8.6 ± 1.2	9.1 ± 1.2
MCV (fl)*	71.0 ± 7.5	65.4 ± 6.7
MCH (pg)	19.4 ± 2.2	18.9 ± 1.4

†Student's t-test was used for statistical analysis.
**P* is significant between the nondeletion form and deletion form groups ($P < 0.005$).

$-\alpha^{2.7}$, $-\alpha^{5.3}$) [25–27]. The deletion junction of $-\alpha^{5.3}$ was known, and we can design the primers located on either side of the junction area to amplify this region to identify it. Although the definite deletion junctions of $-\alpha^{2.7}$ and $-\alpha^{3.5}$ were not clear, we used the differences of nonhomologous regions II and III and the different 3′ end of the α-globin gene, which remained to detect them.

For the nondeletion forms, our method used to detect Hb CS and Hb Quong Sze is easier, eliminates complex procedures, and avoids radioisotopes more than other methods [28,29]. For other nondeletion forms, we can sequence the PCR products of the whole α1- and α2-genes by using the specific primers. The primers are the same as primers used in our previous report [24], but the materials used were DNA, as opposed to RNA.

The clinical data show that the MCV and the occurrence of anemic symptoms and signs in these deletion forms and nondeletion Hb H disease are different. These cases of Hb H with Hb CS have an earlier occurrence of clinical symptoms and may have a poor prognosis relative to the deletion form, and our findings correspond with those of other reports [30,31].

Our method was able to characterize Hb H genotypes more rapidly and could be used not only in the clinical analysis and prenatal diagnosis but also in finding new types of Hb H disease.

ACKNOWLEDGMENTS

This work was supported in part by grants from the National Science Council of the Republic of China and Taipei Institute of Pathology (NSC-82-0412-B196-004-MO2 and TIP 8201).

REFERENCES

1. Weatherall DJ, Clegg JB: "The Thalassemia Syndrome." Oxford: Blackwell, 1981.
2. Bunn HF, Forget BG: "Hemoglobin: Molecular, Genetic, and Clinical Aspects." Philadelphia: WB Saunders. 1986.
3. Breuning MH, Madan K, Verjaal M, Wijnen JT, Meera Khan P, Pearson PL: Human α-globin maps to pter–p13.3 in chromosome 16 distal to PGP. Hum Genet 76:287, 1987.
4. Buckle VJ, Higgs DR, Wilkie AOM, Super M, Weatherall DJ: Localization of human α-globin to 16p13.3-pter. J Med Genet 25:847, 1988.
5. Lauer J, Shen CKJ, Maniatis T: The chromosomal arrangement of human α-like globin genes: Sequence homology and α-globin gene deletions. Cell 20:119, 1980.
6. Proudfoot NJ, Maniatis T: The structure of a human α-globin pseudogene and its relationship to α-globin gene duplication. Cell 21:537, 1980.
7. Hardison RC, Sawada I, Cheng JF, Shen CKJ, Schmid CW: A previously undetected pseudogene in the human α-globin gene cluster. Nucl Acids Res 14:1903, 1986.
8. Higgs DR, Vickers MA, Wilkie AOM, Pretorious IM, Jarman Ap, Weatherall DJ: A review of the molecular genetics of the human α-globin gene cluster. Blood 73:1081, 1989.
9. Embury SH, Lebo RV, Dozy AM, Kan YW: Organization of the α-globin genes in the Chinese α-thalassemia syndromes. J Clin Invest 63:1307, 1979.
10. Zeng YT, Huang SZ: α-Globin Gene organization and prenatal diagnosis of α-thalassemia in Chinese. Lancet 1:304, 1985.
11. Chan V, Chan TK, Cheng MY, Kan YW, Todd D: Organization of the ζ-α genes in Chinese. Br J Haematol 64:97, 1986.
12. Lee HH, Cheung WF, Chang JG, Liu TC, Leung WY, Ng HT, Choo KB: Molecular analysis of hemoglobin H disease in Taiwan. Proc Natl Sci Counc B ROC 12:52, 1988.
13. Peng HW, Han SH, Chow TX, Ho CH, Chin KN, Chiang BN: The molecular basis of Hb H disease in Taiwan. Hum Genet 78:137, 1988.
14. Liu TC, Lin SF, Chen TP, Liu HW, Chang JG: Mutation analysis of the ras gene in myelocytic leukemia by polymerase chain reaction and oligonucleotide probes. J Formosan Med Assoc 90:825, 1991.
15. Chang JG, Lee LS, Lin CP, Chen PH, Chen CP: Rapid diagnosis of α-thalassemia-1 of Southeast type and hydrops fetalis by polymerase chain reaction. Blood 78:853, 1991.
16. Chang JG, Chen CP, Ho HJ, Lin CP, Lee LS, Chen PH: Rapid prenatal diagnosis of Hb Bart's hydrops fetalis in Southeast Asia area by polymerase chain reaction. Int J Hematol 56:155, 1992.
17. Fischel-Ghodsian N, Vickers MA, Seip M, Winichagoon P, Higgs DR: Characterization of two deletions that remove the entire human ζ-α globin gene complex ($--^{Thai}$ and $--^{Fil}$). Br J Hematol 70:233, 1988.
18. Higgs DR, Hill AVS, Bowden DK, Weatherall DJ, Clegg JB: Independent recombination events between the duplicated human α globin genes; implications for their concerted evolution. Nucl Acids Res 12:6965, 1984.
19. Michelson AM, Orkin SH: Boundaries of gene conversion within the duplicated human α globin genes. J Biol Chem 258:15245, 1983.
20. Liebhaber SA, Goossens MJ, Kan YW: Homology and concerted evolution at the α1 and α2 loci of human α-globin. Nature 290:26, 1981.
21. Hess JF, Schmid CW, Shen CKJ: A gradient of sequence divergence in the human adult α-globin duplication units. Science 226:67, 1984.
22. Goossens MJ, Lee KY, Liebhaber SA, Kan YW: Globin structural mutant $\alpha^{125Leu \rightarrow Pro}$ is a novel cause of α thalassemia. Nature 296:864, 1982.
23. Chang JG, Tseng WP, Yang LH, Lee LS, Chen PH, Liu TC: Rapid diagnosis of Hb Constant Spring and Hb E by amplified created restriction sites. Blood 81:565, 1993.
24. Liu TC, Yen JS, Shen JS, Chen YH, Lee LS, Chen PH, Chang JG: Rapid molecular diagnosis of hemoglobin variants by RT-PCR of reticulocyte mRNA and direct sequencing. Hemoglobin 16:379, 1992.
25. Lacerra G, Fioretti G, De Angioletti M, Pagano L, Guarino E, de Bonis C, Viola A, Maglione G, Scarallo A, De Rosa L, Carestia C: $(\alpha)\alpha^{5.3}$: A novel α^{+}-thalassemia deletion with the breakpoints in the α2-globin gene and in close proximity to an Alu family repeat between the ψα2- and ψα1-globin genes. Blood 78:2740, 1991.
26. Kulozik AE, Kar CC, Serjeant GR, Serjeant BE, Weatherall DJ: The molecular basis of α thalassemia in India. Its interaction with sickle cell gene. Blood 71:467, 1988.
27. Zhao JB, Zhao L, Fei YJ, Liu JC, Huisman THJ: A novel α-thalassemia-2 (−2.7kb) observed in a Chinese patient with Hb H disease. Am J Hematol 38:248, 1991.
28. Kropp GL, Fucharoen S, Embury SH: Selective enzymatic amplification of α2-globin DNA for detection of the hemoglobin Constant Spring mutation. Blood 73:1987, 1989.
29. Kropp GL, Fucharoen S, Embury SH: Asymmetrically primed selective amplification/temperature shift fluorescence polymerase chain reaction to detect the hemoglobin Constant Spring mutation. Blood 78: 26, 1991.
30. Bunyaratvej A, Butthep P, Fucharoen S, Saw D: Erythrocyte volume and hemoglobin concentration in hemoglobin H disease: Discrimination between the two genotypes. Acta Haematol 87:1, 1992.
31. Fucharoen S, Winichagoon P, Pootrakul P, Piankijagum A, Wasi P: Difference between two types of Hb H disease, α-thalassemia 1/α-thalassemia 2 and α-thalassemia 1/Hb Constant Spring. Birth Defects 23:309, 1988.

American Journal of Hematology 45:298–303 (1994)

Intravenous Extended Infusion of Recombinant Human Soluble Thrombomodulin Prevented Tissue Factor-Induced Disseminated Intravascular Coagulation in Rats

Mitsunobu Mohri, Michiko Oka, Yoshikazu Aoki, Yasunori Gonda, Sigeto Hirata, Komakazu Gomi, Takao Kiyota, Taisuke Sugihara, Shuji Yamamoto, Torao Ishida, and Ikuro Maruyama

Institute for Life Science Research, Asahi Chemical Industry Co., Ltd, Fuji (M.M., M.O., Y.A., Y.G., S.H., K.G., T.K., T.S., S.Y., T.I.)
Department of Clinical Laboratory Medicine, Kagoshima University School of Medicine, Kagoshima (I.M.), Japan

This study demonstrated that intravenous infusion of recombinant human soluble thrombomodulin (rhs-TM) could inhibit disseminated intravascular coagulation (DIC) caused by 4 hr infusion of tissue factor (TF) in rats. Extended infusion of TF reduced fibrinogen and platelet counts and elevated serum FDP level. Pretreatment and coinfusion of rhs-TM could block changes of these DIC-parameters without prolongation of APTT. Heparin, which is a potent anti-DIC drug, could also inhibit these changes with extra prolongation of APTT and PT. Thus, these results suggest thrombomodulin prevent DIC less bleeding tendency than heparin.

Key words: recombinant human soluble thrombomodulin, DIC, TF, animal model

INTRODUCTION

Thrombomodulin is endothelial cell surface thrombin receptor. Thrombin bound to thrombomodulin loses its procoagulant activities including fibrin formation and platelet aggregation and is accelerated to activate protein C 1,000–2,000 times [1–3]. Activated protein C is a protease and an anticoagulant through its ability to cleave coagulation cofactors Va and VIIIa, and inactivate plasminogen activator inhibitor-1 (PAI-1) [4–5].

Recently we cloned a c-DNA for human thrombomodulin and demonstrated that simian COS cells transfected with the expression vector containing human thrombomodulin c-DNA expressed functionally active thrombomodulin [6]. Human thrombomodulin has five domains, a NH_2 terminal domain (D1), an EGF-like structure domain (D2), an O-glycosilation-rich domain (D3), a transmembrane domain (D4), and a cytoplasmic domain (D5). The minimum essential structure of human thrombomodulin activity is a domain composed of the fourth, fifth, and sixth EGF-like structure of D2 [7,8]. Two forms of recombinant human soluble thrombomodulin consisting of D1, D2, and D3 was reported [9,10]. High molecular analogue had a relatively short half life with heterogeneous chondroitin sulfate chains, and low molecular one had a long half-life with no chondroitin sulfate chains attached [11]. This low molecular recombinant human soluble thrombomodulin (rhs-TM) has the same protein C activating activity as full length native thrombomodulin [12], inhibits thrombin generation through activated protein C pathway [13], delivers bounded thrombin to antithrombin III in vitro [14], and has an antithrombotic activity on thrombin-induced thromboemboli in mice [15]. Recently, it was shown rhs-TM prevented venous thrombosis in a rat model [16], and two forms of rhs-TM (with or without chondroitin sulfate chains) prevented tissue factor induced disseminated intravascular coagulation in a rat model [11]. These studies showed that rhs-TM is an excellent potential drug for the treatment of coagulation disorders. But these previous studies ignored the difference of half lives in vivo between rhs-TM and

Received for publication April 8, 1993; accepted September 22, 1993.

Address reprint requests to Mitsunobu Mohri, First Laboratory for Pharmacological Research, Institute for Life Science Research, Asahi Chemical Industry Co, Ltd, 632-1 Mifuku, Ohito-cho, Tagata-gun, Shizuoka, 410-23, Japan.

heparin for a control drug. In this paper, we demonstrate that infusion of rhs-TM and heparin to maintain a steady concentration of rhs-TM in the blood of rats effectively blocked disseminated intravascular coagulation (DIC) caused by extended infusion of tissue factor. rhs-TM was effective and less prolongation of clotting time at blocking DIC than heparin, which has so far been the most promising drug for treatment of coagulation disorders.

MATERIALS AND METHODS

Materials and Animals

rhs-TM (recombinant human soluble thrombomodulin) was prepared as previously described [15]. Low molecular form of rhs-TM with no chondroitin sulfate chain attached was used in this study. Heparin was obtained from Green Cross, Tokyo, Japan. Rabbit brain tissue factor was obtained from Organon Teknika, Durham, NC. APTT and PT kit were purchased from International Reagents, Kobe, Japan. FDP assay kit was obtained from Teikoku Hormone Mfg., Tokyo, Japan. Fibrinogen assay kit was obtained from Iatron Laboratory, Tokyo, Japan. Sprague-Dawley female rats were purchased from Charles River Japan, Yokohama, Japan.

Tissue Factor Induced DIC Model

Rats (180–270 g) were anesthetized by intraperitoneal injection of 35 mg/kg sodium pentobarbital. Additional three times 17.5 mg/kg of sodium pentobarbital were injected 40–80 min interval in response to the state of rats. Two thirds of the total amount of rhs-TM (0.2, 0.67, and 2.0 mg/kg) or one tenth of the total amount of heparin (10, 30, and 100 U/kg) was injected into the tail vein, and the remaining rhs-TM (0.1, 0.33, and 1.0 mg/kg) or heparin (90, 270, and 900 U/kg) was infused into the same tail vein over the next 4 hr. Following the injection of rhs-TM or heparin, 100 mg/kg of tissue factor was coinfused with rhs-TM or heparin into another tail vein. In this study, the infusions were run at a rate of 1 ml/kg/hr. In the case of rhs-TM, 0.002% Tween-80 was used as an anti-absorption agent. Saline or saline containing 0.002% Tween-80 was infused as vehicle controls in place of heparin, tissue factor and rhs-TM; 4 hr later, blood samples were collected from the abdominal aorta (one tenth of 3.8% trisodium citrate and nine tenths of the blood). Citrated plama samples were obtained by centrifugation and stored at −80°C until assayed. Platelets were counted in duplicate by an auto blood counter, Sysmex M-2000 (Toa Medical Electronics, Kobe, Japan).

Pharmacokinetics

Rats (180–200 g) were anesthetized as described above; 2 mg/kg of rhs-TM or 30 U/kg of heparin was injected, and then 1 mg/kg of rhs-TM or 270 U/kg of heparin and saline was coinfused. After the indicated times, blood samples were collected and centrifuged to obtain plasma. The concentration of rhs-TM and heparin was determined by thrombin clotting time (TCT) using the standard calibration curve of rhs-TM or heparin in rats plasma. A sandwich-type ELISA was performed to determine plasma concentration of rhs-TM antigen.

APTT, PT, and TCT

APTT (activated partial thromboplastin time) and PT (prothrombin time) were measured using kits which utilize conventional coagulometer methods (Heinrich Amelung, Hannover, Germany). TCT was measured as following, 100 μl of 10 or 13 U/ml bovine thrombin (Green cross, Tokyo, Japan) was added into 100 μl of the plasma sample, and then the clotting time was measured at the coagulometer. All assays were performed in duplicate.

Fibrinogen Concentration

Twenty microliters of plasma was diluted with 1 ml of salting-out reagent (0.55 M sodium sulfate, 65.5 mM sodium acetate, and 10 μg/ml of casein), the reaction mixture was incubated for 30 min at 37°C, and then duplicated samples of precipitated fibrinogen were measured at 550 nm with a spectrophotometer. The blank was measured as follows: plasma from hemolysed and nonhemolysed blood was diluted with 1 ml of blank reagent (0.3 M ammonium sulfate, 86 mM sodium acetate), which was measured in a similar fashion.

FDP Concentration

Plasma was treated with the coagulation agents used with the FDP (Fibrinogen or fibrin degradative products) kit, and bovine thrombin was added to avoid incomplete coagulation due to high concentrations of anticoagulants. FDP was measured in the method of latex agglutination according to the manual of the kit.

ELISA for rhs-TM

Two monoclonal antibodies recognized different epitope of rhs-TM were obtained from Balb/c mice immunized with rhs-TM. A conventional sandwich-type ELISA was performed using one antibody and another antibody labelled with horseradish peroxidase. The plasma level of rhs-TM antigen was measured at 492 nm by a plate reader.

RESULTS

Pharmacokinetics of rhs-TM and Heparin

The plasma half-lives of rhs-TM and heparin in rats are about 5 hr and 15 min, respectively (unpublished data). The effects of anticoagulants are thought to be related to their concentrations in plasma, so in an infusion model, it is necessary to maintain plasma adequate concentrations of rhs-TM and heparin. Based on our calculations using a

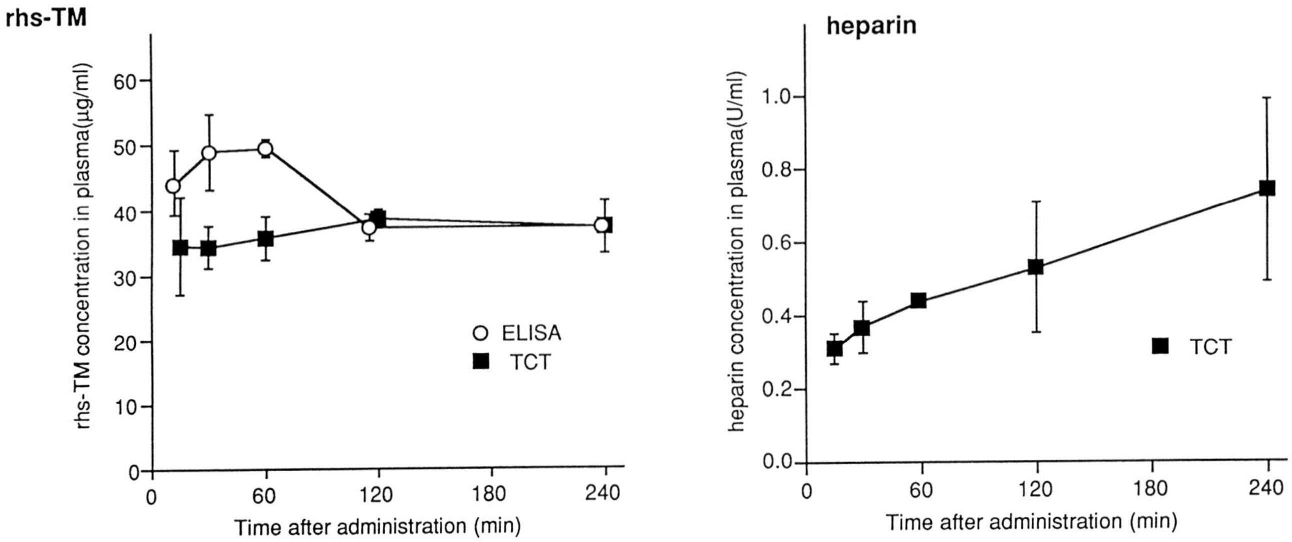

Fig. 1. Plasma levels of rhs-TM and heparin after bolus and during infusion administration in rats. Methods are described in Materials and Methods. Three or four rats were employed for each data points. Symbols and bars represent means and standard deviations.

one compartment model, two thirds of the total amount of rhs-TM or one tenth of the total amount of heparin were bolus injected and one third of the amount of rhs-TM or nine tenths of the amount of heparin were infused over 4 hr to maintain their plasma concentrations.

Figure 1 shows that the concentration of rhs-TM was successfully maintained at about 30–40 µg/ml by TCT method and 30–60 µg/ml by ELISA while infusion at the total dose 3.0 mg/kg of rhs-TM. The plasma concentration of heparin was also maintained between 0.3 U/ml and 0.7 U/ml over 4 hr infusion at the total dose 300 U/kg of heparin. Clinical constitutive infusion of heparin failed to maintain its plasma concentration [17], and apparently in rats, the plasma concentration of heparin gradually increased.

Comparison of the Effects of rhs-TM and Heparin on the Tissue Factor-Induced DIC Model

Intravenous infusion of tissue factor induced decreases in fibrinogen concentration and platelet counts, and elevated APTT, PT, and FDP (Fig. 2, Table I). These results show that administration of TF caused DIC in rats. Coinfusion of rhs-TM or heparin with TF blocked these changes of DIC parameters in a dose-dependent manner; 0.3 mg/kg of rhs-TM and 100 U/kg of heparin caused approximately the same effect in fibrinogen and platelet levels; complete inhibition was observed at 3.0 mg/kg of rhs-TM and 1,000 U/kg of heparin (Fig. 2). Although both drugs blocked TF-induced decrease of fibrinogen and platelet counts and increase of FDP level, highest dose of heparin used (1,000 U/kg) seemed to fail to prevent the prolongation of APTT and PT. The highest dose of rhs-TM used (3.0 mg/kg) completely blocked these changes of DIC-parameter without extra prolongation of APTT and PT (Table I). These results demonstrate that rhs-TM could maintain proper levels of platelets and fibrinogen without increasing clotting time as indicated by APTT and PT.

DISCUSSION

Thrombomodulin possesses two anticoagulant properties, one of which is the direct inhibition of thrombin activity, and the other of which is the down regulation of thrombin generation dependent on activated protein C produced by a thrombin-thrombomodulin complex [1–3]. Since thrombin is a key enzyme in coagulation disorders, one might hypothesize that thrombomodulin would produce activated protein C in proportion to thrombin generated as a result of the disease state. In theory, thrombomodulin may be a safer drug for a treating coagulation disorders because it would have a lower effect on protein C activation in normal and moderate disease states.

Recently, recombinant DNA techniques have enabled the production of recombinant human soluble thrombomodulin (rhs-TM) [7,9,10]; rhs-TM which was expressed in chinese hamster ovarian cells and human 293 cells was produced in two forms: a low molecular weight form with a long half-life and a high molecular weight form with a short half-life [11]. The latter form has AT-III dependent-anticoagulant activity (heparin-like activity) and both types exhibited the ability to inhibit thrombin and activate protein C [9,18]. Nawa et al. also demonstrated that both types of rhs-TM could inhibit

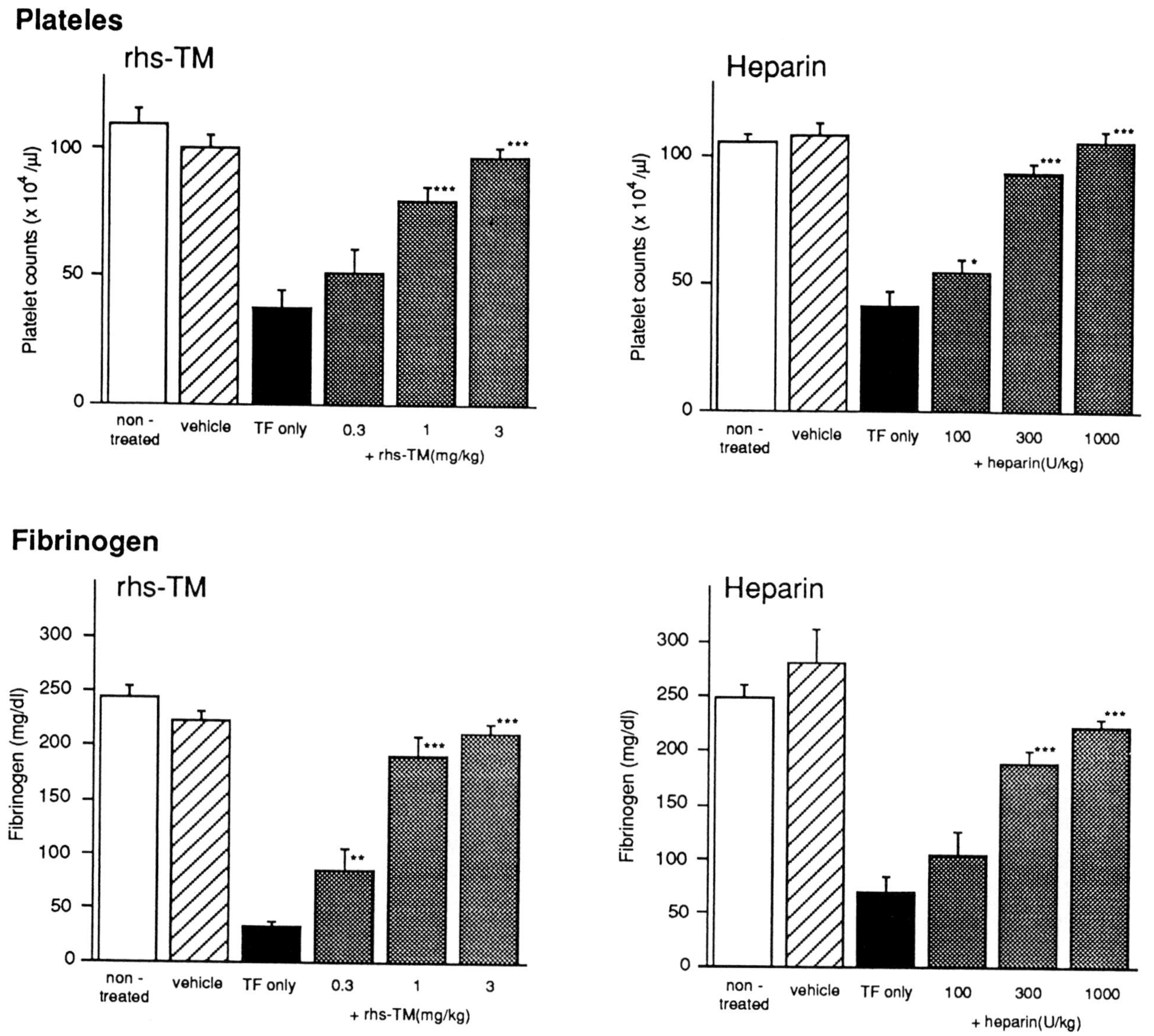

Fig. 2. Effect of rhs-TM and heparin on decrease in fibrinogen and platelets caused by TF infusion in rats. Methods are described in Materials and Methods; 100 mg/kg of rabbit brain TF was infused to cause DIC. Columns and bars represent means and standard errors. Asterisks indicate statistical significance compared to TF only onltrol using the student's t-test, *$P < 0.05$, **$P < 0.01$, ***$P < 0.001$.

decreases in fibrinogen and platelets caused by TF administration in rats and the high molecular weight form of rhs-TM prolonged APTT more than the lower molecular weight form [11].

Heparin has been one of the most useful and popular clinical anticoagulants. Nevertheless, pharmaceutical use of heparin may have some problems, including occasional drops in platelet counts and bleeding [19]. Increases in APTT may be correlated with bleeding. Thus, heparin has been used with careful monitoring clotting time to maintain APTT in the range of 1.5 to 2.5 times normal [20]. Low molecular weight heparin, which more effectively inhibit Xa than normal unfractionated heparin, showed less prolongation of APTT than normal heparin. Therefore it is thought that low molecular weight heparin has less bleeding than normal heparin [21]. In this study, rhs-TM prevented DIC in rats without prolongation of both APTT and PT, but heparin could not. Our unpublished data also demonstrated that rhs-TM blocked DIC caused by infusion of endotoxin without extra prolongation of both APTT and PT [22]. These may be explained by the fact that rhs-TM could work only when thrombin burst is occurred, and activated protein C is produced in proportion to rhs-TM-thrombin complex generated. Heparin inhibit thrombin generation through inhibiting Xa and IXa in proportion to the dose of heparin

TABLE I. Effects of rhs-TM and Heparin on the Elevation of APTT, PT, and FDP by TF Infusion in Rats†

		n	APTT(s) range (median)	PT(s) range (median)	FDP (μg/ml) range (median)
rhs-TM	Nontreated	8	16.6–19.6 (17.4)	14.4–15.6 (14.6)	<2.5
	Vehicle	8	15.8–20.6 (18.0)	14.5–15.9 (15.0)	<2.5
	TF only	8	>150	>150	29–80 (80)
	+0.3 mg/kg	7	33.8–>150 (>150)	16.3–>150 (25.7)*	<2.5–160 (10)
	+1.0 mg/kg	7	23.2–>150 (48.2)*	17.2–19.6 (18.0)**	<2.5–2.5 (<2.5)**
	+3.0 mg/kg	8	38.5–62.3 (48.5)**	18.3–20.2 (18.8)**	<2.5**
Heparin	Nontreated	8	16.9–19.0 (17.6)	14.3–15.3 (15.1)	<2.5
	Vehicle	8	16.3–18.8 (18.0)	14.7–15.8 (15.3)	<2.5
	TF only	8	34.4–>150 (>150)	19.1–>150 (>150)	20–80 (40)
	+100 U/kg	8	30.5–>150 (39.0)*	16.3–>150 (20.4)*	2.5–80 (30)
	+300 U/kg	8	25.3–>150 (>150)	16.1–27.0 (18.5)**	<2.5–2.5 (<2.5)**
	+1,000 U/kg	8	>150	37.8–68.3 (47.6)**	Non-clottable

†Methods are described in Materials and Methods; 100 mg/kg of rabbit brain TF was infused to cause DIC. Asterisks indicate statistical significance compared to TF only control using Wilcoxon's signed rank test.
*P >0.05,
**P >0.01.

used. Thus, rhs-TM may be a much safer drug than heparin for treating coagulation disorders.

This study confirmed previous observations that rhs-TM administered intravenously to rats can prevent tissue-factor-induced DIC without prolongation of clotting time, while equally effective dose of heparin extraordinary prolongs the APTT. Thus, rhs-TM is attractive candidate for inhibiting DIC. Many researchers have suggested that rhs-TM exhibit its anti-coagulant effects through its effects on accelerating protein C generation, but the mechanism in vivo is still unknown. Further study is necessary before the promise becomes reality.

REFERENCE

1. Esmon CT: The roles of protein C and thrombomodulin in the regulation of blood coagulation. J Biol Chem 264:4743, 1989.
2. Dittman WA, Majerus PW: Structure and function of thrombomodulin. Blood 75:329, 1990.
3. Esmon NL: Thrombomodulin. Semin Thromb Haemost 13:454, 1987.
4. Esmon CT: Protein C: Biochemistry, Physiology, and clinical implications. Blood 62:1155, 1983.
5. Marlar RA, Kleis AJ, Griffin JH: Mechanism of activated protein C, a thrombin-dependent anticoagulant enzyme. Blood 59:1067, 1982.
6. Suzuki K, Kusumoto H, Deyashiki Y, Nishioka J, Maruyama I, Zushi M, Kawahara S, Honda G, Yamamoto S, Horiguchi S: Structure and expression of human thrombomodulin, a thrombin receptor on endothelium acting as a cofactor for protein C activation. EMBO J 6:1891, 1987.
7. Zushi M, Gomi K, Yamamoto S, Maruyama I, Hayashi T, and Suzuki K: The last three consecutive epidermal growth factor-like structures of human thrombomodulin comprise the minimum functional domain for protein C-activating cofactor activity and anticoagulant activity. J Biol Chem 264:10351, 1989.
8. Zushi M, Gomi K, Honda G, Kondo S, Yamamoto S, Hayashi T, and Suzuki K: Aspartic acid 349 in the fourth epidermal growth factor-like structure of human thrombomodulin plays a role in its Ca-mediated binding to protein C. J Biol Chem 266:19886, 1991.
9. Parkinson JF, Grinnell BW, Moore RE, Hoskins J, Vlahos CJ, Bang NU: Stable expression of a secretable deletion mutant of recombinant human thrombomodulin in mammalian cells. J Biol Chem 265:12602, 1990.
10. Nawa K, Sakano K, Fujiwara H, Sato Y, Sugiyama N, Teruuchi T, Iwamoto M, Marumoto Y: Presence and function of chondroitin-4-sulfate on recombinant human soluble thrombomodulin. Biochem Biophys Res Commun 171:729, 1990.
11. Nawa K, Itani T, Ono M, Sakano K, Marumoto Y, Iwamoto M: The glycosaminoglycan of recombinant human soluble thrombomodulin affects antithrombotic activity in rat model of tissue factor-induced disseminated intravascular coagulation. Thromb Haemost 67:366, 1992.
12. Suzuki K, Hayashi T, Nishioka J, Kosaka Y, Zushi M, Honda G, and Yamamoto S: A domain composed of epidermal growth factor-like structures of human thrombomodulin is essential for thrombin binding and for protein C activation. J Biol Chem 264:4872, 1989.
13. Ohishi R, Watanabe N, Aritomi M, Gomi K, Kiyota T, Yamamoto S, Ishida T, and Maruyama I: Evidence that the protein C activation pathway amplifies the inhibition of thrombin generation by recombinant human thrombomodulin in plasma. Thromb Haemost 70:423, 1993.
14. Aritomi M, Watanabe N, Ohishi R, Gomi K, Kiyota T, Yamamoto S, Ishida T, and Maruyama I: Recombinant human soluble thrombomodulin delivers bounded thrombin to antithrombin III: Thrombomodulin associates with free thrombin and is recycled to activate protein C. Thromb Haemost 70:418, 1993.
15. Gomi K, Zushi M, Honda G, Kawahara S, Matsuzaki O, Kanabayashi T, Yamamoto S, Maruyama I, Suzuki K: Antithrombotic effect of recombinant human thrombomodulin on thrombin-induced thromboembolism in mice. Blood 75:1396, 1990.
16. Solis MM, Cook C, Cook J, Glaser C, Light D, Morser J, Yu S, Fink L, Eidt JF: Intravenous recombinant soluble human thrombomodulin prevents venous thrombosis in a rat model. J Vasc Surg 14:599, 1991.
17. De Swart CAM, Nijmeyer B, Roelofs JMM, Sixma JJ: Kinetics of intravenously administered heparin in normal humans. Blood 60:1251, 1982.
18. Koyama T, Parkinson JF, Aoki N, Bang NU, Muller-Berghaus G, Preissner KT: Relationship between post-translational glycosylation and anticoagulant function of secretable recombinant mutants of human thrombomodulin. Br J Haematol 78:515, 1991.

19. Gallus AS, Hirsh J: Antithrombotic drugs: part I. Drugs 12:41, 1976.
20. Bain B, Forster T, Sleigh B: Heparin and the activated partial thromboplastin time: A difference between the in-vitro and in-vivo effects and implications for the therapeutic range. Am J Clin Pathol 74:668, 1980.
21. Palm M, Mattsson C, Svahn CM, Weber M: Bleeding times in rats treated with heparin, heparin fragments of high and low anticoagulant activity and chemically modified heparin frgments of low anticoagulant activity. Thromb Haemost 64:127, 1990.
22. Gonda Y, Saitoh K, Hirata S, Aoki K, Mohri M, Gomi K, Sugihara T, Kiyota T, Yamamoto S, Ishida T, Maruyama I: Antithrombotic effect of recombinant human soluble thrombomodulin on endotoxin-induced disseminated intravascular coagulation in rats. Thromb Res 71:325, 1993.

American Journal of Hematology 45:304–309 (1994)

Thrombotic Microangiopathy and Retroviral Infections: A 13-Year Experience

Antonio Ucar, Hugo F. Fernandez, John J. Byrnes, Eric C-Y Lian, and William J. Harrington, Jr.

Division of Hematology-Oncology, Department of Medicine, University of Miami, School of Medicine, Sylvester Comprehensive Cancer Center, Veterans Administration Medical Center, and the William J. Harrington Center for Blood Disease, Miami, Florida

Eleven of fifty serum samples collected from patients with a diagnosis of thrombotic microangiopathy (TMA), from 1979 to 1991, tested positive for antiretroviral antibodies. Seven had human immunodeficiency virus (HIV) infection, and four had human lymphotrophic virus, type I (HTLV-I) infection. All patients were treated with plasma exchange and/or infusion, but only two of the HIV-infected patients obtained a complete response (CR) and one of them died after a few months. Combined results from the literature indicate that most patients with HIV infection survive less than one year from the initial diagnosis of TMA. In the setting of HIV infection, TMA is a treatable condition, but survival for most patients is less than 12 months. Three of the four HTLV-I infected patients with TMA had a CR. These observations strongly suggest that both HIV and HTLV-I infections are associated with TMA, but rigorous epidemiologic studies will be needed to determine the relative risk for each. Retroviral infections should be considered in patients with TMA, especially if the patient has associated risk factors and demographic characteristics.

Key words: TTP (thrombotic thrombocytopenic purpura), HUS (hemolytic uremic syndrome), HIV (human immunodeficiency virus), AIDS (acquired immunodeficiency syndrome), HTLV-I (human T-lymphotrophic virus, type I)

INTRODUCTION

The thrombotic microangiopathies (TMA) are clinical syndromes with considerable overlap, including the hemolytic uremic syndrome (HUS) and thrombotic thrombocytopenic purpura (TTP). TTP is manifested clinically by thrombocytopenia and microangiopathic hemolytic anemia, often with fluctuating neurological signs, fever, and renal abnormalities [1], whereas HUS is characterized by thrombocytopenia, anemia, and more significant renal dysfunction [2]. TMA has diverse potential etiologies, but in most patients no obvious association, underlying disease, or precipitating cause is identified [3]. An association between TMA and the human immunodeficiency virus (HIV) has been recognized since 1984, coinciding with the acquired immunodeficiency syndrome (AIDS) epidemic [4]. In contrast, only an isolated case report of TTP has linked it to human T-lymphotrophic virus, type I (HTLV-I) infection [5]. TMA has been an area of active research at our institution, and serum samples of most patients with this diagnosis evaluated by our service since 1979 had been collected and kept frozen. Miami has one of the highest annual rates of AIDS cases in the United States [6], and due to immigrations from the Caribbean islands, where HTLV-I is endemic [7], infection with HTLV-I is being increasingly diagnosed in our hospitals. The samples collected were tested for retroviral infections to determine their frequency in our population of patients with TMA, and evaluate the possible association between TMA and retroviral infection. We report seven HIV and four HTLV-I infected patients with TMA since 1979 (Table I). Two illustrative cases of HIV and two of HTLV-I-infected patients with TMA are described in detail here.

MATERIALS AND METHODS

From January 1, 1979 to December 31, 1991 serum samples from 50 patients with TTP or HUS were col-

Received for publication May 5, 1993; accepted September 22, 1993.

Address reprint requests to William J. Harrington, Jr., Division of Hematology-Oncology, University of Miami School of Medicine, 1475 N.W. 12th Avenue (D8-4), Miami, FL 33136.

TABLE I. Characteristics of Patients With TMA and Retroviral Infection at Diagnosis

Patient	Diagnosis	Year of diagnosis	Platelet count (per mm^3)	Hematocrit (%)	Creatinine (mg/dl)
HIV+					
1	TTP	1979	18,000	18	2.8
2[a]	TTP	1981	21,000	29	11.4
3	TTP	1984	38,000	16	2.5
4	TTP	1986	25,000	19	1.2
5	TTP	1988	13,000	17	7.6
6	HUS	1990	60,000	18	4.5
7[a]	TTP	1990	21,000	15	2.1
HTLV-I+					
8[a]	TTP	1979	6,000	24	1.7
9	HUS	1981	62,000	21	4.0
10	HUS	1987	32,000	24	11.0
11[a]	TTP	1990	7,000	28	0.6

[a]Cases detailed in this article.

lected at the University of Miami prior to initiation of therapy with plasma infusion or exchange. These samples were obtained either from patients admitted to one of our affiliated hospitals (Jackson Memorial Hospital, Veterans Administration Medical Center and University of Miami Hospitals and Clinics) or sent to us by private physicians in the community. Samples were kept frozen at −70°C until tested in 1992. Specimens were tested for anti-HIV antibodies using enzyme-linked immunosorbent assay (ELISA) (Organon Teknica Corporation, Durham, NC), and positive tests were confirmed by Western blot (Organon Teknica Corporation, Durham, NC). The presence of anti-HTLV-I/II antibodies was initially tested by ELISA (Organon Teknica Corporation, Durham, NC) and then confirmed by Western blot for antibodies to HTLV I/II (Cambridge Biotech Corporation, Worcester, MA). To discriminate between HTLV-I and HTLV-II, three of the four HTLV I/II-positive samples were analyzed on modified immunoblots containing recombinant p21E, an immunodominant epitope of the p21 envelope protein, and two additional recombinant proteins, K55, specific for HTLV-II and, MTA-1, specific for HLTV-I (Diagnostic Biotechnology Ltd, Singapore) (Fig. 1). In one patient, DNA was extracted from peripheral blood lymphocytes, and confirmation of HTLV-I infection was obtained by the polymerase chain reaction (PCR) using primer pairs derived from conserved sequences of the HTLV-I *pol* and *env* genes, as described [8].

Case 3 has been described previously [9] but is described again because of two unique features. She is the earliest diagnosed patient with TMA in this series, and the chronic relapsing course apparently responded to immunosuppressive chemotherapy.

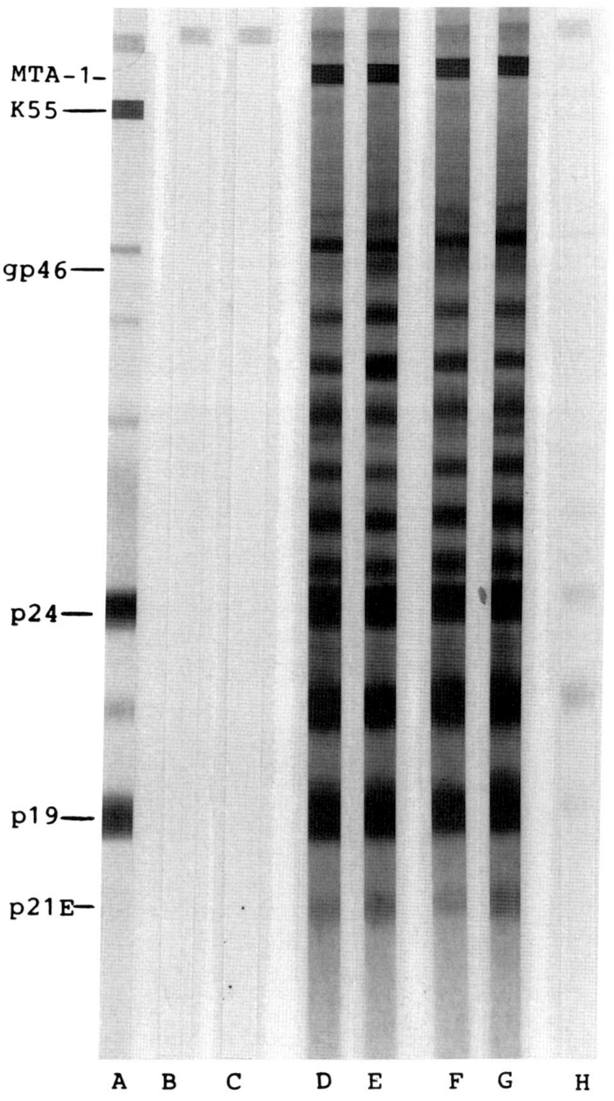

Fig. 1. Patients samples analyzed on human T-cell lymphotrophic virus, type I/II (HTLV-I/II) diagnostic immunoblots. The following samples were reacted with immunoblots at a 1:100 dilution. A: Serum from HTLV-II-infected patient is positive for K55, a recombinant protein that contains an epitope specific for HTLV-II. B,C: Negative control sera. D: Adult T-cell lymphoma positive control sera. E: HTLV-I-associated myelopathy positive control sera. F–H: HTLV-I-infected sera from patients 8, 9, and 10 (Table I) are positive for MTA-1, a recombinant protein that contains an epitope specific for HTLV-I. Channel H appears faint compared to channels F and G, possibly because this sample had been previously thawed.

RESULTS

Serum from 11 of 50 patients with TMA tested positive for a retroviral infection, seven were positive for anti-HIV antibodies and four for anti-HTLV-I antibodies. Three of the HIV and one of the HTLV-I infected patients tested positive during their initial hospital stay, and oth-

TABLE II. Demographic Characteristics of Patients With HIV-Related TMA*

Number	7
Median age	30 (25–35)
Sex	
Male	4
Female	3
Race	
Hispanic	3
Black	2
White	2
Risk factors for HIV infection	
Homosexual	2
IVDU	1
Transfusions	1
IVDU + transfusions	1
Unknown	2
Status of HIV infection	
Asymptomatic	5
ARC	1
AIDS	1

*AIDS, acquired immunodeficiency syndrome; ARC, AIDS-related complex; HIV, human immunodeficiency virus; IVDU, intravenous drug use; TMA, thrombotic microangiopathy.

ers were tested retrospectively. The median age for the HIV infected patients was 30 years old (age range 25–35). There were four men and three women (three hispanic, two black, and two white patients). The demographics and risk factors of these patients appear in Table II. Five of the HIV-positive patients had an asymptomatic infection at presentation, one patient presented with AIDS-related complex (ARC) and one with AIDS (Table II). All four HTLV-I infected patients were black women, who had immigrated from the Caribbean islands (three from Haiti and one from the Bahamas); they were 22, 30, 39, and 62 years of age. Of the seven patients with HIV infection, six presented with TTP and one with HUS. Two of the six patients with TTP had the pentad of thrombocytopenia, microangiopathic hemolytic anemia, renal insufficiency, fever, and neurological abnormalities [1] at clinical presentation (Table III). Of the HTLV-I-positive patients two presented with HUS and two with TTP (Table III). The 11 patients were treated with multiple modalities, but all received fresh frozen plasma (FFP) infusions and eight were also treated with plasma exchange (Table IV). Only two of seven HIV infected patients (both with TTP) and three of four HTLV-I-infected patients achieved a complete response (CR), as defined by ≥1 month of normalization of platelet count, resolution of hemolysis and neurological events. One HIV infected patient achieving CR survived for 11 months from the diagnosis of TMA and the other patient was lost to follow-up after 6 months. All surviving HTLV-I-infected patients were lost to follow up shortly after hospital discharge. The patients not achieving CR died (Table IV).

TABLE III. Clinical Presentation of TMA Patients

	HIV	HTLV-1
Number	7	4
Thrombocytopenic thrombotic purpura	6	2
Microangiopathic hemolytic anemia	6	2
Thrombocytopenia	6	2
Renal insufficiency	5	1
Neurologic abnormalities	4	2
Fever	2	2
Pentad	2	1
Hemolytic-uremic syndrome[a]	1	2

[a]All patients with HUS had renal insufficiency, microangiopathic hemolytic anemia, and thrombocytopenia.

TABLE IV. Treatment Modalities in Patients With TMA

	HIV	HTLV-1
Plasma infusion	7	4
Plasma exchange	6	2
Cryosupernatant infusion	1	0
Corticosteroids	5	2
Vincristine	2	1
Cyclophosphamide	0	1
Aspirin	1	1
Dipyridamole	1	1
Hemodialysis	2	2
Splenectomy	0	1
Response to therapy		
Complete response	2	3
Died	5	1

CASE STUDIES

Case 1 (Patient 2 in Table I)

A 34-year-old black man with history of alcoholism and schizophrenia, was admitted October 10, 1981 to the Miami Veterans Administration Medical Center with three days of nausea, vomiting, diarrhea, and abdominal pain. He had tonic-clonic seizures upon arrival to the emergency room. His blood pressure was 164/110, heart rate 90/min, respiratory rate 18/min, and temperature 99.8°F. He was confused but not in distress. A II/VI ejection murmur was heard, and the neurological examination was abnormal only for confusion. The WBC count was 14,900/mm^3 with 68% neutrophils, 4% bands, 15% lymphocytes, and 13% monocytes; the hematocrit 29%; the platelet count 21,000/mm^3; a disseminated intravascular coagulation (DIC) screen was negative; the BUN 102 mg/dl; the serum creatinine 11.4 mg/dl; the LDH 1,200 U/L (normal <250 U/L), and total bilirubin 3.2 mg/dl with direct fraction of 1.2 mg/dl. Urinalysis showed occult blood. The peripheral smear had numerous schistocytes and polychromasia. The diagnosis of TTP was made. Treatment with FFP infusion, one unit q2h was initiated along with aspirin 300 mg/day and dipyridamole 100 mg q6h. The patient continued seizure activity and Dilantin was started. Clonidine 0.2 mg twice daily was given for blood pressure control. On day (D) 2, his blood pressure was 136/80, he continued confused, the hematocrit was 21%, platelet count 10,000/mm^3, and BUN 117 mg/dl. He was transferred to the Jackson Memorial Hospital intensive care unit (ICU), where plasmapheresis was initiated, supplemented with FFP infusions and hemodialysis. On D 5, the patient's status required endotracheal intubation. The platelet count was 22,000/mm^3, hemoglobin 7.2 g/dl, hematocrit 21%, BUN 72 mg/dl, serum creatinine 5.6 mg/dl, and LDH 956 U/L. A CAT scan of the brain was unremarkable. On D 7, fever of 103.5°F and hypotension developed requiring pressor support and broad spectrum antibiotics. He progressively deteriorated and expired on D 8. A serum specimen tested positive for HIV in 1991.

Case 2 (Patient 7 in Table I)

A 30-year-old black man with history of intravenous drug use (IVDU) and blood transfusion in 1989, was brought to the medical emergency room of Jackson Memorial Hospital, November 18, 1990, after two episodes of tonic-clonic seizures. His mental status rapidly deteriorated, requiring endotracheal intubation for airway protection. His blood pressure was 170/92, pulse 110/min, respiratory rate 12/min, and temperature 98.0°F, which increased to 103°F 4 hr after admission. He was well developed and responsive only to pain; occult fecal blood was present. Laboratory values on admission included a WBC count of 16,900/mm^3 with 50% neutrophils, 22% bands, 24% lymphocytes and 4% monocytes; hematocrit 15%; platelet count 21,000/mm^3; reticulocyte count 16.7%; a DIC screen was negative; BUN 28 mg/dl; serum creatinine 2.1 mg/dl; LDH 5249 U/L (normal <613 U/L); total bilirubin 1.9 mg/dl, with a direct fraction of 0.9 mg/dl; cocaine metabolites were identified in the urine. Urinalysis revealed 2+ protein, 1–5 WBC/high-power field (hpf), and 5–10 red blood cells (RBC)/hpf. The peripheral blood smear had polychromatophilia, and numerous schistocytes. The diagnosis of TTP was made. He was transfused three U of RBCs and antibiotics were initiated. Plasma infusions, one U every three h were started along with IV methylprednisolone 60 mg q6h. On D 2, daily plasma exchange therapy was added. The patient's mental status rapidly improved and on D 3 he was extubated. On D 4, plasmapheresis was stopped and methylprednisolone was replaced by oral prednisone 60 mg/day, which was tapered and discontinued over 2 weeks. At that time, the platelet count was 74,000/mm^3; hematocrit 30%, LDH 1225 U/L, BUN 16 mg/dl, and creatinine 1.2 mg/dl. The patient continued receiving plasma infusions at progressively longer intervals until they were stopped on D 29, when the platelet count was 413,000/mm^3 and LDH 974 U/L. He was seropositive for HIV and was discharged on zidovudine 200 mg 5 times daily. The patient did well until May 20, 1991 when he was admitted to the hospital for *Pneumocystis carinii* pneumonia and oral candidiasis. The platelet count was 250,000/mm^3 and remained stable. He was discharged on bactrim, ketoconazole, and zidovudine but was lost to follow-up.

Case 3 (Patient 8 in Table I)

A 22-year-old black woman from the Bahamas was hospitalized in January 1979 with fever, confusion, and purulent drainage from two recent dental extraction sites. Findings included temperature of 101.3°F and a right central facial paralysis. She moved all extremities equally but had bilateral extensor reflexes. A II/VI ejection murmur was heard at the apex. Initial laboratory values included a WBC count of 5,600/mm^3 with normal differential, hemoglobin 7.2 g/dl, hematocrit 24%, reticulocytes 21%, platelets 6,000/mm^3, negative DIC screen, negative Coombs' test, BUN 10 mg/dl, serum creatinine 1.7 mg/dl, and total bilirubin 1.7 mg/dl. Urine contained 1 to 3 RBC/hpf. Spinal fluid RBC, 153/mm^3; WBC, 3/mm^3; glucose, 62 mg/dl (plasma, 90 mg/dl); and protein, 60 mg/dl. Computerized tomography (CT) of the brain showed left frontal edema. The peripheral blood smear had numerous schistocytes, and the bone marrow examination showed panhyperplasia. The diagnosis of TTP and infectious cerebritis were made and treatment with IV methylprednisolone, 100 mg/day, and penicillin G, 10 million units daily was initiated. Splenectomy was performed on D 3 after the patient develped hematuria and generalized seizures. By D 4, right-sided focal seizures and bloody gastric drainage occurred. The platelet level remained below 10,000/mm^3 and the hematocrit had to be supported with transfusions of RBC. On D 5, plasma infusions were started and by D 7, after 10 U of FFP had been transfused, she was alert and responsive. She was maintained on 3 U/day. On D 13, penicillin was discontinued. Her hematologic parameters were corrected by D 19, and the plasma was stopped, but 4 days later (although her sensorium remained normal) the platelet count had fallen to 61,000/mm^3 and FFP was restarted and the thrombocytopenia resolved. Antiplatelet therapy with aspirin, dipyridamole, and sulfinpyrazone did not prevent hematologic relapse on two subsequent occasions after discontinuation of FFP. On D 48, oral prednisone, 60 mg/day, cyclophosphamide, 100 mg/day, and FFP were started. On D 63, plasma was stopped when the hematocrit reached 36%, reticulocytes 2%, and platelet count 672,000/mm^3. Cyclophosphamide was reduced to 100 mg/day, alternating with 50 mg/day, and the prednisone was tapered to 30 mg/day. On D 71, with the counts stable, she was discharged. One month later, her platelets were 245,000/mm^3. The cyclophosphamide was reduced to 50 mg/day 5 days a week, and the prednisone to 15 mg/day. The patient stopped her medications on her own

4 weeks later, and because the platelet count after 3 further weeks was 345,000/mm^3, the medications were not restarted. She returned to the Bahamas and was lost to follow-up. Her initial serum specimen obtained in 1979 tested positive for HTLV-I in 1991.

Case 4 (Patient 11 in Table I)

A 62-year-old black woman from Haiti with history of hypertension was admitted in 1990 to Jackson Memorial Hospital with dizziness, gum bleeding, weakness, headaches, and mild left-sided chest pain of 5 days' duration. Her blood pressure was 180/100, heart rate 96/min, respirations 16/min, and temperature 100.5°F. She was in no distress, had petechiae in both wrists areas, and had a normal neurological evaluation. Laboratory values on admission included a WBC count of 9,700/mm^3 with 51% neutrophils, 2% bands, 45% lymphocytes, and 2% monocytes; hematocrit 28%; platelet count 7,000/mm^3; reticulocyte count 4.6%; negative DIC screen; negative Coombs' test; BUN 19 mg/dl; serum creatinine 0.6 mg/dl; LDH 4,036 U/L (normal <613 U/L); total bilirubin 1.8 mg/dl with direct fraction of 0.2 mg/dl. Urinalysis revealed 1+ protein, 5–10 RBC/hpf, and 5–10 WBC/hpf. The peripheral blood smear had polychromatophilia and numerous schistocytes. A bone marrow aspirate had adequate megakaryocytes. The diagnosis of TTP was made. A peripheral blood sample was positive for HTLV-I by PCR analysis. On D 2, treatment with oral prednisone 60 mg/day, FFP infusion at 1 unit q3h was initiated. On D 19, the platelet count was 20,000/mm^3 and LDH 2,100 U/L, and the patient developed confusion and left hemiparesis. A CT scan of the brain was unremarkable. Plasma exchange was added to FFP infusions and prednisone. On D 20, her mental status had improved and the left hemiparesis had resolved. On D 37, her platelet count was 122,000/mm^3, LDH 1362 U/L, BUN 56 mg/dl, and creatinine 1.4 mg/dl, plasma exchange was stopped, and FFP infusions along with prednisone 20 mg/day were continued; however, a slow but steady rise in the BUN and serum creatinine occurred. On D 61, the platelet count was 41,000/mm^3, LDH 3,564 U/L, BUN 191 mg/dL, and creatinine 5.2 mg/dl, exchange plasma therapy was restarted and hemodialysis initiated. On D 70, the patient had a fever of 103°F, became hypotensive, and expired 24 hr later, despite broad-spectrum antibiotics.

DISCUSSION

The TMAs are a pathogenically heterogeneous group of disorders. The triggering of intravascular platelet aggregation has been suspected to be the common feature of this syndrome [10]. Multiple associations have been reported, but the association with various infections has led to speculation about their etiologic role [11]. The best-recognized example has been the 0157:H7 strain of *Escherichia coli*, which produces verotoxin, causing platelet aggregation [12]. This strain of *E. coli* is associated with clusters of HUS and with some cases of TTP [13].

Thrombocytopenia frequently occurs in HIV-infected patients [14] and, although immune thrombocytopenia is common [15], thrombotic microangiopathy has to be considered in the differential diagnosis. Since 1988, 37 cases of TMA associated with HIV have been reported [4,16–28], including the seven cases reported here. The incidence of TMA in this setting is unknown as is the mechanism of TMA in HIV infected patients. Despite the fact that five of seven HIV-positive patients in our series presented with asymptomatic HIV infection (Table II) and that plasma exchange and/or infusions were used in all, only two obtained a CR (Table IV). Our results differ with reports from the pooled literature where 20 of 26 (77%) treated patients with TMA and HIV infection achieved CR [4,16–28]. However, four of 30 patients (13%) died prior to the initiation of therapy. Long-term outcomes are unavailable for most of the previously reported patients. In this series, two patients had a CR, one of these survived less than 1 year and the other was lost to follow-up after 6 months but had progressed from asymptomatic HIV infection to AIDS (case 2). Thompson et al. reported that only one of six patients achieving a CR survived more than 1 year after CR [28], suggesting that TMA syndromes occur late in the natural history of HIV infection. It is notable that two of the patients found to be HIV positive in our series developed TMA in 1979 and 1981 (Table I), before the AIDS epidemic, and earlier than the recognition of the association between HIV and TMA [4].

HTLV-I, the first human retrovirus to be discovered [29], is endemic in the Caribbean islands, southwestern Japan, and central Africa [7]. The virus is transmitted by three routes: vertically through breast milk, from blood donor to recipient, and between sexual partners by semen [7]. HTLV-I has been linked to several diseases, most notably adult T-cell leukemia/lymphoma (ATL) [30] and HTLV-I associated myelopathy (HAM) [31]. Many immigrants from the Caribbean reside in South Flordia; therefore, ATL and HAM are increasingly diagnosed in our institutions. This is the second report of the association of HTLV-I and TMA. Although HTLV-I infection in these patients may be coincidental, immunologic abnormalities are associated with TMA [32], and immune dysregulation is increasingly recognized in HTLV-I [33], as well as HIV-infected [34] patients. Three of four HTLV-I-infected patients had a CR to therapy, suggesting that their outcome is not different from that of noninfected patients. Two of the HTLV-I-infected patients were diagnosed with TMA in 1979 (Table I), before the association of HTLV-I and human disease was recognized [29].

Fourteen percent of the TMA patients in this series were HIV infected, and 8 percent had HTLV-I. The 22% incidence of retroviral infections in this group of patients is substantially higher than the incidence of retroviral infection has been in the population served by our institutions [6,35]. Retroviral infections appear to be associated to TMA, but rigorous epidemiologic studies will be needed to determine the relative risk. The operative mechanism is probably not a direct consequence of the retroviral infection but is likely due to the accompanying immune system and cytokine dysregulation that occurs with these infections [7,36]. Conceivably, immune suppression may facilitate infection with other organisms such as *E. coli* 0157:H7 which may be more directly responsible for the onset of the TMA.

REFERENCES

1. Amorosi EL, Ultmann JE: Thrombotic thrombocytopenic purpura: Report of 16 cases and review of the literature. Medicine (Baltimore) 45:139–159, 1966.
2. Shumway CN, Terplan KL: Hemolytic anemia, thrombocytopenia and renal disease in childhood. The hemolytic uremic syndrome. Pediatr Clin North Am 11:577–591, 1964.
3. Lian EC-Y: Thrombotic thrombocytopenic purpura. Annu Rev Med 39:203–212, 1988.
4. Boccia RV, Gelmann EP, Baker CC, Marti G, Longo DL: A hemolytic-uremic syndrome with the acquired immunodeficiency syndrome. Ann Intern Med 101:716–717, 1984.
5. Dixon AC, Kwock D, Nakamura JM, et al.: Thrombotic thrombocytopenic purpura and human T-lymphotrophic virus, type I (HTLV-I). Ann Intern Med 110:93–94, 1989.
6. Parks WP, Lenes BA, Tomasulo PA, et al: Human T-cell lymphotrophic virus infection among blood donors in South Florida. J Acquir Immune Defic Syndr 4:89–96, 1991.
7. Yodoi J, Uchiyama T: Diseases associated with HTLV-I: virus, IL-2 receptor dysregulation and redox regulation. Immunol Today 13:405–411, 1992.
8. Harrington WJ, Sheremata WA, Snodgrass SR, et al: Tropical spastic paraparesis/HTLV-I-associated myelopathy (TSP/HAM): Treatment with an anabolic steroid danazol. AIDS Res Hum Retroviruses 7:1031–1034, 1991.
9. Wallach HW, Oren ME, Herskowtiz A: Treatment of thrombocytopenic purpura with plasma infusions and cyclophosphamide. South Med J 72:1346–1347, 1979.
10. Byrnes JJ, Moake JL: Thrombotic thrombocytopenic purpura and the haemolytic-uraemic syndrome: Evolving concepts of pathogenesis and therapy. Clin Haematol 15:413–442, 1986.
11. Kwaan HC: Miscellaneous secondary thrombotic microangiopathy. Semin Hematol 24:141–147, 1987.
12. Rose PE, Armour JA, Williams CE, et al: Verotoxin and neuraminidase induced platelet aggregating activity in plasma: Their possible role in the pathogenesis of the haemolytic uraemic syndrome. J Clin Pathol 38:438–441, 1985.
13. Cleary TG: Escherichia coli that cause hemolytic uremic syndrome. Infect Dis Clin North Am 6:163–176, 1992.
14. Goldsweig HC, Grossman R, William D: Thrombocytopenia in homosexual men. Am J Hematol 21:243–247, 1986.
15. Walsh CM, Nardi NA, Karpatkin S: On the mechanism of thrombocytopenic purpura in sexually active homosexual men. N Engl J Med 311:635–639, 1984.
16. Jokela J, Flynn T, Henry K: Thrombotic thrombocytopenic purpura in a human immunodeficiency virus (HIV)-seropositive homosexual man. Am J Hematol 25:341–343, 1987.
17. Leaf AN, Laubenstein LJ, Raphael B, et al: Thrombotic thrombocytopenic purpura associated with human immunodeficiency virus type 1 (HIV-1) infection. Ann Intern Med 109:194–197, 1988.
18. Botti AC, Hyde P, DiPillo F: Thrombotic thrombocytopenic purpura in a patient who subsequently developed the acquired immunodeficiency syndrome (AIDS). Ann Intern Med 109:242–243, 1988.
19. Meisenberg BR, Robinson WL, Mosley CA, et al: Thrombotic thrombocytopenic purpura in human immunodeficiency (HIV)-seropositive males. Am J Hematol 27:212–215, 1988.
20. Nair JMG, Bellevue R, Bertoni M, Dosik H: Thrombotic thrombocytopenic purpura in patients with the acquired immunodeficiency syndrome (AIDS)-related complex: A report of two cases. Ann Intern Med 109:209–212, 1988.
21. Platanias LC, Paiusco D, Bernstein S, Murali MR: Thrombotic thrombocytopenic purpura as the first manifestation of human immunodeficiency virus infection. Am J Med 87:699–700, 1989.
22. Segal GH, Tubbs RR, Ratliff NB, Miller ML, Longworth DL: Thrombotic thrombocytopenic purpura in a patient with AIDS. Cleve Clin J Med 57:360–366, 1990.
23. Charasse C, Michelet C, Le Tulzo Y, et al: Thrombotic thrombocytopenic purpura with the acquired immunodeficiency syndrome: A pathologically documented case report. Am J Kidney Dis 17:80–82, 1991.
24. Taff ML, Schwartz IS, Churg J, Boglioli LR: Sudden death due to thrombotic thrombocytopenic purpura and HIV infection. Am J Forensic Med Pathol 12:89–90, 1991.
25. Esforzado N, Poch E, Almirall J, Lopez-Pedret J, Revert L: Hemolytic uremic syndrome associated with HIV infection. AIDS 5:104–105, 1991.
26. Routy J-P, Beaulieu R, Monte M, et al: Immunologic thrombocyotpenia followed by thrombotic thrombocytopenic purpura in two HIV_1 patients. Am J Hematol 38:327–328, 1991.
27. Rarick MU, Espina B, Mocharnuk R, Trilling Y, Levine A: Thrombotic thrombocytopenic purpura in patients with human immunodeficiency virus infection: A report of three cases and review of the literature. Am J Hematol 40:103–109, 1992.
28. Thompson CE, Damon LE, Ries CA, Linker CA: Thrombotic microangiopathies in the 1980s: Clinical features, response to treatment, and the impact of the human immunodeficiency virus epidemic. Blood 80:1890–1895, 1992.
29. Poiez BJ, Ruscetti FW, Gazdar AF, et al: Detection and isolation of type C retrovirus particles from fresh and cultured lymphocytes of a patient with cutaneous T-cell lymphoma. Proc Natl Acad Sci USA 77:7415–7419, 1980.
30. Yamaguchi K, Kiyokawa T, Futami G, et al: Pathogenesis of adult T-cell leukemia from clinical pathologic features. In Blattner WA (ed): "Human Retrovirology: HTLV." New York: Raven Press, 1990, pp 163–171.
31. Gessain A, Barin F, Vernant JC, et al: Antibodies to human T-lymphotrophic virus I in patients with tropical spastic paraparesis. Lancet 2:407–410, 1985.
32. Neame PD: Immunologic and other factors in thrombotic thrombocytopenic purpura (TTP). Semin Thromb Hemosth 6:416–429, 1980.
33. Bowness P, Davies KA, Tosswill J, et al: Autoimmune disease and HTLV-I infection. Br J Rheumatol 30:141–143, 1991.
34. Malatzky-Goshen E, Shoenfeld Y: AIDS and autoimmunity. Autoimmunity 3:201–212, 1989.
35. Centers for Disease Control: HIV/AIDS surveillance report. 1–18, 1992.
36. Zunich KM, Lane HC: Immunologic abnormalities in HIV infection. Hematol Oncol Clin North Am 5:215–228.

American Journal of Hematology 45:310–320 (1994)

Lineage Determination of CD7+ CD5− CD2− and CD7+ CD5+ CD2− Lymphoblasts: Studies on Phenotype, Genotype, and Gene Expression of Myeloperoxidase, CD3ε, and CD3δ

Noriko Yoneda, Eiji Tatsumi, Keisuke Teshigawara, Shigekazu Nagata, Takahiro Nagano, Yuji Kishimoto, Takashi Kimura, Koujiro Yasunaga, and Nobuo Yamaguchi

Department of Laboratory Medicine, Kobe University School of Medicine (N.Y., E.T., N.Y.); Chest Disease Research Institute, Kyoto University (K.T.); Osaka Bioscience Research Institute (S.N.); and First Department of Internal Medicine, Kansai Medical College (T.N., Y.K., T.K., K.Y.)

The gene expression of myeloperoxidase (MPO), CD3ε, and CD3δ molecules, the gene rearrangement of T-cell receptor (TCR) δ, γ, and β and immunoglobulin heavy (IgH) chain, and the expression of cell-surface antigens were investigated in seven cases of CD7+ CD5− CD2− and four cases of CD7+ CD5+ CD2− acute lymphoblastic leukemia or lymphoblastic lymphoma (ALL/LBL) blasts, which were negative for cytochemical myeloperoxidase (cyMPO). More mature T-lineage blasts were also investigated in a comparative manner. In conclusion, the CD7+ CD5− CD2− blasts included four categories: undifferentiated blasts without lineage commitment, T-lineage blasts, T-/myeloid lineage blasts, and cyMPO-negative myeloblasts. The CD7+ CD5+ CD2− blasts included two categories; T-lineage and T-/myeloid lineage blasts.

The 11 cases were of the germ-line gene (G) for TCRβ and IgH. Four cases were G for TCRδ and TCRγ. The others were of the monoclonally rearranged gene (R) for TCRδ and G for TCRγ or R for both TCRδ and TCRγ.

The expression or in vitro induction of CD13 and/or CD33 antigens correlated with the immaturity of these neoplastic T cells, since it was observed in all 11 CD7+ CD5− CD2− and CD7+ CD5+ CD2−, and some CD7+ CD5+ CD2+ (CD3− CD4− CD8−) cases, but not in CD3± CD4+ CD8+ or CD3+ CD4+ CD8− cases.

CD3ε mRNA, but not CD3δ mRNA, was detected in two CD7+ CD5− CD2− cases, while mRNA of neither of the two CD3 molecules was detected in the other tested CD7+ CD5− CD2− cases. In contrast, mRNA of both CD3ε and CD3δ were detected in all CD7+ CD5+ CD2− cases, indicating that CD7+ CD5+ CD2− blasts at least belong to T-lineage.

The blasts of two CD7+ CD5− CD2− cases with entire germ-line genes and without mRNA of the three molecules (MPO, CD3ε, and CD3δ) were regarded as being at an undifferentiated stage prior to their commitment to either T- or myeloid-lineage.

The co-expression of the genes of MPO and CD3ε in a CD7+ CD5− CD2− case or MPO, CD3ε, and CD3δ in a CD7+ CD5+ CD2− case suggested the presence of some overlapping phase for T- and myeloid-lineage commitment during immature stages of differentiation. This helps understand the conversion of some T-ALL/LBL cases to acute myeloblastic leukemia (AML). The detection of CD3ε, but not CD3δ mRNA, in two CD7+ CD5− CD2− cases indicated that the gene expression of CD3ε occurs at a more immature stage of differentiation than that of the CD3δ chain.

Key words: CD7, CD13, peroxidase, CD3ε, CD3δ

INTRODUCTION

Acute lymphoblastic leukemia (ALL) or lymphoblastic lymphoma (LBL) cells of T-lineage have been investigated in terms of cell surface antigen expression [1],

Received for publication June 8, 1993; accepted September 22, 1993.

Address reprint requests to Dr. Eiji Tatsumi, Department of Laboratory Medicine, Kobe University School of Medicine, Kusunoki-Cho, Chuo-Ku, Kobe, 650 Japan.

TABLE I. Clinical Picture of Patients

Case	Age/sex	Date of test	Sample source[a]	Diagnosis	Lymphnode enlargement	Mediastinal mass	Clinical course[b]
1	56M	5/30/'87	PB	ALL	–	–	38M
2	49M	10/17/'89	PB	ALL	–	–	4M
3	43F	12/11/'89	PB	ALL	–	–	22M
4	53M	12/11/'89R[c]	BM	LBL	++	–	26M
5	31M	12/10/'89	BM	LBL[d]	++	+	8M
		7/7/'89	PB				
6	35M	9/27/'88R	PB	ALL	–	–	23M
7	26M	9/28/'88	PB	ALL	–	–	40M
8	32M	10/25/'88	PE	LBL	++	++	
		3/2/'90	PB				19M
9	16M	5/10/'89R	PB	LBL	++	++	21M
10	13M	5/10/'89R	PB	LBL	++	–	38M
11	15F	9/20/'88	PB	LBL	+	–	34M

[a]PB, peripheral blood; PE, pleural effusion; BM, bone marrow.
[b]M, months.
[c]R, relapse.
[d]LBL, lymphoblastic lymphoma.

terminal deoxy-nucleotidyl transferase (TdT) [2], gene rearrangement for T-cell receptors (TCR) [3], and cytoplasmic CD3 or CD3 mRNA [4,5]. It appears, however, that leukemia/lymphoma cells with CD7+ CD5− CD2−, CD7+ CD5+ CD2−, or CD7+ CD5+ CD2+ CD3− CD4− CD8− phenotype have not been investigated sufficiently to determine their exact lineage. Thiel et al. [6] examined phenotypic and genotypic analyses in relation to clinical outcomes in T-ALL/LBL cases, emphasizing that patients with CD7+ CD2− T-ALL/LBL cells had a poor prognosis compared with those with more mature blasts. Hershfield et al. [7] and Kurtzburg et al. [8] emphasized the stem-cell properties of CD7+ CD4− CD8− ALL/LBL cells which were able to differentiate along different lineages in vitro. Expression of CD13 and/or CD33 antigens, which were not tested in these studies [6–8], has been demonstrated in ALL/LBL cells of T- or B-lineage which were negative for cytochemical myeloperoxidase (cyMPO) [9,10]. In addition, Arita et al. [11] have shown that the expression of CD13 antigen or its induction in short-term in vitro culture occurs in immature stage neoplastic T cells with CD7+5−2−, CD7+5+2−, or CD7+5+2+3−4−8− phenotype.

In order to obtain deeper insight into the lineage of neoplastic lymphoblasts with CD7+5−2− and CD7+5+2− phenotypes, CD6 antigen [1,2] was tested additionally, and the expression of CD13 and 33 antigens after short-term in vitro culture was tested. In addition, we investigated the gene expression of myeloperoxidase (MPO) and CD3ε and CD3δ chains, along with gene rearrangement analyses of T-cell receptors (TCR) or δ, γ, and β chain and immunoglobulin heavy chain (IgH). Electron microscope detection of MPO (emMPO) was also performed. Results have shown that the induction in vitro of CD13 and CD33 antigens correlates with the immaturity (CD3− CD4− CD8−) of T-lineage blasts, that MPO mRNA and emMPO can be expressed simultaneously with CD3ε mRNA alone or with both CD3ε and CD3δ mRNA by CD7+5−2− or CD7+5+2− lymphoblasts, and that the CD7+5−2− cases included ones which can be regarded as 'undifferentiated' based upon the absence of MPO, CD3ε, or CD3δ mRNA.

MATERIALS AND METHODS

Patients

Clinical profiles of CD7+ CD5− CD2− and CD7+ CD5+ CD2− patients whose blasts were used for testing in this study are outlined in Table I. All manipulations including cell-surface antigen analyses and inoculations of in vitro cultures were performed within 10 hr after venipuncture, bone marrow, or pleural tap. The more mature neoplastic T-lineage blasts were handled under identical conditions.

Cell Surface Antigen Analysis

Mononuclear cells were separated from heparinized blood, bone marrow aspirate or pleural effusion by Ficoll-Hypacque discontinuous gradient centrifugation [13]. At least 92% of the mononuclear cells obtained were blasts. Cell-surface immunofluorescence analysis was performed using a total of 14 monoclonal antibodies [14]. NUT2 (CD1b), NUT-ER (CD2), NUT3 (CD3), NUTH/I (CD4), NUT-PAN (CD5), NUT-S/C (CD8), NU-B2 (CD20), MCS-2 (CD13), and NU-IA (HLADR) were purchased from Nichirei (Tokyo, Japan); Leu9 (CD7), and Leu12 (CD19) were from Becton-

Dickinson (Mountainview, CA); Mol (CD11b) and My9 (CD33) from Coulter (Hialeah, FL); and ClonabT1 (CD6) was from Biotest (Dreieich, Germany). FITC-conjugated $F(ab')_2$ goat anti-mouse IgG and IgM (Dakopatts, Glostrup, Denmark) were used for indirect immunofluorescence. To block Fc receptors, heat-aggregated (56°C, 30 min) human IgG (50 mg/ml) ('Venilon', Fujisawa, Osaka, Japan) was added to each specimen 10 min prior to each incubation, which was for 30 min at 4°C. The stained cells were assayed with an Epics-C flow cytometer (Coulter).

Short-Term In Vitro Culture

Cells were suspended in RPMI1640 supplemented with 10% fetal calf serum (FCS) (Hy-Clone, Logan, UT) at a cell concentration of 2×10^6/ml in a round bottom tube (2058, Falcon, Oxnard, CA), and cultured in both the absence and presence of 12-0-tetradecanoyl phorbol-13-acetate (TPA) (2.0 ng/ml) (Sigma, St. Louis, MO) in a CO_2 incubator (Tabai, Tokyo, Japan) in an atmosphere of 95% air and 5% CO_2 at 100% humidity for 48 hr. Harvested cells were tested for expression of CD13 and CD33 antigen.

Terminal Deoxynucleotidyl Transferase (TdT)

Indirect immunofluorescence of fixed cytocentrifuged smears using rabbit anti-TdT IgG (Bethesda Research Laboratory, Bethesda, MD) was performed according to previously described methods [2], using a Nikon (Tokyo, Japan) fluorescent microscope equipped with a 100 W mercury bulb.

Detection of Cytoplasmic CD3ε Chain

Cytocentrifuged cell smears were air-dried and fixed with acetone at −20°C for 3 min. Fixed cells were mounted with 10-fold diluted anti-CD3 ε-chain rabbit IgG (Dakopatts, Denmark) for 2 hr at room temperature. Following a wash, fluorescence was developed by overlaying 40-fold diluted FITC-conjugated anti-rabbit-IgG goat IgG (Medical and Biological Labs, Osaka, Japan) on the smear for 30 min. The cells of HL60 [15], HPB-ALL [16], a CD3+ CD4+ CD8+ T-ALL cell-line, and 3N-HPB-ALL, a CD3− CD4+ CD8+ sub-line of HPB-ALL were used as negative and positive control, respectively, and observed with the Nikon fluorescent microscope described above.

Myeloperoxidase (MPO)

Cytochemical myeloperoxidase activity (cyMPO) on blood films was tested according to the method of McJunkin [17]. Briefly, air-dried smears were mounted with 80% methanol containing 0.004% benzidine (Nakarai, Kyoto, Japan) and 0.008% hydrogen peroxide for 30 sec, rinsed with distilled water, and stained with Giemsa stain.

For MPO detection with electron microscopy (em-MPO), 2×10^7 cells were incubated in 3-3′diaminobenzidine and hydrogen peroxide medium for 1 hr, and fixed in 0.5% glutaraldehyde in PBS for 10 min at room temperature. Further processing was performed as previously described [18].

Gene Rearrangement Analysis

High molecular weight DNA was extracted from frozen pellets of the leukemia/lymphoma cells, as previously reported [19,20]. DNA was digested with BamH I (Takara, Kyoto, Japan), EcoRI (Takara), HindIII (Takara), or Bgl II (Toyobo, Osaka Japan). The restriction fragments were size-fractionated on 0.7% agarose gel and transferred to Gene Screen Plus nulon membranes (New England Nuclear, Boston, MA), as described [20]. The probes were labeled with ^{32}P by random priming method or by nick translation (Amersham, Buckinghamshire, England). After hybridizing with the labeled probe, the nylon membranes were washed at an appropriate stringency and autoradiographed.

For T-cell receptor (TCR) β chain gene analysis, a HindIII-EcoRI 3.5 kb fragment recognizing the constant portions of both β1 and β2 chain genes (Cβ1 and Cβ2) were generously provided by Dr. Honjo (Dept. Medical Chemistry, Kyoto University Faculty of Medicine) [21], and used as a Cβ probe. For TCRγ gene analysis, a HindIII-EcoRI 0.7 kb fragment recognizing the joining regions of both γ1 and γ2 chain genes (Jγ1 and Jγ2), a gift from Dr. Rabbitts (MRC, Cambridge, England) [22] was used as a Jγ probe. For testing the Jδ1 region of the TCRδ chain gene, we used an EcoRI 4.5 kb fragment, MH6, isolated by Takihara et al. [23], a gift from Dr. Kawa-Ha (Dept. of Pediatrics, Osaka University School of Medicine), and a Sacl 1.5 kb fragment, JδS16, a gift from Dr. Rabbitts [24]. For testing the Jδ2 and Jδ3 regions of the TCRδ chain gene, we employed a Xbal 1.5 kb fragment, H5, isolated by Takihara et al. [23], and supplied by Dr. Kawa-Ha, recognizing the joining region. For analysis of the immunoglobulin heavy chain (IgH) gene, an EcoRI-HindIII 3.4 kb fragment recognizing the joining region, a gift from Dr. Honjo [25], was used as a Jh probe.

Northern Blot Analysis

Total RNA was extracted from frozen pelleted cells by the guanidinium isothiocyanate method [26]. The RNA was electrophoresed through 1% agarose with formaldehyde and transferred to Gene Screen Plus (New England Nuclear, Boston, MA). After each electrophoresis, we were able to detect clear 28 and 18 S bands. The blots were hybridized with ^{32}P radio-labeled gene probes, and membranes were then autoradiographed.

The MPO cDNA isolated by Morishita et al. [27] was used as a probe for testing gene expression of MPO. Gene

TABLE II. Cell Surface Antigen (%) and TdT Expression*

	T antigens				Myeloid antigens				
Patients	CD7	CD5	CD2	CD6	CD11b	CD13	CD33	HLA-DR	TdT
CD7+ CD5− CD2−									
1	88	2	2	2	2	2 (3,2)[a]	66	80	−
2	63	1	1	1	3	97	77	84	−
3	60	2	2	1	4	2 (3,3)	12 (22,18)	15	−
4	94	3	4	3	2	8 (28,33)	19	76	−
5	83	3	3	3	4	6 (18,28)	20	78	−
	87	8	3	2	8	45 (61,68)	41	77	−
6	79	3	6	3	4	1 (1,1)	47	1	−
7	84	4	7	3	8	18 (22,38)	19 (22,20)	7	+
CD7+ CD5+ CD2−									
8	90	73	6	78	47	8 (28,44)	10 (18,13)	13	−
	82	44	7	72	21	22 (23,70)	13 (24,14)	47	−
9	90	69	6	83	12	10 (35,68)	12 (18,14)	11	+
10	91	63	7	74	71	5 (23,38)	4 (6,4)	6	+
11	93	81	7	86	60	2 (8,25)	19 (24,22)	33	−

*The tested blasts in all cases were CD1− CD3− CD4− CD8− CD10− CD19− CD20− CD24− except for Case 2 (CD10, 27%). The date of sampling is shown in Table I. Terminal deoxy-nucleotidyl transferase. Fluorescence intensity was arbitrarily graded as −, +, or ++. The most intense fluorescence, as observed in Pre-B ALL or lymphoid-type CML (chronic myelogenous leukemia) crisis blasts, corresponds to ++.
[a]In the parenthesis, the positive percentage in the control and TPA-added culture is shown.

probes for testing the expression of CD3ε and CD3δ chains were supplied by Dr. Terhost [28,29] (Dana Farber Cancer Institute, Boston, MA).

Northern blot hybridization was also carried out with β actin probe [30] to ensure that approximately same amount of mRNA was loaded in each lane.

RESULTS

Cases

The brief clinical profiles of 11 CD7+ CD5− CD2− and CD7+ CD5+ CD2− cases are shown in Table I. Lymph-node enlargement was absent in Patients 1, 2, 3, 6, 7, and 10, whereas it was present in Cases 4, 5, 8, 9, and 11. Bone marrow blasts comprised over 80% of the cell population in all patients except for Case 8, in whom the initial involvement was only moderate (22%), but rose to 84% in the later phase of the illness. The diagnosis of lymphoblastic lymphoma (LBL) was made according to the original report [31]. All LBL cases were of the non-convoluted type.

Cell Surface Antigen Analysis

The results of the cell-surface antigen analyses are shown in Table II. Antigens CD1, CD3, CD4, CD8, CD19, CD16, CD20, and CD24 were absent in all 11 cases. The CD10 antigen was negative in all but Case 4, in which CD10 antigen was positive in 27% of the lymph-node blasts. The CD7 antigen was expressed as a sole pan-T antigen in Cases 1 to 7. In Cases 8 to 11, CD7, CD5 and CD6 antigens were expressed. CD13 antigen was expressed by the fresh or 48 hr cultured blasts from Cases 2, 4, 5, and 8 to 11, whereas it was neither expressed by the fresh blasts nor induced in the 48 hr cultured blasts in Cases 1, 3, and 6. The blasts in these three cases expressed CD33 antigen. In Cases 5 and 8, the CD13+ blasts were initially present in 6% and 8%, respectively, but increased to 45% and 22%, when tested again in the later phase of the illness. CD33 antigen was expressed by the fresh and 48 hr cultured cells in all patients except for Case 10. Expression of CD33 antigen was apparently enhanced in the control cultures, but not significantly enhanced by the presence of TPA in some cases (Cases 3, 8, and 11).

For comparison, the overall results of expression or induction of CD13 antigen in more mature T-cell ALL/LBL cases are shown in Table III. In the CD2+ CD5+ CD7+ CD3− CD4− CD8− group, CD13 antigen expression or induction was observed in three of the five cases. Neither CD13 nor CD33 antigen was expressed or induced in any of the 16 CD7+ CD5+ CD2+ cases with CD3− CD4+ CD8+, CD3+ CD4+ CD8+ or CD3+ CD4+ CD8− phenotype.

Detection of Cytoplasmic CD3ε Chain

Cytoplasmic CD3ε chain, as detected with rabbit IgG antibody, was negative in cases 1 to 7, but positive in cases 8 to 11, as shown in Table IV.

Terminal Deoxy-Nucleotidyl Transferase (TdT)

Results are shown in Table II according to an arbitrary grading, marked by −, +, or ++. The most intense fluorescence which was observed in some pre-B ALL blasts or lymphoid type crisis blasts from cases of chronic myelogenous leukemia (CML) were classified as ++.

TABLE III. Expression of CD13 Antigen in CD2+ CD5+ CD7+ T-ALL/LBL Cases*

Pattern of T-cell antigen expression		CD13 antigen expression (positive/total case number)
CD1− CD7+ CD5+ CD2+	CD3− CD4− CD8−	3/5[a]
CD1+[b] CD7+ CD5+ CD2+	CD3− CD4+ CD8+	0/4
CD1+[b] CD7+ CD5+ CD2+	CD3+ CD4+ CD8+	0/7
CD1+ CD7+ CD5+ CD2+	CD3+ CD4+ CD8−	0/1

*CD33 antigen was positive in a CD3− CD4− CD8− CD13− case. CD11b antigen was positive in a CD3− CD4− CD8− CD13+ case.
[a]In one case, 32% of the fresh blasts expressed CD13 antigen. In the other two CD13+ cases, CD13 antigen was induced in vitro in at least 42% of the blasts.
[b]One CD3− CD4+ CD8+ and one CD3+ CD4+ CD8+ case were negative for CD1 antigen.

As shown in Table II, the blasts were positive for TdT in three cases.

Myeloperoxidase (MPO) Detection With Cytochemistry (cyMPO) and With Electron Microscopy (emMPO)

Cytochemical myeloperoxidase activity (cyMPO) was negative in all patients. In Cases 5 and 8, a count of 500 blasts from samples obtained before therapy was negative for cyMPO, whereas 0.3 and 0.8%, respectively, of blasts from the second test (Table I) were positive for cyMPO (Fig. 1).

Electron-microscope studies for MPO (emMPO) were performed in Cases 1, 2, 3, 5, and 8. It was entirely negative in Case 1 (Fig. 2A). One per two hundred blasts in Case 2 had one or two positive granules (Fig. 2B). All blasts in Case 3 had one or two positive granules (Fig. 2C). In Case 5 (in the first sample), all blasts had a few positive granules (Fig. 2D). In the first samples from Case 8, 20% of the blasts had a few positive granules, respectively (Fig. 2E).

Gene Rearrangement Study

When the BamHI or HindIII digests of the DNA extracted from the blasts of each patient were hybridized with a ^{32}P labeled joining region probe (Jh probe) for IgH, only a germ-line gene (G) band was observed, and a monoclonally rearranged gene (R) band was not detected. The TCRβ gene configuration, as tested by hybridizing the EcoRI, BamHI, or HindIII digests with the ^{32}P labeled Cβ probe, was G in all 11 cases. The Southern blot analysis with the EcoRI and BamHI digests using the Jγ probe revealed only two G bands, 3.3 kb/1.8 kb and 21 kb/15 kb, respectively, in all but Patients 6 and 9. In these two patients, two bi-allelic R bands were observed (data not shown).

The Southern blot analysis with the BglII and HindIII digests using Jδ S16 and MH6 probes, respectively, revealed two bi-allelic R bands in Cases 3, 4, 6, and 7, one R and one G band in Cases 5 and 9, one R bands in Case 8, and only a G band in Cases 1, 2, 10, and 11 (Fig. 3A, and B). In these four patients, the EcoRI digests were hybridized with an H5 probe to test the possibility of Jδ 2 and Jδ 3 region rearrangement, but no R band was detected (Fig. 3C).

The overall results are summarized in Table IV. The blasts in Cases 1, 2, 10, and 11 were G for both IgH and TCR. The first samples were tested by Northern blot analysis in Cases 5 and 8.

Gene Expression of Myeloperoxidase (MPO) and CD3ε and CD3δ Chain

The gene expression of myeloperoxidase (MPO), and CD3ε, and CD3δ chains are shown in Figure 4, and summarized in Table IV. It was ensured that the ethydium bromide stain of 28s and 18s rRNA was intact. The signals of β-actin were comparable (data not shown). In Cases 5 and 8, only the first samples were tested. The blasts in Cases 1 and 2 were MPO mRNA− and CD3ε mRNA−δ mRNA−. The blasts in Case 3 were MPO mRNA+ and CD3ε mRNA+δ mRNA−. Case 4 was MPO mRNA− and CD3ε mRNA+δ mRNA−. Case 5 was MPO mRNA+ and CD3ε mRNA−δ mRNA−. Case 8 was MPO mRNA+ and CD3ε mRNA+δ mRNA+. Cases 9 and 10 were MPO mRNA− and CD3ε mRNA+δ mRNA+.

In the three CD7+5+2+ cases in which CD13 and/or 33 antigen expression or induction occurred, CD3ε and CD3δ mRNA were detected, but MPO mRNA was not (data not shown).

DISCUSSION

Although CD7 antigen has been demonstrated to be a reliable marker of neoplastic T cells at the most immature stage of differentiation [32,33], it is known that some cyMPO-positive acute myeloblastic leukemia (AML) cells also express CD7 antigen [34,35]. The expression of CD7 alone cannot, therefore, be used to identify neoplastic cells as being of T-cell lineage. This interpretation is tenable in Cases 1 and 2, in which the blasts were entirely G for IgH and TCR, and had none of the transcripts of MPO, CD3ε, or CD3δ chain genes (Table IV). These two cases can be regarded as acute undifferentiated leukemias in a more strict sense of the term. The other three tested CD7+ CD5−CD2− cases were MPO mRNA+, CD3ε mRNA+ δmRNA−; MPO mRNA−, CD3ε mRNA+δ mRNA−; and MPO mRNA+, CD3ε mRNA− δmRNA−. In contrast, all CD7+ CD5+ CD2− cases can be regarded as belonging to T-lineage at least in terms of the presence of both CD3ε and CD3δ

TABLE IV. Gene Expression of MPO and CD3ϵ and CD3δ Chain, and TCR Gene Rearrangement*

		mRNA Expression			TCR gene rearrangement		
Case	cyCD3ϵ[a]	MPO	CD3ϵ	CD3δ	Jδ	Jγ	Cβ
CD7+ CD5− CD2−							
1	−	−	−	−	G[b]	G	G
2	−	−	−	−	G	G	G
3	−	+	+	−	R/R[b]	G	G
4	−	−	+	−	R/R	G	G
5[c]	−	+	−	−	G/R	G	G
6	−	NT[d]	NT	NT	R/R	R/R	G
7	−	NT	NT	NT	R/R	G	G
CD7+ CD5+ CD2−							
8[c]	+	+	+	+	G/R	G	G
9	+	−	+	+	R/D[b]	R/R	G
10	+	−	+	+	G	G	G
11	+	NT	NT	NT	G	G	G

*IgH gene is G in all cases.
[a]Cytoplasmic CD3ϵ.
[b]G, germ-line genotype; R, monoclonally rearranged genotype; D, deletion.
[c]The sample is the first test.
[d]NT, not tested.

mRNA. Moreover, the CD7+ CD5+ CD2− were always CD6+, whereas the CD7+ CD5− CD2− blasts were always CD6−.

The blasts in 7 of the 11 cases (excepting Cases 1, 3, and 6) expressed CD13 antigen in their fresh state of in in vitro culture in the presence of TPA (2.0 ng/ml) after 48 hr (Table II). CD13 antigen was expressed or induced in vitro in three out of the five CD7+ CD5+ CD2+ CD3− CD4− CD8− cases (Table III). In contrast, CD13 antigen was neither expressed nor induced in vitro in the CD3− CD4+ CD8+, CD3+ CD4+ CD8+, or CD3− CD4+ CD8+ cases. Thus, when neoplastic T cells are sufficiently immature, the expression or induction of CD13 antigen is frequent. The expression or induction of CD13 antigen can, therefore, define immaturity of neoplastic T cells.

The expression or in vitro induction of CD13 antigen by T-ALL or LBL cells has already been reported [9,10], although not in some reports studying immature stage neoplastic T cells [6,8,36]. The report by Arita et al. [11] and the results shown in the current study indicate that in vitro short-term culture in the presence of TPA is useful and meaningful, not only for induction and expression of CD13 antigen, but also to demonstrate that it is absent and not inducible in some blasts. Frequently, a major proportion of the cultured cells were induced to express CD13 antigen in the absence of TPA (Cases 4, 5, 8, 9, and 10) (Table II). The recent isolation of the gene encoding the CD13 antigen [37], and its identification as aminopeptidase N [38] will help to further clarify the behavior of this antigen molecule, which is sometimes simply

A

B

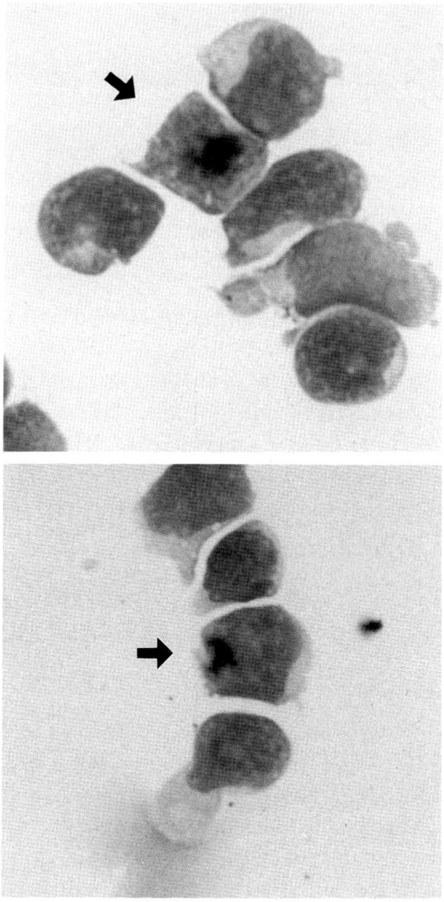

Fig. 1. cyMPO(+) cells on cytocentrifuged smears. A: Case 5 blasts in the second test (0.3% positive). B: Case 8 blasts in the second test (0.8% positive).

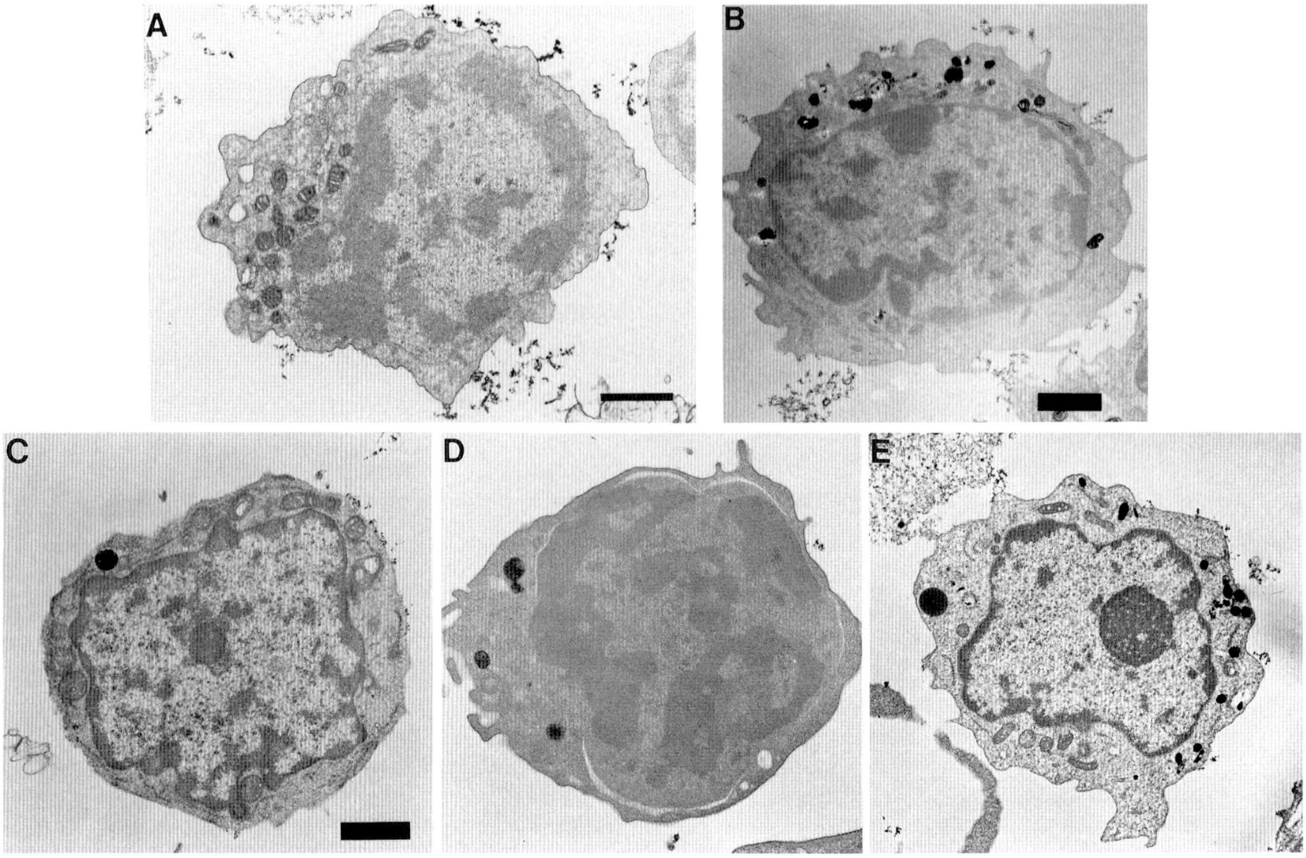

Fig. 2. emMPO. The scale represents 1.0 μ. A: Case 1, No blasts have MPO-positive granules. B: Case 2, One of 200 blasts has MPO-positive granules. C: Case 3, all blasts have one or two MPO-positive granules. D: Case 5, All blasts have MPO-positive granules in the first test. E: Case 8, Twenty percent of the blasts had a few MPO-positive granules.

referred to as "myeloid antigen," based upon its cellular distribution.

CD11b antigen was expressed in all CD7+ CD5+ CD2− cases and in one of eight CD7+ CD5+ CD2+ CD3− CD4− CD8− cases (Table III), but not in the other T-ALL/LBL or the CD7+ CD5− CD2 cases. This fact should be noted in phenotyping neoplastic T-cell subsets accurately.

During this study, we attempted to examine blasts from two cases with CD7+ CD5− CD2+ phenotypes which had been included in reports by others [3], but materials for Northern or Southern blot analyses were not available.

MPO gene expression was detected in Cases 3, 5, and 8 (Fig. 4, Table IV). The blasts in Case 3 had CD3ε, but not CD3δ RNA, and were R for TCRδ and G for TCRγ and TCRβ chains. These results can be interpreted to place the lineage of Case 3 blasts in a quite immature location in the T-cell differentiation pathway, close to or overlapping with myeloid lineage. The blasts from Case 5 had neither CD3ε nor CD3δ chain genes, and was R for the TCRδ chain and G for the TCRγ and TCRβ chains. The clinical diagnosis of Case 5, in which systemic lymph-node enlargement, a mediastinal mass and bone marrow involvement were present, was LBL. The cyMPO was negative after counting 500 blasts during the initial presentation. The exclusive expression of the MPO gene and the possible lack of significance of the R of TCRδ in Case 5 make it difficult to distinguish the Case 5 blasts from tumor-forming CD7+ AML cases despite the typical clinical appearances as LBL.

In Case 8, the co-expression of MPO, CD3ε, and CD3δ chain genes is more strongly indicative of the existence of an overlapping phase of myeloid and T-cell differentiation pathways during immature stages than is the co-expression of MPO and the CD3ε gene in Case 3. In this sense, Case 8 is the most representative in this series of patients.

The two patterns of gene expression of the two CD3 chains, the CD3ε chain alone in the most immature stage and both CD3ε and CD3δ chains in more mature stages, suggests a hierarchial order of expression of these two CD3 molecules. This hierarchy has not been clearly reported in human neoplastic T cells but has previously

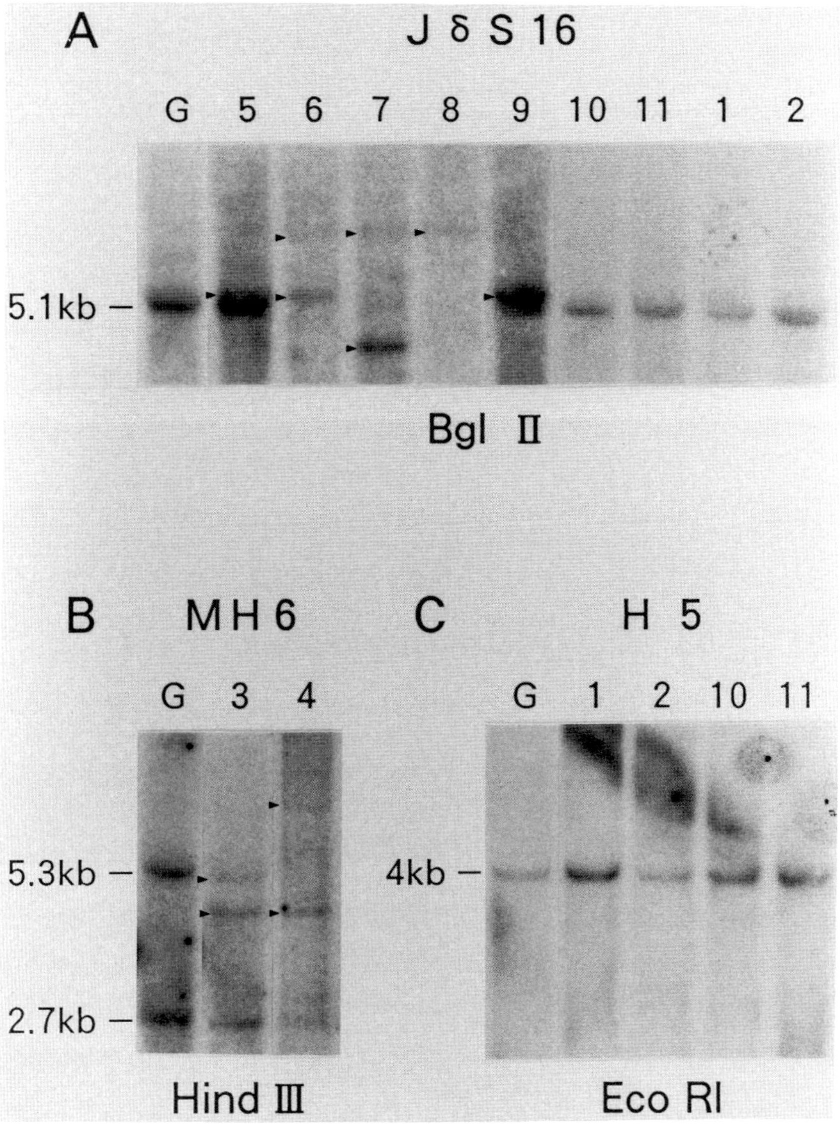

Fig. 3. Southern blot analysis for TCRδ gene. Lane number corresponds to the case numbers in Tables I and II. In Lane G, the DNA extracted form the cells of a pre-B ALL line is loaded. A: BglII digests hybridized with a Jδ S16 probe. Only a germ-line gene (G) band (5.1 kb) is observed in Cases 10, 11, 1, and 2. One G band and a monoclonally rearranged gene (R) band are observed in Cases 5 and 9. One R band is present in Case 8. Two (biallelic) R bands are observed in Cases 6 and 7. B: HindIII digests hybridized with an MH6 probe. Two R bands are observed in Cases 3 and 4. C: EcoRI digests hybridized with H5 probe. Only a G band is observed in Cases 1, 2, 10, and 11.

been described in some IL-2 dependent natural-killer-like clones of normal cell origin [39,40]. The gene expression of CD3ε and CD3δ chains has been shown to occur prior to TCRγ and TCRβ chain gene rearrangement [4]. Their occurrence prior to TCRδ chain gene rearrangement, as revealed in Case 10, is a new finding.

CD3ε mRNA and cytoplasmic CD3ε has always been detected in a co-existing manner in previous reports [4,5,36]. In Cases 3 and 4, cytoplasmic CD3ε was not detected despite the presence of CD3ε mRNA. The method of fixation used in this report may be responsible, although it was adopted as the optimum after testing several other techniques [4,5,36]. Alternatively, cytoplasmic CD3ε chains may be difficult to detect in the cytoplasm, when not accompanied by CD3δ chain. Notably, mRNA of both CD3ε and CD3δ chains has always been detected in the materials studied up until now [4,5,36]. The last possibility is that the presence of CD3ε mRNA may not signify the production of the CD3ε molecule. Cytoplasmic CD3ε chain was not mentioned in the reports in which the natural-killer-like clones expressed only CD3ε mRNA [39,40].

The results of emMPO (Fig. 2) were in accord with those of MPO mRNA in all tested cases. In Case 2, only

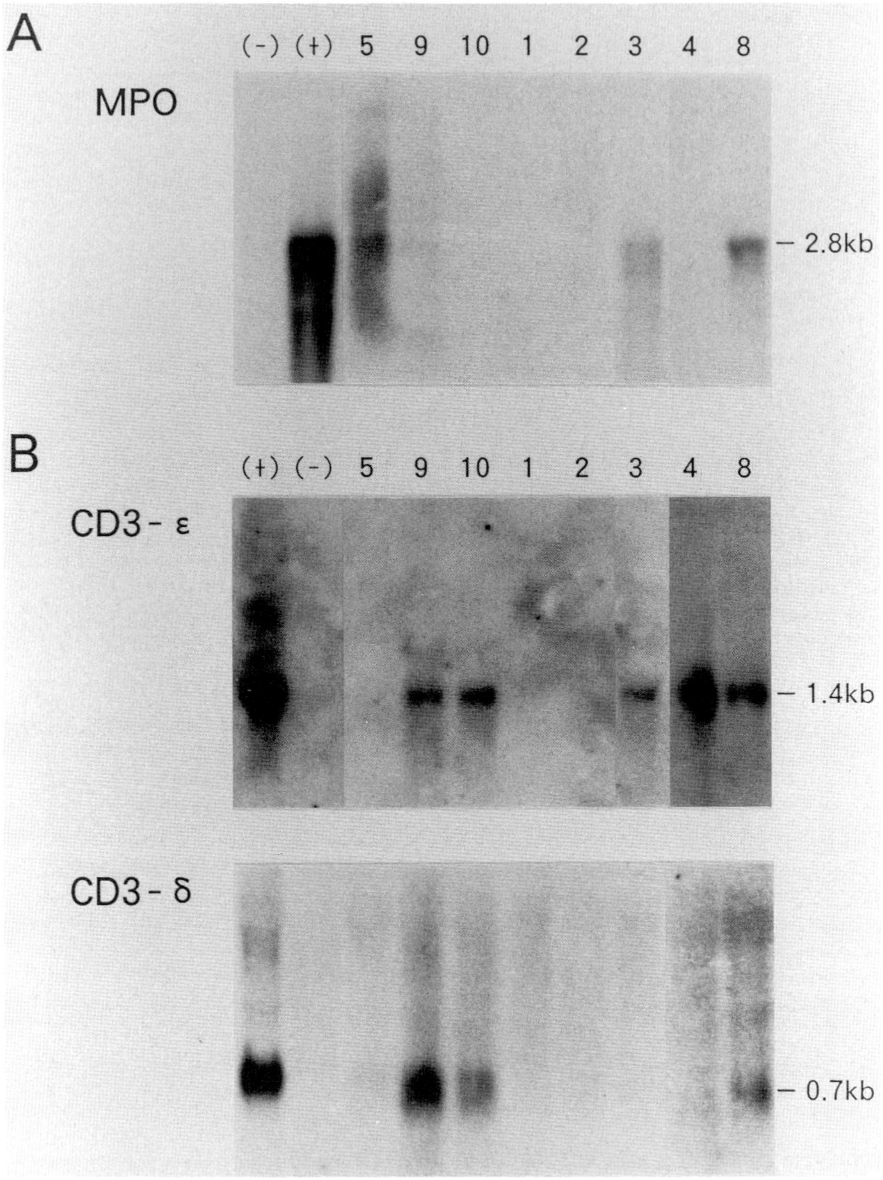

Fig. 4. Northern blot analyses with the MPO (A) gene probe and with the CD3ε and CD3δ (B) gene probes. Lane numbers correspond to case numbers in Tables I and II. The RNA extracted from the HL-60 cells is loaded in Lane (+) in A and in Lane (−) in B. The RNA extracted from the HPB-ALL cells is loaded in Lane (−) in A and Lane (+) in B.

one per two hundred cells had MPO-positive granules, and this was interpreted as negative. Each of the Case 3 blasts had one or two MPO-positive granules. In this case, the Northern blot study detected MPO transcript.

The co-existance of emMPO, MPO mRNA, and CD3ε mRNA or both CD3ε mRNA and CD3δ mRNA is particularly intriguing when considering cyMPO+ AML conversion of LBL or T-ALL [41]. This was reported shortly after the initial descriptions of LBL [31] and has since been repeatedly confirmed [42–45]. In Cases 5 and 8, the MPO mRNA+ blasts were cyMPO− after counting 500 blasts obtained during the initial presentation, and 0.3 and 0.8% of the blasts, respectively, became cyMPO+ in the sample taken after several courses of chemotherapy (Fig. 1). Chemotherapy might be responsible for the slight but significant manifestation of cyMPO in Cases 5 and 8. Since the blasts in Case 3, 5 and 8 expressed MPO mRNA before therapy, some inherent capacity for multilineage differentiation, as reported by Kurtsburg et al. [8] may be responsible. Their cases, in which CD13 induction in vitro or the gene expression of MPO and CD3 molecules was not investigated, seem to share some properties with our cases.

Further studies of the gene structure and expression of the key molecules in immature leukemia/lymphoma celles are necessary to clearly define the immature stages of human hematopoietic cell differentiation, and to document molecular events associated with undifferentiatedness or lineage promiscuity [46], as exemplified in this series of cases.

ACKNOWLEDGMENTS

This study was supported by a Grant-in-Aid for General Scientific Research (No. 01571269, 1989), the Ministry of Education, Science and Culture, Japan and by the Clinical Pathology Research Fund (1989).

Thanks are due to Dr. J. Raff (University of Louisville School of Medicine, Louisville, KY) for the critical reading of this manuscript, and to Ms. K. Doi and S. Suda for their excellent technical assistance.

We wish to express our appreciation for supplying patient materials and clinical data to Dr. N. Nesumi and Dr. Y. Toyokawa (Case 1) (Kansai Denryoku Hospital, Osaka); Dr. T. Kobayashi (Case 2) (North Shinshu General Hospital, Nagano); Dr. H. Sakoda (Case 3) (Sumitomo Hospital, Osaka); Dr. K. Ohno, Dr. R. Ogawa, Dr. T. Natazuka, Dr. T. Matsui, Dr. Nakao, and Dr. T. Fujita (Cases 4, 5, and 8) (Third Dept. Internal Medicine, Kobe University School of Medicine, Kobe); Dr. H. Yabe, Dr. K. Nagai, and Dr. S. Nakayama (Kobe Municipal Hospital, Kobe); Dr. H. Konishi (Case 7) (Kurashiki Chuo Hospital, Kurashiki); Dr. Y. Kiriyama and Dr. T. Tsutsui (Cases 9 and 10) (Dept. Pediatrics, Kobe Municipal Hospital), and to Dr. Kosaka, Dr. K. Sano, Dr. R. Murakami, and Dr. H. Nakamura (Case 11) (Dept. Pediatrics, Kobe University School of Medicine).

REFERENCES

1. Foon KA, Todd RF: Immunologic classification of leukemia and lymphoma. Blood 68:1, 1986.
2. Bollum FJ: Terminal deoxynucleotidyl transferase as a hematopoietic cell marker. Blood 54:1203, 1979.
3. Felix CA, Wright JJ, Poplak DG, Reaman GH, Cole D, Goldman P, Korsmeyer SL: T-cell receptor α-, β- and γ-genes in T cell and pre-B cell acute lymphoblastic leukemia. J Clin Invest 80:545, 1987.
4. Van Dongen JJM, Krissansen GW, Wolvers-Tettero ILM, Comans-Bitter WM, Hooijkaase H, Van Wering ER, Terhost C: Cytoplasmic expression of the CD3 antigen as a diagnostic marker for immature T-cell malignancies. Blood 71:603, 1988.
5. Pittaluga S, Uppenkamp M. Cossman J: Development of T3/T cell receptor gene expression in human pre-T neoplasms. Blood 69:1062, 1987.
6. Thiel E, Kranz BR, Raghavachar A, Bartram CR, Loffler H, Messener D, Ganser A, Ludwig W-D, Buchner T, Hoelzer D: Prethymic phenotype and genotype of pre-T (CD7+/ER−)-cell leukemia and its clinical significance within adult acute lymphoblastic leukemia. Blood 73:1247, 1989.
7. Hershfield MS, Kurtzberg J, Harden E, Moore JO, Whang-Peng J, Haynes BF: Conversion of a stem cell leukemia from a T-lymphoid to a myeloid phenotype induced by the adenosine deaminase inhibitor.2′-deoxycoformycin. Proc Natl Acad Sci USA 81:253, 1984.
8. Kurtzburg J, Waldmann TA, Daney MP, Bigner SH, Moore JO, Hershfield MS, Haynes BF: CD7+, CD4−, CD8− acute leukemia: A syndrome of malignant pluripotent lymphohematopoietic cells. Blood 73:381, 1989.
9. Sobol RE, Mick R, Royston I, Davery FR, Ellinson RR, Newman R, Cuttner J, Griffin JD, Collins H, Nelson DA, Bloomfield CD: Clinical importance of myeloid antigen expression in adult acute lymphoblastic leukemia. N Eng J Med 316:1111, 1987.
10. Drexler HG, Sagawa K, Menon M, Minowada J: Reactivity pattern of "myeloid monoclonal antibodies" with emphasis on MCS-2. Leuk Res 10:17, 1986.
11. Arita Y, Kita K, Nasu K, Doi S, Fukuhara S, Nishikori M, Miwa S, Tatsumi E, Nosaka T, Hatanaka M, Uchino H: Frequent expression of myeloid antigen (CD13) on immature T cells in culture. Acta Hematol Jpn 53:21, 1990.
12. Knowles RW: Immunochemical analysis of the T-cell specific antigens. Reinherz EL, Haynes BE, Nadler LM, Bernstein ID. New York: Springer, 1986 pp 259–288.
13. Böym A: Separation of leucocytes from blood and bone marrow. Scand J Clin Lab Invest 21: 77, 1968.
14. McMichael AJ: (1987) Leucocyte Typing White Cell Differentiation Antigens. Oxford: Oxford Press, 1,050 pp.
15. Collins SJ, Gallo RC, Gallagher RE: Continuous growth and differentiation of human myeloid leukemia cells in suspension culture. Nature 270:347, 1977.
16. Morikawa S, Tatsumi E, Baba M, Harada T, Yasuhira K: Two E-rosette forming lymphoid cell lines. Int J Cancer 21:166, 1978.
17. McJunkin FA: A benzidine-polychrome stain for blood. JAMA 74:17, 1920.
18. Kishimoto Y, Nagano T, Kimura T, Adachi M, Tatsumi E, Ryo R, Yamaguchi N, Yasunaga K: Ultrastructural analysis of megakaryoblasts by simultaneous detection of platelet peroxidase and platelet glycoprotein. Act Hematol Jpn 52:102, 1989.
19. Southern EM: Detection of specific sequences among DNA fragments separated by gel electrophoresis. J Mol Biol 98:503, 1975.
20. Maniatis T, Fritsch EF, Sambrook J: 1982. "Molecular Cloning. A Laboratory Manual." New York: Cold Spring Harbor Laboratory, 545 pp.
21. Ikuta K, Ogura T, Shimizu A, Honjo T: Low frequency of somatic mutation in β chain variable region genes of human T-cell receptors. Proc Natl Acad Sci USA 82:7701, 1985.
22. Lefranc MP, Rabbitts TH: Two tandemly organized human genes encoding the T-cell γ constant region sequences show multiple rearrangement in different T-cell types. Nature 316:464, 1985.
23. Takihara Y, Tkachuk D, Michalpoulus E, Champagne E, Reiman J, Minden M, Mak TW: Sequence and organization of the diversity, joining, and constant region genes of the human T-cell δ-chain locus. Proc Natl Acad Sci USA 85:6097, 1988.
24. Boehm T, Baer R, Lavenir I, Forster A, Waters JJ, Nacheva E, Rabbitts TH: The mechanism of chromosomal translocation t(11;14) involving the T-cell receptor Cδ locus on human chromosome 14q11 and a transcribed region of chromosome 11p15. EMBO J 7:385, 1988.
25. Takahashi N, Nakai S, Honjo T: Cloning of human immunoglobulin μ gene and comparison with mouse μ gene. Nuc Acid Res 8:5983, 1980.
26. Glisin VR, Crkvenjakov R, Byus C: Ribonucleic acid isolated by cesium chrolide centrifugation. Biochemistry 13:2633, 1974.
27. Morishita K, Kubota N, Asano S, Kaziro Y, Nagata S: Molecular cloning and characterization of cDNA for human myeloperoxidase. J Biol Chem 262:3844, 1987.
28. Van den Eisen P, Shepley B-A, Borst J, Cligan JE, Markham AF,

Orkin S, Terhost C: Isolation of cDNA clones encoding the 20k T3 glycoprotein of human T-cell receptor complex. Nature 312:413, 1984.

29. Gold DP, Puck JM, Pettey CL, Cho M, Coligan J, Woody JN, Terhost C: Isolation of cDNA clones encoding the 20k non-glycosylated polypeptide chain of the human T-cell receptor/T3 complex. Nature 321: 431, 1986.
30. Ponte P, Gumming P, Blau H, Kedes L: Human actin genes are single copy for α-skeletal and α-cardiac actin but multicopy for β- and γ-cytoskeletal genes: 3′ untranslated regions are isotype specific but are conserved in evolution. Mol Cell Biol 3:1783, 1983.
31. Nathwani BM, Rappaport H: Malignant lymphoma, lymphoblastic. Cancer 38:946, 1976.
32. Link M, Warnke R, Finlay J, Amylon M, Miller R, Dilley J, Levy R: A single monoclonal antibody identifies T-cell lineage of childhood lymphoid malignancies. Blood 62:722, 1983.
33. Pittalgua S, Raffeld M, Lipford EH, Cossman J: 3A1(CD7) expression precedes Tβ gene rearrangements in precursor T (lymphoblastic) neoplasms. Blood 68:133, 1986.
34. Zutter MM, Martin PJ, Hanke D, Kidd PG: CD7+ acute non-lymphocytic leukemia: Evidence for an early multipotential progenitor. Leuk Res 14:23, 1990.
35. Lo Coco FL, Rossi GD, Pasqualetti D, Lopez M, Diverio D, Latalgiata R, Fenu S, Mandelli F: CD7 positive acute myeloid leukemia: A subtype associated with cell immaturity. Br J Hematol 73:480, 1989.
36. Van Dongen JJM, Quertermous T, Bartram CR, Gold DP, Wolves-Tettero ILM, Commans-Bitter WM, Hooilkaas H, Adriaansen HJ, DeKlein A, Raghavachar A, Ganser A, Duby AD, Seidman J, Van den Eisen P, Terhost C: T-cell receptor-CD3 complex during early T cell differentiation: Analysis of immature T cell acute lymphoblastic leukemia (T-ALL) at DNA, RNA and cell membrane level. J Immunol 138:1260, 1987.
37. Look AT, Peiper SC, Rebetinsch MB, Ashmun RA, Russel MF Lemons RS, LeBeau MM, Rubin CM, Sherr CJ: Molecular cloning, expression and chromosomal localization of the gene encoding a human myeloid membrane antigen (gp150). J Clin Invest 78:914, 1986.
38. Ashmun RA, Look AT: Metalloprotease activity of CD13/aminopeptidase N on the surface of human myeloid cells. Blood 75:462, 1990.
39. Ciccone E, Viale O, Pende D, Malnati M, Blassoni R, Melioli G, Moretta A, Long EO, Moreta R: Specific lysis of allogeneic cells after activation of CD3-lymphocytes in mixed lymphocyte culture. J Exp Med 168:2403, 1988.
40. Biassoni R, Ferrini S, Prigione I, Moretta A, Long EO: CD3 negative lymphokine-activated cytotoxic cells express CD3ε gene. J Immunol 140:1685, 1988.
41. Kjeldsberg CR, Nathwani BN, Rappaport H. Acute myeloblastic leukemia developing in patients with mediastinal lymphoblastic lymphoma. Cancer 44:2316, 1979.
42. Herrman R, Han T, Barcos MP, Lok S, Henderson ES: Malignant lymphoma of pre-T-cell type terminating in acute myeloblastic leukemia. Cancer 46:1383, 1980.
43. Posner MR, Said J, Pinkus GS, Nadler LM, Hardy R, Flatow F, Skarin AT: T-cell lymphoma with subsequent acute non-lymphocytic leukemia. Cancer 50:118, 1980.
44. Murphy SB, Stass S, Kalwinsky D, Rivera G: Phenotypic conversion of acute leukemia form T-lymphoblastic to myeloblastic induced by therapy with 2′-deoxycoformycin. Br J Haematol 55:285, 1983.
45. Nosaka T, Ohno H, Doi S, Fukuhara S, Miwa H, Kita K, Shirakawa S, Honjo T, Hatanaka M: Phenotypic conversion of T lymphoblastic lymphoma to acute biphenotypic leukemia composed of lymphoblasts and myeloblasts: Molecular genetic evidence of the same clonal origin. J Clin Invest 81:1824, 1988.
46. Greaves MF, Chan LC, Furlry AJW, Watt SM, Molgaard HV: Lineage promiscuity in hematopoietic differentiation and Leukemia. Blood 67:1, 1986.

American Journal of Hematology 45:321–324 (1994)

Prevalence of Antithrombin Deficiency in Healthy Blood Donors: A Cross-Sectional Study

Philip S. Wells, Morris A. Blajchman, Penny Henderson, Michael J. Wells, Christine Demers, Ron Bourque, and Ann McAvoy

The Canadian Red Cross Society and the Departments of Pathology and Medicine McMaster University, Hamilton, Ontario, Canada

The prevalence of antithrombin (AT) deficiency in the general population has been variously estimated to be between 0.05 and 5 per 1,000 in the population; 2,491 blood donors were screened in an attempt to clarify this issue using plasma samples taken from the blood donor units. From this initial population, 122 individuals were identified as having plasma AT levels lower than 2 standard deviations below the normal mean. Twenty-two samples had evidence that thrombin had been generated during blood collection and the remaining cohort of 100 blood donors were asked to return but only 59 complied. The data obtained from these 59 were compared with that from 51 age- and sex-matched control blood donors. Both groups of subjects were assessed for previous evidence, or family history, of thrombotic events, as well as exposure to risk factors associated with the development of deep vein thrombosis (DVT). All had venous blood samples taken from which the supernatant plasma was immediately removed and quick frozen for later assaying. Only 6 of the 59 subjects with initial low AT levels had repeat AT-Xa levels below 0.80 units/ml (normal range 0.94 ± 0.14). Upon repeating the AT-Xa determinations on new samples from these six individuals, only three were found again to be low. One was found to have a type 3 AT deficiency (an Arg47Cys substitution). The other two with a low AT level had mean functional AT-Xa levels of 0.61 and 0.71 units/ml, respectively, with correspondingly low AT:Ag levels consistent with a type 1 AT deficiency. Two of these three subjects has been in high risk situations without evidence of having developed DVT and none had evidence of venous reflux on Doppler venography. In addition, none had personal or family histories of previous thrombotic events. These present data indicate that the prevalence of AT deficiency in our blood donor population is 2 per 1,000 (95% confidence intervals: 0.7–6/1,000).

Key words: antithrombin, antithrombin deficiency, blood donors, prevalence, thrombin

INTRODUCTION

It is well known that individuals with antithrombin (AT) deficiency represent a particular group at increased risk for thromboembolic events. Such individuals were thought to have an increased risk estimated to be approximately 1% per year; however, a recent prospective cross-sectional study of a large AT deficient kindred (Ala382Thr) indicates that the risk of thrombosis in such AT-deficient individuals may be much lower than previously estimated [1,2]. The previously overestimated risk of thrombosis may be related to the fact that such patients are often identified as having AT-deficiency only after the thromboembolic event had occurred. Thus, the derivation of estimates of risk from such individuals probably represents selection bias. To appreciate the true risk of thrombosis in AT-deficient subjects it would be useful also to know the prevalence of AT-deficiency in the general population. This prevalence has been generally estimated to be 0.2/1,000; however, recent studies suggest that the prevalence of AT deficiency may be as high as 5/1000 [3–5]. Similar low estimates of the prevalence of protein C deficiency existed until a recent study indicated that the true prevalence of protein C deficiency in the general population to be as high as 17/1,000 [6]. Our studies of the prevalence of AT-deficiency in healthy blood donors from Southwestern Ontario reveal the prev-

Received for publication June 29, 1993; accepted September 22, 1993.

Address reprint requests to Dr. M.A. Blajchman, Department of Pathology, Room 2N31, McMaster University Health Sciences Centre, 1200 Main Street West, Hamilton, Ontario, L8N 3Z5, Canada.

alence of AT-deficiency to be approximately 2/1,000, that immediate processing of the blood sample is necessary to avoid false low results, and that repeat testing of putative AT-deficient subjects is essential.

MATERIALS AND METHODS

Antithrombin Assays

Functional AT assays were performed, using either factor Xa or thrombin (IIa) as the substrate, on an automated machine (ACL-300 from Instrumentation Laboratory, Fisher, Mississauga, ON) [7]. For the factor Xa based AT assay (AT-Xa), unknown plasma was diluted 1/20, to which was added bovine factor Xa (1 unit/ml), from Diagnostica Stago (obtained from Welmark Diagnostic, Guelph, ON), chromogenic substrate CBS 31.39 (3.5 mM/l) also from Diagnostica Stago and sodium heparin (3 units/ml). The normal range (mean ± 2 SD) for the AT-Xa assay, based on the results from 100 consecutive blood donors, was 0.80 to 1.08 units/ml. For the thrombin-based AT assay (AT-IIa), the unknown plasma sample was diluted 1 in 40 to which was added human thrombin (15 units/ml) and the chromogenic substrate CBS 34.47 (1.8 mM/l); both from Diagnostica Stago. The normal range for the AT-IIa assay was 0.82 to 1.15 units/ml (mean ± 2 SD). The AT antigen (AT-Ag) assay was performed by the Mancini technique using rabbit antibodies to human AT from Atlantic Antibodies (obtained from NCS Diagnostic, Mississauga, ON) and run on a 1% seakem (LE) agarose gel. The normal range (mean ± 2 SD) for the AT-Ag assay was 0.78 to 1.06 units/ml.

Blood Donors

The initial assessment of AT levels involved all blood donors who presented to selected Canadian Red Cross Society Blood Donor Clinics in communities within 200 km of Hamilton, Ontario, between June 1990 and December 1990. These clinics tend to attract blood donors with a demographically similar distribution to that of the population, but with an imposed age limit of 17 to 70. Initial plasma samples for AT assay were taken from blood donor units, rather than directly from the donors. These blood samples were therefore anticoagulated with citrate phosphate dextrose and adenosine (CPDA-1), refrigerated immediately after collection at 4°C, and the supernatant plasma removed 24 to 48 hr later. This approach was used for all 2,491 blood donor samples obtained initially. For the subsequent testing of study subjects, between June 1991 and May 1992, whole blood was drawn directly into vacutainer tubes (Becton-Dickinson) containing 0.102 M buffered citrate. These samples were immediately centrifuged at 3,000g for 15 min, the supernatant plasma separated, quick frozen at −40°C, and kept frozen until batch assayed for AT functional and antigenic activity at a later date.

Subject Assessment

From the original 2,491 blood donors (960 females and 1,531 males), a cohort of putative AT-deficient individuals was identified. This cohort, together with an age/sex-matched control group of blood donors was asked to return for a second round of testing. All putative AT-deficient and control subjects were evaluated by two physicians, who were blinded as to diagnostic category, employing a standard questionnaire to ascertain the presence of a previous history of pulmonary embolism (PE), deep vein thrombosis (DVT), or superficial phlebitis. The questionnaire also evaluated whether the subject had been in a situation at high risk for venous thrombosis, whether there was a family history of thrombosis, and whether there were concomitant conditions that might result in acquired AT-deficiency. All study subjects were also examined by Doppler ultrasound (5 mHz) for evidence of venous reflux. This was performed on the common femoral, superficial femoral, popliteal, and posterior-tibial veins. Reflux was considered to be present if retrograde venous flow was demonstrated reproducibly over a vein segment of at least 5 cm. Venous flow was assessed after the patient performed a Valsalva manoeuvre and also after rapid manual occlusion above a venous segment. Manual occlusion of superficial veins was done if reflux was detected, in order to exclude false positive results.

RESULTS

The functional AT-Xa levels in the original groups of 2,491 blood donors generated a curve skewed to the left. Thus, 122 blood donors were found to have functional AT-Xa values lower than 2 SD below the mean of the level in the 2,491 blood donors, whereas only 62 would have been expected from a normal distribution. This unexpected finding indicated there may have been a problem with sample procurement. Indeed within this group of 122 putative AT-deficient subjects there were 22 samples that were clearly shown to have a prolonged thrombin clotting time, which indicated that thrombin had been generated either during blood collection or sample handling. We thus identified 100 putative AT-deficient subjects, who were recalled for re-testing. Upon recall,these putative AT-deficient subjects were compared to a cohort of age- and sex-matched control blood donors (n = 51), that were previously untested for AT, but randomly selected from the Hamilton Centre's blood donor registry. Blood samples from both the putative AT-deficient and control subjects were collected by the more rigorous technique, as described above in the methods. The results of the AT-Xa, AT-IIa and AT-Ag concentrations in the 51 control subjects is shown below in Table I. The reproduc-

TABLE I. Antigenic and Functional Antithrombin Levels in 51 Normal Blood Donors

	Mean[a] (units/ml)	Range (units/ml)
AT'Ag	0.92 ± 0.14	0.80–1.16
AT-Xa	0.94 ± 0.14	0.83–1.08
AT-IIa	0.96 ± 0.16	0.83–1.15

[a]Mean ± 2 SD.

ibility of both the AT-Xa and the AT-IIa assays was determined using samples from 33 additional subjects (known AT-deficient and normal). The mean values obtained by two technologists for these 33 samples were 0.86 and 0.85 units/ml respectively with $r = 0.97$ and 0.98, respectively.

From the initial group of 100 putative AT-deficient blood donors only 59 agreed to be reevaluated. Only six of these were found to have a functional AT-Xa level below the established lower limit of normal (<0.80 units/ml). The other 53 subjects had AT-Xa levels that were well within the normal range. The six individuals with low At-Xa results were recalled a third time. On this occasion the AT-Xa level was found to be within the normal range in three. Because the mean AT-Xa levels using the three results available were in the normal range, AT deficiency was considered to have been excluded in these three subjects. Three other subjects again had low AT-Xa levels. The first was a 20-year-old male who had a mean AT-Xa level of 0.45 units/ml, with the AT-Xa results being 0.44, 0.45, and 0.45 units/ml on the three plasma samples available. His mean (of three values) plasma AT-Ag level was 1.0 units/ml. The mutant AT allele of this subject has been sequenced and shown to be an Arg47Cys substitution. The second putative AT-deficient blood donor was a 66-year-old male who was found to have a mean plasma AT-Xa level of 0.61 units/ml (from the three determinations of 0.56, 0.61, and 0.66 units/ml, respectively). This individual has ten children, three of whom have also been found to have low functional and antigenic AT activity. His mean (of three values) plasma AT-Ag level was 0.60 units/ml. The third putative AT-deficient blood donor is a 67-year-old male whose plasma AT-Xa levels, based on four determinations (the fourth determination was from a later visit to a blood donor clinic), were 0.77, 0.65, 0.78, and 0.66 units/ml, respectively, for a mean value of 0.71 units/ml. His mean AT-Ag level (from the four samples) was 0.76 units/ml. This subject refused to allow his family members to be tested, but as acquired causes of AT deficiency have been ruled out he is presumed to have an inherited AT-deficiency. In the three AT-deficient patients, the difference between the mean AT-Xa and the AT-IIa results assays were statistically significant ($P < 0.001$ by the two-tailed t-test for paired samples), with the AT-Xa values always lower than the AT-IIa values and more in line with the AT-Ag levels.

Thus, two individuals in this study are considered to have a type 1 AT deficient allele, defined as the absence of the mutant AT gene product in the plasma [8]. Another is considered to have a type 3 AT deficient allele, defined as due to a mutant AT gene affecting the heparin-binding domain of the AT molecule [8]. None of the three individuals found to have AT-deficiency have either a personal or family history of a venous thromboembolic event. Moreover, none have evidence of a previous DVT as determined by Doppler examination. Both putative type 1 AT-deficient individuals have been exposed to risk factors for thrombosis. The individual with type 3 AT-deficiency has not yet been exposed to a situation generally associated with increased risk for thrombosis. Thus, as 3 of the 59 putative AT-deficient individuals that returned for testing were found to be AT-deficient, we can extrapolate that five of the 100 putative AT-deficient patients would have been deficient. Using a denominator of 2,520 subjects tested (i.e., 2,491 − 22 + 51), this gives an estimated prevalence of AT-deficiency in healthy blood donors of 2/1,000 individuals. From this estimated prevalence, the 95% confidence intervals has been estimated as 0.7/1,000 to 6/1,000.

DISCUSSION

Antithrombin (AT) is one of the key plasma inhibitors of the coagulation pathway. Although AT inhibits several activated serine clotting proteins, its primary biologic activity appears to relate to its ability to inhibit thrombin [9]. In unselected patients presenting with recurrent venous thromboembolic events, up to 5% have been found to be AT-deficient [1]. A recent prospective study, however, indicates the prevalence of AT-deficient individuals in such patients to be 2.8% [10]. Reports in the literature, up until 1988, suggest that the prevalence of AT-deficiency in the general population may be as high as 0.2/1,000 or as low as 0.05/1,000 [1,3]. A recent report, however, suggests that the prevalence may be as high as 5/1,000 [5]. Importantly, in this latter study there were no repeat AT determinations in those individuals who were found to have low functional AT activities. This appears to be crucial, as recent evidence suggests that AT levels may decrease during stress [11], and as suggested by the present study, one AT level is not necessarily definitive. A second publication, reporting a prevalence of AT-deficiency of approximately 4/1,000, has only been published in abstract form and provides insufficient detail to allow critical evaluation [4].

The data from our previous investigations indicate that functional AT determinations using factor Xa as the substrate (AT-Xa) represents a better discriminating test than an assay based on thrombin (AT-IIa) for the detection of individuals with AT-deficiency [12]. First, the AT-Xa levels and the immunologic (AT-Ag) levels correlate more closely than they do with the AT-IIa levels. Secondly, the range of normal levels of functional AT in normal controls is higher with the AT-IIa assay than with the AT-Xa assay. Thirdly, the number of abnormal results obtained in AT-deficient subjects with the AT-Xa assay are lower and more clearly abnormal than are the results with the AT-IIa assay [12]. This was also seen in this present study. We recommend therefore that the AT-Xa be the assay of choice for determining whether a particular individual has AT-deficiency.

Based on our cohort of blood donors, we estimate the overall prevalence of AT-deficiency to be approximately 2/1,000. In addition, we have identified several important issues, which had not previously been noted about functional AT determinations. The need for repeat testing is striking! Initial testing suggested that the prevalence of AT-deficiency in our blood donor population might be as high as 40/1,000. However, based on the evidence of thrombin generation in 22 of the initial samples and previously reported prevalences, we suspected that this might be an overestimate. To ensure inclusion of all true AT-deficient subjects we attempted to retest all subjects who had an initial AT level less than 2 SD below the normal mean. Of the 100 putative AT-deficient subjects identified only 59 made themselves available for follow-up. Of these 59, 6 were found to have functional AT-Xa levels 2 SD deviations below the mean. These six subjects were retested yet again and three were found to have persistently low AT levels. These three individuals are clearly AT-deficient with functional AT-Xa levels more than 3 SD below the normal mean. One of these subjects has been identified as having a type 3 AT-deficiency (Arg47Cys). The other two have been putatively classified as having type 1 AT-deficiency [8]. Studies are underway to try to define the molecular pathology of the mutant AT alleles in these latter two individuals.

ACKNOWLEDGMENTS

These studies were supported, in part, by the Canadian Red Cross Society R&D fund. Dr. P.S. Wells is the recipient of a McLaughlin scholarship from the University of Ottawa, and M.J. Wells is a recipient of a research fellowship from the Heart and Stroke Foundation of Ontario.

REFERENCES

1. Hirsh J, Piovella F, Pini M: Congenital Antithrombin III deficiency: Incidence and clinical features. Am J Med 87(Suppl 38):34S–38S, 1989.
2. Demers C, Ginsberg JS, Hirsh J, Henderson P, Blajchman MA: Thrombosis in antithrombin-III deficient persons: Report of a large kindred and literature review. Ann Int Med 116:754–761, 1992.
3. Odegard OR, Fagerhol ML, Mette L: Heparin cofactor activity and antithrombin III concentration in plasma related to age and sex. Scan J Haematol 17:258–262, 1976.
4. Tait RC, Walker ID, Perry DJ, Carrell RW, Islam SIA, McCall F, Mitchell R: Prevalence of antithrombin III deficiency subtypes in 4000 healthy blood donors. Thromb Haemost 65:839, 1991 (abstract).
5. Meade TW, Dyer S, Howarth DJ, Imeson JD, Stirling Y: Antithrombin III and procoagulant activity: Sex differences and effects of the menopause. Br J Haemat 74:77–81, 1990.
6. Miletich J, Sherman L, Broze G Jr: Absence of thrombosis in subjects with heterozygous protein C deficiency. N Engl J Med 317:991–996, 1987.
7. Kahle LH, Schipper HG, Jenkins CS, tenCate JW: Antithrombin III. 1. Evaluation of an automated antithrombin III method. Thromb Res 12:1003–1014, 1978.
8. Blajchman MA, Austin RC, Fernandez-Rachubinski F, Sheffield WP: Molecular biology of inherited human antithrombin deficiency. Blood 80:2159–2171, 1992.
9. Ofosu FA, Hirsh J, Esmon CT, Modi GJ, Smith LM, Anvari N, Buchanan MR, Fenton JW, Blajchman MA: Unfractionated heparin inhibits thrombin-catalysed amplification reactions of coagulation more efficiently than those catalysed by factor Xa. Biochem J 257: 143–150, 1989.
10. Pabinger I, Brücker S, Kyrle PA, Schneider B, Korninger HC, Niessner H, Lechner K: Hereditary deficiency of antithrombin III, protein C and protein S: Prevalence in patients with a history of venous thrombosis and criteria for rational patient screening. Blood Coag Fibrinol 3:547–553, 1992.
11. Canevari A, Tacconi F, Zucchella M, Pacchiarini L, Soffiantino F, Grignani G: Antithrombin III biological activity and emotional stress in patients with coronary artery disease. Haematologica 77:180–182, 1992.
12. Demers C, Henderson P, Blajchman M, Wells MJ, Mitchell L, Johnson M, Ofosu FA, Fernandez-Rachubinski F, Andrew M, Hirsh J, Ginsberg JS: An antithrombin III assay based on factor Xa inhibition provides a more reliable test to identify congenital antithrobin III deficiency than an assay based on thrombin inhibition. Thromb Haemost 69:231–235, 1993.

American Journal of Hematology 45:325–329 (1994)

Disseminated *Mycobacterium avium*-Intracellulare Infection in a Patient With Myelodysplastic Syndrome (Refractory Anemia)

Hiroko Tsukada, Takaaki Chou, Yasuo Ishizuka, Osamu Ogawa, Takako Saeki, Satoshi Ito, Masaya Wakabayashi, Naoki Hayashi, and Masaaki Arakawa

Department of Medicine (II), Niigata University Medical School (H.T., T.C., Y.I., O.O., T.S., S.I., M.W., M.A.), and Division of Internal Medicine, Niigata Cancer Center Hospital (N.H.), Niigata, Japan.

A 31-year-old woman presented with fever and arthralgia. Despite treatment with antimicrobials and corticosteroids, her symptoms persisted. A diagnosis of myelodysplastic syndrome (MDS)-refractory anemia (RA) was made by pancytopenia, dysplasia, and trisomy 8. Cultures of bone marrow, blood, and gastric juice showed *Mycobacterium avium*-intracellulare (MAI). She was treated with antimycobacterial drugs and recombinant human G-CSF/M-CSF and showed an initial response, but spike fever recurred and pancytopenia progressed. Hepatosplenomegaly and marked retroperitoneal lymphadenopathy were revealed, indicating further dissemination of MAI. Treatment with recombinant human GM-CSF and very-low-dose cytosine arabinoside, was started but was not effective. This case showed significant reduction in peripheral blood T-lymphocytes, especially the CD4^{+} population, and low immunoglobulin levels. Immunodeficiency state associated with long-term steroid therapy and MDS seemed to contribute to the development of the disseminated infection with MAI.

Key words: disseminated mycobacterial infection, immunological abnormality, colony-stimulating factor, MDS-RA, steroid therapy

INTRODUCTION

Disseminated *Mycobacterium avium*-intracellulare (MAI) infection was very rare until 1982, when it began to appear in patients with human immunodeficiency virus (HIV) infection [1,2]. Except in patients with acquired immunodeficiency syndrome (AIDS), very few cases have been reported, and more than one-half of patients were known to be compromised hosts [3–6]. We report here the development of systemic MAI infection in a female patient with myelodysplastic syndrome (MDS)-refractory anemia (RA) with marked immunological abnormalities.

CASE REPORT

A 31-year-old woman was almost well until March, 1991, when she began to experience fever, fatigue, and arthralgias. In May, 1991, she was admitted to a hospital for evaluation. Despite treatment with empirical antimicrobials, oral prednisone (daily dosage from 40 to 80 mg), and steroid pulse therapy, symptom persisted and she was transferred to our department for further evaluation in September, 1991.

On admission, the temperature was 36.6°C, the pulse 84 beats/min, and the blood pressure 96/56 mmHg. Examinations of the lungs, the heart, and the abdomen were normal. There was no lymphadenopathy or hepatosplenomegaly. The laboratory data are summarized in Table I. The bone marrow was normocellular, with trilineage dysplasia and no increment of blastic cells. The chromosomal analysis of bone marrow cells revealed karyotype 46, XY, with partial (8.3%) trisomy of chromosome 8. A diagnosis of MDS-RA was made based on the disease criteria [7]. Decrease of CD4^{+}T cells in peripheral blood and serum immunoglobulin level revealed her immunodeficiency state, but human immunodeficiency virus

Received for publication December 3, 1992; accepted June 30, 1993.

Address reprint requests to Takaaki Chou, MD, Department of Medicine (II), Niigata University Medical School, 1-757 Asahimachidori, Niigata City, 951 Japan.

TABLE I. Laboratory Data

Peripheral blood		GOT	80 I.U./liter	(8–25)	Lymphocyte subset	
RBC	526 × 10^4/μl	GPT	165 I.U./liter	(3–23)	CD3	69.2%
Hb	14.1 g/dl	ALP	310 I.U./liter	(80–180)	CD4	23.3%
Ht	44.6%	LAP	102 I.U./liter	(39–57)	CD8	43.6%
WBC	3500/μl	LDH	1,049 I.U./liter	(225–434)	CD57	12.8%
Band	7%	T-B	0.9 mg/dl	(0.3–1.1)	CD19	0.5%
Seg	80%	ChE	5,415 I.U./liter	(4,950–8,900)	CD25	0.8%
Bas	0%				HLA-DR	30.0%
Eos	1%	T-P	6.2 g/dl	(6.6–8.0)	CD4/CD8	0.53%
Lym	9%	Alb	59.5%			
Mon	3%	α_1	5.8%		Lymphocyte blast formation test	
Plt	9.9 × 10^4/μl	α_2	7.4%		(uptake of ^{3}H-thymidine; CPM)	
		β	14.9%		PHA 23,130	(45,000–53,200)
Bone marrow		γ	12.4%		ConA 16,438	(23,458–63,250)
NCC	11 × 10^9/μl				PWM 7,834	(16,670–42,450)
MgK	31/μl	BUN	21 mg/dl	(8–20)		
		CRN	0.5 mg/dl	(0.6–1.1)	ADCC activity 63% (41–72)	
Myeloid series		Na	143 mEq/liter	(140–147)		
Blast	0.5%	K	3.7 mEq/liter	(3.6–4.7)	NK activity 70% (18–40)	
Promy	3.0%	Cl	103 mEq/liter	(101–110)		
Myelo	6.4%	T-C	236 mg/dl	(141–248)	Granulocyte function test	
Meta	7.2%				Phagocytic activity 78.0% (70–90)	
Band	4.2%	CEA	3.8 ng/dl	(<4.0)		
Seg	19.0%	CA19-9	17 ng/dl	(<35)	Bacteriocidal activity	
Eos	3.2%	NSE	6.8 ng/ml	(<8.0)	(H_2O_2 production) 94.3% (>70)	
Baso	0.4%	SCC	<1.0 ng/ml	(<1.0)		
Erythroid series						
Pro	0.2%	ESR	7 mm/hr		HIV antigen (−)	
Mac-poly	0.4%	CRP	2.3 mg/dl		Anti-HIV antibody (−)	
Nor-baso	1.0%	RA	<10 I.U./dl		DNA analysis of BM-MNC	
Nor-poly	0.4%	ANA	(−) I.U./dl		monoclonal rearrangement of	
Nor-orth	34.0%	IgG	940.0 mg/dl		TCR or lg gene (−)	
Lymph	11.2%	IgA	116.4 mg/dl		Urinalysis	
Mono	0.2%	IgM	258.6 mg/dl		U-protein (−)	
Retic.	0.4%	IgD	1.0 mg/dl		U-glucose (−)	
Plasma	1.8%	IgE	<31 mg/dl		occult blood (−)	
					Tuberculin test 0 × 0/0 × 0 mm	

(HIV) antigen and antibody against HIV were negative. A PPD skin test was negative. PWM-, ConA-, and PHA-induced lymphoproliferation was impaired in comparison to healthy controls. Natural killer (NK) cell activity, antibody-dependent cellular toxicity (ADCC), neutrophil phagocytosis, and its bacterial killing were within normal range.

Soon after admission, high fevers again persisted following the withdrawal of the oral prednisone, and pancytopenia progressed (Fig. 1). Although no significant bacterial pathogen was detected by regular surveillance culture, clot section of bone marrow aspiration specimen showed acid-fast bacilli, without granulomas and necrosis (Fig. 2). Chest X-ray showed bilateral diffuse nodular infiltrates. Transbronchial lung biopsy was performed in September, 1991, revealing diffuse thickening of the alveolar walls, moderate infiltrations of mononuclear cells, and no granulomas. Later, cultures of bone marrow, peripheral blood, gastric juice, and the lung biopsy specimen grew MAI, confirming the diagnosis of systemic dissemination of MAI infection.

Therapy was begun with isoniazid, streptomycin, rifampin, ciprofloxacin, tobracin, ethambutol, cycloserine, and erythromycin. Subcutaneous injections of the recombinant human (rh)G-CSF and intravenous injection of M-CSF were also started. She showed an initial response, and liver dysfunction improved, but spike fevers recurred and pancytopenia refractory to rhG-CSF and M-CSF administration again progressed. In December, 1991, computed tomographic scanning of the abdomen showed hepatosplenomegaly and marked retroperitoneal lymphadenopathy (Fig. 3). Percutaneous needle aspiration of the retroperitoneal lymph nodes revealed a necrotic tissue with abundant acid-fast bacilli, indicting further progression of systemic MAI dissemination. As her pancytopenia has also gradually progressed despite the treatment with G-CSF and M-CSF, treatment with rhGM-CSF and very low-dose cytosine arabinoside for

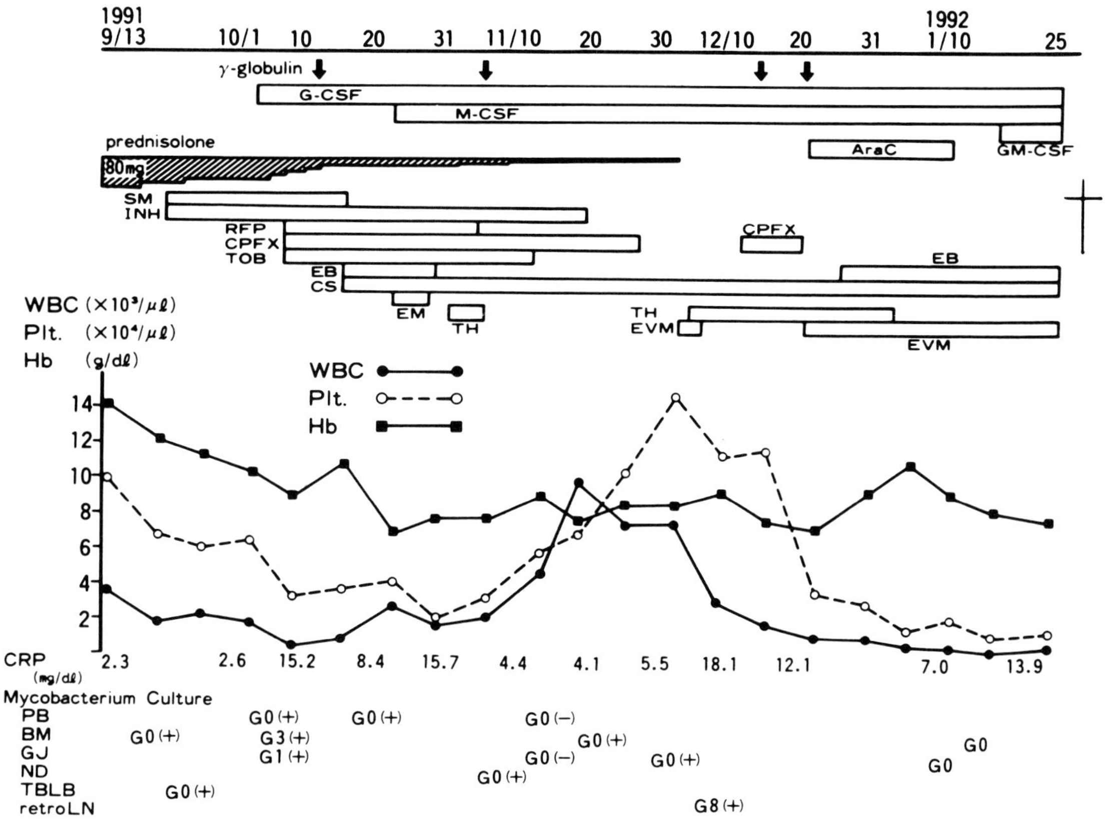

Fig. 1. Clinical course of the patient. Culture, results of mycobacterial culture; PB, peripheral blood; BM, bone marrow; GJ, gastric juice; G, Gaffky number; TBLB, transbronchial lung biopsy specimen; NC, nasal cavity; retroLN, retroperitoneal lymph nodes.

her MDS-RA was started, and ethionamide and enviomycin were added to her antimycobacterial regimen. Despite these treatments, the patient's condition deteriorated rapidly, and the serum total bilirubin level was elevated to 24.5 mg/dl and a direct bilirubin to 20.0 mg/dl, without elevation of GOT, GPT, NH3, or alkaline phosphatase levels, and she died in January, 1992.

Postmortem examination revealed marked cholestasis in the liver, and acid-fast stain-positive, rod-shaped organisms without granulomas in multiple sites, bone marrow, retroperitoneal lymphnodes, lung, liver, spleen, and pulmonary hilar lymph nodes. Cultures of these organs grew exclusively MAI.

DISCUSSION

In the present case, a diagnosis of MDS was made from the following findings: 1) pancytopenia, 2) normocellular marrow, 3) no evidence of other hematological disorders associated with pancytopenia (acute leukemia, myelofibrosis, nutritional deficiency, aplastic anemia, hypersplenism, etc.), 4) trilineage dysplasia (dyserythropoiesis: megaloblastic changes, nuclear fragments; dysgranulopoiesis: pseudo-Pelger anomaly, marked hypogranular PMN, ringed nuclei; dysmegakaryopoiesis: round mononuclear megakaryocytes, large platelets), and 5) chromosomal abnormality in BM (trisomy 8).

Disseminated atypical mycobacterial infection is known to be associated with a high incidence of hematological abnormalities, such as leukemoid reactions, myelofibrotic changes, the hemophagocytic syndrome, polycythemia, and pancytopenia [8–10]. The hypothesis that myelosuppressive effects of *Mycobacterium* bring on pancytopenia has been supported by cases in which recovery of peripheral blood counts with antimycrobacterial therapy has been accepted as evidence of a normal bone marrow [11,12]. In our case, the chromosomal abnormality (trisomy 8), frequently seen in the MDS [13,14], suggests that her myelodysplasia might be primary rather than secondary to the MAI infection.

Although transformation to acute leukemia has been reported with variable frequency, infection is one of the major causes of death in patients with MDS [15,16]. The majority of infections were bacterial, and the causative organisms were typical of those associated with infections in patients with deficient neutrophil defenses (neutropenia and/or neutrophil dysfunction) [16–19]. On the other hand, to our knowledge, no cases of association of

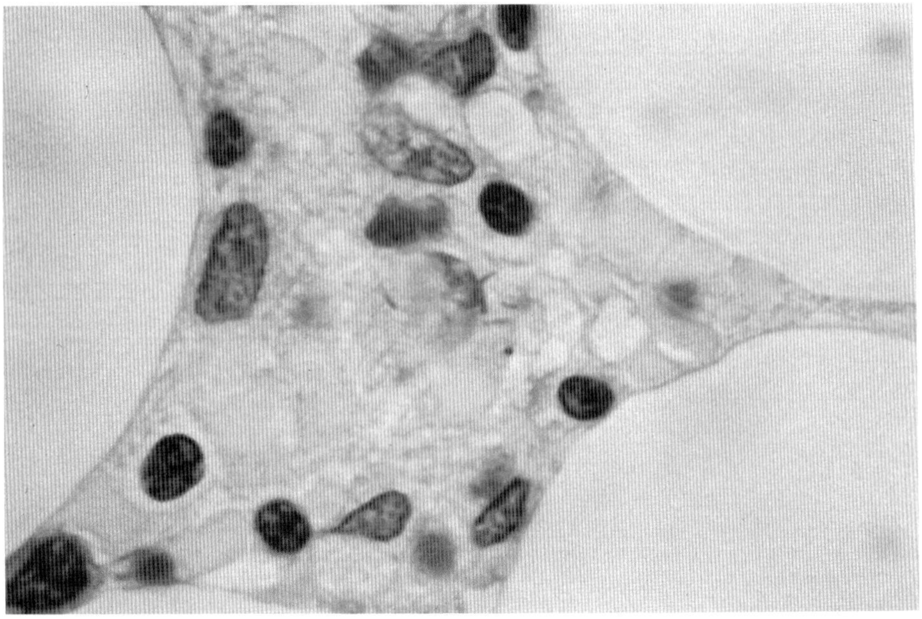

Fig. 2. Ziehl-Neelsen stain of a clot section of bone marrow, showing acid-fast bacilli without granulomas nor necrosis. ×400.

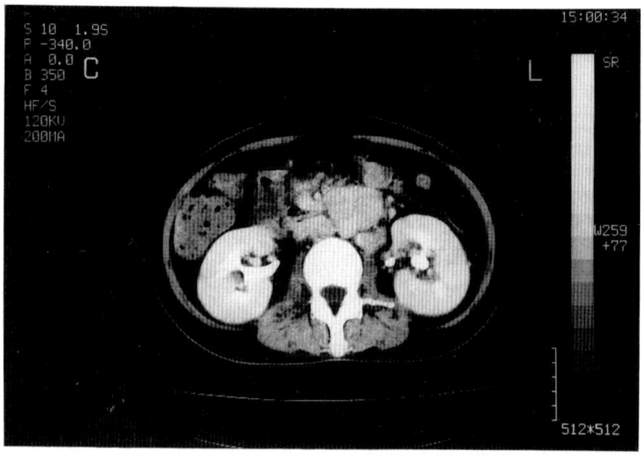

Fig. 3. Computed tomographic scan through the level of the kidneys discloses enlarged retroperitoneal lymph nodes.

disseminated MAI infection and the MDS similar to our case have been reported.

In the bone marrow biopsy specimen from this patient, aggregates of macrophages filled with organisms were associated with absent granulomatous reaction and necrosis. This appearance seems to be a characteristic finding in AIDS patients infected with MAI [1,20]. Furthermore, the patient also showed significant reduction in peripheral blood T lymphocytes, low serum immunoglobulin levels, and impaired lymphocyte functions even after withdrawal of corticosteroids. From these findings, we have considered, in addition to the extended course of corticosteroids, some defects in cellular immunity that may have contributed significantly to the development of the disseminated infection of MAI. The possibility of HIV infection and some lymphoid malignancy, common predisposing conditions in disseminated MAI infection [1,2,4,5], which are known to be a cause of immune deficiency, was excluded in this case.

Recent reports have shown that there are serious defects in the lymphoid systems in addition to the abnormalities in the myeloid populations of MDS patients, such as decreased absolute numbers of T lymphocytes, markedly decreased ratio of $CD4^+/CD8^+$, and selective NK cell defect [21,22]. Monoclonal gammopathy, polyclonal increases, or decreases in serum immunoglobulins also have recently reported [23–25]. The immunological abnormalities of our patient may be considered to be accompanied by MDS.

While the possibility that mycobacterial infection itself might bring alterations in immunity could not be excluded, Skvor and Trnka [26] and Edwards and Kirkpatrick [27] confirmed the diminished presence of T cells in patients with tuberculosis and further demonstrated that the extent of the T cell reduction correlated with duration and extent of disease. Untreated patients with reduced cells had normal concentrations of T cells after 4–6 week of therapy [26,27]. Decreased in vitro lymphocyte proliferation has also been described in tuberculosis and atypical mycobacterial infections [28,29]. In that very few drugs are known to be effective in MAI infection under such immunosuppressive conditions [5,20,30], we considered that she could not recover with only the administration of the antimycobacterial agents.

Thus we started treatment intended to restore or potentiate host-defense mechanism in combination with variable antimycobacterial agents. First, rhG-CSF and M-CSF were given to increase the number of granulocytes and to activate monocyte/macrophage-lymphocyte system [31–33]. Finally, we attempted to improve her immunological abnormalities with very-low-dose cytarabine [34] and rhGM-CSF treatment [35] for the MDS, by killing the pathological clone and restoring the residual normal hematopoietic stem cell clone, if it existed. Despite these extensive treatments, she died, and postmortem examinations showed minimal or absent granulomatous response similar to her condition on admission.

Finally, the case presented here draws attention to the importance of disseminated atypical *Mycobacterium* infection in patient with MDS. Further investigation of the immunological abnormalities as well as bacteriological surveillances in MDS patients should be used for early diagnosis and treatment.

ACKNOWLEDGMENTS

We thank Dr. Y. Kita, Department of Internal Medicine, Kinki Chu-oh Hospital, and Dr. F. Kuze, Department of Internal Medicine, Institute of the Chest, Kyoto University, for identification and characterization of MAI and for helpful suggestions with this case.

REFERENCES

1. Wallace JM, Hannah R: *Mycobacterium avium* complex infection in patients with the acquired immunodeficiency syndrome. Chest 93: 926, 1988.
2. Horsburgh CR, Selik RM: The epidemiology of disseminated nontuberculous mycobacterial infection in the acquired immunodeficiency syndrome (AIDS). Am Rev Respir Dis 139:4, 1989.
3. Saito H, Tasaka H, Osasa S, Tamura T, Fukuhara T, Yamada A: Disseminated *Myco-bacterium intracellulare* infection. Am Rev Respir Dis 109:572, 1974.
4. Weinstein RA, Glomb HM, Grumet G, Gelman E, Schechter GP: Hairy cell leukemia: Association with disseminated atypical mycobacterial infection. Cancer 48:380, 1981.
5. Horsburgh CR, Mason UG, Farhi DC, Iseman MD: Disseminated infection with *Myco-bacterium avium*-intracellulare: A report of 13 cases and a review of the literature. Medicine 64:36, 1985.
6. Nunez JM Monteagudo I, Lopez-Longo FJ, Cobeta JC, Rivera J: Disseminated *Mycobacterium avium*-intracellulare infection in a patient with polymyositis. Arthritis Rheum 32:934, 1989.
7. Bennett JM, Catovsky D, Daniel MT, Flandrin G, Galton DAG, Gralnick HR, Sultan C: Proposals for the classification of the myelodysplastic syndromes. Br J Haematol 51:189, 1982.
8. Engstrom PF, Dewey GC, Barrett O: Disseminated *Mycobacterium kansasii* infection: Successful treatment of a patient with pancytopenia. Am J Med 52:533, 1972.
9. Hunt BJ, Andrews V, Pettingale KW: The significance of pancytopenia in miliary tuberculosis. Postgrad Med J 63:801, 1987.
10. Weintraud M, Siegman-Ingra Y, Josiphov J, Rahmani R, Liron M: Histiocytic hemo-phagocytosis in miliary tuberculosis. Arch Intern Med 144:2055, 1984.
11. Mangion PB: Disseminated tuberculosis complicated by pancytopenia. Proc R Soc Med 64:1000, 1971.
12. Rosenberg MJ, Rumans LW: Survival of a patient with pancytopenia and disseminated coagulation associated with miliary tuberculosis. Chest 73:536, 1978.
13. Second International Workshop on Chromosomes in Leukemia, 1979: Chromosomes in preleukemia. Cancer Genet Cytogenet 2:108, 1980.
14. Heim S, Mitelman F: Chromosome abnormalities in the myelodysplastic syndromes. Clin Haematol 15:1003, 1986.
15. Weidorf DJ, Oken MM, Johnson GJ, Rydell RE: Chronic myelodysplastic syndrome: Short survival with or without evolution to acute leukemia. Br J Haematol 55:691, 1983.
16. Pomeroy C, Oken MM, Rydell RE, Filice GA: Infection in the myelodysplastic syndromes. Am J Med 90:338, 1991.
17. Boogaerts MA, Nelissen V, Roelant C, Goosens W: Blood neutrophil function in primary myelodysplastic syndromes. Br J Haematol 55: 217, 1983.
18. Martin S, Baldock SC, Ghoneim ATM, Child JA: Defective neutrophil function and microbicidal mechanisms in the myelodysplastic disorders. J Clin Pathol 36:1120, 1983.
19. Williamson PJ, Oscier DG, Mufti GJ, Hamblin TJ: Pyogenic abscesses in the myelodysplastic syndrome. Br Med J 299:375, 1989.
20. Fraser RG, Peter-Pare JA, Pare PD, Fraser RS, Genereux GP (eds): Nontuberculous *Mycobacteria*. In: "Diagnosis of Diseases of the Chest, 3rd ed." Philadelphia: W.B. Saunders Company, 1989, p 933.
21. Bynoe AG, Scott CS, Ford P, Roberts BE: Decreased T helper cells in the myelodysplastic syndrome. Br J Haematol 54:97, 1983.
22. Kerndrup G, Meyer K, Ellegaard J, Hokland P: Natural killer (NK)-cell activity and antibody-dependent cellular cytotoxicity (ADCC) in primary preleukemic syndrome. Leukemia Res 8:239, 1984.
23. Economopoulos T, Economidou J, Giannopoulos G, Terzoglou C, Papageorgiou E, Dervenoulas J, Arseni P, Hadjioannou J, Raptis S: Immune abnormalities in myelodysplastic syndromes. J Clin Pathol 38:908, 1985.
24. Mufti GJ, Figes A, Hamblin TJ, Oscier DG, Copplestone JA: Immunological abnormalities in myelodysplastic syndromes: I. Serum immunoglobulins and autoantibodies. Br J Haematol 63:143, 1986.
25. Colombat PH, Renoux M, Lamagnere J, Renoux G: Immunologic indices in myelodyslastic syndrome. Cancer 61:1075, 1988.
26. Skvor J, Trnka L: Immunoprofile studies in patients with pulmonary tuberculosis. I. Correlation of pretherapy cellular tests with characteristics of the disease. Scand J Respir Dis 60:161, 1979.
27. Edwards D, Kirkpatrick CH: The immunology of mycobacterial disease. Am Rev Respir Dis 134:1062, 1986.
28. McMurray DN, Echeverri A: Cell-mediated immunity in anergic patients with pulmonary tuberculosis. Am Rev Respir Dis 118:827, 1978.
29. Mason UG III, Kirkpatrick CH. Modulation of immunologic response in nontuberculous mycobacterial infections with indomethacin. J Clin Immunol 4:112, 1984.
30. Banks J, Jenkins PA: Combined versus single antituberculosis drugs on the in vitro sensitivity patterns of non-tuberculous mycobacteria. Thorax 42:838, 1987.
31. Yoh A, Kitagawa S, Okabe T, Urabe A, Komatsu Y, Itoh S, Takaku F: Recombinant human granulocyte colony-stimulating factor repairs the abnormalities of neutrophils in patients with myelodysplastic syndromes and chronic myelogenous leukemia. Blood 70:404, 1987.
32. Negrin RS, Haeuber DH, Nagler A, Kobayashi Y, Sklar J, Donlon T, Vincent M, Greenberg PL: Maintenance treatment of patients with myelodysplastic syndromes using recombinant human granulocyte colony stimulating factor. Blood 76:36, 1990.
33. Motoyoshi K, Takaku F, Mizoguchi H, Miura Y: Purification and some properties of colony-stimulating factor from normal human urine. Blood 52:1012, 1978.
34. Worsley A, Mufti GJ, Copplestone JA, Oscier DG, Hamblin TJ: Very low-dose cytarabine for myelodysplastic syndromes and acute myeloid leukemia in the elderly. Lancet 26:966, 1986.
35. Hoffkin K, Overkamp F, Stirbu J, Grothey A, Flasshove M, Hoelzer D, Ganzer A: Recombinant human granulocyte-macrophage colony-stimulating factor and low-dose cytosine-arabinoside in the treatment of patients with myelodysplastic syndromes. Onkologie 13:33, 1990.

American Journal of Hematology 45:330–334 (1994)

Deep Vein Thrombosis in a 13-Year-Old Boy With Hereditary Protein S Deficiency and a Review of the Pediatric Literature

A. Blanco, M. Bonduel, L. Peñalva, M. Hepner, and M. Lazzari

Departamento de Hemostasia y Trombosis, Instituto de Investigaciones Hematológicas, Academia Nacional de Medicina (A.B., L.P., M.L.); and Servicio de Hematología y Oncología, Hospital de Pediatría "Prof. Dr. Juan P. Garrahan," (M.B., M.H.), Buenos Aires, Argentina

We report a 13-year-old boy with hereditary deficiency of protein S, who developed a deep vein thrombosis of the lower limb after a varicella with severe cutaneous lesions.

Hereditary protein S deficiency is an established cause of thrombophilia; however thrombotic events are seldom described in pediatric patients. A review of previous literature revealed 35 cases, 16 girls and 19 boys, with a first episode below of the age of 18 years old (x = 10y). The 57% of the patients had venous thrombosis, 20% arterial thrombosis, and 14% both and in 9% the type of thrombosis was not reported. Predisposing factors were referred in only 12 cases. The deficiencies can be classified as type I in 25 patients and type III in 8.

Key words: blood coagulation disorders, glycoproteins, pediatrics, thrombophlebitis

INTRODUCTION

Protein S, a vitamin K dependent cofactor of protein C, plays an important role in the anticoagulant system limiting thrombus formation [1–5]. Hereditary deficiency has been associated with venous and arterial thrombosis, coumarin-induced skin necrosis and neonatal purpura fulminans [6–14].

CASE REPORT

In 1990, a 13-year-old boy was admitted to the hospital. Twenty days earlier he developed a varicella with severe cutaneous lesions, fever, weight loss, and progressive tumefaction of the left lower limb 4 days after the first eruption. The laboratory evaluation revealed hemoglobin level of 10.4 g/dl, white blood cell count 14.5×10^9/L, platelet count 550×10^9/L, prothrombin time 65% (normal range 70–120%), activated partial thromboplastin time 48 sec (normal range 35–50 sec), thrombin time 18 sec (normal value 18 sec), and negative fibrinogen degradation products. Factor assays showed FII 65 U/dl, FV 86 U/dl, FVII-X 60 U/dl, fibrinogen 498 mg/dl. Hepatic and renal function studies were normal. Negative results of antinuclear antibodies, rheumatoid factor. Cultures of blood, urine, and throat were negative. X-ray film of the chest, electrocardiogram, echocardiographic study, and computed tomographic scan of the abdomen were normal. A Doppler study and a contrast angiography confirmed the diagnosis of deep vein thrombosis (DVT) of the left common femoral vein. Intravenous heparin and acenocumarol were started and the former was discontinued on the 7th day. He was maintained on oral anticoagulation (INR: 2–2.5) without thrombohemorrhagic complications.

No history of personal clinical antecedents was noticed. The parents and a sister of 10-year-old had no history of thrombotic events. However, an episode of probable DVT of a lower limb was presumably referred to a maternal aunt who underwent prolonged immobilization after trauma. According to the family history a thrombophilic hereditary defect was suspected.

Received for publication January 15, 1992; accepted September 28, 1993.

Address reprint requests to Alicia Blanco, Departamento de Hemostasia y Trombosis, Instituto de Investigaciones Hematológicas, Academia Nacional de Medicina, Pacheco de Melo 3081, 1425 Buenos Aires.

TABLE I. Levels of Protein S

	Protein S Antigen (U/dl)		Protein S activity (U/dl)	C4bp (U/dl)
	Total	Free		
Propositus[a] 1	70	38	—	—
2	72	45	50	85
Mother	70	47	50	83
Father	95	107	110	150
Sister	76	94	114	86
Aunt	62	35	43	80
Normal value	60–130	60–120	60–120	65–120

[a]1, first sample, 2, second sample.

MATERIALS AND METHODS

Venous blood samples were collected with sodium citrate; platelet poor plasma was immediately processed or stored at −20°C. Immunologic determinations of protein C, protein S (total and free), antithrombin III, plasminogen, and C4b-binding protein were determined by Laurell's technique [15] using polyclonal rabbit antibodies against the respective antigens (ASSERA Protein C, ASSERA PLG and ASSERA C4bBP, Diagnostica Stago, Asnières, France; Protein S and Antithrombin III, Dakopatts, Denmark). Free protein S was obtained by treatment of plasma with 25% polyethylene glycol (PEG 8000) for 30 min at 4°C, followed by electroimmunoassay. Results were expressed respect to a normal pool of plasma and a normal pool of plasma after precipitation with PEG for free protein S. Functional activities were determined by coagulation assay for protein C [16] and S (STACLOT Protein S, Diagnostica Stago, Asnières, France) and by chromogenic substrate assays for antithrombin III (IMMUNOCHROM ATIII, Immuno AG, Wien) and plasminogen (COATEST Plasminogen, KabiVitrum, Stockholm, Sweden). The normal pool of plasma was calibrated against the Blood Coagulation Factors Plasma Reference code 89/592 (4th British Standard) from the National Institute for Biological Standards and Control, London, United Kingdom. The sample of the patient was drawn at 3 and 20 months after the acute episode. Both parents, his sister and his maternal aunt were also studied. Other members of his family were not available for testing.

RESULTS

Table I showed protein S results in the available members of the family. Low value of free protein S antigen and decreased functional activity were found in the propositus, his mother, and his aunt. The father and the sister had normal results. Antithrombin III, protein C, and plasminogen levels were normal (Table II). Neither the propositus nor his parents showed a vitamin K deficiency (Table III). The results were confirmed in the second sample.

TABLE II. Levels of Protein C, Antithrombin III, and Plasminogen

	Protein C (U/dl)		Antithrombin III (U/dl)		Plasminogen (U/dl)	
	Antigen	Activity	Antigen	Activity	Antigen	Activity
Propositus	93	94	107	90	97	98
Mother	98	90	115	120	116	110
Father	93	82	125	145	120	128
Sister	78	85	97	107	120	110
Aunt	82	80	85	99	115	94
Normal value	60–120	60–120	80–120	80–120	80–140	80–140

TABLE III. Coagulation Tests*

	Normal values	Propositus 1	Propositus 2	Mother	Father	Sister	Aunt
Platelet count (10^9/L)	150–300	295	263	318	252	228	235
APTT (sec)	35–50	46	42	48	36	41	47
PT (%)	70–120	70	70	75	100	75	80
TT (sec)	18	19	18	18	18	18	18
FII (U/dl)	70–120	70	70	70	100	80	80
Fibrinogen (mg/dl)	200–400	200	216	260	200	212	331
FDG (μg/ml)	<11	<11	<11	<11	<11	<11	<11

*APTT, activated partial thromboplastin time; PT, prothrombin time; TT, thrombin time; FII, factor II; FDP, fibrin(ogen) degradation products. 1: first sample; 2: second sample.

TABLE IV. Thrombotic Episodes Prior to the Age of 18 Years in Patients With Protein S Deficiency†

						Protein S		
Patient	Age	Sex	Thrombotic event	Risk factor	Hereditary deficiency	Free	Total	Reference
1	14y	M	DVT	Negative	+	ND*	13%	6
	15y		DVT/PE	Negative				
	16y		DVT	Negative				
2	15y	M	DVT	Trauma	+	ND*	18%	6
3	5y	F	PVT	Negative	+	ND	35%	18
	10y		DVT	Surgery				
	>10y		SVT ●	Negative				
4	12y	F	SVT ●	Negative	+	ND	44%	19
	14y		DVT	Pneumonia				
5	3y	F	DVT	Burn	+	ND	49%	20
	14y		DVT	Surgery				
6	2y	F	DVT	Tonsillar angina	±	ND	49%	21
7	4m	M	Stroke	Negative	+	38%	110%	22
8	14y	F	DVT	Trauma	+	R	33%	23
	18y		DVT	Trauma				
9	18y	M	DVT	Negative	+	R*	17%	24
10	10y	M	DVT	?	+	ND	58%	25
11	12y	M	Stroke	Negative	−	ND	50%	26
12	6m	M	Stroke DVT	?	+	<10%	54%	26
	15y		DVT	Negative				
13	16y	F	LAT	Negative	ND	36%	93%	26
14	18y	F	Stroke	?	ND	R	N	27
15	12y	M	Stroke	Negative	+	ND	8 mg/L	28
	12y		PE/DVT					
16	15y	F	DVT	Negative	+	8%@	58%	29
17	17y	M	DVT	?	+	ND	ND	29
18	17y	M	T ●	Negative	+	4%@*	32%	29
19	6y	F	DVT ●	Lymphoadenopathy	+	<12%	34%	30
20	7y	M	Sinus T DVT	Negative	+	<12%	79%	30
21	15y	M	SVT ●/DVT ● PE	?	±	1.8 mg/L	12 mg/L	31
22	11y	F	DVT ●	Measles	+	21%	25%	32
23	3y	F	DVT	Nephroblastoma	−	42%	109%#	33
24	6y	M	DVT/PE	Nephrotic syndrome	−	24%	13%#	34
25	12y	M	Stroke	Negative	ND	ND	50%	35
26	5m	M	Stroke/VT	Negative	ND	<10%	54%	35
27	1m	F	Stroke/VT	Negative	ND	38%	73%	35
28	16y	F	LAT/VT	Negative	ND	36%	93%	35
29	13y	F	T	?	+	3%@	72%	36
30	17y	F	T	?	ND	1%@	60%	36
31	5y	F	PH/DVT	Negative	−	ND	6%	37
32	13y	M	DVT	Salmonella Typhimurium	−	1) * 2) Normal activity		38 33
	6y	M	LAT	Infection	+	1) 0% 2) 55%	0% 0%	39
34	2y	M	Sinus T DVT	Pneumonia	+	15%*	5%	40
35	11y	M	DVT/SVT PE	Varicella	−	1) <0.06U/mL* 2) N	0.14U/mL N	41

†m, month; y, year; F, female; M, male; T, thrombosis; DVT, deep vein thrombosis; LAT, leg arterial thrombosis; PE, pulmonary embolism; PVT, portal vein thrombosis; SVT, superficial venous thrombosis; VT, venous thrombosis; PH, pulmonary hypertension; (●), recurrent; ND, no data; N, normal; R, reduce; (*), low functional activity; (@), percent normal total protein S concentration; #, combined with other hemostatic disorder; (^), during oral anticoagulation; 1), during infection; 2), after infection; (+), certain; (±), uncertain; (−), unlikely

DISCUSSION

The association between hereditary protein S deficiency and thrombosis has been demonstrated and the underlying pathophysiology involving protein C pathway is relatively well understood [6–14,17]. However, it is unclear, why only some members of the families suffer thrombotic diseases, spontaneously or associated with some predisposing conditions [8]. The homozygous protein S deficiency is associated with neonatal purpura fulminans; cutaneous, ocular and central nervous system lesions are similar to those found in protein C deficiency [13,14]. Although a high percentage of adults who are heterozygous for protein S deficiency have thrombotic episodes, these complications are seldom described in pediatric patients. As it has been reported in adults, the protein S deficiency is mainly associated with venous thrombosis [8,10]. A review of previous literature revealed that 35 cases have been described (Table IV), 16 girls and 19 boys [6,18–41]. The first thrombotic episode was observed as earlier as 1 month old and up to 18 year old (x = 10y). In pediatric patients 57% (n = 20) suffered venous thrombosis, 20% (n = 7) had only arterial episodes and 14% (n = 5) presented both kinds of thrombosis. In three cases the type of thrombosis was not mentioned. The association of the first thrombotic event with risk factors has been clearly referred in 12 out of 28 patients; no data was available in 7 cases. This is similar to the data in adults, which showed that more than 50% of the thrombotic episodes were not preceded by precipitating conditions [8]. The type of deficiency is difficult to evaluate due to the evolution of the assays for protein S. However, considering the published results 25 patients can be classified as type I (i.e., both total and free antigen reduced) and 8 patients as type III (i.e., normal total antigen and reduced free antigen) [17]. A low molecular weight variant in plasma and platelets was described in a patient with a type I deficiency [24]. An hereditary deficiency was identified in 20 patients (57%) and two patients (6%) had familiar thrombotic antecedents without biochemical confirmation; in six cases (17%) the deficiency could be acquired and in seven patients (20%) no data were available. No sex differences were found respect to the age of presentation of the symptoms, kind of thrombosis or type of deficiency.

In addition, acquired deficiencies of protein S have been described as being related to infection [42]. Acquired purpura fulminans with selective consumption of protein C and protein S has been reported [43,44]; so has a case of a boy with streptococcal throat infection, purpura fulminans and a protein S deficiency due to a temporary protein S antibody [47]. Interestingly, the most frequent viral infection associated with acquired purpura fulminans is varicella [42]. In two patients with this illness, reduced levels of protein C and protein S have been detected during the acute phase that became normal in the convalescence [45,46]. Recent reports have described a boy with varicella, purpura fulminans, a lupus anticoagulant and transitory severe protein S deficiency [48], and the occurrence, during recovery from varicella, of severe thromboembolic disease in a boy with a transient isolated deficiency of protein S due to the presence of a circulating autoantibody to protein S [41]. The propositus had a low level of free protein S antigen. Besides, the functional activity was also decreased. The other blood coagulation inhibitors were present in normal amount. Similar results were obtained in his mother and his aunt suggesting heterozygous state for type III deficiency, in accordance with the autosomal dominant hereditary pattern of this defect. Clinical and laboratory findings in the propositus can be explained by protein S deficiency. However, it is interesting to remark that 20 days before the thrombotic episode, the patient presented a varicella with severe cutaneous lesions. Considering that acquired protein S deficiency has been associated with varicella, it is tempting to speculate that viral infection might as well have played a role in predisposing for the development of thrombosis in this boy with hereditary protein S deficiency.

REFERENCES

1. Di Scipio RG, Hermodson MA, Yates SG, Davie EW: A comparison of human prothrombin factor IX (Christmas factor), factor X (Stuart factor) and Protein S. Biochemistry 16:698–708, 1977.
2. Walker FJ: Protein S and the regulation of activated protein C. Sem Thromb Hemost 10:131–138, 1984.
3. de Fouw NJ, Haverkate F, Bertina RM, Koopman J, van Wijngaarden A, van Hinsbergh VW: The cofactor role of protein S in the acceleration of whole blood clot lysis by activated protein C in vitro. Blood 67:1189–1192, 1986.
4. Dahlbäck B: Inhibition of protein Ca cofactor function of human and bovine protein S by C4b-binding protein. J Biol Chem 261:12022–12027, 1986.
5. D'Angelo A, Lockhart MS, D'Angelo SV, Taylor FB: Protein S is a cofactor for activated protein C neutralization of an inhibitor of plasminogen activation released from platelets. Blood 69:231–237, 1987.
6. Comp PC, Nixon RR, Cooper MR, Esmon CT: Familial protein S deficiency is associated with recurrent thrombosis. J Clin Invest 74: 2082–2088, 1984.
7. Schwarz HP, Fischer M, Hopmeier P, Batard MA, Griffin JH: Plasma protein S deficiency in familial thrombotic disease. Blood 64:1297–1300, 1984.
8. Engesser L, Broekmans AW, Briët E, Brommer EJ, Bertina RM: Hereditary protein S deficiency: Clinical manifestations. Ann Int Med 106:677–682, 1987.
9. Bertina RM: Hereditary protein S deficiency. Haemostasis 15:241–246, 1985.
10. Allaart CF, Aronson DC, Ruys Th, Rosendaal FR, van Bockel JH, Bertina RM, Briët E: Hereditary protein S deficiency in young adults with arterial occlusive disease. Thromb Haemost 64:206–210, 1990.
11. Proby CM, Chitolie A, Bevan DH, Mortimer PS: Cutaneous necrosis associated with protein S deficiency. J R Soc Med 83:646–647, 1990.

12. Berkompas DC: Coumadin skin necrosis in a patient with a free protein S deficiency: Case report and literature review. Indiana Med 84:788–791, 1991.
13. Mahasandana C, Suvatte V, Chuansumrit A, Marlar RA, Manco Johnson MJ, Jacobson LJ, Hathaway WE: Homozygous protein S deficiency in an infant with purpura fulminans. J Pediatr 117:750–753, 1990.
14. Pegelow CH, Ledford M, Young J, Zilleruelo G: Severe protein S deficiency in a newborn. Pediatrics 89:674–676, 1992.
15. Laurell CB: Quantitative estimation of proteins by electrophoresis in agarose gel containing antibodies. Anal Biochem 15:45–52, 1966.
16. Francis RB, Patch MJ: A functional assay for protein C in human plasma. Thromb Res 32:605–613, 1983.
17. Bertina RM: Hereditary deficiencies of protein C and S. In Aznar J, España F (eds): "Protein C Pathway." Barcelona: Springer-Verlag Iberica, 1991, pp 111–120.
18. Sas G, Blaskó G, Petrö I, Griffin JH: A protein S deficient family with portal vein thrombosis. Thromb Haemost 54:724, 1985.
19. Rose PG, Essig GF, Vaccaro PS, Brandt JT: Protein S deficiency in pregnancy. Am J Obstet Gynecol 155:140–141, 1986.
20. Mannucci PM, Tripodi A, Bertina RM: Protein S deficiency associated with "juvenile" arterial and venous thrombosis. Thromb Haemost 55: 440, 1986.
21. De Stefano V, Leone G, Ferrelli R, Marietti G, Tortorolo G, Bizzi B, Bertina RM: Severe deep vein thrombosis in a 2 year-old child with protein S deficiency. Thromb Haemost 58:1089, 1987.
22. Israels SJ, Seshia SS: Childhood stroke associated with protein C or S deficiency. J Pediatr 111:562–564, 1987.
23. Bezeaud A, Venisse L, Conard J, Horellou MH, Salomon JL, Lebaleur A, Samama M, Guillin MC: Hereditary protein S deficiency and recurrent venous thrombosis: Study of a family. Presse Med 16:1895–1897, 1987.
24. Schwarz HP, Heeb MJ, Lottenberg R, Roberts H, Griffin JH: Familial protein S deficiency with a variant protein S molecule in plasma and platelets. Blood 74:213–221, 1989.
25. Ploos van Amstel HK, Reitsma PH, Hamulyak K, de Die-Smulders CEM, Mannucci PM, Bertina RM: A mutation in the protein S pseudogene is linked to protein S deficiency in a thrombophilic family. Thromb Haemost 62:897–901, 1989.
26. Sié P, Boneu B, Biermé R, Wiesel ML, Grunebaum L, Cazenave JP: Arterial thrombosis and protein S deficiency. Thromb Haemost 62: 1040, 1989.
27. Sacco RL, Owen J, Mohr JP, Tatemichi TK, Grossman BA: Free protein S deficiency: A possible association with cerebrovascular occlusion. Stroke 20:1657–1661, 1989.
28. Whitlock JA, Janco RL, Phillips JA: Inherited hypercoagulable states in children. Am J Pediatr Hematol Oncol 11:170–173, 1989.
29. Woodhams BJ, Matthews KB, Lee CA, Kernoff PB: Functional protein S assay shows improved correlation with clinical symptoms in hereditary deficiency. Thromb Res 57:651–657, 1990.
30. Pan EY, Gomperts ED, Millen R, Gilsanz V: Bone mineral density and its association with inherited protein S deficiency. Thromb Res 58:221–231, 1990.
31. Cros D, Comp PC, Beltran G, Gum G: Superior sagittal sinus thrombosis in a patient with protein S deficiency. Stroke 21:633–636, 1990.
32. Girolami A, Simioni P, Lazzaro AR, Pontara E, Ruzza G: Heterozygous protein S deficiency: A study of a large kindred. Acta Haematol 84:162–168, 1990.
33. Demarmels F, Lüthy AR, Hirt A, Furlan M, Lämmle B: Inferior vena cava thrombosis in a child with nephroblastoma and combined deficiency of antithrombin III and free protein S. Blut 61:295–297, 1990.
34. Garbrecht F, Gardner S, Johnson V, Grabowski E: Deep venous thrombosis in a child with nephrotic syndrome associated with a circulating anticoagulant and acquired protein S deficiency. Am J Pediatr Hematol Oncol 13:330–333, 1991.
35. Wiesel ML, Borg JY, Grunebaum L, Vasse M, Levesque H, Bierme R, Sie P: Influence of protein S deficiency on the arterial thrombosis risk. Presse Med 20:1023–1027, 1991.
36. Malm J, Laurell M, Nilsson IM, Dahlbäck B: Thromboembolic disease. Critical evaluation of laboratory investigation. Thromb Haemost 68:7–13, 1992.
37. O'Sullivan J, Chatuverdi R, Bennett MK, Hunter S: Protein S deficiency: Early presentation and pulmonary hypertension. Arch Dis Child 67:960–961, 1992.
38. Ceyhan M, Kanra G, Benderlioglu B, Secmeer G, Hicsönmez G, Kirazli S: Transient protein S deficiency with deep venous thrombosis during *Salmonella typhimurium* infection. Arch Dis Child 68:138–139, 1993.
39. Horowitz IN, Galvis AG, Gomperts ED: Arterial thrombosis and protein S deficiency. J Pediatr 121:934–937, 1992.
40. Prats JM, Garaizar C, Zuazo E, Lopez J, Piñan MA, Aragües P: Superior sagittal sinus thrombosis in a child with protein S deficiency. Neurology 42:2303–2305, 1992.
41. D'Angelo A, Della Valle P, Crippa L, Pattarini E, Grimaldi L, D'Angelo S: Autoimmune protein S deficiency in a boy with severe thromboembolic disease. N Engl J Med 238:1753–1757, 1993.
42. Francis RB: Acquired purpura fulminans. Sem Thromb Hemost 16: 310–325, 1990.
43. Powars DR, Rogers ZR, Patch MJ, McGehee WG, Francis RB: Purpura fulminans in meningococcemia: Association with acquired deficiencies of protein C and S. N Engl J Med 317:571–572, 1987.
44. Madden RM, Gill JC, Marlar RA: Protein C and S levels in two patients with acquired purpura fulminans. Br J Haematol 75:112–117, 1990.
45. Dominey A, Kettler A, Yiannias J, Tschen J: Purpura fulminans and transient protein C and S deficiency. Arch Dermatol 124:1442–1443, 1988.
46. Phillips WG, Marsden JR, Hill FG: Purpura fulminans due to protein S deficiency following chickenpox. Br J Dermatol 127:30–32, 1992.
47. Bergmann F, Hoyer PF, D'Angelo SV, D'Angelo A, Mazzola G, Oestereich C, Barthels M: Protein S deficiency due to a temporary protein S antibody in a boy with purpura fulminans. Thromb Haemost 69:556, 1993 (abstract).
48. Manco-Johnson M, Lefkowitz J, Nuss R, Hays T: Purpura fulminans in a child with varicella, a lupus anticoagulant and severe protein S deficiency. Thromb Haemost 69:1229, 1993 (abstract).

American Journal of Hematology 45:335–340 (1994)

Myelomonocytic Crisis With t(5;17) and a p53 Mutation in a Patient With Chronic Myelogenous Leukemia

Hitoshi Nakagawa, Hiroshi Fujii, Hiroyuki Nakai, Johji Inazawa, and Shinichi Misawa
Kyoto First Red Cross Hospital (H.N., H.F.), Third Department of Medicine (H.N., S.M.), and Department of Hygiene (J.I.), Kyoto Prefectural University of Medicine, Kyoto, Japan

We report a 64-year-old Japanese man with chronic myelogenous leukemia (CML) who expired with myelomonocytic crisis. Cytogenetic analyses of chronic phase (CP) and accelerated phase (AP) cells revealed a Philadelphia chromosome and an isochromosome for the long arm of chromosome 17, i(17q). This karyotype was replaced by another karyotype in blast crisis (BC), resulting in near triploidy with t(5;17) (p15;p11) and loss of chromosome 17pter→p11. Interphase fluorescent in situ hybridization studies with a chromosome 17 specific alpha satellite DNA probe confirmed the presence of a clonal change in BC. In addition, single-strand conformation polymorphism analysis and PCR-direct sequencing of BC cells revealed a point mutation at codon 203 of the p53 gene, GTG to GAG (Val to Glu), and loss of the normal allele. In contrast, no alterations of the p53 gene were found in CP and AP cells. Therefore, progression of CML in this patient appeared to be related to loss of 17p, as well as a mutation in the p53 gene.

Key words: myelomonocytic crisis, CML, t(5;17),p53 gene

INTRODUCTION

Most patients with chronic myelogeneous leukemia (CML) progress from a relatively indolent chronic phase (CP), to an aggressive accelerated phase (AP) and blast crisis (BC) during the course of their disease. Blast cells during BC usually display myeloid or lymphoid phenotypes, and myelomonocytic crises have rarely been reported [1,2]. Cytogenetic studies have shown various chromosomal changes in addition to t(9;22) (q34;q11), as the disease progresses to AP or BC [3]. One of the most frequent additional chromosome aberrations is an isochromosome for the long arm of chromosome 17, i(17q), although its role in disease progression is not understood [4]. The p53 gene, a tumor suppressor gene located on 17p13 [5], has recently been implicated in the progression of CML [6,7].

We report here a case of CML myelomonocytic crisis, in which one clone with i(17q) in CP and AP is replaced by another clone in BC with a karyotype in near triploidy der(5)t(5;17). We show that single-strand conformation polymorphism (SSCP) analysis and PCR directed sequencing reveal a point mutation of p53 at codon 203 only in the BC phase sample.

CASE REPORT

A 64-year-old Japanese man presented in August 1989 with a history of general malaise and leukocytosis. Physical exam showed bilateral axillary and inguinal adenopathy, as well as hepatosplenomegaly. The hematocrit was 33.8%, platelet count was 587 $\times$ 10^{12}/L, and leukocyte count was 13.4 $\times$ 10^{12}/L with a differential of 0.5% blast, 4.5% promyelocyte, 5.5% myelocyte, 11.0% metamyelocyte, 36.0% stabs, 31.0% segments, 2.0% lymphocyte, 5.5% basophil, and 0.5% monocyte. The bone marrow aspirate revealed a markedly hypercellular specimen with increased myeloid elements. Blast cells were 2.8% of nucleated cell counts. The alkaline phosphatase score of the mature granulocytes was 55 (normal range; 150–250). Chromosome analysis revealed a 46,XY, t(9;22) (q34;q11) karyotype. A diagnosis of CML was made.

Received for publication May 1, 1993; accepted September 22, 1993.

Address reprint requests to Dr. Hitoshi Nakagawa, Kyoto First Red Cross Hospital, Higashiyama-ku, Kyoto 605, Japan.

The patient received 2 mg busulfan daily, followed by 0.5–0.75 mg esquinone daily until January 1991. Subsequent maintenance therapy consisted of 500 million units alpha interferon (OPC-18) s.c. daily. Bilateral inguinal adenopathy recurred and femoral bone pain appeared in February 1991, followed by high fevers, splenomegaly, and progressive anemia. Blast cells were 5.4% in a repeat bone marrow aspirate. Cytogenetic study revealed a new i(17q) in addition to the previously noted t(9;22)(q34;q11). Ranimustine 50–100 mg was administrated weekly for this AP. Clinical symptoms improved, but high fevers and splenomegaly rapidly progressed again in May 1991. Monoblastoid cells increased in peripheral blood, and the alkaline phosphatase score in mature granulocytes was increased to 310. The bone marrow was now replaced by monoblastoid cells approaching 99% of the nucleated cell counts, and they were positive for peroxidase. Fourteen percent were positive for N-chloroesterase, 67% positive for alpha-N butyrate esterase, and 7% positive for both. Serum and urine lysozyme were elevated to 251 and 1,840 u/ml, respectively. A diagnosis of myelomonocytic crisis was therefore made. The disease was now refractory to chemotherapy, and the patient died of intestinal bleeding and pneumonia on June 3, 1991, 22 months after the initial diagnosis of CML was made.

TABLE I. Summary of Karyotypic Analyses

Clinical phase	Date	Karyotype
Chronic phase	8/29/1989	46,t(9;22) (q34;q11) [42][a]
	4/ 3/1990	46,XY,t(9;22) (q34;q11) [10] /46,idem,i(17q) [1]
	1/14/1991	46,XY,t(9;22) (q34;q11) [23] /46,idem,i(17q) [21]
Accerelated phase	3/ 4/1991	46,XY,t(9;22) (q34;q11) [29] /46,idem,i(17q) [20] /46,XY [1]
	3/29/1991	46,XY,t(9;22) (q34;q11) [42] /46,idem,i(17q) [7] /46,idem,−16,+der(6)t(1;16) (q23;q22),i(17q) [1]
	4/24/1991	46,XY,t(9;22) (q34;q11) [8] /46,idem,i(17q) [2]
Blast crisis	6/ 3/1991	46,XY,t(9;22) (q34;q11) [1] /62–70,XY,+1,+1,+2,+2,+3, +4,+der(5)t(5;17) (p15;p11) +6,+6,+7,+8,+8,+9,+9, t(9;22) (q34;q11)×2,+10, +12,+13,+14,+15,+18,+19, +19,+20,+21,+der(22)t(9;22) (q34;q11) [cp11][b]

[a]The number of analized metaphase cells are shown in the square brackets.
[b]cp is the abbreviation of a composite karyotype, according to the ISCN (1991) [9].

MATERIALS AND METHODS

Cytogenetics

Chromosome analyses were performed according to a short-term culture method [8]. After chromosome banding with the Trypsin-Giemsa method, well-spread metaphase cells were photographed, and karyotyped according to the ISCN (1991) [9].

Fluorescence In Situ Hybridization (FISH)

The method of FISH has been described previously [10,11]. The chromosomal DNA was denatured on glass slides in 70% formamide and 22× SSC at 70°C for 90 sec. A biotinylated chromosome 17-specific alpha satellite DNA probe, p17H8 (Oncor, U.S.A.), was dissolved in formamide and denatured at 75°C for 10 min. Following hybridization, the slides were washed sequentially in 50% formamide/2×SSC, 2×SSC, and 1×SSC. Fluorescent signal amplification and detection were carried out as previously described [11]. Counterstaining was carried out with propidium iodide. Two humdred interphase cells were observed and the number of fluorescence signals in each nucleus were counted up to 200 cells under a fluorescence microscope (NIKON).

PCR-SSCP and DNA Sequencing

High molecular weight DNA was extracted from bone marrow samples obtained in CP (8/29/1989), AP (3/4/1991), and BC (6/3/1991) according to Maniatis et al. [12]. One hundred nanograms of DNA was amplified by PCR in the presence of [α-P^{32}]dCTP, by 12 sets of primers covering the entire coding region of the p53 gene [13–15]. The PCR products were denatured and loaded onto a 6% nondenaturing polyacrylamide gel with or without 10% glycerol, followed by electrophoresis at room temperature. The gel was dried and exposed to Kodak X-Omat film at −80°C.

One sample displayed aberrant bands, and 1 μg of DNA from this sample was amplified by asymmetric PCR. Following purification, dideoxy-mediated chain-termination reactions were carried out, followed by electrophoresis on an 8% polyacrylamide gel with 7 M urea.

RESULTS

Cytogenetics

The karyotypes are summarized in Table I. An i (17q) chromosome was first seen in 1 of 11 metaphases in CP (4/3/1991). This karyotype was replaced by a more complex karyotype in near triploidy, including triple Ph and an unbalanced t(5;17) leading to loss of the 17p terminal. The i(17q) was no longer detected. A representative karyotype from BC is shown in Figure 1.

Fluorescent In Situ Hybridization

In situ hybridization of a chromosome 17-specific alpha-satellite DNA probe to a BC metaphase cell is shown

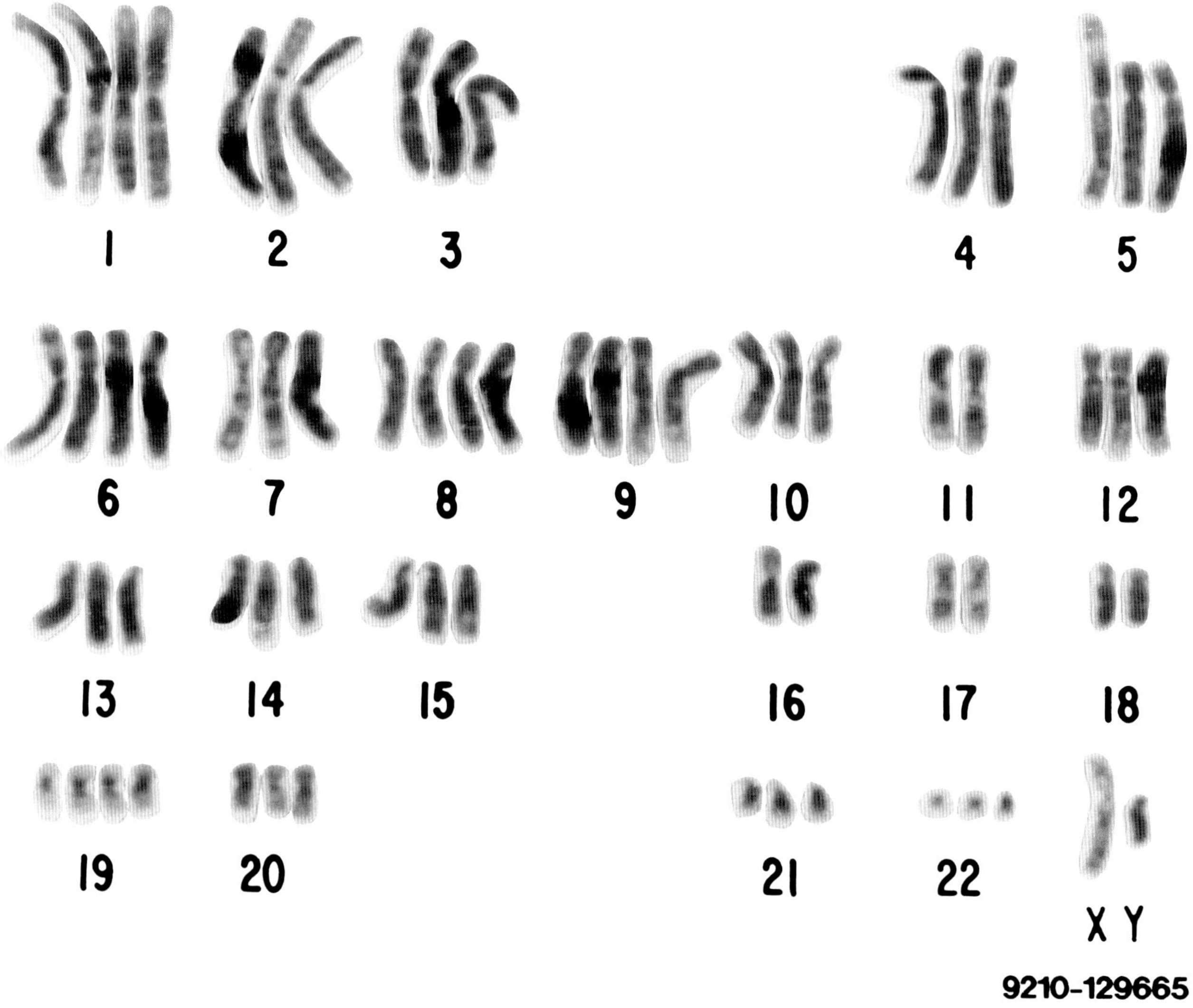

Fig. 1. Karyotype of CML blast crisis in a 64-year-old patient.

in Figure 2. Fluorescent signals are seen at the centromere of two apparently normal chromosome 17s, and also on the short arm of a marker chromosome. The marker chromosome was determined to be a deriverative of chromosome 5 by G-banding. The centromeric region and long arm of chromosome 17 had therefore been translocated to the short arm of chromosome 5.

The fluorescent sites in each nucleus were compared between samples from AP and BC. Single sites were seen in 8% of 200 AP nuclei, two sites were seen in 90.5%, and three sites in 1.5% of AP cells. No cells had more than four sites. The corresponding results for BC cells as follows: 0% (single site), 12.5% (two sites), 82% (three sites), and 5.5% (four fluorescent sites). In situ hybridization to interphase cells confirmed this clonal alteration at the time of BC (Fig. 3).

p53 Gene Mutation

Although no aberrant bands were observed by PCR-SSCP analysis of CP and AP samples, BC samples displayed abnormal SSCP pattern of exon 6 (Fig. 4a). Subsequent DNA revealed a T:A to A:T conversion at codon 203, resulting in substitution of glutamic acid for valine (Fig. 4b). Normal bands were not detectable on autoradiography, indicating loss of the wild type p53 allele. DNA sequencing of exon 6 from CP and AP samples revealed no mutations.

DISCUSSION

We report a case of CML myelomonocytic crisis, in which serial karyotypic studies and p53 sequences were

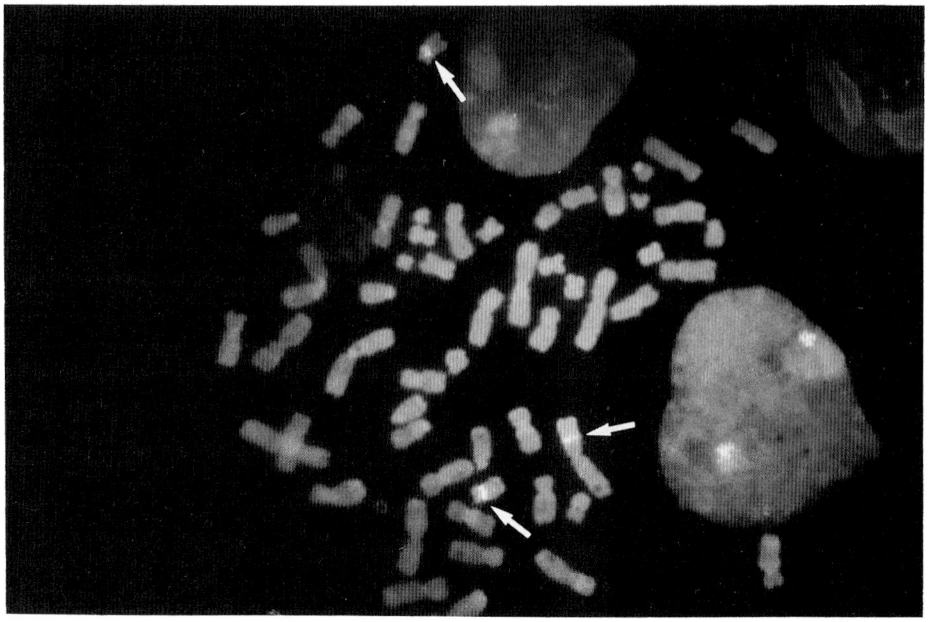

Fig. 2. In situ hybridization of a metaphase BC cell with a chromosome 17-specific alpha satellite DNA probe. Arrows indicate three fluorescent sites; two at the centromeric regions of the normal chromosome 17s, and one on the short arm of a marker chromosome.

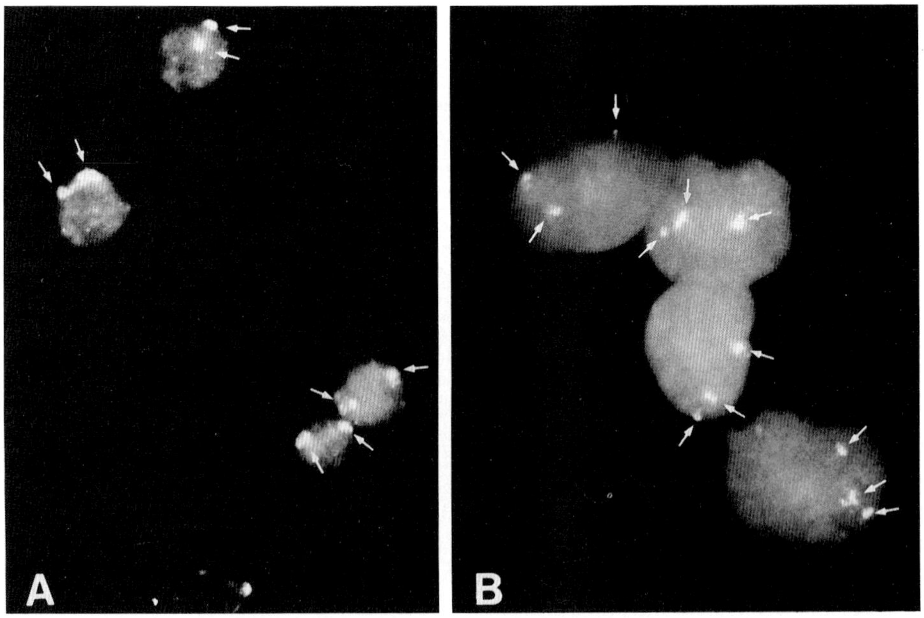

Fig. 3. In situ hybridization of interphase AP (A) and BC (B) cells. Most AP cells have two fluorescent sites related to chromosome 17, while BC cells have three fluorescent sites.

monitored. CP and AP cells displayed i(17q) in 9–48% metaphase cells, but no alterations of the p53 gene were detected. In contrast, the i(17q) clone was replaced by a t(5;17) clone in BC, which also led to loss of 17p13. This clone also had a p53 gene mutation and loss of the normal allele. The patient died following an aggressive BC clinical course. The absence of normal bands in PCR-SSCP analysis indicates that both normal 17s carry the p53 mutation. This would imply mitotic instability with endoreduplication of at least 17 but probably a number of other chromosomes.

In situ hybridization studies utilizing a chromosome specific centromere probe made it possible to detect chromosome aberrations in interphase nuclei. Chromosome

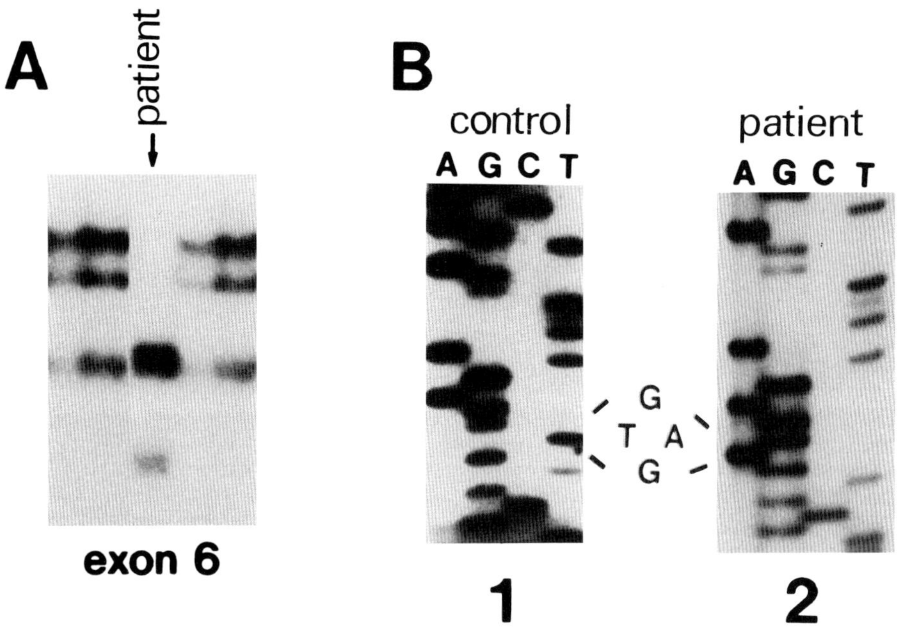

Fig. 4. PCR-SSCP analysis and DNA sequencing of exon 6 from the p53 gene in BC cells. A: A sample from the patient (arrow) exhibits aberrantly migrating bands. B: Sequencing of exon 6 reveals a point mutation at codon 203 (GTG→GAG).

17-specific alpha-satellite DNA probe was utilized to confirm the clonal change between AP and BC. The majority of cells in AP displayed two fluorescent sites, indicating two normal chromosome 17s or one normal chromosome 17 and an i(17q). These cells were replaced by cells with three fluorescent sites in BC.

The 5/17 translocation chromosome found in BC has a dicentric structure. The centromere originated from chromosome 17 must be non functional. It is interesting that in Figure 3B one of the three signals appears to be smaller than the other two. This may imply a small all centromere of reduced size which could make it non-functional and would also confirm the total loss of 17p.

P53 gene mutations have been reported in a variety of human malignancies [16]. For example, Fenaux et al. have noted frequent p53 gene mutations in acute myeloid leukemias with loss of the short arm of chromosome 17 (17p-) [17]. Point mutations of one p53 allele combined with the loss of the other p53 allele seems to be the leading cause of inactivation of both normal p53 alleles [18,19]. These data support the model of recessive tumor suppression by the p53 gene.

A p53 gene mutation appears to be implicated in the evolution of CML from CP to BC in our patient reported here. One p53 gene was lost in AP due to the presence of the isochromosome. This may well be a "pre-mutation" making the cells susceptible to a second mutation at the p53 locus leading to BC. Nonrandom changes involving a 17p have previously been reported in approximately a third of myeloid blast crises [20]. Ahuja et al. have detected structural alterations of the p53 gene in 11 of 54 BC cases, which were rarely seen in CP (1 of 44) [21]. We have also previously reported frequent association of chromosome 17p- and p53 gene mutations in BC [13].

Therefore, a consecutive study of p53 and chromosome 17p alterations was undertaken during the entire course of CML in a single patient, not previously reported. We show that a change of 17p and a p53 mutation were clearly related to disease progression of CML in this patient. The clinical significance of these 17p- and p53 mutations in the course of CML will be further elucidated by investigating a larger number of patients.

REFERENCES

1. Leder LD, Mischke W, Garbrecht M, Stolzenbach G: Terminal Ph[1]-positive monocytic crisis in chronic myeloid leukemia providing evidence for the promyelocytic origin of monocytes. Klin Wschr 67:237–43, 1979.
2. Rodgers GM, Carrera CJ, Ries CA, Bainton DF: Blastic transformation of a well-differentiated monocytic leukemia: Changes in cytochemical and cell surface markers. Leukemia Res 6:613–622, 1982.
3. Krulik M, Smadja N, Gramont A, Gonzales-Canali G, Audebert AA, Dray C, Brissaud P, Debray J: Sequential karyotype study on Ph-positive chronic myelocytic leukemia. Cancer 60:974–979, 1987.
4. Sandberg AA: The chromosomes in human cancer and leukemia. 2nd edition. New York, Elsvier, 1990, pp 458–475.
5. Isobe M, Emanuel BS, Givel D, Oren M, Croce CM: Localization of gene for human p53 tumor antigen to band 17p13. Nature 320:84, 1986.
6. Kelman Z, Prokocimer M, Peller S, Kahn Y, Rechavi G, Manor Y, Cohen A, Rotter V: Rearrangements in the p53 gene in Philadelphia

chromosome positive chronic myelogenous leukemia. Blood 74:2318–2324, 1989.
7. Ahuja H, BarEli M, Advani SH, Benchimoe S, Cline MJ: Alterations in the p53 gene and the clonal evolution of the blast crisis of chronic myelocytic leukemia. Proc Natl Acad Sci USA 86:6783–6787, 1989.
8. Misawa S, Horiike S, Taniwaki M, Abe T, Takino T: Prefixation treatment of ethidium bromide for high resolution banding analysis of chromosomes from cultured human bone marrow cells. Cancer Genet Cytogenet 22:319–329, 1986.
9. ISCN: Guidelines for Cancer Cytogenetics, Supplement to An International System for Human Cytogenetic Nomenclature. Mitelman F (ed). Basel: Karger, 1991.
10. Laurence JB, Villnave Singer RH: Sensitive, high-resolution chromatin and chromosome mapping in situ: Presence and orientation of two closely integrated copies of EBV in a lymphoma line. Cell 52:51–61, 1988.
11. Nakagawa H, Inazawa J, Horiike S, Misawa S: Detection of an i(17q) in CML with fluorescent in situ hybridization using chromosome 17 specific alpha satellite DNA probe. Cancer Genet Cytogenet 62:140–143, 1992.
12. Sambrook J: Isolation of high molecular-weight DNA from mammalian cells. In: Fritsch EF, Maniatis T (eds) "Molecular Cloning," Ed. 2. Cold Spring Harbor, NY: Cold Spring Harbor Laboratory Press, 1989, pp 9.14–9.23.
13. Orita M, Suzuki Y, Sekiya T, Hayashi K: Rapid and sensitive detection of point mutations and DNA polymorphisms using the polymerase chain reaction. Genomics 5:874–879, 1989.
14. Toguchida J, Yamaguchi T, Dayton SH, Beauchamp RL, Herrera GE, Ishizaki K, Yamamuro T, Meyers PA, Little JB, Sasaki MS, Weichselbaum RR, Yandell DW: Prevalence and spectrum of germline mutations of the p53 gene among patients with sarcoma. N Engl J Med 326:1301–1308, 1992.
15. Nakai H, Misawa S, Toguchida J, Yandell DW, Ishizaki K: Frequent p53 gene mutations in blast crisis of chronic myelogenous leukemia, especially in myeloid crisis harboring loss of a chromosome 17p. Cancer Res 52:6588–6593, 1992.
16. Fromentel C, Soussi T: TP53 tumor suppressor gene: A model for investigating human mutagenesis. Genes Chrom Cancer 4:1–15, 1992.
17. Fenaux P, Jonveaux P, Quiquandon I, Lai JL, Pignon JM, Loucheux-Lefebre MH, Bauters F, Berger R, Kerckaert JP: P53 gene mutations in acute myeloid leukemia with 17p monosomy. Blood 78:1652–1657, 1991.
18. Baker SJ, Fearon ER, Nigro JM, Hamilton SR, Preisinger AC, Jessup JM, Van Tuinen P, Ledbetter DH, Barker DF, Nakamura Y, White R, Vogelstein B: Chromosome 17 deletions and p53 gene mutations in colorectal carcinomas. Science 246:491, 1989.
19. Varley JM, Brammar WJ, Lane DP, Swallow JE, Dolan J, Walker R: Loss of chromosome 17p13 sequences and mutation of p53 in human breast carcinomas. Oncogene 6:413, 1991.
20. Fleischman EW, Prigogina EL, Volkova MA, Frenkel MA, Zakhartchenko NA, Konstantinova LN, Puchkova GP, Balakirev SA: Correlations between the clinical course, characteristics of blast cells, and karyotype patterns in chronic myeloid leukemia. Human Genet 58:285–293, 1981.
21. Ahuja H, Bar Eli M, Arlin Z, Advani S, Allen SL, Goldman J, Snyder D, Foti A, Cline M: The spectrum of molecular alterations in the evolution of chronic myelocytic leukemia. J Clin Invest 87:2042–2047, 1991.

American Journal of Hematology 45:341–344 (1994)

Impact of Reinduction Regimens for Relapsed and Refractory Acute Lymphoblastic Leukemia in Adults

Jeanna L. Welborn
Department of Internal Medicine, Division of Hematology and Oncology, University of California, Davis, California

The clinical outlook for adults with acute lymphoblastic leukemia (ALL) has improved with the use of intensive chemotherapy. Complete remissions (CR) are achieved in 80% of adults but the majority relapse on maintenance chemotherapy and a few exhibit primary resistance to induction therapy. This report compares the various salvage treatments and provides guidance in selecting a regimen with the optimum clinical outcome. Regimens using high-dose ara-C (HDAC) in combination with mitoxantrone, amsacrine, or idarubicin are superior to HDAC alone or with L-asparaginase. The sequential administration of methotrexate and L-asparaginase is equally effective. The duration of second CR is short for all chemotherapeutic regimens.

Key words: acute lymphoblastic leukemia, treatment, reinduction regimens, remission

INTRODUCTION

The clinical outlook for adults with acute lymphoblastic leukemia (ALL) has improved over the past two decades with the use of intensive chemotherapy regimens and the prophylactic treatment of the central nervous system. The treatment of ALL in adults is modeled after the pediatric regimens which report cure rates of 50–75% in childhood ALL. A complete remission (CR) can be achieved in over 80% of adults, but only 20% of these patients will remain disease free. Most adults relapse on maintenance chemotherapy, whereas a few exhibit primary resistance to induction chemotherapy.

Once a patient fails to achieve or maintain a complete remission, salvage chemotherapy regimens are used in hopes of achieving a stable remission or as preparation for bone marrow transplantation. This report compares the various salvage treatments in order to provide some guidance in selecting the regimen with the optimum clinical outcome as well as suggest areas for further investigation.

MATERIALS AND METHODS

The literature was reviewed for the clinical reports of chemotherapeutic regimens of adults with relapsed or refractory ALL for the period 1978–1992. Abstracts and regimens utilizing bone marrow transplantation were not considered for this analysis. All patients were resistant to or had relapsed after prior chemotherapy as reported by the authors. Each published regimen was reviewed for the number of patients, drug regimen for induction, consolidation and maintenance, percentage of patients who died during chemotherapy, the percentage of patients who achieved a CR and their median survival. The median age of the patients, immunophenotype, and karyotype of the leukemic cells, white blood cell (WBC) count, and median duration of the previous CR were used to determine the composite of high-risk patients in each study.

RESULTS

A total of 44 chemotherapy regimens involving 861 adult patients with relapsed and refractory ALL are summarized in Table I for the period 1978–1992. The study size ranged from 3–68 patients with an average of 20 patients per regimen. Only 15 of the 44 regimens had more than the requisite 15 patients necessary to detect a statistical difference as a result of the treatment regimen. The median age of the entire patient population was 26 years. There was no correlation between the median age of the patients and the rate of CR or duration of CR. All

Received for publication June 3, 1993; accepted September 22, 1993.

Address reprint requests to Dr. Jeanna L Welborn, Hematology and Oncology, University of California Davis Medical Center, 1508 Alhambra Blvd., Room 320, Sacramento, CA 95816.

TABLE I. Summary of the Treatment Regimens for Relapsed and Refractory Acute Lymphoblastic Leukemia in Adults*

Ref.	First investigator	Regimen	Schedule for HDAC in doses	C/M Given	#Pt	Age	%CR	Duration of CR (mo)	Treatment deaths (%)
1	Kantarjian	HDAC	3g/m2 × 4-12	−/−	30		27	3	14–57
2	Rohatiner	HDAC	2g/m2 × 12	−/−	10	39	33	2	10
3	Early	HDAC	2-3g/m2 × 10-12	−/−	5		0		
4	Herzig	HDAC	3g/m2 × 12	−/−	4		25		
5	Takaku	HDAC	2-3g/m2 × 10-12	−/−	5		0		
6	Rudnick	HDAC	3g/m2 × 3-4	−/−	3	34	0		
7	Morra	HDAC	3g/m2 × 12	+/−	15	36	73	5	0
8	Barnett	HDAC	2g/m2 × 12	+/−	12		42		
9	Willemze	HDAC	3g/m2 × 12	−/+	3	18	67	3.5	
10	Hiddemann	HDAC,mitox	3g/m2 × 8	−/−	11	31	64	2.3	27
11	Kantarian	HDAC,mitox	3g/m2 × 6	−/−	25	25	36	2	32
12	Lejeune	HDAC,mitox	2g/m2 × 8	+/+	20		50	6	15
13	Hiddemann	HDAC,mitox	3g/m2 × 8	−/−	24	31	50	3.5	25
14	Arlin	HDAC,mitox	3g/m2 × 5	+/+	10	38	80	3	20
15	Milpied	HDAC,mitox,PE	1g/m2 × 10	−/+	43	28	70	3	12
16	Peters	HDAC,amsa,PE	1g/m2 × 12	+/−	13	24	77		
17	Zittoun	HDAC,amsa	3g/m2 × 4-12	−/−	14	28	21		17
18	Arlin	HDAC,amsa	3g/m2 × 5	−/−	40	23	72	4	8
19	Stryckmans	HDAC,amsa	1g/m2 × 12	+/+	4		50		
20	Marit	HDAC,amsa	3g/m2 × 4	−/−	7		43	2	
21	Giona	HDAC,ida	3g/m2 × 6	+/+	57	27	54	6	
22	Arcese	HDAC,ida	1-3g/m2 × 6-12	+/−	168	17	64	2.5	8
8	Barnett	HDAC, V,P	2g/m2 × 12	+/−	6		67		
23	Willemze	HDAC,V,P,D	1g/m2 × 12	+/−	3		67		
24	Capizzi	HDAC, asp	3g/m2 × 4	−/−	6	26	30	12	9
25	Amadori	HDAC, asp	3g/m2 × 8	−/−	10	14	30	4.5	40
26	Capizzi	mtx, asp		−/−	10	22	80		
27	Yap	mtx, asp		−/+	26	25	58	4.3	8
27	Yap	mtx, asp, ifos		−/+	11	24	55	3.5+	18
28	Esterhay	mtx, asp, V, Decadron		+/+	14	30	79	7.5	11
29	Terebelo	mtx, asp, V,P		−/+	36	32	25	5	8
30	Woodruff	D, asp, V,P		−/+	23	22	69	2	17
31	Bostrom	D, asp, V,P		−/+	40	10	65	6	17
32	Freund	D, asp, Vn,P		+/+	33	26	64	3.6	12
33	Elias	DVP		−/+	10		50	3.8	
34	Early	DAVP		−/−	14	22	57		21
35	Paciucci	mitox, V,P		−/−	14	35	57	5.5	21
20	Marit	mitox, E		−/−	5		60	6	
36	Paciucci	mitox		−/+	10	35	50	5	
37	Liso	epi, V		−/−	14	37	25	5.5	
38	Ryan	dox, ifos		−/+	9		89		0
39	Sanz	VM-26, ara-c		+/−	19	18	42	2	26
40	Legha	amsa		−/+	20	26	5	1.5	
41	Bickers	rubidazone		+/+	15		27	4	3

*C/M, consolidation/maintenance; CR, complete remission; amsa, amsacrine; asp, L-asparaginase; D, daunorubicin; dox, doxorubicin; epi, epirubicin; E, etoposide; HDAC, high-dose ara-C; ida, idarubicin; ifos, ifosfamide; mtx, methotrexate; mitox, mitoxantrone; P, prednisone; V, vincristine; Vn, vindesine.

the studies reported the rate of CR, but only two-thirds of the studies reported the duration of CR. No postremission therapy was given in 18 trials, most of which used HDAC as the induction chemotherapy. Treatment related mortality averaged 15% with a range of 0–57%. Most of these reports are based on small numbers of patients and useful prognostic factors were rarely described such as presenting white cell count, immunophenotype and karyotype of the leukemic clone, and the duration of the previous CR.

HDAC as a single agent was used in nine studies involving 87 patients [1–9]. The CR rate ranged from 0 to 73% with an overall rate of 34%. Toxicity was not reported. The median duration of CR was 3.6 months in five studies. The combination of HDAC with mitoxantrone, amsacrine, idarubicin, or vincristine plus steroids yielded a 60% CR rate among 442 patients and a 12% treatment-related death rate [8,10–23]. The median duration of CR of 3.4 months is similar to that achieved with single agent HDAC. The combination of L-asparaginase with HDAC in 16 patients gave similar results as HDAC alone with a CR rate of 30%, which is inferior to the other HDAC combination regimens [24,25].

Several studies using sequential methotrexate and L-asparaginase had a combined CR rate of 51% in 97 patients and a median duration of 5.2 months [26–29]. This regimen was well tolerated with an average of 10% treatment-related deaths.

A variety of regimens using combinations of anthracyclines, vinca alkaloids and antimetabolites were studied in 171 patients [20,30–35,37–39]. Some patients were included who relapsed after bone marrow transplantation [31]. These regimens resulted in a combined CR of 61% and a median duration of 4 months. Treatment related deaths were 17%. The combination of ifosfamide and doxorubicin yielded a CR rate of 89% in nine patients with minimal toxicity but the duration of CR and risk parameters of the patients were not reported [38]. Single-agent chemotherapy in three small studies yielded few remissions [36,40,41].

DISCUSSION

Treatment of adults with relapsed and refractory ALL is generally based on the encouraging experience with childhood ALL. However, the clinical and biologic features which are predictive of a good prognosis in childhood ALL are uncommon in adult ALL and may contribute to the poor outcome in adults with this disease [42,43]. This has important implications in designing reinduction regimens that should address high-risk patients with resistant disease. These patients are often treated with salvage chemotherapy which is reminiscent of the treatment for acute nonlymphocytic leukemia, a disease common in adults and for which there is vast experience in treating high risk patients [44]. Most patients will respond to reinduction with a variety of standard regimens or newer non-cross-resistant regimens, but none appears to offer lasting remission.

The most encouraging remission rates are achieved with HDAC in combination with mitoxantrone, amsacrine, or idarubicin and are superior to HDAC alone or with L-asparaginase. However the duration of remission is short and additional effective therapy such as bone marrow transplantation will be necessary for long term survival. Clinical trials of high-dose chemotherapy with methotrexate and 6-mercaptopurine have shown promising results in childhood ALL and should be evaluated in adult ALL treatment protocols [45].

The sequential administration of methotrexate and L-asparaginase is effective in most patients and could be considered as an alternative to HDAC combinations. It does appear to be less toxic but the duration of CR is similar and offers no advantage in that respect.

The most extensive experience in salvage chemotherapy for adult ALL is with vincristine, prednisone, and anthracycline-type agents. Remission rates of around 60% are consistently obtained but are of 3–4 months in duration, with or without postinduction therapy. Even patients who relapse shortly after bone marrow transplantation are likely to respond in a similar manner [31]. The combination of ifosfamide and doxorubicin was very effective in a single study involving 9 patients and should be explored in a larger trial with well-described high-risk patients [38].

Published clinical trials can best be interpreted and compared to other regimens when the study patients are well described by the known risk parameters for ALL, such as age, presenting WBC count, time to response, prior CR duration, cytogenetics, and immunophenotype of the leukemic cells. The data reported in these studies were not sufficient to correlate the clinical outcomes with high-risk patients. In addition, most of these reports involved less than 20 patients and the failure to detect a real improvement among the treatment regimens may be due to an inadequate number of patients. Randomized trials are needed to compare high-dose regimens with standard dose regimens in defined subsets of patients and to devise strategies to achieve durable remissions in adult ALL patients.

REFERENCES

1. Kantarjian HM, Estey EH, Plunkett W, et al: Phase I-II clinical and pharmacologic studies of high-dose cytosine arabinoside in refractory leukemia. Am J Med 81:387–394, 1986.
2. Rohatiner A, Slevin ML, Dhaliwal HS, Malpas JS, Lister TA: High-dose cytosine arabinoside: response to therapy in acute leukemia and non-Hodgkin's lymphoma. Cancer Chemother Pharmacol 12:90–93, 1984.
3. Early AP, Preisler HD, Slocum H, et al: A pilot study of high-dose 1-B-D-arabinofuranosylcytosine for acute leukemia and refractory lymphoma: Clinical response and pharmacology. Cancer Res 42: 1587–1594, 1982.
4. Herzig RH, Wolff SN, Lazarus HM, Phillips GL, Karanes C, Herzig GP: High-dose cytosine arabinoside therapy for refractory leukemia. Blood 62:361–369, 1983.
5. Takaku F, Urabe A, Mizoguchi H, et al: High-dose cytosine arabinoside in the treatment of resistant acute leukemia. Semin Oncol 12(suppl 3):144–150, 1985.
6. Rudnick SA, Cadman ED, Capizzi RL, et al: High-dose cytosine arabinoside in refractory acute leukemia. Cancer 44:1189–1193, 1979.
7. Morra E, Lazzarino M, Inverardi D, et al: Systemic high-dose ara-C for the treatment of meningeal leukemia in adult acute lymphoblastic leukemia and non-Hodgkin's lymphoma. J Clin Oncol 4:1207–1211, 1986.
8. Barnett MJ, Rohatiner AZS, Ganesan TS, Richards MA, Miller A, Lister TA: A phase II study of high-dose cytosine arabinoside in the treatment of acute leukaemia in adults. Cancer Chemother Pharmacol 19:169–171, 1987.
9. Willemze R, Zwaan FE, Colpin G, Keuning JJ: High dose cytosine arabinoside in the management of refractory acute leukemia. Scand J Haematol 29:141–146, 1982.

10. Hiddemann W, Kreutzmann H, Straif K, et al: High-dose cytosine arabinoside in combination with mitoxantrone for the treatment of refractory acute myeloid and lymphoblastic leukemia. Semin Oncol 14:73–77, 1987.
11. Kantarjian HM, Walters RL, Keating MJ, et al: Mitoxantrone and high-dose cytosine arabinoside for the treatment of refractory acute lymphocytic leukemia. Cancer 65:5–8, 1990.
12. Lejeune C, Tubiana N, Gastaut JA, et al: High-dose cytosine arabinoside and mitoxantrone in previously-treated acute leukemia patients. Eur J Haematol 44:240–243, 1990.
13. Hiddemann W, Buchner Th, Heil G, et al: Treatment of refractory acute lymphoblastic leukemia in adults with high dose cytosine arabinoside and mitoxantrone (HAM). Leukemia 4:637–640, 1990.
14. Arlin ZA, Feldman EJ, Finger LR, et al: Short course high dose mitoxantrone with high dose cytarabine is effective therapy for adult lymphoblastic leukemia. Leukemia 5:712–714, 1991.
15. Milpied N, Gisselbrecht C, Harousseau J-L, et al: Successful treatment of adult acute lymphoblastic leukemia after relapse with prednisone, intermediate-dose cytarabine, mitoxantrone, and etoposide (PAME) chemotherapy. Cancer 66:627–631, 1990.
16. Peters WG, Willemze R, Colly LP: Intermediate and high-dose cytosine arabinoside-containing regimens for induction and consolidation therapy for patients with acute lymphoblastic leukemia and lymphoblastic non-Hodgkin's lymphoma: The Leyden experience and review of the literature. Semin Oncol 14:86–91, 1987.
17. Zittoun R, Bury J, Stryckmans P, et al: Amsacrine with high-dose cytarabine in acute leukemia. Cancer Treat Rep 69:1447–1448, 1985.
18. Arlin ZA, Feldman E, Kempin S, et al: Amsacrine with high-dose cytarabine is highly effective therapy for refractory and relapsed acute lymphoblastic leukemia in adults. Blood 72:433–435, 1988.
19. Stryckmans P, de Witte T, Bitar N, et al: Cytosine arabinoside for induction, salvage, and consolidation therapy of adult acute lymphoblastic leukemia. Semin Oncol 14:67–72, 1987.
20. Marit G, Cony P, Duclos F, et al: Treatment of relapsed or refractory acute leukemia: Comparison of two different regimens. Hamatol Bluttransfus 33:614–618, 1990.
21. Giona F, Testi AM, Amadori S, et al: Idarubicin and high-dose cytarabine in the treatment of refractory and relapsed acute lymphoblastic leukemia. Ann Oncol 1:51–55, 1990.
22. Arcese W, Meloni G, Giona F, et al: Idarubicin plus ara-c followed by allogeneic or autologous bone marrow transplantation in advanced acute lymphoblastic leukemia. Bone Marrow Transplant 7:38, 1991.
23. Willemze R, Peters WG, Colly LP: Short-term intensive treatment (V.A.A.P.) of adult acute lymphoblastic leukemia and lymphoblastic lymphoma. Eur J Haematol 41:489–495, 1988.
24. Capizzi RL, Poole M, Cooper MR, et al: Treatment of poor risk acute leukemia with sequential high-dose ara-C and asparaginase. Blood 63:694–700, 1984.
25. Amadori S, Papa G, Avvisati G, et al: Sequential combination of high dose ara-C (HiDAC) and asparaginase (ASP) for the treatment of advanced acute leukemia and lymphoma. Leuk Res 8:729–735, 1984.
26. Capizzi RL, Keeser LW, Sartorelli AC: Combination chemotherapy: Theory and practice. Semin Oncol 4:227–253, 1977.
27. Yap B-S, McCredie KB: L-Asparaginase and methotrexate combination chemotherapy in relapsed acute lymphoblastic leukemia in adults. Cancer Treat Rep 65(suppl 1):83–87, 1981.
28. Esterhay RJ, Wiernik PH, Grove WR, Markus SD, Wesley MN: Moderate dose methotrexate, vincristine, asparaginase, and dexamethasone for treatment of adult acute lymphocytic leukemia. Blood 59:334–345, 1982.
29. Terebelo HR, Anderson K, Wiernik PH, et al: Therapy of refractory adult acute lymphoblastic leukemia with vincristine and prednisone plus tandem methotrexate and L-asparaginase; Results of a Cancer and Leukemia Group B study. Am J Clin Oncol 9:411–415, 1986.
30. Woodruff RK,Lister TA, Paxton AM, et al: Combination chemotherapy for hematological relapse in adult acute lymphoblastic leukaemia. Am J Hematol 4:173–177, 1978.
31. Bostrom B, Woods WG, Nesbit ME, et al: Successful reinduction of patients with acute lymphoblastic leukemia who relapse following bone marrow transplantation. J Clin Oncol 5:376–381, 1987.
32. Freund M, De Boben M, Diedrich H, et al: Treatment of relapsed acute lymphocytic leukemia in adults. Hamat Bluttransfus 33:432–436, 1990.
33. Elias L, Shaw MT, Raab SO: Reinduction therapy for adult acute leukemia with adriamycin, vincristine and prednisone: A Southwest Oncology Group study. Cancer Treat Rep 63:1413–1415, 1979.
34. Early AP, Preisler HD, Gottlieb AJ, Lanchant NA: Treatment of refractory adult acute lymphocytic leukaemia and acute undifferentiated leukaemia with an anthracycline antibiotic and cytosine arabinoside. Br J Haematol 48:369–375, 1981.
35. Liso V, Specchia G, Pavone V, Capalbo S, Dione R: Continuous infusion chemotherapy with epirubicin and vincristine in relapsed and refractory acute leukemia. Acta Haematol 83:116–119, 1990.
36. Paciucci PA, Keaveney C, Cuttner J, Holland JF: Mitoxantrone, vincristine, and prednisone in adults with relapsed or primarily refractory acute lymphocytic leukemia and terminal deoxynucleotidyl transferase positive blastic phase chronic myelocytic leukemia. Cancer Res 47: 5234–5237, 1987.
37. Paciucci PA, Ohnuma T, Cuttner J, Silver RT, Holland JF: Mitoxantrone in patients with acute leukemia in relapse. Cancer Res 3919–3922, 1983.
38. Ryan DH, Bickers JN, Vial RH, et al: Doxorubicin and ifosfamide combination chemotherapy in previously treated acute leukemia in adults: A Southwest Oncology Group pilot study. Cancer Treat Rep 64:869–872, 1980.
39. Sanz GF, Sanz MA, Rafeeas FJ, Martinez JA, Martin-Aragones G, Marty ML: Tenoposide and cytarabine combination chemotherapy in the treatment of relapsed adolescent and adult acute lymphoblastic leukemia. Cancer Treat Rep 70:1321–1323, 1986.
40. Legha SS, Keating MJ, McCredit KB, Bodey GP, Freireich EJ: Evaluation of AMSA in previously treated patients with acute leukemia: Results of therapy in 109 adults. Blood 60:484–490, 1982.
41. Bickers J, Benjamin R, Wilson H, Eyre H, Hewlett J, McCredie K: Rubidazone in adults with previously treated acute leukemia and blast cell phase of chronic myelocytic leukemia: A Southwest Oncology Group study. Cancer Treat Rep 65:427–430, 1981.
42. Hoelzer D: High-dose chemotherapy in adult acute lymphoblastic leukemia. Semin Hematol 28:84–89, 1991.
43. Arlin ZA, Feldman EF, Finger L, et al.: "Quality" remissions: A new target of induction therapy in acute leukemia and the next step in developing curative treatment. Semin Hematol 28(suppl 4):44–47, 1991.
44. Mauer AM: Adult and childhood acute lymphocytic leukemia: Are they different diseases? Am J Hematol 42:127–131, 1993.
45. Welborn JL, Lewis JP, Meyers FJ: Impact of reinduction regimens on the clinical course of adult acute nonlymphocytic leukemia. Leukemia 2:711–716, 1988.
46. Hoelzer D, Gale RP: Acute lymphoblastic leukemia in adults: Recent progress, future directions. Semin Hematol 24:27–39, 1987.

American Journal of Hematology 45:345–346 (1994)

Two Different Mutations in Codon 68 Are Observed in Hb G-Philadelphia Heterozygotes

T.P. Molchanova, D.D. Pobedimskaya, Z. Ye, and T.H.J. Huisman

Laboratory of Protein Chemistry, Department of Biochemistry and Molecular Biology, Medical College of Georgia, Augusta, Georgia

Through sequencing of amplified DNA containing the appropriate α-globin genes we have identified the base substitution leading to the formation of Hb G-Philadelphia [α68(E17)Asn Lys]. Three subjects (~25% Hb G) had an AAC AA*A* change at codon 68 of the α2-globin gene; the chromosome with this mutation carried two α genes (αα). Six subjects (~33% Hb G) had an AAC AA*G* change at the same codon of the α2α1 hybrid gene on a chromosome with the 3.7 kb deletion ($-\alpha^{3.7}$). These results indicate two independent mutations which likely occurred in different populations; increase in the level of Hb G is primarily dependent upon the loss of one or more α-globin genes.

Key words: α-thal, α gene deletion, α2 mutation, α1 mutation, PCR, sequencing, quantities G-Phil

INTRODUCTION

The level of Hb G-Philadelphia [$\alpha_2$68(E17)Asn Lysβ_2] [1] in heterozygotes varies greatly and four different percentages have been reported: ~25%, ~35%, ~45%, and 100%. Some 10 to 20 years ago it was determined that heterozygotes with ~25% had four α-globin genes ($\alpha^G\alpha/\alpha\alpha$ or $\alpha\alpha^G/\alpha\alpha$), those with ~35% had three ($-\alpha^G/\alpha\alpha$), those with ~45% had two ($-\alpha^G/-\alpha$), while a few subjects with Hb G and Hb H disease had only the α^G gene ($-\alpha^G/--$) [for review and references, see Refs. 2–4]. Hb G heterozygotes with ~25% Hb G were mainly Caucasian and those with the higher percentages were Black. Unexplained was the relationship between the 25% heterozygotes with a Hb G mutation on one of the two α-globin genes and those carrying the Hb G mutation on the α2α1 hybrid gene which is characteristic for the $-\alpha^{3.7}$ kb deletion [5]. Here, we provide data for nine Hb G heterozygotes showing that those with ~25% Hb G have an AAC AA*A* mutation in their α2-globin gene, while a different mutation (AAC AA*G*) is present in the α2α1 hybrid gene of those with ~35% Hb G.

MATERIALS AND METHODS

Blood samples were collected in vacutainers with EDTA as anticoagulant. Hematological data were obtained with an automated cell counter. Hb G [i.e., α^G hemoglobin (Hb) components] was quantified by cation exchange high performance liquid chromatography (HPLC) [6]. DNA was extracted from the white cells with the method of Poncz et al. [7]. α-Globin gene typing was by gene mapping [8] or with a polymerase chain reaction (PCR) based technique [9]. Sequencing of the α2- and α1-globin genes was with methodology used in earlier studies [9]; amplification primers were specific for either the α2- or the α1-globin genes as well as the α2α1 hybrid gene of the $-\alpha^{3.7}$ kb deletion [9].

RESULTS AND DISCUSSION

Sequence analysis of the nine amplified DNA samples identified an AAC AA*G* change at codon 68 of the α2α1 hybrid gene of six individuals, and an AAC AA*A* change at the same location in the α2 gene of the remaining three subjects. Both mutations result in an Asn Lys replacement at α68. Table I summarizes all data including the Hb G percentages, the number of α-globin genes, the codon 68 mutations, and the proposed genotypes. Two infants (M.L. and D.C.) were heterozygous for an

Received for publication August 26, 1993; accepted September 22, 1993.

Address reprint requests to Dr. Titus H.J. Huisman, Department of Biochemistry and Molecular Biology, Medical College of Georgia, Augusta, GA 30912-2100.

TABLE I. Data for the Nine Subjects Participating in This Study

Case[a]	Sex-Age	Hb G %[b]	Number of α genes[c]	Codon 68 mutation	Genotype
E.L.	M-55	25.8	4	α2:AAC AAA	$\alpha^G\alpha/\alpha\alpha;\beta^A/\beta^A$
M.L.	M-newborn	33.2	3	α2:AAC AAA	$\alpha^G\alpha/-\alpha^{3.7};\beta^A/\beta^S$
S.M.	F-19	25.1	4	α2:AAC AAA	$\alpha^G\alpha/\alpha\alpha;\beta^A/\beta^A$
T.C.	F-adult	34.3	3	$\alpha^{3.7}$:AAC AAG	$-\alpha^G(3.7)/\alpha\alpha;\beta^A/\beta^A$
D.C.	M-1½	33.8	3	$\alpha^{3.7}$:AAC AAG	$-\alpha^G(3.7)/\alpha\alpha;\beta^A/\beta^C$
1016	M-newborn	33.1	3	$\alpha^{3.7}$:AAC AAG	$-\alpha^G(3.7)/\alpha\alpha;\beta^A/\beta^A$
2005	M-newborn	28.5	3	$\alpha^{3.7}$:AAC AAG	$-\alpha^G(3.7)/\alpha\alpha;\beta^A/\beta^A$
2060	F-newborn	32.8	3	$\alpha^{3.7}$:AAC AAG	$-\alpha^G(3.7)/\alpha\alpha;\beta^A/\beta^A$
2186	F-newborn	32.7	3	$\alpha^{3.7}$:AAC AAG	$-\alpha^G(3.7)/\alpha\alpha;\beta^A/\beta^A$

[a]E.L. is the father of M.L.; T.C. is the mother of D.C.; S.M. participated in a high school testing program; the remaining four newborn babies are unrelated and were selected when their slowly moving Hb FG and Hb G were detected in an ongoing newborn testing program.

[b]Hb G = Hb G ($\alpha_2{}^G\beta_2$) + Hb FG ($\alpha_2{}^G\alpha_2$) + Hb G_2 ($\alpha_2{}^G\delta_2$) + Hb SG ($\alpha_2{}^G\beta_2{}^S$) + Hb CG ($\alpha_2{}^G\beta_2{}^C$); all these Hb components were resolved and quantitated by cation exchange HPLC [6].

[c]By gene mapping or agar gel electrophoresis of the PCR product of DNA amplified with primers specific for the 3.7 kb deletion [9].

additional β chain variant (Hb S and Hb C, respectively). E.L., his newborn son, and S.M. carried the AA*C* AA*A* mutation at codon 68 of the α2-globin gene. E.L. and S.M. had a Hb G value of 25–26%, as expected. The newborn M.L. had a Hb G percentage of 33.2%; the increase results from an α-thal-2 ($-\alpha^{3.7}$) chromosome in trans which he inherited from his mother (data not shown). The remaining six subjects were heterozygotes for the $-\alpha^{3.7}$ α-thal-2 deletion. The α2α1 hybrid gene carried the AA*C* AA*G* mutation at codon 68, while the Hb G value varied between 28.5 and 34.3%, with an average of 32.5%.

These results suggest the existence of two independent mutations leading to the same amino acid replacement in the α chain. The AA*C* AA*A* mutation occurred in the major α2-globin gene, perhaps in an Italian population (E.L. and S.M. are members of army families with an Italian background), while the AA*C* AA*G* mutation is specific for the α2α1 hybrid gene observed in the Black population. Increases in the levels of Hb G are the result of a deletion of one or more α-globin gene(s).

ACKNOWLEDGMENTS

This study was supported by the United States Public Health Services research grant HLB-05168.

REFERENCES

1. Baglioni C, Ingram VM: Abnormal human haemoglobins. V. Chemical investigation of Haemoglobins A, G, C, X from one individual. Biochim Biophys Acta 48:253, 1961.
2. Baine RM, Rucknagel DL: Variation in the number of alpha loci found in heterozygotes for Hemoglobin G Philadelphia (α68 Asn Lys). Am J Hum Genet 27:15A, 1975 (abstract).
3. Milner PF, Huisman THJ: Studies on the proportion and synthesis of Haemoglobin G Philadelphia in red cells of heterozygotes, a homozygote, and a heterozygote for both Haemoglobin G and α thalassaemia. Br J Haematol 34:207, 1976.
4. Sciarratta GV, Sansone G, Ivaldi G, Felice AE, Huisman THJ: Alternate organization of α G-Philadelphia globin genes among U.S. Black and Italian Caucasian heterozygotes. Hemoglobin 8:537, 1984.
5. Higgs DR, Vickers MA, Wilkie AOM, Pretorius I-M, Jarman AP, Weatherall DJ: A review of the molecular genetics of the human α-globin gene cluster. Blood 73:1081, 1989.
6. Bissé E, Wieland H: High-performance liquid chromatographic separation of human haemoglobins: Simultaneous quantitation of foetal and glycated haemoglobins. J Chromatogr 494:95, 1988.
7. Poncz M, Solowiejczyk D, Harpel B, Mory Y, Schwartz E, Surrey S: Construction of human gene libraries from small amounts of peripheral blood: Analysis of β-like globin genes. Hemoglobin 6:27, 1982.
8. Gu YC, Landman H, Huisman THJ: Two different quadruplicated α globin gene arrangements. Br J Haematol 66:245, 1987.
9. Molchanova TP, Pobedimskaya DD, Postnikov YuV: A simplified procedure for sequencing amplified DNA containing the α2- or α1-globin gene. Hemoglobin, in press.

American Journal of Hematology 45:347–353 (1994)

LETTERS AND CORRESPONDENCE

Letters and correspondence submitted for possible publication must be identified as such. Text length must not exceed 500 words and five bibliographic references. A single concise figure or table may be included if it is essential to support the communication. Letters not typed double-spaced will not be considered for publication. Letters not meeting these specifications will not be returned to authors. Letters to the Editor *are utilized to communicate a single novel observation or finding.* Correspondence *is to be used to supplement or constructively comment on the contents of a publication in the journal and cannot exceed the restrictions for Letters to the Editor. The Editor reserves the right to shorten text, delete objectional comments and make other changes to comply with the style of the journal. Permission for publication must be appended as a postscript. Submissions must be sent to Marcel E. Conrad, M.D., Associate Editor, American Journal of Hematology, USA Cancer Center, Mobile, Alabama 36688 to permit rapid consideration for publication.*

Rearrangement of the BCR/ABL and TCR-β Genes in Lymph Node Blast Crisis Diagnosed of Chronic Myeloid Leukemia

To the Editor: We read with interest Tittley et al.'s letter to the editor entitled "Occurrence of T-cell lymphoma in a patient with Philadelphia chromosome-positive chronic myelogenous leukemia with rearrangements of *bcr* and *TCR*β genes in lymph nodes" [1]. We recently had the opportunity to examine a similar patient [2]. In our case, *bcr/abl* gene rearrangements were obtained in lymph node, peripheral blood, and bone marrow samples, the bands obtained being the same in all the samples. In the study of the *TCR*-β, *TCR*-γ, and *JH* rearrangements in lymph node, peripheral blood, and bone marrow, *TCR*-β rearrangements were found only in the lymph node cells.

On diagnosing the lymph node infiltration, the peripheral blood and bone marrow were in the chronic phase of chronic myeloid leukemia (CML). However, 3 weeks later, the existence of blastic infiltration by cells having morphology, cytochemical, immunophenotype, and rearrangements identical to those of the lymph node was demonstrated in the bone marrow.

The existence of rearrangement of the *bcr/abl* gene in the lymph node neoplastic cells shows that such cells present a reciprocal translocation between the *abl* protooncogene located on chromosome 9 and the *bcr* major region located on chromosome 22, this being the molecular alteration of the Philadelphia chromosome in CML [3]. Thus the lymph node cells originate from the clone responsible for the CML, and the correct diagnosis in this case would be lymph node blast crisis of CML with a T-cell lymphoid phenotype more than that of a T-cell lymphoma in a patient with CML. The patient was treated with vincristine, daunoblastine, and prednisone, leading to remission of the blast crisis and return to the chronic phase of the disease.

In the case presented by Tittley et al., there was a lack of *bcr/abl* rearrangements with the *Bam*HI enzyme in the peripheral blood, while this rearrangement is present in lymph nodes with the same enzyme. It is of interest that the bands obtained in the lymph node and peripheral blood with the *Bgl*II and *Eco*RI enzymes are similar.

In our opinion, this discordance in the results between the peripheral blood and nymph nodes with only the *Bam*HI restriction enzyme has no logical explanation, since, if this was a change in the rearrangement of the *bcr/abl* gene in the clone that has arisen from the lymph node, this should appear with *Bgl*II and *Eco*RI enzymes. We believe that the case of Tittley et al. corresponds to a lymph node blast crisis (lymphoblastic T) of CML, as has been reported in other cases in the literature [2,4-6]. A follow-up study of the patient would have been interesting, since the lymph node infiltration generally occurs shortly after the medullar and peripheral blood infiltration in cases of lymph node blast crisis of CML.

A. Villegas
F.A. González
Servicio de Hematología y Hemoterapia, Hospital Universitario San Carlos, Professor Martín Lagos s/n, Madrid, Spain

References

1. Tittley P, Trempe JM, Van der Jagt R, Drouin J, Huebsch L, McLeish B, Cheng G: Occurrence of T-cell lymphoma in patient with Philadelphia chromosome-positive chronic myelogenous leukemia with rearrangements of BCR and TCR-β genes in Lymph nodes. Am J Hematol 42:229-230,1993.
2. González FA, Villegas A, Ferro MT, Cabello P, Morales D, Perez J, Martínez R: Usefulness of the rearrangement of the bcr/abl gene in extramedullary (lymph nodes) blast crisis diagnosed of chronic myeloid leukemia. Br J Haematol 84:341-342, 1993.
3. Heisterkamp N, Stam K, Groffen J, de Klein A, Grosveld G: Structural organization of the bcr gene and its role in the Ph' translocation. Nature 315:758-760, 1985.
4. Giannone L, Whitlock JA, Kinney MC, Wolff SN, Dev VG: Use of the BCR probe to demonstrate extramedullary recurrence of CGL with a T cell lymphoid phenotype following bone marrow transplantation. Bone Marrow Transplant 3:631-635, 1988.
5. Hirose Y, Tachibana J, TaKiguchi T, Tatsumi E, Kondo S: T-lymphoblastic transformation of chronic myelocytic leukemia following T-lymphoblastic and myeloblastic biphenotypic crisis in the lymph nodes with rearrangement of bcr and TCR-β genes. Eur J Haematol 45:282, 1990.
6. Djulbegovic B, Hadley T, Yen F: Occurrence of high grade T-cell lymphoma with Philadelphia chromosome negative chronic myelogenous leukemia with breakpoint cluster region rearrangement: Case report and review of the literature. Am J Hematol 36:63, 1991.

Gaucher's Disease and Acquired Coagulopathy

To the Editor: Acquired coagulation factor deficiency developing in the adult is most often caused by liver disease, vitamin K deficiency, or consumption coagulopathy. Other less common reported associations include autoantibodies, multiple myeloma, and Gaucher's disease. We recently cared for a 39-year-old woman with idiopathic, symptomatic splenomegaly, who underwent a diagnostic and therapeutic splenectomy. Preoperative laboratory evaluation showed multiple coagulation factor deficiencies, without evidence of liver disease. Pathologic examination of the spleen showed Gaucher's disease. All coagulation laboratory abnormalities were resolved postsplenectomy. The combination of acquired coagulation factor deficiency and splenomegaly might be a useful clue to the diagnosis of Gaucher's disease.

TABLE I. Coagulation Laboratory Results

Test	Normal range	Presplenectomy	Postsplenectomy
Prothrombin time (sec)	10.4–12.6	14.9	11.5
Partial thromboplastin time (sec)	24.8–37.2	41.9	34.0
Factor VIII (U/dl)	45–145	26	149
Factor IX (U/dl)	62–126	83	138
Factor XI (U/dl)	53–113	36	104

The patient had been in excellent health until 4 months prior to admission, when she noted progressive abdominal fullness and early satiety. The patient's family history was significant for severe hemophilia A in one son, two brothers, and one nephew. Physical examination showed massive splenomegaly without any adenopathy. Bone marrow examination and liver function studies were within normal limits. Her packed cell volume was 0.26, with a platelet count of 49×10^9/liter. Preoperative coagulation study results are shown in Table I. She received 280 ml fresh frozen plasma and 2 units packed red cells and platelet concentrates, then underwent splenectomy without complications. Pathologic examination of the spleen was consistent with Gaucher's disease.

The patient recovered promptly postoperatively and was seen again 1 month later for follow-up. Repeat coagulation study results are shown in Table I. All detected factor deficiencies had been completely resolved. Although she was a carrier for hemophilia A, her factor VIII level 1 month postoperatively was not decreased. A normal level of factor VIII activity in carriers of hemophilia A is not unusual, perhaps due to the great variability of factor VIII activity in individuals and to lyonization. No previous reports of association between hemophilia A and Gaucher's disease could be found in the literature.

The association of coagulation factor deficiencies and Gaucher's disease has been observed previously [1–5]. Although various mechanisms have been postulated to account for this observation, adsorption of the factors by accumulated sphingolipid (glucocerebroside) appears the most likely, but this is yet to be proven. The reported association of factor XI deficiency and Gaucher's disease is, at least in many cases, a coincidence of two disorders more commonly observed in those of Ashkenazi Jewish descent [2,4]. This patient was not of Ashkenazi Jewish descent.

In some of the previous reports, significant or complete correction of the coagulation factor defect was observed following splenectomy [3,5], but correction may be incomplete or delayed [1]. The defect in Gaucher's disease, glucocerebrosidase deficiency, leads to accumulation of glucocerebroside in macrophages in many organs besides the spleen. Therefore, if the accumulation of glucocerebroside plays a role in this development of these factor deficiencies, it should not be surprising that the deficiencies may be only partially or temporarily corrected by splenectomy. Whether treatment of patients with enzyme replacement will lead to correction of the coagulation abnormalities has not been determined.

In patients with known Gaucher's disease, it appears to be advisable to consider screening for the presence of coagulation factor deficiencies and correcting them prior to splenectomy. In patients such as the one presented here, the coincidence of splenomegaly and factor deficiencies in the absence of liver disease or a consumptive coagulopathy might be a useful clue to the diagnosis of Gaucher's disease.

ACKNOWLEDGMENTS

J.E.H. is supported by Physician Scientist Award HL02592. The authors express their appreciation for the excellent technical support provided in the performance of the coagulation factor assays by Mary N. Acker, MT(ASCP)SH.

JOHN E. HUMPHRIES
CHARLES E. HESS
Departments of Internal Medicine and Pathology, University of Virginia Health Sciences Center, Charlottesville, Virginia

REFERENCES

1. Sawitsky A, Boklan BF: Gaucher's disease and coagulation factors (letter). Ann Intern Med 77:150–151, 1972.
2. Seligsohn U, Zitman D, Many A, Klibansky C: Coexistence of factor XI (plasma thromboplastin antecedent) deficiency and Gaucher's disease. Israel J Med Sci 12:1448–1452, 1976.
3. Yates P, Morse C, Standen GR: Gaucher's disease and acquired coagulopathy. Clin Lab Haematol 14:331–334, 1992.
4. Berrebi A, Malnick SDH, Vorst EJ, Stein D: High incidence of factor XI deficiency in Gaucher's disease (letter). Am J Hematol 40:153–161, 1992.
5. Vreeken J, Meinders AE, Keeman JN, Feltkamp TEW: A chronic clotting defect with some characteristics of excessive intravascular coagulation in a patient with Gaucher's disease. Folia Med Neerl 10:180–185, 1967.

Megadose Methyprednisolone for Pure Red Cell Aplasia

To the Editor: Garcia Vela et al. briefly presented an adult patient with pure red cell anemia (PRCA) treated successfully with cyclosporine A (CSA) [1]. They mentioned Raghavachar's conclusion that "CSA seems to be the most efficient treatment of PRCA, with an overall response rate of 65%."

I would emphasize that all 12 children with congenital and two with acquired PRCA responded to megadose methylprednisolone (MDMP; 30–100 mg/kg/day), which was tapered gradually until hemoglobin reached 11 g/dl, then continued 1 mg/kg for 6–12 months [2–4]. It is administered orally (it is given once before 9 AM) in recently treated patients as efficiently as with the intravenous route [5,6]. Since MDMP is much less expensive and has been 100% effective in our hands, it should be used comparatively on an international scale to determine the most effective treatment for PRCA.

ŞINASI ÖZSOYLU
Department of Pediatrics, Hacettepe University Medical Faculty, and Hacettepe Children's Hospital, Ankara, Turkey

REFERENCES

1. Garcia Vela JA, Monteserin MC, Onci F, Barea LM, Lastra A, Perez V: Cyclosporine used as a single drug in the treatment of pure red cell aplasia associated with thymoma. Am J Hematol 42:238, 1993.
2. Özsoylu Ş: High dose intravenous corticosteroid for a patient with Diamond-Blackfan syndrome refractory to classical prednisolone treatment. Acta Haematol 71:207, 1984.
3. Özsoylu Ş: High dose intravenous corticosteroid treatment for patient with Diamond-Blackfan syndrome resistant or refractory to conventional treatment. Am J Pediatr Hematol Oncol 10:210, 1988.
4. Özsoylu Ş: High dose intravenous methylprednisolone (HIVMP) in hematologic disorders. Hematology Rev 4:197, 1990.
5. Özsoylu Ş: Megadose methylprednisolone for pure red cell aplasia. Br J Hematol 81:625, 1992.
6. Özsoylu Ş, Albayrak D, Güler E, Duru F: Oral megadose methylprednisolone for Diamond-Blackfan anemia. Eur J Pediatr 151:629, 1992.

Essential Thrombocythemia and Pregnancy

To the Editor: We read with interest the article by Chow et al. "Essentia thrombocythemia in pregnancy: Platelet count and pregnancy outcome" [1]. Essential thrombocythemia (ET) has often been described in youn adults and is usually associated with a long, benign course. We had a opportunity to follow four women with ET through a total of seven preg nancies. All four were diagnosed as having ET according to criteria of the Polycythemia Vera Study Group [2]. Two were diagnosed during pregnancy; the other two were found through incidental blood counts, and all four were asymptomatic. They had thrombocyte counts ranging between 700×10^9/liter and $1,000 \times 10^9$/liter during their pregnancies, except for one patient with a count of 250×10^9/liter who had just completed 3 months of busulfan before pregnancy. Three of them did not receive treatment during pregnancy; the fourth was given low-dose aspirin because of a missed twin. There was one missed abortion, one missed twin, and six successful deliveries. All four were treated after delivery wioth hydroxyurea or busulfan for short periods, with lowering of the thrombocyte count, and subsequent pregnancies in two of the patients were uneventful. Chow et al. [1] observed a progressive decline in platelet count during pregnancy, with a rebound thrombocytosis after delivery. Only in one patient did we observe this phenomenon; the thrombocyte count decreased from 980×10^9/liter to 570×10^9/liter, with a rebound thrombocytosis of 935×10^9/liter after delivery. On the contrary, the thrombocyte count in the patient who started her pregnancy with 250×10^9/liter rose to 776×10^9/liter and necessitated further treatment after delivery. ET has an expected course and can be associated with thromboembolic events or bleeding due to high thrombocyte counts and abnormal platelet function. The question of management of patients with ET and pregnancy is important to allow a normal pregnancy and delivery. Our experience demonstrates that pregnancy can have a normal outcome even with high thrombocyte counts and no treatment. The role of aspirin in these patients remains to be determined.

Naomi Rahimi-Levene
Zion Hagay
Uriel Elchalal
Alain Berrebi

Hematology Institute, Department of Gynecology and Obstetrics, Kaplan Hospital, Rehovot, Israel

References

1. Chow EY, Haley LP, Vickars LM: Essential thrombocythemia in pregnancy: Platelet count and pregnancy outcome. Am J Hematol 41:249, 1992.
2. Murphy S, Hand H, Rosenthal D, Laszio J: Essential thrombocythemia: An interim report. The Polycythemia Vera Study Group. Semin Hematol 23:177, 1986.

Hodgkin's Disease in a Patient With Neurofibromatosis

To the Editor: Von Recklinghausen's disease, or neurofibromatosis, is associated with a number of neoplasms, including pheochromocytoma, Wilms tumor, neuroblastoma, meningioma, glioma, fibrosarcoma of bone, leukemia, and lymphoma [1]. However, malignant lymphoma is rare in patients with neurofibromatosis, and the nature of the association between neurofibromatosis and malignant lymphoma is unknown. To the best of our knowledge, neither has been reported to coexist with Hodgkin's disease. We describe a case of Hodgkin's disease developing in a patient with neurofibromatosis.

On March 2, 1990, a 70-year-old man was admitted for evaluation of facial and right upper arm edema. Multiple café-au-lait spots were noted on the trunk and limbs. Lymph nodes were palpable in the right supraclavicular area. The liver and spleen were not palpable. A chest X-ray and whole-body computed tomographic scan disclosed lymphadenopathy in the mediastinum and right pleural effusion. Specimens obtained by lymph node biopsy showed lymphocyte depletion, and a diagnosis of Hodgkin's disease was made. Lymphadenopathy in the mediastinum gradually increased, and the patient complained of dyspnea. He was treated with radiation therapy (3,000 rads to the mediastinum) and five courses of chemotherapy with nitrogen mustard, vincristine, procarbazine, and prednisone (MOPP). All evidence of Hodgkin's disease disappeared, and for 7 months there was no clinical evidence of recurrence. However, on November 26, 1990, the patient was readmitted because of vertigo and stupor. Lymphadenopathy was not detected, and Hodgkin's disease was thought not to have recurred. The patient died on November 27, 1990.

Neurofibromatosis is an autosomal dominant disorder characterized by proliferation of cellular elements embryologically derived from the neural crest. Clinical manifestations include multiple café-au-lait spots and neurofibromas on the trunk [3]. This disease is frequently complicated by neoplasms of neural crest origin. Rarely, malignant disease of other than neural crest origin occurs, including malignant lymphoma and leukemia [2–6]. The relationship between neurofibromatosis and malignant lymphoma is not understood. Berman et al. [3] speculated that long-term antigenic stimulation may provoke the neoplastic conversion, and Kaplan et al. [6] suggested that genetic factors are strongly implicated. To date, reported malignant lymphomas in patients with neurofibromatosis have all been non-Hodgkin's disease. In the case described here, we were unable to discern a relationship between the Hodgkin's disease and the neurofibromatosis.

Hideyo Natori
Ken Tanaka
Kaori Shiraishi
Seishi Osabe
Hiroto Jojima
Junichi Honda
Kazuhiko Matsuo
Osamu Nakashima
Kotaro Oizumi

First Department of Internal Medicine and Department of Pathology, Kurume University School of Medicine, Fukuoka, Japan

References

1. Hope DG, Mulvihill JJ: Malignancy in neurofibromatosis. Adv Neurol 21:33, 1981.
2. Bader JL, Miller RW: No maternal effect in childhood leukaemia with neurofibromatosis. Lancet 1:503, 1979.
3. Berman BW, Binder RA, Cornfield DB: Burkitt lymphoma in patient with neurofibromatosis and pheochromocytoma. Am Med Assoc 237:993, 1977.
4. Cushing B, Kaplan J, Bhaya N, Roskamp J: Multiple incidence of thymic lymphoblastic lymphoma in a family with neurofibromatosis. Proc Am Assoc Cancer Res 19:362, 1978.
5. Radi MT, Foucar E, Palmer CH, Gooding RA: Malignant lymphoma arising in a large congenital neurofibroma of the head and neck. Cancer 61:1667, 1988.
6. Kaplan J, Cushing B, Chang C-H, Poland R, Roscamp J, Perrin E, Bhaya N: Familial T-cell lymphoblastic lymphoma: Association with Von Recklinghausen neurofibromatosis and Gardner syndrome. Am J Hematol 12:247, 1982.

Splenic Infiltrates in Acute Lymphoblastic Leukemia

To the Editor: Leukemia can infiltrate any organ of the body [1]. A patient can have persistent leukemic activity in extramedullary organs while being in "complete remission" [2–5]. Central nervous system (CNS), testis, ovary, and rarely orbit are considered to be the sanctuary sites for acute lymphoblastic leukemia (ALL) [6]. We present here two cases of ALL, one having persistent splenomegaly and leukemic infiltrates in the spleen and the other having isolated relapse in the spleen. To the best of our knowledge, the latter is the first such case report in the literature.

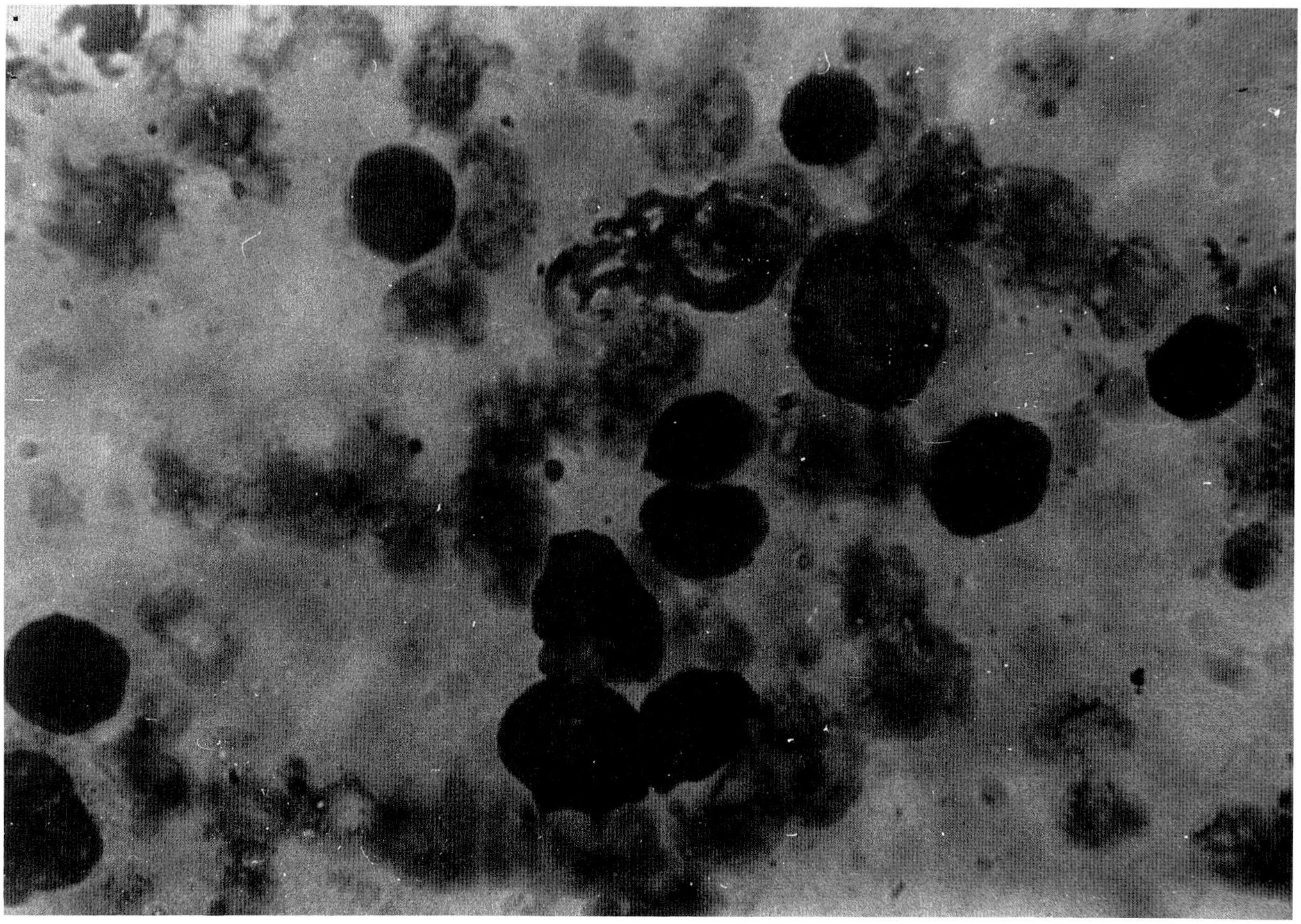

Fig. 1. Microphotograph (hematoxylin and eosin stain ×100) of splenic fine-needle aspiration cytology smear showing lymphoblasts.

Case 1

A 14-year-old boy was shown to have acute lymphoblastic leukemia, L_1 type, in July, 1992. At presentation he had generalized lymphadenopathy and hepatosplenomegaly. After induction chemotherapy using National Cancer Institute Protocol MCP 841 (vincristine 1.4 mg/M^2 i.v. every week for four doses, intrathecal methotrexate 12 mg every week for four doses, L-asperaginase 6,000 units/M^2 subcutaneously on alternate days for ten doses, oral prednisolone 40 mg/M^2 daily for 1 month, and daunorubicin 30 mg/M^2 i.v. on days 8,15, and 29), he had normal bone marrow, cerebrospinal fluid (CSF), and hemogram. The lymphadenopathy and hepatomegaly abated, but splenomegaly persisted. A fine-needle aspiration cytologic study of the spleen showed numerous blast cells. He was continued on the chemotherapy protocol and is in complete remission, and his spleen is no longer palpable.

Case 2

A 42-year-old woman was shown to have ALL, L_1 type, in March, 1990. She entered complete remission after induction chemotherapy with vincristine 1.4 mg/M^2 i.v. every week for four doses, intrathecal methotrexate 12 mg every week for four doses, oral prednisolone 40 mg/M^2 daily for 1 month, and doxorubicin 30 mg/M^2 iv. on days 8, 15, and 29. In July, 1992, while on maintenance chemotherapy, she was admitted for fever with rigor. She had splenomegaly, and her bone marrow and CSF cytology were normal. A splenic fine-needle aspiration cytologic study showed numerous blast cells (Fig. 1). She remained well on the chemotherapy until December, 1992, when she developed bone marrow relapse. She had persistent splenomegaly.

Acute leukemia can infiltrate almost any organ of the body [1]. A patient with acute leukemia is said to be in remission if bone marrow, CSF cytology, and hemogram are normal. The presence of extramedullary infiltrates in a patient with ALL who is otherwise in complete remission is well documented in the literature [2–5].

A patient with ALL can relapse in bone marrow, testis, ovary, central nervous system, and rarely orbit [6]. Patients who present with testicular relapse are often shown to have leukemic infiltrates in abdominal nodes, spleen, and liver [6]. Cases resembling case 1 have been described in the literature [2–5]. Patients with extramedullary infiltrates have a poor prognosis even if they are treated with additional systemic chemotherapy [4]. Additional local radiotherapy has been shown to have no overall survival advantage, although it does clear extramedullary infiltrates [7]. Therefore, we opted to treat this patient without any change in the protocol, and his spleen regressed to the normal size.

Case 2, to the best of our knowledge, is the first case report of relapse related to the spleen. This patient had been on maintenance chemotherapy for 1 year when she developed splenomegaly due to leukemic infiltrates. Bone marrow, CSF, and hemogram reports were normal. Thus this is a case of isolated splenic relapse in ALL. Testis, ovary, and CNS act as sanctuary sites due to difficult accessibility of the organs to the chemotherapeutic agents. It is difficult to consider the spleen as a sanctuary site because of the rich blood supply and easy access to chemotherapeutic agents to it. Two cases similar to this case have been reported in which lymph node involvement preceded bone marrow involvement by months [3]. She had persistent splenomegaly, and 5 months later she developed bone marrow relapse. We opted to continue this patient on chemotherapy because splenic irradiation has not been shown to be curative [4,8].

Combination systemic chemotherapy and local radiotherapy is the standard treatment for isolated testicular and CNS relapses. Similar combinations might have been better in these cases also.

ACKNOWLEDGMENTS

We are thankful to our patients, without whom this publication would not have been possible. We also thank the director of our institute for his permission to publish this paper.

ASHWIN P. PATEL
KIRTI M. PATEL
SHILIN N. SHUKLA
BIPIN N. SAVANI
N. GOPAL
KETAN N. BAVISHI
P.L. MADAN
ASHA ANAND
BHARAT J. PARIKH
PANKAJ M. SHAH
Departments of Medicine and Pathology, The Gujarat Cancer and Research Institute, Asarwa, Ahmedabad, India

REFERENCES

1. Henderson ES: Acute leukemia: General considerations. In McGraw-Hill, Williams WJ, Beutler E, Erslev AJ, Lichtman MA (eds): "Hematology." 4th Ed. McGraw-Hill, 1991, p 243.
2. Sharp HL, Nesbit ME, White G, Krivit W: Renal and hepatic pathology following initial remission of acute leukemia induced by prednisolone. Cancer 20:1395–1402, 1967.
3. Nies BA, Bodey GP, Thomas LB, Brecher G, Freireich EJ: The persistence of extra-medullary leukemic infiltrates during bone marrow remission of acute leukemia. Blood 26:133–141, 1965.
4. Mathe G, Schwarzenberg L, Mery AM, Cattan A, Schneider M, Amiel JL, Schumberger JR, Poisson J, Wajcner G: Extensive histological and cytological survey of patients with acute leukemia in "complete remission." Br Med J 1:640–642, 1966.
5. Simone JV, Holland E, Johnson W: Fatalities during remission of childhood luekemia. Blood 39:759, 1972.
6. Ninane J, Taylor D, Day S: The eye as a sanctuary in acute lymphoblastic leukaemia. Lancet i:452–453, 1980.
7. Baum E, Heyn R, Nesbit M: Occult abdominal involvement with apparently isoalted testicular relapse in children with acute lymphocytic leukemia. Am J Pediatr Hematol Oncol 6:343–346, 1984.
8. Sharp HL, Nesbit ME, D'Angio GJ, Krivit W: Addition of local radiation after bone marrow remission in acute leukemia in children. Cancer 20:1403–1404, 1967.

Aspergilloma Formation in a Pneumatocele in a Patient With Acute Lymphoblastic Leukemia

To the Editor: Pneumatoceles are commonly seen as a sequelae of staphylococcal pneumonia in infants and young children [1,2], and are infrequent in adults with pneumonia [3]. They usually resolve spontaneously and completely over several weeks or months, although spontaneous pneumothorax has been increasingly reported [4] in acquired immunodeficiency syndrome (AIDS) patients with *Pneumocystis carinii* pneumonia (PCP).

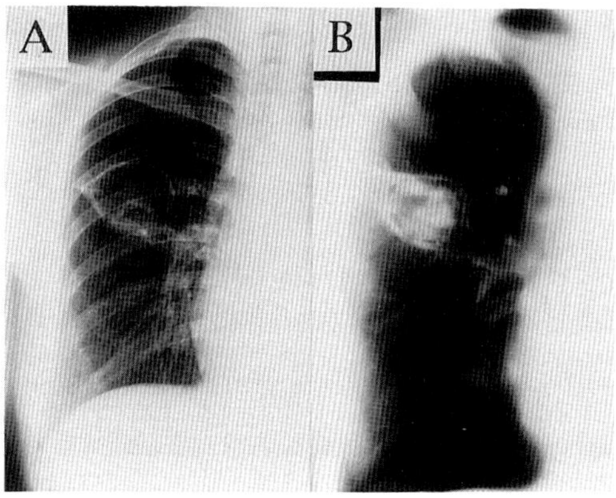

Fig. 1. A: Chest roentgenogram showing a pneumatocele in right upper lobe. B: Tomogram showing a fungus ball formation in a lumen of the pneumatocele.

We describe an adult patient with acute lymphoblastic leukemia complicated by a postpneumonic pneumatocele in which refractory aspergilloma occurred.

A 31-year-old woman was admitted to our hospital because of fever in November 1990. Physical examination showed generalized lymphadenopathy and hepatosplenomegaly. Laboratory studies revealed a leukocyte count of 327×10^9/L with 74% blasts, a hemoglobin concentration of 71 g/L, and platelet count of 59×10^9/L. Bone marrow examination confirmed the diagnosis of acute lymphoblastic leukemia (FAB classification: L2). The radiograph of the chest was normal. The patient achieved a complete remission with a combination chemotherapy consisting doxorubicin, vincristine, and prednisolone, and a subsequent re-induction therapy with high-dose cytosine-arabinoside and mitoxantrone. During a severely granulocytopenic phase after the second chemotherapy, the patient experienced persistent fever; at that time, the chest radiograph revealed a peripheral infiltrative shadow in the right upper lobe. Cultures of pharyngeal swab and blood were negative. Antibiotics were prescribed; the patient had been defervesced, coinciding with recovery of the granulocytopenia. The chest radiograph showed thin-walled cavitation of the infiltrates, compatible with a pneumatocele; at that time, the level of serum C-reactive protein returned to normal. During a granulocytopenic phase following another consolidation, the patient became febrile again. The chest roentgenogram showed a fungus ball formation in the pneumatocele (Fig. 1).Repeated sputum cultures grew Aspergillus spp. Although the patient had been intensively treated with parental amphotericin B and miconazol, the aspergilloma exacerbated repeatedly in granulocytopenia after intensive antileukemic chemotherapies. The patient experienced an overt relapse of leukemia in August 1991; her clinical course progressive deteriorated and the patient died of respiratory failure in May 1992. Autopsy revealed fulminant aspergillosis in the lung.

Postpneumonic pneumatoceles generally have self-limited and favorable prognosis; pneumatoceles have been increasingly described in patients with AIDS associated with PCP [4,5]. Although subsequent pneumothorax is not an unusual complication, secondary infectious complications within a pneumatocele have not been reported previously. In this case, prolonged immunosuppression, which has resulted from both the repeated episodes of granulocytopenia and the long-term administration of prednisolone, may have contributed to the unusual aspergilloma formation in the lumen of the pneumatocele. Considering the increasing frequency of pneumatoceles in AIDS patients with PCP, there is a possibility of secondary fungal infection developing in the pneumatoceles occurring in the setting.

KEN SATOH
AKIHIKO CHUBACHI

Hidetaka Niitsu
Takashi Nimura
Akira B. Miura
Third Department of Internal Medicine, Akita University School of Medicine, Akita, Japan

References

1. Meyers HI, Jacobson G: Staphylococcal pneumonia in children and adults. Radiology 72:665–681, 1959.
2. Hendren WH, Haggerty RJ: Staphylococcic pneumonia in infancy and childhood. JAMA 168:6–16, 1958.
3. McGarry T, Giosa R, Rohman M, Huang CT: Pneumatocele formation in adult pneumonia. Chest 92:717–720, 1987.
4. Goodman PC, Daley C, Minagi H: Spontaneous pneumothorax in AIDS patient with *Pneumocystis carinii* pneumonia. AJR 147:29–31, 1986.
5. DeLorenzo LJ, Huang XT, Maguire GP, Stone DJ: Roentgenographic patterns of *Pneumocystis carinii* pneumonia in 104 patients with AIDS. Chest 91:323–327, 1987.

Acute Monoblastic Leukemia (M5a) Presenting Numb Chin Syndrome

To the Editor: Numb chin syndrome is paresthesia restricted to the distribution of the mental nerve. Although a rare and apparently harmless symptom, its presence is sometimes ominous, reflecting hidden malignancy. While the syndrome was initially described in 1930 by Charles Bell [1], its importance in malignant diseases was established only recently. Isolated mental neuropathy was not recognized in a large survey of 5,778 patients with lymphoma and leukemia in the late fifties [2]. Since Calverley and Mohnac aroused the underlying malignancy in such an innocuous symptom, a variety of neoplasms have been shown to cause the syndrome [2–4]. The syndrome appears to be caused more often by a metastatic or infiltrating malignancy of the jaw than by direct involvement of the nerve. There is no well-documented report of hematological disorders except for Burkitt's lymphoma and L3 ALL [5]. Once a patient develops numb chin, the prognosis is usually grim [1–5]. Here we describe the successful chemotherapeutic management of a case of acute monoblastic leukemia (M5a) initially presenting with numb chin syndrome.

A 32-year-old female was admitted to our hospital because of paresthesia of the lower lip and chin, persisting fever and purpura lasting for 3 weeks. She was anemic and feverish, and had scattered purpura on her forehead and extremities. Neither superficial lymphadenopathy nor hepatosplenomegaly was observed. Gums were not swollen or spongy. Neurologically, there was no abnormality except for bilateral paresthesia and hypesthesia to all modalities of stimulation found over the distribution of mental nerve. Laboratory findings disclosed severe thrombocytopenia ($2.4 \times 10^4/\mu l$), anemia (Hb 8.2 g/dl), leukocytopenia (2,200/μl) with erythroblastosis, and elevated serum LDH and lysozyme. Five sternal bone marrow aspirations attempted were dry taps. Smears were made from the fluid adhering to the tip of the needle only. Normal components of hematopoietic cells in the bone marrow were replaced by proliferating monoblastoid cells (>99%), which were negative for peroxidase, periodic acid-Schiff and naphthol AS-D chloracetate esterase, but positive for α-naphthyl butylate esterase. Radiographic and computerized tomographic examination of the mandible were normal. Lumbar puncture revealed no abnormality. She was diagnosed with acute monoblastic leukemia (M5a). Complete remission was achieved with the disappearance of numb chin after the multiagent chemotherapy. Thereafter, she was treated with intermittent consolidation chemotherapy and has been free of disease for more than 3 years without neurological deficits.

Numb chin syndrome may be produced by any pathological process involving the mental nerve, the mandibular nerve, or even the mandibular trunk [2]. In this case, the bone marrow was supposed to be closely packed with a huge number of the neoplastic cells, because the five attempts at sternal marrow aspirations were dry taps. The symptom appeared bilaterally and disappeared equally in both sides during chemotherapy. The compression of the mental nerve at the stenotic mental foramen by the proliferating neoplastic cells in the bone marrow was the most likely cause of the syndrome in this case.

Tatsuharu Ohno
Yuzuru Yasuda
Hiroo Furukawa
Hematology Unit, Neurology Unit, Department of Internal Medicine, Ohtsu Red Cross Hospital, Nagara, Ohtsu, Japan

References

1. Furukawa T: Charles Bell's description of numb chin syndrome. Neurology 38: 331, 1988.
2. Bruyn RPM, Boogerd W: The numb chin. Clin Neurol Neurosurg 93:187, 1991.
3. Calverley JR, Mohnac AM: Syndrome of the numb chin. Arch Intern Med 112: 819, 1963.
4. Massey EW, Moore J, Schold SCJr: Mental neuropathy from systemic cancer. Neurology 31:1277, 1981.
5. Kuroda Y, Fujiyama F, Ohyama T, Watanabe T, Endo C, Neshige R, Kakigi R: Numb chin syndrome secondary to Burkitt's cell acute leukemia. Neurology 41: 453, 1991.

Hirulog® Therapy for Heparin-Associated Thrombocytopenia and Deep Venous Thrombosis

To the Editor: We read with interest the report by Dr. Nand regarding the treatment of deep venous thrombosis with Hirulog® (Biogen, Inc, Cambridge, MA) in a patient with heparin-associated thrombocytopenia [1]. Thrombin inhibitors such as Hirulog® appear to be effective anticoagulants and are not associated with thrombocytopenia, making them ideal candidates for the treatment of patients with a history of heparin-associated thrombocytopenia.

We wish to point out a discrepancy between the title and text of the report and the actual drug used in the patient described by Dr. Nand. The title and text of the paper refer to the use of recombinant hirudin in the patient described, yet the author provides the reference to Hirulog® as the proprietary name of the commercial source of recombinant hirudin. Recombinant hirudin and Hirulog® are not synonymous. Recombinant hirudin is a protein of 65 amino acids [2] and is derived from cloning of the hirudin gene [3] from the medicinal leech, *Hirudo medicinalis*. Hirulog®, a 20 amino acid peptide, is a synthetic analogue of recombinant hirudin [4] constructed from knowing the residues essential for the binding of recombinant hirudin to thrombin. Though both recombinant hirudin and Hirulog® are potent inhibitors of thrombin, they differ in their inhibition kinetics [4,5] and pharmacology. Neither drug is commercially available in the United States.

Preliminary reports of clinical trials in humans have suggested that both Hirulog® and recombinant hirudin may be effective in preventing and treating deep venous thrombosis, prevention of reocclusion after angioplasty or thrombolytic therapy, and in the treatment of unstable angina. Because clinical experience with these agents has not matured, it is not yet possible to determine if either of these agents will demonstrate a greater clinical advantage over the other. These potent thrombin antagonists may be more effective than heparin because, unlike heparin, they appear to inhibit clot-bound thrombin, do not require anti-thrombin III, and have not been associated with thrombocytopenia.

Thomas Reid II
Barbara M. Alving
Division of Medicine, Department of Hematology, Coagulation Laboratory, Walter Reed Army Institute of Research, Washington D.C.

REFERENCES

1. Nand S: Hirudin therapy for heparin-associated thrombocytopenia and deep venous thrombosis. Am J Hematol 43:310–311, 1993.
2. Bagdy N, Barabas É, Gráf L, Peterson TE, Magnusson S: Hirudin: Methods Enzymol 45:669–678, 1976.
3. Courtney M, Loison G, Lemoine Y, Riehl-Bellon N, Degrysse E, Brown SW, Cazenave J-P, Defreyn G, Delebassee D, Bernat A, Maffrand J-P, Roitsch C: Production and evaluation of recombinant hirudin. Sem Thromb Hemost 15:288–292, 1989.
4. Maraganore JM, Bourdon P, Jablonski J, Ramachandran KL, Fenton JW: Design and characterization of hirulogs: A novel class of divalent peptide inhibitors of thrombin. Biochemistry 29:7095–7101, 1990.
5. Stone SR, Hofsteenge J: Kinetics of the inhibition of thrombin by hirudin. Biochemistry 25:4622–4628, 1986.

Author's Reply

Response to the Editor: I agree with Dr. Reid and Dr. Alving that Hirulogs are synthetic analogues of recombinant Hirudin. Though similar in their inhibitory effect on thrombin, there are pharmacologic differences between the two compounds.

We were provided this agent under the name "Hirulog" by Biogen Incorporated, Cambridge, MA. I was very keen to use a generic term for this drug. After some thought, I chose the term "Hirudin" for the title and specified in the text that a hirulog was used to treat this patient.

Like Dr. Reid and Dr. Alving, I believe that the Hirudins are a promising group of agents. Comparative studies of Hirudins vs. the Heparins, and recombinant Hirudin vs. Hirulogs will be necessary to find out the more effective and safer anticoagulant.

SUCHA NAND

Loyola University Medical Center, Section of Hematology/Oncology, Maywood, Illinois

Author Index to Volume 45

Abe, Kazuhiro, 181
Adams, Paul C., 146, 260
Adams, Robert J., 279
Adekile, A.D., 51
Al-Batniji, Fatma, 142
Altisent C., 103
Alving, Barbara M., 352
Anand, Asha, 349
Aoki, Yoshikazu, 298
Arakawa, Masaaki, 325
Arruda, V.R., 96
Ashihara, Eishi, 262

Balaban, Ed, 193
Baldini, Luca, 25
Barbieri, Sergio, 25
Barbone, Ersilia, 270
Bartram, Claus, 79
Bavishi, Ketan N., 349
Baynes, Roy D., 288
Baysal, E., 51, 91
Bell, William R., 1
Berberana, M., 237
Berrebi, Alain, 348
Bertrand, Jean Claude, 252
Bhavnani, M., 192
Binder, Bernd R., 16
Blajchman, Morris A., 321
Blanco, A., 330
Blumberg, Neil, 189
Bobbio-Pallavicini, Enrico, 99
Bockenstedt, Paula L., 248
Bolling, Steven F., 248
Bonduel, M., 330
Bothwell, Thomas H., 288
Bourque, Ron, 321

Brandão-Néto, José, 1
Brody, Judith, 39
Burns, C. Patrick, 98
Byrnes, John J., 304

Cámara, R., 237
Canellos, George P., 283
Cao, Antonio, 81
Carl, Elizabeth, 279
Carpo, Marinella, 25
Carvalho, M.H., 96
Castillo, Ricrado, 109
Cesana, Bruno, 25
Cesar, Jesus M., 109
Chan, J.K.C., 275
Chang, Jan-Gowth, 293
Charles, Linda A., 128
Chen, Pao-Huei, 293
Chen, Tyen-Po, 293
Chiou, Shyh-Shin, 293
Chorba, Terence L., 112
Chou, Takaaki, 325
Chubachi, Akihiko, 271, 351
Chung, J.S.L., 275
Clarke, Matthew J., 112
Clary, Anthony, 279
Colman, Robert W., 73
Cook, James D., 288
Costa, F.F., 96
Cottler-Fox, M., 269
Cro, Lilla, 25

Damilano, Isabella, 25
Dean, Mark, 205
Deguchi, Katsumi, 232
Demers, Christine, 321
Dennig, Dieter, 63
Dhodapkar, Madhav, 187
Dimovski, A.J., 51
Distenfeld, Ariel, 167
Dittmar, Klaus, 39
Divoky, V., 51
Duru, Feride, 94
Dutcher, Janice P., 224

Elchalal, Uriel, 348
Elford, H.L., 136
Espinosa, José I., 109
Evatt, Bruce L., 112
Exner, Tom, 205

Favaloro, Emmanuel J., 205
Felber, Norbert, 39
Fernandes, D., 96
Fernandez, Hugo F., 304
Fernández-Rañada, J.M., 237
Firpo, Meri, 63
Fischereder, Michael, 258
Flowers, Mary E.D., 240
Follett, Kenneth A., 98
Freiberg, Richard, 156
Frenkel, Eugene P., 193
Friedman, Brian M., 288
Frogheri, Laura, 81, 265
Fujii, Hiroshi, 335
Fujii, Hisaichi, 185
Fujioka, Seitoku, 122
Fujita, Naohisa, 262
Fukumoto, Manabu, 88
Furukawa, Hiroo, 244, 352

García, Vicente Vicente, 10
García-Avello, Angel, 109
Garr, Susan B., 85
Gasparetto, Cristina, 63
Geissler, Klaus, 79
Gertz, Morie A., 187
Gesteira, F., 96
Gillio, Alfred P., 63
Gilman, John G., 265
Girolami, Antonio, 270
Gitel, Sanford, 217
Glueck, Charles J., 156
Glueck, Helen I., 156
Gohchi, Kengo, 196
Goldberg, Stuart L., 187
Goldsmith, Jonathan C., 142
Gomi, Komakazu, 298
Gonçalves, M.G., 96
Gonda, Yasunori, 298
González, F.A., 347
Gopal, N., 349
Gordon, Erlinda M., 142
Goto, Hideo, 262
Gotoh, Moritaka, 196
Graninger, Wolfgang, 79
Grelac, Françoise, 252
Griffin, James D., 283
Griggs, Jennifer J., 177
Grispo, Linda, 205
Guffanti, Andrea, 25
Guiso, Luciana, 81, 265
Güler, Ertu rul, 94
Guyotat, Denis, 252
Gyorkey, Ferenc, 272

Haas, Oskar, 79
Hagay, Zion, 348
Hamer, Tracey, 156
Hanabusa, 196
Harrington, William J., Jr., 304
Hashimoto, K., 94
Hayashi, Naoki, 325
Heal, Joanna Mary, 189
Henderson, Clyde, 156
Henderson, Penny, 321
Henley, Susan E., 177
Hepner, M., 330
Hess, Charles E., 347
Hirai, Hisamaru, 194
Hirata, Sigeto, 298
Hirata, Toshiyuki, 262
Hirono, Akira, 185
Holman, Robert C., 112
Honda, Junichi, 349
Hughes, Graham R.V., 193
Huisman, T.H.J., 51, 91, 345
Humphries, John E., 347

Ibáñez, A., 103
Ijima, Hiroko, 58
Ikeda, Kazuma, 212
Imamura, Nobutaka, 181
Inaba, Tohru, 262
Inagaki, Minoru, 196
Inazawa, Johji, 335
Inoue, Hirofumi, 274
Irino, Shozo, 212
Ishibashi, Takafumi, 244
Ishida, Torao, 298
Ishino, Takako, 271
Ishizuka, Yasuo, 325
Ito, Satoshi, 325
Iwahashi, Masahito, 273

Jaeger, Ulrich, 79
Jaffe, Jeffrey P., 258
Jojima, Hiroto, 268, 349

Kane, William H., 128
Kaneko, Toshihiro, 232
Ka ifo lu, Mehmet Ali, 94
Katakami, Hideki, 88
Kawanishi, Koichi, 212
Kawano, Seiji, 150
Keller, Frank G., 128
Kenmotsu, Naomi, 189
Khamashta, Munther A., 193
Kimura, Takashi, 310
Kirschmann, Chava, 201
Kishimoto, Yuji, 310
Kita, Kenkichi, 88
Kiyota, Takao, 298
Kobayashi, Nobuyuki, 273
Kohno, Isao, 16
Koutts, Jerry, 205
Kroll, Michael H., 272
Kubota, Kazuo, 191
Kuramoto, Atsushi, 181
Kuroume, Takayoshi, 58
Kutlar, Abdullah, 279

Lamana, M., 237
Lazzari, M., 330
Lechner, Klaus, 79
Levy, Mark, 156
Lian, Eric C-Y, 304
Liang, Raymond, 100
Lichtenberg, Robert, 63
Lin, Jen H., 39
Lin, Sheng-Fung, 293
Liu, Jin Cai, 279
Liu, Ta-Chih, 293
Lobos, José C., 109
Loewy, Gabriel, 167
Longinotti, Maurizio, 81, 265
López, J., 237
Loudianos, Georgios, 81

Ma, S.K., 275
Macik, B. Gail, 128
Madan, P.L., 349
Magallón, M., 103
Maiolo, Anna T., 25
Manca, Laura, 265
Mano, Hiroyuki, 194
Marcom, P. Kelly, 128
Martin-Villar, J., 103
Martinowitz, Uri, 217
Maruyama, Ikuro, 298
Masala, Bruno, 265
Mathew, Anna, 167
Matsuda, Juzo, 196
Matsumoto, Makoto, 273
Matsuo, Kazuhiko, 349
Matsushima, Takafumi, 191
Matulonis, Ursula A., 283
McAvoy, Ann, 321
McKie, Kathleen, 279

McKie, Virgil, 279
Meyer, Theo E., 288
Mills, Letha E., 240
Minamikawa, Kouzou, 232
Minden, Mark D., 194
Miranda, S.R.P., 96
Misawa, Shinichi, 335
Mismetti, Patrick, 252
Miura, A.B., 94
Miura, Akira B., 271, 351
Miura, I., 94
Miwa, Shiro, 185
Mohri, Mitsunobu, 298
Molchanova, T.P., 91, 345
Monteagudo, J., 103
Monteagudo, Juán, 109
Moore, Malcolm A.S., 63
Moraleda, José M., 10
Mrowiec, Zbigniew, 224
Murakami, Hirokazu, 191
Murphy, Charles, 171

Nagai, Masami, 212
Nagano, Takahiro, 310
Nagata, Shigekazu, 310
Najfeld, Vesna, 195
Nakagawa, Hitoshi, 335
Nakagawa, Masao, 262
Nakai, Hiroyuki, 335
Nakase, Tsutomu, 232
Nakashima, Osamu, 349
Nakaya, Ryusuke, 232
Nakayama, Shiro, 185
Nand, Sucha, 353
Nascimento, M.L., 96
Natori, Hideyo, 268, 349
Navarro, José L., 109
Nichols, Fenwick T., 279
Niitsu, H., 94
Niitsu, Hidetaka, 351
Nimura, T., 94
Nimura, Takashi, 351
Nishinari, T., 94
Nobile-Orazio, Edoardo, 25
Nomiyama, Jun, 274

O'Reilly, Richard J., 63
Oeda, Eiichi, 274
Ogawa, Osamu, 325
Oggiano, Lina, 81
Ohiwa, Michiaki, 232
Ohno, Tatsuharu, 244, 352
Oizumi, Kotaro, 268, 349
Oka, Michiko, 298
Okabe, Hiroaki, 16
Okajima, Kenji, 16
Oku, Naritoshi, 262
Okuma, Minoru, 244
Okuno, Yoshiaki, 88
Oldham, H. Newland, Jr., 128
Oleksowicz, 224
Olson, JOhn D., 98
Ortel, Thomas L., 128
Osabe, Seishi, 268, 349
Ota, Hiromi, 181
Otero, M.J., 237
Otsuka, Maki, 273
Özsoylu, Sinasi, 96, 348

Pace, B.S., 136
Panzer, Simon, 79
Parikh, Bharat J., 349
Patel, Ashwin P., 349
Patel, Kirti M., 349
Pennell, Beverly J., 98
Peñalva, L., 330
Pérez, G., 237
Petit, José, 271
Pirastu, Mario, 81
Pistidda, Paola, 81, 265
Pobedimskaya, D.D., 91, 345
Porta, Camillo, 99
Purucker, M.E., 269
Puszkin, Elena, 224

Qin, W.-B., 91
Queiroz, I.L., 96

Radaszkiewicz, Thaddaeusz, 79
Rahimi-Levene, Naomi, 348
Randi, Maria Luigia, 270
Rao, A. Koneti, 73
Reid, Thomas III, 352
Reynaud, Jacqueline, 252
Riba, J., 103
Rimini, Elena, 81
Rivera, José, 10
Rodgers, George M., 85
Rodríguez-Pérez, A., 103
Rowe, Jacob M., 177, 189
Rubin, Ronald N., 73
Rumbaut, Rolando E., 272
Russ, Sheryl A., 97

Saad, S.O.T., 96
Saeki, Takako, 325
Saitoh, Noriko, 196
Sánchez-Roig, María J., 10
Santinga, John T., 248
Sasaki, Kazunori, 212
Sasaki, Yutaka, 88
Satoh, Ken, 351
Satoh, Noriko, 271
Savani, Bipin N., 349
Sawamura, Morio, 191
Schafer, Andrew I., 272
Schulman, Sam, 217
Schultz, John C., 32
Seaborg, Barbara J., 98
Seidler, Christopher W., 240
Shah, Pankaj M., 349
Shahidi, Nasrollah T., 32
Shalmon, Lea, 201
Sharma, S., 91
Sheehan, Richard, 193
Shibuya, Tsunefumi, 88
Shimazaki, Chihiro, 262
Shimotakahara, Shigemi, 273
Shinohara, Kenji, 274
Shinohara, Masahiko, 191
Shiraishi, Kaori, 268, 349
Shirakawa, Shigeru, 232
Shitara, Toshiji, 58
Shukla, Shilin N., 349
Sivakumaran, M., 192
Small, Trudy, 63
Smith, Clay, 63
Soe, Gilbu, 16

Solomon, Alan, 171
Sonati, M.F., 96
Sosa, Felix, 156
Sotomatu, Manabu, 58
Stamatoyannopoulos, G., 136
Steegmann, J.L., 237
Strine, Tara W., 112
Stroop, Davis, 156
Sugihara, Taisuke, 298
Sugiyama, Tateo, 244
Sullivan, Keith M., 240
Sun, Tsieh, 39
Susin, Myron, 39
Suzuki, Akira, 88

Takahara, Jiro, 212
Takahashi, Takayuki, 88
Takatsu, H., 94
Takatsuki, Kiyoshi, 16
Tamura, Jun'ichi, 191
Tanaka, Ken, 268, 349
Tange, Tsuyoshi, 194
Tardy, Bernard, 252
Tardy-Poncet, Brigitte, 252
Tasaka, Taizo, 212
Tatsumi, Eiji, 150, 310
Tefferi, Ayalew, 187
Teichberg, Saul, 39
Teshigawara, Keisuke, 310
Tracy, Trent, 156
Tseng, Wen-Ping, 293
Tsukada, Hiroko, 325
Tsukamoto, Miyo, 196
Tsuyuoka, Reiko, 88
Tuncer, Murat, 94
Tusell, J., 103

Ucar, Antonio, 304

Verma, Ram S., 196
Villalta Fernández, M.J., 237
Villegas, A., 347
Volc-Platzer, Beatrix, 79
Vreugdenhil, Gerard, 192

Wada, Hideo, 232
Wakabayashi, Masaya, 325
Wakita, Yoshihiro, 232
Walsh, Peter N., 73
Weiner, Robert, 39
Weiss, Deborah T., 171
Welborn, Jeanna L., 341
Welch, Michael, 156
Wells, Michael J., 321
Wells, Philip S., 321
Westerman, M.P., 194
Wilson, J.B., 91
Wong, K.F., 91, 275

Yamada, Teruo, 122
Yamagata, Noboru, 262
Yamaguchi, A., 94
Yamaguchi, Nobuo, 150, 310
Yamamoto, Shuji, 298
Yasada, Yuzuru, 352
Yasunaga, Koujiro, 310
Yazaki, Yoshio, 194
Ye, Z., 345
Yetgin, Sevgi, 94
Yoneda, Noriko, 150, 310
Yugami, Shin-ichiroh, 58
Yumen, Omar H., 97

Zaizov, Rina, 201
Zuckerman, Dina, 224

Subject Index to Volume 45

Acute lymphoblastic leukemia, 341
Acute megakaryoblastic and promegakaryocytic leukemia, 181
Adhesion molecule, 262
Adverse effects, 189
African siderosis, 288
Aγ gene, 136
$^{A}\gamma^{T}$, 265
AIDS (acquired immunodeficiency syndrome), 304
AIDS, 112
All-*trans*-retinoic acid, 177
α gene deletion, 345
α-globin genes, 201
α-interferon, 248
α-thal, 345
α-thalassemia, 91
α1 mutation, 345
α2 mutation, 345
α_2-plasmin inhibitor, 16
Anemia, 136
Animal model, 298
Anticoagulation, 85
Antifibrinolytic therapy, 16
Antithrombin, 321
Antithrombin deficiency, 321
APL, 212
$(AT)_X(T)_Y$ motif, 51
Autoantibody, 244
Autoimmune thrombocytopenia, 244
Autotransplants, 283

-globin gene, 51
-thal mutations, 51
-thalassemia, 265
-thromboglobulin, 224

Blast crisis, 283
Bleeding, 142
Bleeding tendency, 16
Blood cell lineages, 122
Blood coagulation disorders, 330
Blood donors, 321
Blood platelets, 189
Blood transfusion, 189
BMT, 237
Bovine thrombin, 128

CD13, 310
CD21 antigen, 150
CD3δ, 310
CD3ε, 310
CD36(OKM5), 181
CD59 expression, 122
CD7, 310
Cell culture, 181
Chronic graft versus host disease, 240
Clotting, 128, 142
CML, 283, 335
Collagen binding assay, 205
Colony-stimulating factor, 325
Combined immune deficiency, 63
Concentrates, 217
Congenital neutropenia, 63
Cytokine combinations, 63
Cytokines, 58

DDAVP, 205
Dermis, 167
Desmopressin, 205
DIC, 232, 298
Dimethylsulfoxide toxicity, 187
Disseminated intravascular coagulation, 325
Disseminated mycobacterial infection, 325
Drug toxicity, 258
Dyshypoprothrombinemia, 103

Encephalopathy, 187
Epstein-Barr virus, 150
Erythrocyte ghost, 1
Erythropoietin, 237
Extramedullary hematopoiesis, 167

F reticulocytes, 136
Factor V, 128
Factor VIII, 217
Factor VIII inhibitors, 240
Ferritin, 146
Fetal hemoglobin, 51
Fibrin and fibrinogen degradation products, 16
Flow cytometric analysis, 181
Flow cytometry, 122

γ globin, 136
G6PD deficiency, 185
Gene deletion, 201
Globin, 136
Globin gene, 91
Glycoprotein Ib, 10
Glycoproteins, 330

Hairy cell leukemia, 39
Hb H disease, 201, 293
Hb Q-India, 91
Hb Q-Thailand, 91
Hematopoiesis, 167
Hematopoietic suppression, 32

Hemochromatosis, 288
Hemolysis, 237
Hemolytic anemia, 187
Hemophilia, 103, 112, 142
Hemophilia A, 217
Hepatic iron, 146
Hepatotoxicity, 258
HIV, 112
HIV (human immunodeficiency virus), 304
HLA types, 237
HLA typing, 260
HTLV-I (human T-lymphotrophic virus, type I), 304
HUS (hemolytic uremic syn drome), 304
Hypercalcemia, 88
Hypofibrinolysis, 156

Idiopathic hypereosinophilic syndrome, 248
IgE plasma cell leukemia, 262
IgG monoclonal gammopathy, 171
Immune hemolysis, 237
Immunoglobulin molecule, 171
Immunologic phenomena, 79
Immunological abnormality, 325
Immunology, 189
Interferon-α, 262
Interferon-γ, 32
Interleukin-2, 224
Iron, 260
Iron absorption, 146

Liver cirrhosis, 10
Loeffler's syndrome, 248
Low-grade B-cell lymphoma, 39
Low-molecular-weight heparin, 252
Lp(a), 156

MAG-antibodies, 25
Malignant histiocytosis, 244
MDS-RA, 325
Megakaryocytes, 258
MoAb FVIII, 142
Monoclate-P, 142
Monoclonal gammopathies of undetermined significance, 25
Mortality, 112
Multiple myeloma, 88
Mutation, 185
Myelodysplastic syndrome, 79
Myelofibrosis, 167
Myelomonocytic crisis, 335

Neoplasms, 189
Normal individuals, 1
Novel $\delta^{+}27$ $\beta^{\circ}39$ thalassemia allele in cis, 81

Osteonecrosis, 156

p53 gene, 335
Paroxysmal nocturnal hemoglobinuria, 122
PCR, 293, 345
Pediatrics, 330
Pentosan polysulfate, 252
Peripheral blood stem cell trans plant, 187
Peripheral neuropathy, 25
Peroxidase, 310
Plasma cell, 171
Plasminogen activator inhibitor, 156
Platelet, 224
Platelet aggregation, 224
Platelet factor 4, 224
Platelets, 258
PML, 212
Polymorphic pattern, 51
Prevalence, 321
Proteinuria, 171
Prothrombin time, 85
Pseudocyst, 103
PTH-rP, 88

Quantities G-Phil, 345

Recombinant human granulocyte colony-stimulating factor, 58
Recombinant human soluble thrombomodulin, 298
Reinduction regimens, 341
Remission, 341
Restriction enzyme digestion, 293

Secondary iron overload, 260
Sequencing, 345
Sequential VAD-MP chemo therapy, 262
Serum transferrin receptor, 288
Severe congenital neutropenia, 58
Sickle cell disease, 279
SLE, 79
Soluble interleukin-2 receptor, 58
Southeast Asia, 293
Splenic lymphoma, 39
Stability, 217
Stem cell, 167
Stem cells, 283
Steroid therapy, 325
Stroke, 279
Systemic fibrinogenolysis, 16

t(15;17), 212
t(5;17), 335
T-lineage neoplasms, 150
TF, 232
TF, 298
Thalassemia, 265, 279
Thrombin, 321
Thrombocytopenia, 252
Thrombophlebitis, 330
Thromboplastin, 85
Thromboxane B2, 224
Thymic stage, 150
Tissue plasminogen activator, 156
TNF-α, 32
Trace elements, 1
Transferrin saturation, 146
Treatment, 189, 341
Trisomy 8, 212
TTP (thrombocytopenic purpura), 304
Two-gene deletion, 201

Undifferentiated acute myelogenous leukemia, 177

Variant, 187
Venous thrombosis, 252
Villous lymphocytes, 39
von Wilebrand factor, 205
von Willebrand's disease, 205

Wäldenstrom's macroglobulinemia, 25

Zinc binding sites, 1